Unwanted effects of cosmetics and drugs used in dermatology

UNWANTED EFFECTS OF COSMETICS AND DRUGS USED IN DERMATOLOGY

Third edition

Anton C. de Groot, M.D., Ph.D.
Department of Dermatology
Carolus-Liduina Hospital
's-Hertogenbosch
The Netherlands

J. Willem Weyland, Ph.D.
Food Inspection Service
Cosmetics Department
Enschede
The Netherlands

Johan P. Nater, M.D., Ph.D.
formerly Department of Dermatology
Academic Hospital
State University of Groningen
The Netherlands

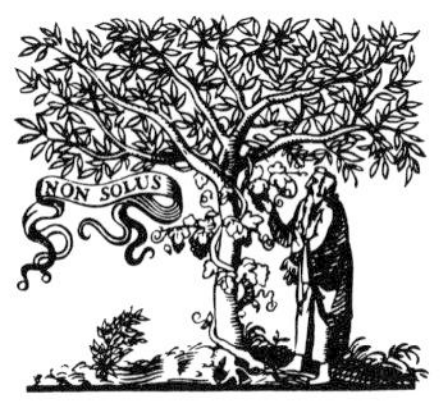

1994
ELSEVIER - Amsterdam - London - New York - Tokyo

ISBN 0 444 89775 5

This book is printed on acid-free paper.

Published by:
Elsevier Science B.V.
P.O. Box 211
1000 AE Amsterdam
The Netherlands

Printed in The Netherlands

Preface to the Third Edition

This 3rd Edition provides updated information on side effects of cosmetic products, topical and systemic drugs used in dermatology, and other dermato-therapeutic modalities including PUVA therapy and (new in this edition) dermal implants, laser therapy, chemical face peels and cryotherapy. The format of the book has remained essentially the same. We like to consider it to be a reference work with the following characteristics: comprehensiveness, easy to use, easy location of relevant information, copiously referenced, and up to date.

Although it has become a cliché to state in the preface of new editions of any book that "there has been an explosion of new knowledge since the last edition" (the second edition of this book was published eight years ago), the addition of over 1500 new references and 200 pages attests to the validity of this statement.

The section on cosmetics has largely been rewritten and extended, testifying to the special interest in this subject of two of the authors, Anton de Groot who wrote his 1988 thesis on "Adverse reactions to cosmetics" and our new co-author, Willem Weyland, who is the head of the Dutch "Food and Drug Administration", department of cosmetics.

The section on side effects of systemic drugs used in dermatology (Chapter 19) has also been expanded and now includes a full review of the side effects of the retinoids, and the newcomers itraconazole, terbinafine and cyclosporin A. Also, information on side effects are now provided in a standardized format with subheadings for each organ system, which makes searching for specific adverse reactions easier and quicker.

The patch test concentrations and vehicles throughout the text have been made in accordance with those advised in the book *Patch Testing* (second Edition, 1994) written by the senior author.

In the text, many cross-references to other sections have been deleted. Instead, the index of drugs has been made comprehensive.

We hope that this book — even better than the previous editions — will help solve the problems of the practising physician who is confronted with an adverse reaction to a cosmetic or drug, and also aid those who are scientifically interested by providing access to recent relevant literature.

Anton C. de Groot
J. Willem Weyland
Johan P. Nater

Table of contents

1. Contact dermatitis

INTRODUCTION

1.1 Dermatitis and eczema are names used to indicate a certain inflammatory state of the skin; when caused by external agents, this reaction is termed contact dermatitis or contact eczema.

Contact dermatitis may be classified as follows:

- Acute toxic contact dermatitis (§ 2)
- Irritant contact dermatitis (§ 2)
- Allergic contact dermatitis (§ 3)
- Phototoxic contact dermatitis (§ 6)
- Photoallergic contact dermatitis (§ 6)

MORPHOLOGICAL ASPECTS OF CONTACT DERMATITIS

1.2 An *acute allergic* contact dermatitis is characterized by polymorphy of the eruption; in the acute phase the skin reddens, clusters of minute papules, non-umbilicated vesicles and swelling occur, as well as weeping and exudation leading to the formation of crustae. The eruption is usually accompanied by itching, which may vary from moderate to quite severe. In cases of strong reactions the process may be noted to spread. In the subacute phase the polymorphy of the eruption diminishes: the skin becomes dry and scaly and fissures may be noted.

When the eruption becomes chronic, areas of the epidermis thicken, with deepening of the normal skin lines (lichenification); erythema and papules are less prominent. Multiple excoriations indicate the process to itch.

Irritant contact dermatitis often starts with dryness, itching and scaliness of the skin; papules and vesicles may develop later. In many cases it is impossible, on clinical examination, to distinguish between acute irritant dermatitis and acute allergic contact dermatitis.

2. Toxic and irritant contact dermatitis

ACUTE TOXIC CONTACT DERMATITIS

2.1 Acute toxic contact dermatitis may be provoked by single or repeated contacts with strongly toxic substances. The association between the injury and the toxic substance is usually quite obvious from the patient's history.

This type of reaction occurs frequently as a result of, mostly accidental, contacts with acids, alkalis, cleansers, solvents, etc.; only very rarely, however, is it caused by drugs (§ 8) [44].

IRRITANT CONTACT DERMATITIS

2.2 Irritant contact dermatitis is a term used to describe a localized, superficial, exudative, non-immunological inflammation of the skin, which is due to the direct influence of one or more external factors [15]. Many substances, including drugs, may after repeated contact with the skin cause irritant dermatitis by direct action. This occurs without previous sensitization; immunological processes are not involved.

During and after the first contacts no visual alterations may be observed. After repeated contact, the skin gradually becomes erythematous; drying and cracking occurs, and later, an eczematous reaction with papules and vesicles may develop.

An irritant substance will cause dermatitis if it is permitted to act in sufficient intensity and quantity and for a sufficient length of time. Irritant reactions may develop in all persons, though the individual susceptibility varies greatly. This probably depends on the thickness of the epidermis. Certain areas such as the eyelids and the scrotum are particularly susceptible to irritation [10]. Irritant reactions are more easily provoked under occlusion, e.g. under adhesives and polyethylene, or in skin folds.

Differential diagnosis

2.3 The condition of an already eczematized skin (from whatever cause) is quickly worsened by the application of a mild irritant medicament; the resulting exacerbation may be mistaken for an allergic reaction. In such cases irritant and allergic reactions are often difficult to distinguish. The differential diagnosis between irritant and allergic contact dermatitis must be made by means of patch testing. This is sometimes rather difficult, as patch tests with mild irritants (if insufficiently diluted) may cause false positive patch test reactions, especially when they are performed on patients with an eczematous eruption elsewhere on the skin. In such circumstances even standard test substances in routine concentrations may elicit false positive reactions. The problem of false positive reactions is further discussed in § 3.12.

Topical drugs that have caused irritant dermatitis are listed in § 2.4.

2.4 Irritant dermatitis due to topical drugs and cosmetics ingredients

Drug	Use	Ref.
6-aminonicotinamide	psoriasis therapy	29
ammonium persulfate	hair bleaches	7
benzalkonium chloride	antiseptic	9
benzoyl peroxide	acne therapy	18
cantharidin	wart treatment	6
carmustine (BCNU)	topical cytostatic drug	39
cetrimonium bromide (cetrimide)	antiseptic	42
chrysarobin	psoriasis therapy	11
citral	fragrance material	35
clioquinol	antiseptic	12
colchicine	treatment of condylomata acuminata	26
diethyl toluamide (DEET)	insect repellent	41
dimethyl sulfoxide (DMSO)	solvent	14
dinitrochlorobenzene (DNCB)	treatment of alopecia areata and warts	16
dithranol (cignolin, anthralin)	psoriasis therapy	30, 33
ether	solvent	17
5-fluorouracil	topical cytostatic drug	10
glyceryl thioglycolate	permanent wave	45
hexachlorophene	antiseptic	2, 28
hydroquinone	skin bleaching agent	24
6-hydroxy- 1,3-benzoxathiol-2-one	psoriasis therapy	22
iodine tincture	antiseptic	13
lindane (γ-benzene hexachloride)	treatment of scabies	43
mechlorethamine hydrochloride	treatment of mycosis fungoides	38
mesulfen	scabicide	31
monobenzone (monobenzyl ether of hydroquinone)	skin bleaching agent	23
phenol	antipruritic	4, 21
podophyllum resin	treatment of condylomata acuminata	25
propylene glycol	vehicle constituent	34, 36
povidone-iodine	antiseptic	27
quaternary ammonium compounds	antiseptics	9
resorcinol	antipruritic, peeling agent	3
salicylic acid	keratolytic drug	11
sulfur	treatment of scabies	43
selenium sulfide	dandruff therapy	1
sodium lauryl sulfate	vehicle constituent	8, 32
tar	psoriasis and eczema therapy	20
tretinoin (retinoic acid)	acne therapy	19, 40
urea	keratolytic drug, enhances penetration of chemicals through the skin	5, 37

2.5 REFERENCES

1. Albright, S.D. and Hitch, J.M. (1966): Rapid treatment of tinea versicolor with selenium sulfide. *Arch. Dermatol., 93*, 460.
2. Baker, H., Ive, F.A. and Lloyd, M.J. (1969): Primary irritant dermatitis of the scrotum due to hexachlorophene. *Arch. Dermatol., 99*, 693.
3. Becker, S.W. and Obermayer, M.E. (1947): *Modern Dermatology and Syphilology, 2nd Edition.* J.B. Lippincott Co., Philadelphia, London, Montreal.
4. Björnberg, A. (1968): *Skin Reactions to Primary Irritants in Patients with Hand Eczema.* O. Isacsons Tryckeri, Gothenburg.
5. Colin Hindson, M.T. (1971): Urea in the topical treatment of atopic eczema. *Arch. Dermatol., 104,* 284.
6. Dilaimy, M. (1975): Lymphangitis caused by cantharidin. *Arch. Dermatol., 111,* 1073.
7. Fisher, A.A. and Dooms-Goossens, A. (1976): Persulfate hair bleach reactions. *Arch. Dermatol., 112,* 1407.
8. Novak, E. and Francom, S.F. (1984): Inflammatory response to sodium lauryl sulfate in aqueous solutions applied to the skin of normal volunteers. *Contact Dermatitis, 10*, 101–104.
9. Gall, H. (1979): Toxisches Kontaktekzem auf die quaternäre Ammonium-Verbindung Benzalkoniumchlorid. *Dermatosen Beruf Umw., 27,* 139.
10. Shelley, W.B. and Shelley, E.D. (1988): Scrotal dermatitis caused by 5-fluorouracil (Efudex). *J. Am. Acad. Dermatol., 19*, 929–931.
11. Goodman, L.S. and Gilman, A. (Eds.) (1970): *The Pharmaceutical Basis of Therapeutics, 4th Edition.* The MacMillan Co., London, Toronto.
12. Kero, M., Hannuksela, M. and Sothman, A. (1979): Primary irritant dermatitis from topical clioquinol. *Contact Dermatitis, 5*, 115.
13. Kirchmayr, W. (1957): Zum Problem der sogenannten Jodüberempfindlichkeit. *Wien. klin. Wschr., 69*, 578.
14. Kligman, A.M. (1965): Topical pharmacology and toxicology of dimethylsulfoxide. Part 1 and 2. *J. Am. Med. Assoc., 193*, 769 and 923.
15. Malten, K.E. (1981): Thoughts on irritant contact dermatitis. *Contact Dermatitis, 7,* 238.
16. The Merck Index: *An Encyclopedia of Chemicals and Drugs, 9th Edition* (1976): Merck and Co., Inc., Rahway, U.S.A.
17. Michel, P.J. (1952): Les dermites de l'éther. *J. Méd. Lyon, 33,* 741.
18. Pace, W.E. (1965): Benzoyl peroxide-sulfur cream for acne vulgaris. *Can. Med. Assoc. J., 93,* 252.
19. Weiss, J.S., Ellis, C.N., Headington, J.T., Tincoff, T., Hamilton, T.A. and Voorhees, J.J. (1988): Topical tretinoin improves photoaged skin. *J. Am. Med. Assoc., 259*, 527–532.
20. Rothenborg, H.W. and Hjorth, N. (1968): Allergy to perfumes from toilet soaps and detergents in patients with dermatitis. *Arch. Dermatol., 97,* 417.
21. Rubin, M. B. and Pirozzi, D.J. (1973): Contact dermatitis from carbolated vaseline. *Cutis, 12,* 52.
22. Schoefinius, H.H. (1972): Kontaktdermatitis mit erhöhter Körpertemperatur unter Behandlung von Psoriasis vulgaris capitilii mit einem Benzoxathiol-Derivat. *Z. Haut-u. Geschl.kr., 47,* 227.
23. Spencer, M.C. (1962): Leukoderma following monobenzylether of hydroquinone bleaching. *Arch. Dermatol., 86,* 615.
24. Spencer, M.C. (1965): Topical use of hydroquinone for depigmentation. *J. Am. Med. Assoc., 194,* 962.
25. Sullivan, M. and King, L.S. (1947): Effects of resin of podophyllum on normal skin, condylomata acuminata and verrucae vulgares. *Arch. Dermatol. Syphilol., 56,* 30.
26. Von Krogh, G. and Rudén, A.K. (1980): Topical treatment of penile condylomata acuminata with colchicine at 48–72 hour intervals. *Acta. derm.-venereol. (Stockh.), 60,* 87.
27. Okano, M. (1989): Irritant contact dermatitis caused by povidone-iodine. *J. Am. Acad. Dermatol., 20*, 860.
28. Watt, T.L. and Baumann, R.R. (1972): Primary irritant dermatitis caused by pHisohex. *Cutis, 10,* 363.
29 Zackheim, H.S. (1975): Treatment of psoriasis with 6-amino-nicotinamide. *Arch. Dermatol., 111,* 880.
30. Puschmann, M. and Schmersahl, P. (1983): Untersuchungen zur Frage der Nebenwirkungen von Anthralin und seinen beiden Hauptveruntreinigungen an der gesunden Haut. *Z. Hautkr., 58,* 410.
31. Meneghini, C.L., Vena, G.A. and Angelini, G. (1982): Contact dermatitis to scabicides. *Contact Dermatitis, 8,* 285.
32. Bruynzeel, D.P., van Ketel, W.G., Scheper, R.J. and von Blomberg-van der Flier, B.M.E. (1982): Delayed time course of irritation by sodium lauryl sulfate: Observations on threshold reactions. *Contact Dermatitis, 8,* 236.

33. Kingston, T. and Marks, R. (1983): Irritant reactions to dithranol in normal subjects and psoriatic patients. *Br. J. Dermatol., 108,* 307.
34. Andersen, K.E. and Storrs, F.J. (1982): Hautreizungen durch Propylenglykol. *Hautartz, 33,* 12.
35. Rothenborg, H.W., Menné, T. and Sjølin, K.-E. (1977): Temperature dependent primary irritant dermatitis from lemon perfume. *Contact Dermatitis, 3,* 37.
36. Trancik, R.J. and Maibach, H.I. (1982): Propylene glycol: irritation or sensitization? *Contact Dermatitis, 8,* 185.
37. Cramers, M. and Thormann, J. (1981): Skin reactions to an urea-containing cream. *Contact Dermatitis, 7,* 189.
38. Goday, J.J., Aguirre, A., Ratón, J.A. and Diaz-Pérez, J.L. (1990): Local bullous reaction to topical mechlorethamine (mustine). *Contact Dermatitis, 22*, 306–307.
39. Zackheim, H.S., Epstein, E.H. and Crain, W.R. (1990): Topical carmustine (BCNU) for cutaneous T cell lymphoma: A 15-year experience in 143 patients. *J. Am. Acad. Dermatol., 22,* 802–810.
40. Thomas, J.R. III and Doyle, J.A. (1981): The therapeutic uses of topical vitamin A acid. *J. Am. Acad. Dermatol., 4,* 505.
41. Reuveni, H. and Yagupsky, P. (1982): Diethyltoluamide-containing insect repellent. *Arch. Dermatol., 118,* 582.
42. Mercer, D.M. (1983): Cetrimide burn in an infant. *Postgrad. Med. J., 59*, 472–473.
43. Farkás, J. (1983): Irritative contact dermatitis to scabicides as a sort of postscabies dermatitis. *Dermatosen, 31*, 189–190.
44. Jackson, E.M. and Goldner, R. (1990): *Irritant Contact Dermatitis*. Marcel Dekker, New York.
45. Rapaport, M. (1983): Irritant contact dermatitis to glyceryl monothioglycolate. *J. Am. Acad. Dermatol., 9*, 739–742.

3. Allergic contact dermatitis (general aspects)

IMMUNOLOGICAL ASPECTS

3.1 In the last two decades our understanding of the basic mechanisms underlying induction, expression and regulation of allergic contact dermatitis has rapidly increased. Several excellent recent papers on the subject have been published, to which the reader is referred [4,22,28,74–76,95].

THE TECHNIQUE OF PATCH TESTING [12,23,29,73]

3.2 The process of sensitization leads to a specific hypersensitivity of the skin. This can be demonstrated by the application of the causative substance(s) to a normal skin site, which is usually done under occlusion. This procedure, named patch testing, is used for diagnosing allergic contact dermatitis. Although its purpose is primarily the positive identification of a contact allergic reaction and the establishment of its cause(s), negative patch test results are nevertheless of similar importance in that allergic contact dermatitis *from the tested substances* can then be ruled out and other possibilities should be considered.

The technique of patch testing has been standardized [23]. Present standard methods include a device and test material. The Al-test was the standard method of applying antigens for years and is still widely used. In this method filter paper discs are fixed to a strip of plastic-coated aluminum foil. In the past few years, this method has been largely supplanted by aluminum or polypropylene plastic chambers and cups. Most allergens, incorporated in a petrolatum vehicle, are applied to the filter paper discs or cups, and fixed with tape to the upper part of the back and left in place for 48 hours. Contemporary tapes are made of nonwoven textile material and an acrylate adhesive, to which allergic reactions are rare.

The TRUE test [134] is a ready-to-apply test method that uses polyester patches coated with allergens in hydrophilic vehicles.

The test materials are removed after 2 days and the reactions are scored 20 minutes and 1 or 2 days later according to the following scheme:

+? = doubtful reaction, possibly caused by a weak irritant effect: the reaction shows only a weak erythema without infiltration
+ = erythema with infiltration
++ = erythema, infiltration, papules
+++ = the same with formation of vesicles
++++ = strong positive reaction with marked edema and confluent vesicles/ bullae

– = negative
IR = irritant reaction
NT = not tested.

As patch testing in patients with an acute and/or widespread dermatitis may worsen the existing eruption and may furthermore lead to false-positive reactions, this procedure should be performed only after the eruption has subsided. The site chosen for patch testing must have been free from dermatitis preferably for at least four weeks, in order to avoid false-positive reactions. For other causes of false-positive patch test reactions, see § 3.12. For further details on the technique of patch testing, the reader is referred to the relevant literature [12,23,29,31,73].

PATCH TESTING WITH TOPICALLY APPLIED MEDICAMENTS AND COSMETICS

3.3 Allergic contact dermatitis from topically applied drugs or cosmetics can be caused by:
1. The active ingredient
2. The vehicle constituents
3. The additives.

Additives are substances added to the vehicle in order to enhance the quality and tenability. They include preservatives, antioxidants, stabilizers, emulsifiers, solubilizers, colouring agents and perfume ingredients.

The first problem for the dermatologist, in cases of suspected contact allergy to topical drugs, is to obtain full information about the composition of the medicament or cosmetic. The identification of a sensitizer in a locally applied preparation can be relatively easy if this sensitizer is already known in the literature and/or is part of routine patch test batteries.

Difficulties occur when a particular substance has never been reported to induce contact allergic reactions. This may happen with materials which have a low sensitizing capacity or with newly developed drugs, constituents or additives. In such cases the physician has to answer the following questions before adequate patch testing with the drug or cosmetic can be performed:
1. Which concentration of the substance should be used for patch testing (i.e. a non-irritating concentration)?
2. Which vehicle should be used?
3. Are other test methods indicated, e.g. photopatch tests?

THE TEST CONCENTRATION

3.4 Approximately 300 patch test materials are commercially available from Hermal (Reinbeck/Hamburg, Germany) and Chemotechnique (Malmö, Sweden). For other chemicals and products, the investigator must decide how to apply them as a patch test. Chemicals usually need to be diluted, and it is of the utmost importance to use an appropriate patch test concentration. The ideal patch test concentration of an allergen is that which induces a moderately strong reaction in a sensitized individual, does not cause irritant reactions and does not induce patch test sensitization. Unfortunately, due to interindividual variations in susceptibility to irritation and in degree of sensitization, 'ideal' patch test concentrations which never cause either false-positive or false-negative reactions do not exist. Recommended test concentrations are available in several textbooks [24,89,93,94,135] and in this book. For chemicals or products for which insufficient information is available, the advice of the International Contact Dermatitis Research Group and the North American Contact Dermatitis Group may be followed [12]: "To avoid irritant reactions, an open test with different concentrations should be used first. If the result is negative, a patch test can be performed with a 10–100 times lower concentration. A suitable concentration for patch-testing for most substances is 0.1–1%." A positive allergic test reaction with a new substance must be validated by negative controls (minimum of 20 subjects). In still unclear cases, a repeated open application test according to the method of Hannuksela and Salo should be performed [136,137], and serial dilution tests are often very helpful.

THE VEHICLE TO BE USED FOR PATCH TESTING

3.5 The vehicles for patch test allergens are currently being reinvestigated and reevaluated [23]. For certain allergens, aqueous solutions or solvents such as ethanol, acetone, methyl ethyl ketone, and ethyl ether are recommended [24,89,93, 94,135]. Stability is low and these solutions are difficult to handle and preserve. A semisolid vehicle overcomes these problems to some extent. White petrolatum is currently the standard vehicle. Unfortunately, bioavailability of incorporated allergens may be low, resulting in false-negative reactions. 'Softisan', a hydrophilic lanolin substitute, showed promise as a vehicle, but has been little tested so far [138]. Hydrophilic gels, used as vehicle for the TRUE test, are good alternatives [134].

Attention should be paid to the bioavailability of the substance in the material made up for patch testing, in order to avoid false-negative results.

PHOTOPATCH TESTING

3.6 Photopatch tests are indicated when photosensitivity is suspected. This adverse effect should be considered in all patients with a dermatitis occurring on sun-exposed areas.

In photopatch testing a standard patch test with the suspected agent, suitably diluted, is applied to the skin for a period of 24 hours. The area is subsequently exposed to UV radiation (e.g. sunlight) and the reaction is read after 24 to 48 hours. Appropriate non-UV-exposed control tests are necessary to compare the degree of the reaction and the influence of the UV radiation. Phototoxic patch test reactions must be differentiated from photoallergic ones. A phototoxic reaction is a sunburn type of reaction occurring within six hours, and consists of erythema only. A photoallergic reaction has eczematous features (papules, vesicles etc.); combinations occur frequently. Characteristics of phototoxic and photoallergic reactions are listed in § 3.7.

When only the irradiated test site is positive, the diagnosis of photosensitivity is made. When the non-irradiated site is also positive but far less positive than the irradiated site, both contact allergy and photosensitivity are present. If both test sites are equally positive there is an allergic contact sensitivity without photosensitization. Numerous techniques and light sources for photopatch testing have been described (see Chapter 6). Drugs having caused phototoxic and/or photoallergic reactions are listed in Chapter 6.

3.7 Some characteristics of phototoxic and photoallergic reactions [27]

Feature	Photoallergy	Phototoxicity
prevalence	low	high
latency between first exposure and response	present	absent
dosage	low	high
action spectrum	wide	narrow, usually short-wave UV radiation
recurrence requires:	– 'light' + photosensitizer, *or* – 'light' alone, *or* – photosensitizer alone.	'light' + photosensitizer
lesion morphology	various forms	intensified sunburn
skin flare-up	*a:* at an unirradiated site *b:* at previously affected area	absent
results of photopatch testing	*a:* allergic morphology and histology, response delayed *b:* retested, response more immediate	limited to area of contact, and response more immediate
cross-reactions	may occur to chemically related compounds	–

THE INTERPRETATION OF PATCH TEST RESULTS

Irritant versus allergic patch test reactions

3.8 In order to differentiate between irritant and allergic patch test reactions the following characteristics of both types of reactions may be taken into account:

Irritant reactions	Allergic reactions
– relatively oligomorphous	– frequently more polymorphous
– reaction not spreading	– reaction spreading beyond the test site borders
– sharp delimitation	– vaguely delimited
– commonly no inclination to increase in size and severity after removal: commonly 'decrescendo' course (with exceptions)	– frequently greater and stronger reaction the days after removal: commonly a 'crescendo' course in the days after removal
– smarting	– itching

Irritant reactions usually develop fully earlier than allergic responses. However, it has been shown [80] that some irritant responses are at their maximum after two days, and are consequently very similar to allergic patch test reactions. This makes differentiation more complicated. Frequently, even after a careful examination, a decisive answer about the character of an observed patch test reaction remains impossible. This is especially the case when low-strength (?+ or +) reactions are obtained. Unfortunately, these are the reactions most frequently observed in the practice of patch testing. In such cases a punch biopsy of the patch test area may be of some (unfortunately limited) help. The following characteristics of the histopathology of allergic and irritant dermatitis may be useful for differentiation between them [25]:

3.9 Distinctive histological criteria between allergic and irritant patch test reactions in man

	Allergic reactions	Irritant reactions
Epidermis:		
spongiosis	+ to +++	+ or –
exocytosis	+ to +++	+++
vesicles	+ (spongiotic)	+ (not spongiotic)
formation of bullae	facultative (spongiotic)	facultative (rarely spongiotic)
pustules	–	+ or –
necrosis of epidermal cells	–	+ to +++
acantholysis of epidermal cells	–	+ or –
distribution of the infiltrate in the epidermis	focal	diffuse
Dermis:		
perivascular infiltrate	mononuclear	mononuclear or mixed (mononuclear + neutrophils)
eosinophilic leukocytes	+ or –	–
dilatation of lymphatic vessels	+ or –	–
dilatation of blood capillaries	+ or –	+ or –
edema	+ or –	very unusual

It must be stressed that even these histological criteria often are insufficient, again especially in low-strength (?+ or +) reactions. Other reported methods for differentiation (e.g. the lymphocyte transformation test) may be useful in individual cases. For routine daily practice they are generally too costly and time-consuming. As yet, the best method to differentiate between allergic and irritant patch test reactions is to test a number of healthy volunteers with the incriminated test substance and to perform serial dilution tests on the patient with the suspected allergen.

Multiple positive patch test reactions

3.10 When more than one patch test is positive, the following possibilities should be considered:

1. Concomitant sensitization: this means sensitization to two or more substances present in the same product.
2. Simultaneous sensitization: this means sensitization to two or more substances present in different products. A special form of simultaneous sensitization is the so-called 'Ampliative medicament allergy' [82]. It is well-known that patients with chronic venous stasis leg ulcers have a tendency, in the course of time, to develop contact sensitivities to multiple locally applied medicaments [81]. In some leg ulcer patients a propensity may be noted to develop, within a short period of time, contact allergic reactions to a whole series of locally applied immunologically innocuous medicaments. This state has been called ampliative medicament allergy [82]. Probably the dense lymphocytic infiltrate around the ulcers, in combination with the condition of the surrounding skin and the occlusive effect of bandages, provides a good receptor site for the rapid induction of sensitization, even to low-grade allergens in topical medications.
3. Cross-sensitivity: this implies that a secondary allergen, chemically related to the primary allergen, also produces a positive patch test reaction. Cross-sensitivity can only be assumed when the sensitized person has not been in contact with the secondary allergen previously.
4. One allergen is present in different products or substances (e.g. positive reactions to several balsams may be caused by one and the same allergen present in these substances).
5. One or more patch tests are false-positive (§ 3.12).

False-positive and false-negative patch test reactions [128,132,133]

3.11 One of the main problems in contact allergy is the occurrence of false-positive or false-negative reactions to patch tests. A false-positive reaction is a positive patch test reaction in the absence of contact allergy. A false-negative reaction is a negative patch test reaction in the presence of contact allergy. These reactions are especially to be expected when materials are tested for which no proper test concentration and vehicle has been established. False-positive reactions are caused by weakly irritant materials.'Typical' irritant reactions caused by strong irritants are easily recognized. They are characterized by:

- a sharply defined vivid erythema, which quickly (in about 24 hours) fades away
- an erosion
- the formation of a bulla corresponding to the size of the test material.

However, problems occur with mild irritant reactions, which are often characterized by a slightly elevated erythema without a clear infiltration. This kind of reaction is not easily distinguishable from a true but weak allergic reaction.

Causes of false-positive reactions to patch tests

3.12 Several situations may lead to false-positive reactions:

1. The drug has (also) an irritant action and the test concentration has been too

high. This has been reported, for instance, in patch testing with clioquinol [20].

2. The vehicle (e.g. powder or pieces of powderized pills) causes false-positive traumatic reactions.
3. The drug is unevenly dispersed in the vehicle or on the patch tester.
4. The allergen has degraded (e.g. oxidized) into an irritant substance.
5. The vehicle used for testing is an irritant.
6. The diluent is (too) volatile and thus the concentration of the drug on the patch tester becomes higher than intended.
7. The drug is a potent sensitizer, but the patient is not allergic at the moment of patch testing. Sometimes a late reaction (after one or two weeks) to a patch test is noted in such situations, which may indicate that active sensitization by patch testing has taken place.
8. The test is read too quickly after removal of the patch tester. Redness and edema occurring within a few minutes after removal of the adhesive and the patch tester are mistaken for a true positive reaction.
9. The presence of an irritant or allergic dermatitis in an acute phase elsewhere on the skin may increase non-specific reactivity to some (but not all) mild irritants [3].
10. The presence of a severe reaction to adhesive tape makes a reliable reading difficult. The skin in the region of the test has become highly irritated and may elicit reactions to normally correctly diluted but potentially irritating substances
11. One or more positive patch test reactions may cause false-positive reactions to other patch tests. This condition has been termed ‘angry back’ [38], but as the phenomenon is not restricted to the back, it is preferable to use the name ‘excited skin syndrome’ (ESS) [83,88]. Weak positive patch test reactions, concomitant to other weak or strong positive reactions may lose their reactivity in up to 45% when retested [88]. Allergens which are marginal irritants, e.g. formaldehyde, frequently cause weak positive reactions in the ESS, which are lost at retesting. False-positive reactivity is often found at the proximity of strong reactions (‘spill-over’).
12. Patch tests with salts of metals (nickel, copper, arsenic, mercury) may produce a non-specific reaction characterized by small pustules, each with a small erythematous areola. The reaction differs clinically and histopathologically from a true positive patch test reaction.
13. Localized scratching or rubbing over a patch test site may cause a dermographism reaction mimicking a positive patch test [84].

Causes of false-negative reactions to patch tests

3.13 The following situations may lead to false-negative reactions:

1. The amount of the drug tested is too small.
2. The concentration of the allergen in the test substance or in the proprietary preparation is too low. It is sometimes necessary to increase the patch test concentration with a factor of 10 or more to obtain positive allergic patch test reactions. This is for instance the case with neomycin, methyl(chloro)isothiazolinone and corticosteroids.
3. The allergen is degraded or oxidized during storage.
4. The allergic dermatitis has been caused by a photoallergen.

5. The allergen is volatile.
6. The diluent is volatile, rapid evaporization decreases the possibility of penetration of the allergen into the epidermis.
7. The allergen is poorly absorbed. The bioavailability of the allergen in the patch test vehicle (e.g. petrolatum) may be considerably lower than in the original proprietary drug.
8. A 'quenching effect' has occurred: a contact sensitizing substance no longer causes contact sensitization in combination with another substance [42]. This phenomenon has thus far only been observed in the maximization test with the sensitizing aldehydes phenylacetaldehyde, citral and cinnamic aldehyde. This phenomenon probably is of no importance as a cause of false-negative reactions, and the whole concept of 'quenching' has actually been challenged [19,127].
9. A compound allergy has occurred: a mixture of substances causes an allergic reaction, but the individual ingredients react negatively. Thus the 'allergen' is a combination of more than one ingredient [7]. Some cases of compound allergy may actually indicate inadequate testing, e.g. using the wrong vehicle for patch testing [139].
10. Corticosteroids present in the medication tested decrease the extent as well as the strength of the reaction. It is possible that low-grade patch test reactions are completely masked [126].
11. The skin of the patient is still in a refractory state immediately after a severe allergic contact dermatitis (presumably all available T-lymphocytes are involved in the clinical reaction).
12. The patient is under corticosteroid treatment. It is generally assumed that doses of 15 mg prednisolone or more may suppress weak positive patch test reactions.
13. The skin has recently been treated with a potent corticosteroid preparation. In view of the fact that a depot of steroid is formed in the skin an interim period of one week is considered necessary in order to obtain trustworthy patch test results. Otherwise, weak positive reactions may be diminished in size and strength, or even completely suppressed. Intermediate-strength topical steroids are said *not* to prevent the detection of contact allergy by patch testing [91, 92].
14. Immunosuppressive drugs inhibit the patch test reaction.
15. There is a slow development of the patch test reaction — the test is read too quickly, e.g. as seen with neomycin and corticosteroid testing (positive reactions may sometimes only be noted after several days) [125].
16. The sensitivity to the tested substance is a low-grade one. This may occur in patch tests with cross-reacting substances.
17. The permeability of the skin in the test area is low compared with the site of clinical exposure. Nail polish may cause dermatitis of the face and the neck, whilst the hands are not affected, and the patch tests on the skin of the back remain negative.
18. Technical problems, e.g. insufficient occlusion of the patch tests.
19. The product to be tested has to be diluted to avoid irritant reactions (e.g. shampoos, cutting oils). In (necessarily) doing so, the allergen is rendered too dilute to react.
20. Some women may be hyporeactive before their menstruation [129].

21. UV-B light suppresses the elicitation of allergic contact dermatitis, and some positive reactions may be missed when patch testing during summertime in northern latitudes [56,130].
22. Impaired cell-mediated immunity prevents a positive patch test reaction, e.g. in coeliac disease [131].

The relevance of true positive patch test reactions

3.14 Patch tests are performed primarily to establish the cause of an allergic contact dermatitis. However, a causal relationship between the allergen thus demonstrated and the eruption is not always clear, especially when the patient apparently has not been exposed to the allergen (at least according to his medical history).

The following situations may occur:

1. The patient does not know or does not *remember* having been in contact with the allergen previously.
2. The patient's history is incomplete, e.g. important details concerning his work or his hobbies have been overlooked. Exact and detailed information may provide a satisfactory explanation and subsequently the solution to the cure of the patient's skin problem.
3. The observed patch test reaction is caused by a compound cross-reacting to the allergen that has caused the eruption, but the actual causative allergen has not been tested, and therefore remains unknown. In this case, the patient may rightly deny contact with the allergen demonstrated. In such situations it would be useful to know to which compound(s) the positively reacting substance has been reported to cross-react. as this may possibly indicate the actual causative allergenic substance.
   An alphabetical listing of substances that are known to cross-react is provided in § 3.15, and for every substance the possible primary sensitizer is stated. It must, however, be pointed out that not all reactions listed are true cross-reactions; sometimes the compound mentioned forms part of (or is an ingredient of) the primary sensitizer (see Point 4).
4. The observed patch test reaction is caused by a compound which is an ingredient of the preparation that has caused the contact allergic reaction. When both the patient and the physician are unaware of this, and the sensitizing preparation has not been tested (or the preparation failed to elicit a positive reaction due to the low concentration of the allergen), the significance of the positive patch test reaction may be overlooked.
5. The observed patch test reaction is caused by a complex preparation (e.g. balsam Peru) which contains several allergenic compounds, but the patient has been sensitized by one of its ingredients from *another source*. Again, the patient may (apparently) rightly deny previous contact with the allergen demonstrated by patch testing.

On the other hand, not every positive patch test reaction may be considered relevant to the existing dermatosis, even when the patient has apparently been exposed to the allergen thus demonstrated.

The following possibilities must be kept in mind:

1. The observed positive reaction is a secondary, complicating and aggravating

factor, but not the primary cause of the eruption. This may be seen especially with topical drugs.
2. The reaction is caused by an allergen to which the patient has been exposed in the past, but is not relevant to the present situation.
3. The patient has been in contact with the allergen, but the observed patch test reaction represents a cross-reaction to the actual causative allergen.
4. The patient is allergic to several chemicals, and the allergen demonstrated is unrelated to the eruption.

3.15 List of (pseudo) cross-reactions

Compound cross-reacting to the primary sensitizer, or forming part of it	Primary sensitization to	See §
abietic acid	dihydroabietyl alcohol	5.14
	rosin (colophony)	5.38
abietic alcohol	rosin (colophony)	5.38
alcohols	other alcohols	5.7
amantadine	tromantadine	5.41
ambutyrosin	neomycin	5.23
amikacin	neomycin	5.23
3(aminomethyl)-pyridine	butoxyethyl nicotinate	5.41
aminophylline	ethylenediamine dihydrochloride	5.20
aminosydin	neomycin	5.23
ammonium thioglycolate	glyceryl thioglycolate	26.14
amodiaquin	clioquinol	5.7
α-amylcinnamic alcohol	α-amylcinnamic aldehyde	5.14
α-amylcinnamic aldehyde	α-amylcinnamic alcohol	5.14
amylocaine	tetracaine	5.18
antazoline sulfate	ethylenediamine dihydrochloride	5.20
	tripelennamine	5.28
antidiabetics (para-compounds)	sulfonamide	5.23
aryl salicylates	phenyl salicylate	23.53
atranorin	oak moss	5.14
azo-dyes	p-aminobenzoic acid	29.19
	diacetazotol	5.41
	other azo-dyes	
bacitracin	neomycin (?)	5.23
	polymyxin-B sulfate	5.23

(continued)

§ **3.15** *(continuation)*

Compound cross-reacting to the primary sensitizer, or forming part of it	Primary sensitization to	See §
balsam Peru	balsam Tolu	5.14
	beeswax	5.38
	benzaldehyde	5.14
	benzoin tincture	5.38
	benzyl benzoate	5.40
	benzyl cinnamate	5.14
	benzyl salicylate	5.14
	cinnamic acid	
	cinnamic alcohol	5.14
	cinnamic aldehyde	5.14
	cinnamon oil	5.14
	coniferyl alcohol	5.14
	coumarin	5.14
	diethylstilbestrol	5.41
	2-ethoxyethyl-*p*-methoxycinnamate	29.19
	eugenol	5.14
	farnesol	5.14
	isoeugenol	5.14
	methyl cinnamate	
	propanidid (?)	5.18
	propolis	5.41
	rosin (colophony)	5.38
	storax	5.38
	tiger balm	5.41
balsam Peru/rosin/turpentine oils/ wood tars	(some) perfume ingredients	5.10
balsam Tolu	balsam Peru	5.14
	benzyl benzoate	5.40
benzalkonium chloride	benzethonium chloride	5.7
	benzoxonium chloride	5.7
	cetalkonium chloride (?)	5.7
	cetrimonium bromide	
benzestrol	diethylstilbestrol	5.41
benzocaine	butethamine	5.18
	glyceryl PABA	29.19
	old orthoform	5.18
	parabens	5.7
benzoic acid	balsam Peru	5.16
	propolis	5.41
benzoin	balsam Peru	5.14
	storax	5.38

(continued)

§ **3.15** *(continuation)*

Compound cross-reacting to the primary sensitizer, or forming part of it	Primary sensitization to	See §
benzyl alcohol	balsam Peru	5.14
	benzoin tincture	5.38
	propolis	5.41
benzyl benzoate	balsam Peru	5.16
	propolis	5.43
benzyl cinnamate	benzoin tincture	5.38
	2-ethoxyethyl-*p*-methoxycinnamate	29.19
	propolis	5.41
benzyl ferulate	propolis	5.41
benzyl isoferulate	propolis	5.41
benzyl nicotinate	butoxyethyl nicotinate	5.41
benzyl paraben	diethylstilbestrol	5.41
benzyl penicillin	penethamate hydriodide	5.43
p-benzylphenol	diethylstilbestrol	5.41
bisphenol-A	diethylstilbestrol	5.41
	monobenzyl ether of hydroquinone	5.41
2-bromo-2-nitropropane-1,3-diol (bronopol)	formaldehyde	5.7
	other formaldehyde donors	
brompheniramine	dexchlorpheniramine maleate	5.28
bupivacaine	lidocaine	5.18
butirosin	neomycin	5.23
butylene glycol	propylene glycol	5.20
cananga oil	benzyl salicylate	5.14
carvacrol	thymol	5.7
cera flava	propolis	5.41
cetrimonium bromide	benzalkonium chloride	5.7
ω-chloroacetophenone	chlorphenoxide	5.30
chloramphenicol	azidamfenicol	5.23
p-chloro-*m*-cresol	chloroxylenol	5.7
chlorofluoromethane	freon 11/12	5.20
chloroxylenol	*p*-chloro-*m*-cresol	5.7
chlorpheniramine	dexchlorpheniramine maleate	5.28

(continued)

§ **3.15** *(continuation)*

Compound cross-reacting to the primary sensitizer, or forming part of it	Primary sensitization to	See §
chlorpromazines	chlorprothixene	5.43
chlorquinaldol	clioquinol	5.7
cinnamates	balsam Peru	5.14
cinnamic acid	balsam Peru	5.14
	propolis	5.41
cinnamic alcohol	balsam Peru	5.14
	cinnamic acid	5.14
	cinnamic aldehyde	
	propolis	5.41
cinnamic aldehyde	cinnamic alcohol	5.14
	cinnamon oil	
cinnamon oil	propanidid	5.18
cinnamyl alcohol	2-ethoxyethyl-*p*-methoxycinnamate	29.19
cinnamyl cinnamate	propolis	5.42
citronellal	hydroxycitronellal	5.14
clindamycin	lincomycin	5.23
clioquinol	dibucaine (?)	5.18
	quinine sulfate (?)	5.43
clotrimazole	other imidazoles (?)	5.30
cocamide DEA	lauramide DEA	26.2
cocamidopropyl betaine	cocobetaine	26.2
cocarboxylase	thiamine (vitamin B1)	5.43
colistin	bacitracin	5.23
coniferyl benzoate	propolis	5.41
cresols	phenol	5.37
croconazole	other imidazoles	5.30
cycloheximide	neomycin (?)	5.23
DC yellow 10	DC yellow 11	27.16
dehydroabietic acid	rosin (colophony)	5.38
demethylchlortetracycline	chlortetracycline	5.23
dextropimaric acid	rosin (colophony)	5.38
diazolidinyl urea	formaldehyde	5.7
	imidazolidinyl urea	5.7

(continued)

§ **3.15** *(continuation)*

Compound cross-reacting to the primary sensitizer, or forming part of it	Primary sensitization to	See §
diazolidinyl urea (continued)	other formaldehyde donors	
5,7-dibromo-8-hydroxyquinoline (DBO)	clioquinol	5.7
dibucaine	lidocaine	5.18
dichlorophene	hexachlorophene	5.7
dienestrol	diethylstilbestrol	5.41
diethanolamine	ethylenediamine	5.20
diethazine hydrochloride	chlorpromazine	5.43
diethylenetetramine	ethylenediamine dihydrochloride	5.20
diethylstilbestrol	monobenzone (monobenzylether of hydroquinone) (?)	5.41
diglyceryl dithioglycolate	glyceryl thioglycolate	26.14
dihydralazine	hydrazines	5.43
dihydroabietic acid	rosin (colophony)	5.38
dihydrostreptomycin	streptomycin	5.23
diisopropyl fluorophosphate	epinephrine chloride (?)	5.41
dimercaprol (BAL)	thioglycerol	5.20
N,N′-dimethyl piperazine	piperazine	5.43
p-dinitrobenzene	chloramphenicol (?)	5.23
dinitrochlorobenzene	chloramphenicol (?) pyrrolnitrin (?)	5.23 5.30
dioxybenzone	oxybenzone	29.19
diphenhydramine	dexchlorpheniramine maleate	5.28
diphenylamine	*N*-phenyl-*p*-phenylenediamine	26.6
diuretics (para-compounds)	sulfonamide	5.23
DMDM hydantoin	formaldehyde MDM hydantoin other formaldehyde donors	5.7 5.7
dodecyl gallate	propyl gallate	29.3
domiphen bromide	benzoxonium chloride	5.7
econazole	other imidazoles	5.30
enilconazole	other imidazoles	5.30

(continued)

§ **3.15** *(continuation)*

Compound cross-reacting to the primary sensitizer, or forming part of it	Primary sensitization to	See §
epinephrine borate	epinephrine chloride	5.41
essential oils	balsam Peru	5.14
	propolis	5.42
	wood tars	5.37
ethopropazine hydrochloride	chlorpromazine	5.43
ethyl aminobenzoate	parabens	5.7
ethyl chloride	chlorofluoromethane (?)	5.20
ethylenediamine hydrochloride	aminophylline	5.43
	antazoline	5.28
	edetic acid (EDTA)	5.7
	piperazine	5.43
	promethazine hydrochloride	5.28
	triethanolamine	5.20
	zinc pyrithione (?)	26.2
ethylenediamine dihydroiodide	ethylenediamine dihydrochloride	5.20
eugenol	balsam Peru	5.14
	benzoin tincture	5.38
	isoeugenol	5.14
	propanidid	5.18
evernic acid	oak moss	5.14
farnesol	propolis	5.42
flufenamic acid	etofenamate (?)	5.41
formaldehyde	aryl-sulfonamide resin	28.2
	2-bromo-2-nitropropane-1,3-diol (bronopol)	5.7
	DMDM hydantoin	5.7
	diazolidinyl urea	5.7
	glutaraldehyde (?)	5.7
	imidazolidinyl urea	5.7
	quaternium-15	5.7
framycetin	neomycin	5.23
fumarprotocetraric acid	oak moss	5.14
gentamicin	neomycin	5.23
	sisomycin	13.40
geranium	geranial	5.16
glyceryl isostearate	isostearyl alcohol	27.16

(continued)

§ **3.15** *(continuation)*

Compound cross-reacting to the primary sensitizer, or forming part of it	Primary sensitization to	See §
glyceryl ricinoleate	zinc ricinoleate	29.13
halogenated quinolines	other halogenated quinolines	5.7
halogenated salicylanilides	bithionol	5.7
	trichlorocarbanilide	5.7
hexachlorophene	bithionol	5.7
	dichlorophene (?)	5.7
	halogenated salicylanilides (usually photo-cross-reactions)	
hexamethonium bromide	benzalkonium chloride	5.7
hexamethylene tetramine	ethylenediamine	5.20
hexestrol	diethylstilbestrol	5.41
hexylene glycol	butylene glycol	5.20
	propylene glycol	5.20
hexylresorcinol	resorcinol	5.37
homatropine	atropine sulfate	13.40
4-homosulfanilamide	parabens	5.7
hydralazine	hydrazines	5.43
hydrochlorothiazide	dibenzthione	5.30
hydrogenated castor oil	zinc ricinoleate	29.13
hydroquinone	phenol (?)	5.37
	pyrocatechol	26.6
	resorcinol	5.37
hydroxycitronellal	citronellal	5.14
	geranial	5.14
	linalool (?)	5.14
	methoxycitronellal	5.14
hydroxyhydroquinone	resorcinol	5.37
hydroxyzine	zinc pyrithione (?)	26.2
ibuproxam	ketoprofen	5.41
imidazolidinyl urea	diazolidinyl urea	5.7
	other formaldehyde donors	5.7
iodine	povidone-iodine	5.7
isobutyl-*p*-aminobenzoate	old orthoform	5.18

(continued)

§ **3.15** *(continuation)*

Compound cross-reacting to the primary sensitizer, or forming part of it	Primary sensitization to	See §
isoconazole	other imidazoles	5.30
isoeugenol	eugenol	5.14
isoniazid (INH)	hydrazines	5.43
4-isopropylaminodiphenylamine	*N*-phenyl-*p*-phenylenediamine	26.6
isopropyl dibenzoylmethane	butyl methoxydibenzoylmethane	27.16
isostearyl alcohol	glyceryl isostearate	27.16
jasmin oil	benzyl salicylate	5.14
kanamycin	dihydrostreptomycin	5.23
	framycetin (?)	5.23
	gentamicin sulfate	5.23
	neomycin	5.23
	streptomycin	5.23
	tobramycin	5.23
ketoconazole	other imidazoles	5.30
ketoprofen	ibuproxam	5.41
lanolin	eucerin	5.20
	lanette N	5.20
	lanette wax	5.20
lavender oil	geranial	5.14
levamisole	tetramisole hydrochloride	5.43
levopimaric acid	rosin (colophony)	5.38
linalool (?)	hydroxycitronellal	27.8
lincomycin	clindamycin	5.25
mafenide	parabens	5.7
maleopimaric acid	colophony	5.38
menadione (vitamin K3)	vitamin K4	5.43
mepacrine	chloroquine diphosphate	5.43
mepivacaine hydrochloride	lidocaine	5.18
meprylcaine	benzocaine	5.18
mepyramine maleate	dexchlorpheniramine maleate (?)	5.28
	ethylenediamine hydrochloride	5.20
mercurials (anorganic, organic, metallic mercury)	other anorganic and organic mercurials, and metallic mercury	5.7

(continued)

§ **3.15** *(continuation)*

Compound cross-reacting to the primary sensitizer, or forming part of it	Primary sensitization to	See §
metabutethamine	benzocaine	5.18
meta-dihydroxybenzenes	resorcinol	5.37
methacycline	oxytetracycline	5.23
methyl abietate	rosin (colophony)	5.38
methyl cinnamate	2-ethoxyethyl-*p*-methoxycinnamate	29.19
methyl heptine carbonate	methyl octine carbonate	5.14
methyl octine carbonate	methyl heptine carbonate	5.14
methyl-2-piperazine	piperazine	5.43
N-methylpiperazine	piperazine	5.43
metoprolol	alprenolol	5.43
miconazole	other imidazoles	5.30
monobenzone (monobenzylether of hydroquinone)	diethylstilbestrol hydroquinone	5.41
morphine	apomorphine	5.43
moskene	musk ambrette	5.14
neoabietic acid	rosin (colophony)	5.38
neomycin	dihydrostreptomycin	5.23
	framcyetin	5.23
	gentamicin	5.23
	streptomycin	5.23
nerilidol	propolis	5.41
p-nitrobenzoic acid	chloramphenicol	5.23
nitrofuran derivatives (?)	nitrofurazone (?)	5.23
nitrofurazone	furazolidone	5.43
nitrofurylaminothiadiazoles	2-(5-nitro-2-furyl)-5-amino-1,3,4-thiadiazole	5.37
	ichthyol (?)	5.7
octoxynol-9	nonoxynols	5.20
octyl gallate	propyl gallate	29.3
orthoform, new	orthoform, old	5.18
orthoform, old	orthoform, new	5.18
oxiconazole	other imidazoles	5.30

(continued)

§ **3.15** *(continuation)*

Compound cross-reacting to the primary sensitizer, or forming part of it	Primary sensitization to	See §
oximetazole chlorhydrate	imidazole chlorhydrate	5.41
oxprenolol	propranolol	5.43
oxybenzone	dioxybenzone	29.19
palustric acid	rosin (colophony)	5.38
parabens	other parabens	5.7
	monobenzone	5.40
	para-compounds	
para-compounds	3-(aminomethyl)pyridine/pyridyl salicylate	5.41
	benzidine	5.42
	benzocaine	5.18
	codeine (?)	5.43
	diacetazotol	5.41
	glyceryl PABA	29.19
	mafenide	5.23
	parabens	5.7
	procaine	5.18
	promethazine hydrochloride	5.28
	sulfonamides	5.23
	tetracaine hydrochloride	5.18
paromomycin	framycetin (?)	5.23
	neomycin	5.23
PEG 400 ricinoleate	zinc ricinoleate	29.13
perfume ingredients (some)	balsam Peru/rosin/ turpentine oil/wood tars/	
pheniramine	dexchlorpheniramine maleate	5.28
phenol	resorcinol	5.37
phenothiazines	chlorpromazine	5.43
	promethazine hydrochloride	5.28
	tripelennamine	5.28
phenyl-benzimidazole sulfonic acid	witisol	29.19
phenylbutazone	oxyphenbutazone	5.41
p-phenylenediamine	*p*-aminobenzoic acid	29.19
	diphenylamine (?)	5.20
	parabens	5.7
	para-compounds	
β-phenylethylhydrazine	hydrazines	5.43

(continued)

§ **3.15** *(continuation)*

Compound cross-reacting to the primary sensitizer, or forming part of it	Primary sensitization to	See §
phenylhydrazine	hydrazines	5.43
phenylmercuric acetate	*p*-chloromercuriphenol	5.7
pheprazone	oxyphenbutazone	5.41
α-pinene	benzoin tincture	5.38
piperazine citrate	ethylenediamine hydrochloride	5.20
	zinc pyrithione (?)	26.2
polyethylene glycols	other polyethylene glycols	5.20
polymyxin	polymyxin-B sulfate	5.23
polymyxin-B sulfate	bacitracin	5.23
potassium iodide (?)	clioquinol	5.7
prilocaine	lidocaine	5.18
pristinamycin	virginiamycin	5.23
procaine	*p*-aminobenzoic acid	29.19
	butethamine	5.18
	parabens	5.7
promethazine hydrochloride	chlorpromazine	5.43
	ethylenediamine hydrochloride	5.20
	triethanolamine (?)	5.20
	tripelennamine	5.28
propolis	balsam Peru	5.14
propranolol	oxprenolol	5.43
propylene glycol	butylene glycol	5.20
	hexylene glycol	5.20
pyridine derivatives	nicotinic acid	5.43
pyridoxine HCl	pyridoxine dioctanoate	26.14
pyrimidine analogs (brominated, chlorinated)	idoxuridine	5.41
pyrocatechol	resorcinol	5.37
pyrogallol	resorcinol	5.37
quaternium-15	formaldehyde	5.7
	other formaldehyde donors	
quinine	clioquinol	5.7
reindeer lichen	oak moss	5.14

(continued)

§ **3.15** *(continuation)*

Compound cross-reacting to the primary sensitizer, or forming part of it	Primary sensitization to	See §
resoquine	clioquinol	5.7
resorcinol	phenol	5.37
resorcinol acetate	resorcinol	5.37
ribostamycin	neomycin tobramycin	5.23
risocaine	old orthoform	5.18
rosin (colophony)	balsam Peru dihydroabietyl alcohol wood tars	5.14 5.14 5.37
sisomicin	neomycin tobramycin	5.23
sodium salicylate	methyl salicylate	5.41
sodium stearate	stearic acid	27.3
sodium sulphoricinate	zinc ricinoleate	29.13
sorbic acid	potassium sorbate	5.7
sorbitan mono-oleate	sorbitan sesquioleate (Arlacel 83®)	5.20
sorbitan monostearate	sorbitan sesquioleate (Arlacel 83®)	5.20
spectinomycin	neomycin	5.23
spiramycin	tylosin	5.43
storax	diethylstilbestrol tincture of benzoin	5.41 5.38
streptomycin	dihydrostreptomycin framycetin (?) neomycin (?)	5.23 5.23 5.23
sulconazole	other imidazoles	5.30
sulfated castor oil	zinc ricinoleate	29.13
sulfapyridine	tripelennamine	5.28
sulfonamides	*p*-aminobenzoic acid aryl-sulfonamide resin other sulfonamides para-compounds	29.19 28.2 5.23
suxibenzone	oxyphenbutazone	5.41
sweetening agents (para-compounds)	other para-compounds sulfonamide	 5.23

(continued)

§ **3.15** *(continuation)*

Compound cross-reacting to the primary sensitizer, or forming part of it	Primary sensitization to	See §
TEA-oleyl polypeptide	potassium coco-hydrolyzed animal protein	26.2
tetracycline	oxytetracycline	5.23
tetraethylenetetramine	ethylenediamine	5.20
tetrahydroabietic acid	rosin (colophony)	5.38
tetramethylthiuram disulfide	tetraethylthiurammonosulfide	5.43
	tetraethylthiuramdisulfide	5.43
thiazinamium	chlorpromazine	5.43
tioconazole	other imidazoles	5.30
tobramycin	neomycin	5.43
tocopheryl nicotinate	tocopheryl acetate	29.3
tree moss	oak moss	5.14
triazine-antihypertensive drugs	dibenzthione (?)	5.30
triethanolamine	promethazine hydrochloride (?)	5.28
triethylenetetramine	ethylenediamine	5.20
trifluorthymidine	idoxuridine	5.41
trimethylpsoralen	8-methoxypsoralen	5.37
triphenylmethane dyes	other triphenylmethane dyes	5.7
turpentine	rosin (colophony)	5.38
turpentine oil	lemon oil	5.14
tylosin	spiramycin (?)	5.43
undecylenic acid	zinc undecylenate	5.30
ung. alc. lanae B.P.	xanthocillin (?)	5.23
usnic acid	oak moss	5.14
vanilla	balsam Peru	5.14
	benzoin tincture	5.38
	coumarin	5.14
vanillin	coumarin	5.14
	propolis	5.42
virginiamycin	pristinamycin	5.23
vitamin K4	menadione (vitamin K3)	5.43
witisol	phenyl-benzimidazole sulfonic acid (?)	29.19

(continued)

§ **3.15** *(continuation)*

Compound cross-reacting to the primary sensitizer, or forming part of it	Primary sensitization to	See §
wool alcohols	Amerchol	
	eucerin	5.20
	lanette N	5.20
	lanette wax	5.20
	laureth-4 (?)	5.20
	other wool alcohol derivatives	
ylang-ylang oil	benzyl salicylate	5.14
	geranial	5.14
zinc oxide	zinc sulfate	5.20
zinc undecylenate	undecylenic acid	5.30

RISKS OF PATCH TESTING FOR THE PATIENT

3.16 Patch testing may be considered a fairly innocent method of investigation. Occasionally however the patient is exposed to some serious hazards and inconveniences. Therefore, in every case in which patch testing appears to be indicated, the advantages and disadvantages of this method of investigation should be taken into account. The following problems may present themselves:

A: The patient develops a strong skin reaction to the adhesive. A large part of the skin of the back becomes red and irritated. Apart from the inconvenience to the patient the results of the test are less reliable. Causes of skin reactions to the adhesive are:

- trauma of removal
- irritation
- retention of sweat
- disturbance of bacterial flora
- contact allergic reactions to constituents of the adhesive. The adhesive may contain rosin (colophony), rubber chemicals, dammar, lanolin, antiseptics, preservatives, acrylates [18].

Currently used adhesives rarely induce allergic reactions.

In most European and US centres patch tests are left in place for a period of 48 hours. When, despite previous testing with different brands of adhesives, irritation is to be expected, an application period of 24 hours should be used. In hot climates a patch test application period of 24 hours generally is to be preferred.

B: Patch tests are performed with a substance which acts as an irritant in the concentration tested. This danger presents itself when materials of unknown composition are tested. Unknown substances presented for patch testing should therefore be investigated carefully and literature data should be collected before the material is applied to the skin. Subsequently, the correct concentration and vehicle for patch testing has to be established. In the first phase of this investigation the substance must be tested in several concentrations, in order to obtain data about the correct non-irritant patch test concentration. These preliminary tests should preferably be performed on the skin of the investigator himself. These tests are not entirely without risk, and the investigator should consider to stop his experiment at once as soon as untoward effects (severe itching or burning, pain) become manifest. In the next phase, patch tests with the substance in this concentration must be performed on a group of at least 20 healthy volunteers. In the correct concentration the allergen will elicit a moderate reaction in the sensitized person, whilst controls will remain negative.

C: Patch testing induces contact allergy to the tested substance. Examples of substances with a strong contact sensitizing capacity are: mafenide (*p*-amino-methylbenzenesulfonamide), other azo-compounds, and some natural products from trees or plants. Of course, patch testing with well-known contact sensitizers such as 2,4-dinitrochlorobenzene (DNCB) and mechlorethamine carries the same risk.

D: Contact urticarial reactions may be observed occasionally during and due to patch testing [79]. Anaphylactoid reactions greatly endangering the patients have occurred with the application of several allergens. See Chapter 7 on Contact urticaria.

E: Strong (++++) patch test reactions are often very troublesome to the patient. These reactions may be controlled by application of a corticosteroid preparation. Pigmentation or depigmentation may subsequently develop and constitute a major cosmetic problem.

F: Patch tests with the relevant allergen may induce a recurrence or an exacerbation of the dermatitis [55].

G: In patients with psoriasis or lichen ruber, a Koebner phenomenon may occur.

H: Very infrequently, keloid formation after patch tests may be noted [54].

I: Systemic symptoms may occur occasionally. A case of respiratory symptoms presumably due to a patch test with piperazine has been documented [78]. The patient was strongly allergic to piperazine, and had experienced eczema and respiratory symptoms when being exposed to this chemical. Gastrointestinal symptoms related to patch tests with hydroxyethylmethacrylate [96] and fatigue, headache, irregular menstruation and gastrointestinal upset from patch testing with UV curable acrylic monomers [97] have been observed.

J: Occasionally lymph node enlargement has been reported in association with a strongly positive patch test reaction [86].

K: An extensive purpuric eruption with papulonodular lesions, lesions en cocarde and bullae with a tendency to necrose was seen in a patient who had a very strong patch test reaction to Frullania [87]. The vasculitis was presumably due to an immune complex reaction.

THE USE OF PATCH TESTS IN DRUG ERUPTIONS

3.17 The value of patch tests with drugs that have caused skin eruptions after systemic administration is sometimes doubted. It is pointed out that positive reactions are only to be expected in cases of Type IV allergic reactions, which constitute a minority. Also, the allergic rash may be caused by a metabolite rather than by the drug itself, which may cause false-negative reactions to patch tests with the drug.

Nevertheless, we think that performing patch tests in patients who have suffered from drug eruptions is worthwhile and may assist is making a proper diagnosis [117]:

1. The patient has developed a systemic eczematous contact-type dermatitis medicamentosa. This possibility is surveyed in Chapter 17.
2. In some cases of fixed drug eruption, patch tests with the incriminated drug are positive, provided they are performed at the site of the fixed eruption [46]. The most well-known cause of this type of reaction is phenolphthalein.
3. In eruptions caused by certain systemic drugs, the value of patch testing has been proven by clinical experience. This is apparently especially the case in maculopapular and urticarial rashes due to penicillin or its derivatives [50,58]. Other drug eruptions caused by systemic administration, in which patch testing has yielded positive allergic patch test reactions relevant to the diagnosis, are summarized in § 3.18. In patients with urticaria and anaphylaxis from pyrazolones, contact urticarial patch test reactions are frequently observed [11].

3.18 Patch testing in drug eruptions

Drug	Patch test conc. and vehicle	Cross-reactions	Comment	Ref.
amantadine	pure		*photo*patch test positive	72
aminophenazone	10% in DMSO 40%			57
aminophylline	2.5% pet.	ethylenediamine		63
amitriptyline	?			1
amoxicillin	pure	other penicillins		50,52,58
ampicillin	pure	other penicillins		50,58
benzydamine	0.1–1% aqua		positive *photo*patch test	104
benzylpenicillin	pure	other penicillins		50,58
carbamazepine	1% and 5% pet.		also *photo*patch test positive [8]	8,17, 100
carbimazole	pure			66
carbromal	?			1
carprofen	5%–10%–20% pet.		*photo*patch test positive	62
captopril	10% aqua			108
cefuroxime	10% aqua	cephalothin, cephaloridine *not* to penicillins		3

(continued)

§ **3.18** *(continuation)*

Drug	Patch test conc. and vehicle	Cross-reactions	Comment	Ref.
cephalexin	1% o.o. and pure	*not* to penicillin		121
cephalosporin	20% pet. and pure	penicillins		50,58,64
chloramphenicol	50%?			67
cimetidine	100 mg/ml aqua			120
clobazam	pure		generalized drug rash from patch testing	55
clomipramine	0.1%–5% pet.	possibly to chlorpromazine	patch test and *photo*-patch test positive	100
cloxacillin		other penicillins		50,58
codeine	0.01% aqua	other opioids		119
diclofenac	2.5% pet.	not to other NSAIDs	urticaria after oral administration; anafylactic shock after i.m. administration	45
dimethyl sulfoxide	10% pet.		the drug had been administered in the bladder	100
diphenhydramine	1% pet.			61
dipyrone	pure	aminophenazone	contact urticarial patch test reaction	71
ephedrine hydrochloride	5% aqua			16
ethylenediamine	1% pet.	aminophylline		63
feneticillin	pure	other penicillins		50,58
flucloxacillin	powder pure	other penicillins		52
hydrochlorothiazide	1% pet.		*photo*patch test positive	68
hydromorphone	pure and 0.2% aqua			2
isoniazid (INH)	1% pet.		pustular drug eruption, and pustular patch test	21
ketoconazole	pure	bifonazole ? econazole	*scratch* test positive	66
			patch test positive in ref. 15 but dubious report	15
metamizole	pure		urticarial drug eruption	99

(continued)

§ **3.18** *(continuation)*

Drug	Patch test conc. and vehicle	Cross-reactions	Comment	Ref.
methyl dopa	? in pet.		positive *photo*patch test	102
methylprednisolone acetate	comm. prep.	other corticosteroids		115
neomycin and other aminoglycosides	?			1
nitrofurantoin	1% alc.			98
nystatin	30,000 I.U./g PEG	not to amphotericin B		59
penicillins	pure	cephalosporins other penicillins		50,58
phenacetin	10% in DMSO 40%			57
phenazone	5% pet.		EEM-like eruption	60
phenobarbital	0.1% aqua			107
phenol	1% aqua			70
phenothiazine	?		*photo*patch test positive	34
phenylbutazone	pure	amidopyrine metamizol oxyphenbutazone propyphenazone	urticarial drug eruption	99
piroxicam	1% and 10% pet.	thiosalicylic acid	patients with photosensitive drug rashes from piroxi-cam are allergic (*not* photo-allergic) to the thiosalicylic part of thimerosal	116
practolol	10% and 50% pet.			9
prednisolon	pure	methylprednisolon		113
prednisolon succinate	comm. prep.	prednisolon	pustular allergic drug eruption	114
propranolol	pure			51
propyphenazone	pure	aminophenazone dipyrone phenylbutazone,	contact urticarial patch test reaction	71
pseudoephedrine HCl	1% pet.	norephedrine HCl		109
pyrazinamide	1%–10% alc.			106
quinidine sulfate	1% saline sol.	quinidine	*photo*patch test positive	13,65

(continued)

§ **3.18** *(continuation)*

Drug	Patch test conc. and vehicle	Cross-reactions	Comment	Ref.
sodium metabisulfite	5% pet.		antioxidant in local anesthetic, administered per injection	111
sulfonamide	?			1
tetrazepam	1% aqua		tetrazepam is a benzodiazepine	105
thioridazine	?		thioridazine is a phenothiazine; positive *photo*patch test	101
tiaprofenic acid	pure		positive *photo*patch tests. It is uncertain whether the reactions observed are phototoxic or photo-allergic in nature	103
vitamin K (phytonadione)	commercial preparation	*not* to menadiol	reactions tend to occur in patients with liver disease and may rarely progress to a scleroderma-like phase	53

However, in order to exclude non-specific reactions, a series of control tests on a panel of healthy volunteers remains imperative, as many medicaments applied without dilution and under occlusion in patch test conditions act as mild irritants.

Patch testing in drug eruptions has been reviewed [117,118].

THE PERSISTENCE OF ACQUIRED EPIDERMAL SENSITIVITY

3.19 The course of an acquired epidermal sensitivity is a matter of great practical importance. The results of the investigations on this subject published thus far have been rather contradictory. The relevant literature on the persistence of positive patch test reactions is summarized in § 3.20. The scarceness of available data makes it impossible to restrict this survey to topically applied drugs. Unfortunately, the available reports are difficult to compare due to methodological differences. Some early investigators [14] found that if the offensive agent was removed, the hypersensitivity subsided, or disappeared completely in a large proportion of cases. The results of another investigation [47] led to a more pessimistic view. In ten patients, patch test reactions to clioquinol (vioform) were still unchanged positive after an average interval of 6 years, even though these patients had scrupulously avoided the allergen and related chemicals. The more recent study of Keczkes et al. [77] in which only 14% of patch test reactions were negative after a period of 10–12 years (although admittedly, probably in a biased population) also seems to indicate that allergic contact sensitivity tends to persist for many years, although a proportion of patients show diminution of their sensitivity over the years. The persistence probably does not only depend on renewed contact with the allergen or related substances but also on the nature of the allergen, and possibly the intensity of the acquired hypersensitivity.

The possibility also remains that those cases with negative results on re-patch testing may have been false-positive reactions the first time [33,122]. In one report, however, sensitization was assured, as was total avoidance of the allergen [123]. Of 31 patients who had been treated more than 7 years previously with DNCB for alopecia areata, 23 (74%) still reacted to a patch test. Of 35 patients who had been treated with squaric acid dibutyl ester, 24 (69%) were still allergic after 3 years of complete avoidance of the allergen [123]. Finally, the possibility should be kept in mind that a negative (repeat) patch test does not necessarily exclude (subthreshold) sensitization [41].

3.20 The persistence of positive patch test reactions

Allergen	Interval in patch testing (years)	Number of patients	Negative on re-patch testing (%)	Ref.
turpentine	1–3.5	106	3	14
nickel	1.5–11	54	43	39
balsam Peru		18	16	
nickel	4.2 (average)	9	22	6
turpentine		12	66	
balsam Peru		9	44	
nickel	13.5 (average)	11	18	40
turpentine		29	62	
nickel	2–5	40	10	90
bichromate	3–10	20	45	10
p-phenylenediamine	3–10	50	8	
nickel	5.5–7.6	27	4	30
turpentine			6	
chromate	16	?	25	26
parabens			74	
nickel	2	21	38	44
nickel	1.2–5	36	41	37

(continued)

§ **3.20** *(continuation)*

Allergen	Interval in patch testing (years)	Number of patients	Negative on re-patch testing (%)	Ref.
turpentine nickel balsam Peru	2–15	105	64 32 50	48
22 allergens	1–3	208	25	35
bichromate	4–7	48	21	49
clioquinol	6	10	0	47
46 allergens	10–12	100	14	77
ethylenediamine	10	16	25	124
wool alcohols	0.5–6	37	59	33

3.21 REFERENCES

1. Agrup, G. (1972): Patch testing in drug allergy. In: *Mechanisms in Drug Allergy*. Editors: C.H. Dash and H.E.H. Jones. Churchill Livingstone, Edinburgh.
2. de Cuyper, C. and Goeteyn, M. (1992): Systemic contact dermatitis from subcutaneous hydromorphone. *Contact Dermatitis, 27*, 220–223.
3. Romano, A., Pietrantonio, F., di Fonso, M. and Venuti, A. (1992): Delayed hypersensitivity to cefuroxime. *Contact Dermatitis, 27*, 270–271.
4. Bergstresser, P.R. (1989): Contact allergic dermatitis. Old problems and new techniques. *Arch. Dermatol., 125*, 276–279.
5. Brian, R.G. and Nater, J. P. (1973): Ulcus cruris en contacteczeem. *Ned. T. Geneesk., 117,* 561.
6. Bülow, K. (1954): En efterundersögelse of eczempatienter med positive lappepröver. *Ugeskr. Laeg., 18,* 245.
7. Kellett, J.K., King, C.M. and Beck, M.H. (1986): Compound allergy to medicaments. *Contact Dermatitis, 14,* 45–48.
8. Terui, T. and Tagami, H. (1989): Eczematous drug eruption from carbamazepine: coexistence of contact and photocontact sensitivity. *Contact Dermatitis, 20*, 260–264.
9. Felix, R.H. and Comaish, J.S. (1974): The value of patch tests and other skin tests in drug eruptions. *Lancet, 1,* 1017.
10. Fisher, A.A., Pelzig, A. and Kanof, N.B. (1958): The persistence of allergic eczematous sensitivity and the cross-sensitivity pattern to paraphenylenediamine. *J. Invest. Dermatol., 30,* 9.
11. Maucher, O.M. and Fuchs, A. (1986): Der Hauttest zur Verifizierung der Pyrazolonallergie. *Allergologie, 9*, 305–314.
12. Fregert, S. (1981): *Manual of contact dermatitis, 2nd Edition,* Munksgaard, Copenhagen, Denmark.
13. Ljunggren, B., Hindsén, M. and Isaksson, M. (1992): Systemic quinine photosensitivity with photoepicutaneous cross-reactivity to quinidine. *Contact Dermatitis, 26*, 1–4.
14. Gomez-Orbaneja, J. and Barrientos, E. (1938): Funktionelle Nachuntersuchungen bei Ekzematikern. *Schweiz. Med. Wschr., 24,* 694.
15. Garcia-Bravo, B., Mazuecos, J., Rodriguez-Pichardo, A., Navas, J. and Camacho, F. (1989): Hypersensitivity to ketoconazole preparatons; study of 4 cases. *Contact Dermatitis, 21*, 346–347.
16. Audicana, M., Urrutia, J., Echechipia, S., Munoz, D. and Fernandez de Corres, L. (1992): Sensitization to ephedrine in oral anticatarrhal drugs. *Contact Dermatitis, 24*, 223.

17. Romaguera, C., Grimalt, F., Vilaplana, J. and Azob, A. (1989): Erythroderma from carbamazepine. *Contact Dermatitis, 20*, 304–305.
18. Jordan, W.P. (1975): Cross-sensitization patterns in acrylate allergies. *Contact Dermatitis, 1,* 13.
19. Ford, R.A. (1992): Studies of the quenching phenomenon. *Contact Dermatitis, 27*, 60–61. (D. Basketter and F. Allenby, Reply).
20. Kero, M., Hannuksela, M. and Sothman, A. (1979): Primary irritant dermatitis from topical clioquinol. *Contact Dermatitis, 5,* 115.
21. Holdiness, M.R. (1986): Contact dermatitis to antituberculosis drugs. *Contact Dermatitis, 15*, 282–288.
22. Baadsgaard, O. (1990): Immunologic mechanisms of contact dermatitis. In: *Exogenous Dermatoses: Environmental Dermatitis.* Editors: T. Menné and H.I. Maibach. CRC Press, Boca Raton. pp. 3–20.
23. Fischer, T. and Maibach, H.I. (1990): Improved, but not perfect, patch testing. *Am. J. Contact Dermatitis, 1*, 73–90.
24. De Groot, A.C. (1994): *Patch Testing. Test Concentrations and Vehicles for 2800 Allergens, 2nd Edition.* Elsevier, Amsterdam.
25. Lachapelle, J.M. (1992): Histopathological and immuno-histopathological features of irritant and allergic contact dermatitis. In: *Textbook of Contact Dermatitis.* Editors: R.J.G. Rycroft et al. Springer, Heidelberg. Chapter 3, pp. 91–104.
26. Lakaye, G. and Lapière, M. (1961): Evolution des eczémas de contact professionel. *Arch. Belges Dermatol., 17,* 130.
27. Magnus, I.A. (1976): *Dermatological Photobiology.* Blackwell Scientific Publications, Oxford. p. 255.
28. Abel, E.A. and Wood, G.S. (1986): Mechanisms in contact dermatitis. *Clin Rev. Allergy, 4*, 339–352.
29. Wahlberg, J.E. (1992): Patch testing. In: *Textbook of Contact Dermatitis.* Editors: R.J.G. Rycroft et al. Springer, Heidelberg. Chapter 10, pp. 241–268.
30. Marcussen, P. (1959): Specificity of patch tests with 5% nickel sulphate. *Acta derm.-venereol. (Stockh.), 39,* 187.
31. Fischer, T. and Maibach, H.I. (1990): Patch testing in allergic contact dermatitis. In: *Exogenous dermatoses: Environmental Dermatitis.* Editors: T. Menné and H.I. Maibach. CRC Press, Boca Raton. pp. 86–102.
32. Marzulli, F.N. and Maibach, H.I. (Eds.) (1977): In: *Advances in Modern Toxicology, Vol. 4: Dermatotoxicology and Pharmacology.* Hemisphere Publishing Corporation, Washington-London; John Wiley and Sons, New York-London-Sydney-Toronto.
33. Carmichael, A.J., Foulds, I.S. and Bransbury, D.S. (1991): Loss of lanolin patch-test positivity. *Br. J. Dermatol., 125*, 573–576.
34. Matsuo, I., Ozawa. A., Niizuma, K. and Ohkido, M. (1979): Lichenoid dermatitis due to chlorpromazine phototoxicity. *Dermatologica (Basel) 159,* 46.
35. Meneghini, C.L. and Angelini, G. (1977): Behaviour of contact allergy and new sensitivities on subsequent patch tests. *Contact Dermatitis, 3*, 138.
36. Meneghini, C.L., Rantuccio, F., Riboldi, A. and Hofmann, M.F. (1967): Beobachtungen über das Persistieren der experimentellen ekzematösen Kontaktsensibilisierung auf einige chemische Substanzen beim Menschen. *Berufsdermatosen, 15,* 103.
37. Meneghini, C.L., Rantuccio, F. and Lomuto, M. (1971): Modelli sperimentali della ipersensibilità di tipo ritardato da contatto: Implicazioni cliniche nelle dermatiti eczematose. *Folia allerg. 18,* 317.
38. Mitchell, J.C. (1975): The angry back syndrome: eczema creates eczema. *Contact Dermatitis, 1*, 193.
39. Morgan, J.K. (1953): Observations on the persistence of skin sensitivity with reference to nickel eczema. *Brit. J. Dermatol. 65,* 84.
40. Nielsen, J.P. and Bang, K. (1954): On the persistenee of acquired hypersensitivity, illustrated by re-examination and repetition of standardized patch tests on eczematous patients. *Acta derm.-venereol. (Stockh.), 34,* 110.
41. Shuster, S. (1992): Patch-test sensitivity and reproducibility in individuals and populations. *Am. J. Contact Dermatitis, 3*, 74–78.
42. Opdyke, D. (1976): Inhibition of sensitization reactions induced by certain aldehydes. *Food Cosm. Toxicol., 14,* 197.
43. Pevny, I., Mahr, E. and Schröpl, F. (1974): Toxische Hautreaktionen beim Epikutantest mit tricyclischen Psychopharmaka. *Hautarzt, 25,* 430.
44. Rhodes, E.I. and Warner, J. (1966): Contact eczema, follow-up study. *Brit. J. Dermatol. 79,* 640.
45. Schiavino, D., Papa, G., Nucera, E. et al. (1992): Delayed allergy to diclofenac. *Contact Dermatitis, 26*, 357–358.

46. Schulz, K.H. and Schmidt, P. (1967): Fixe Exantheme durch drei verschiedene Arzneimittel mit getrennter Lokalisation. Beitrag zur Frage der Barbituratallergie. *Z. Haut.- u. Geschl. kr., 42,* 561.
47. Soesman-van Waadenoyen Kernekamp, A. and Van Ketel, W. G. (1980): Persistence of patch test reactions to clioquinol (vioform) and cross-sensitization. *Contact Dermatitis, 6,* 455.
48. Te Lintum, J.C.A. and Nater, J.P. (1973): On the persistence of positive patch test reactions to balsam of Peru, turpentine and nickel. *Brit. J. Dermatol., 89,* 629.
49. Thormann, J., Jespersen, N.B. and Joensen, H.D. (1979): Persistence of contact allergy to chromium. *Contact Dermatitis, 5,* 261.
50. de Haan, P., Bruynzeel, D.P. and van Ketel, W.G. (1986): Onset of penicillin rashes: relation between type of penicillin administered and type of immune reactivity. *Allergy, 14,* 75–78.
51. Van Ketel, W.G. and Soesman, A. (1977): Een op de ziekte van Lyell gelijkende eruptie door Propranolol. *Ned. T. Geneesk., 121,* 1475.
52. Kennedy, C., Stolz, E. and van Joost, Th. (1989) Sensitization to amoxycillin in Augmentin®. *Contact Dermatitis, 20,* 313–314.
53. Sanders, M.N. and Winkelmann, R.U. (1988): Cutaneous reactions to vitamin K. *J. Am. Acad. Dermatol., 19,* 699–704.
54. Calnan, C.D. (1981): Keloid formation after patch tests. *Contact Dermatitis, 7,* 279.
55. Machet, L., Vaillant, L., Dardine, V. and Lorette, G. (1992): Patch testing with clobazam: relapse of generalized drug eruption. *Contact Dermatitis, 26*: 247–348.
56. Veien, N.K., Hattel, T. and Laurberg, G. (1992): Is patch testing a less accurate tool during the summer months? *Am. J. Contact Dermatitis, 3,* 35–36.
57. Heise, H. and Mattheus, A. (1982): Dimethylsulfoxid (DMSO) als Vehikel zur perkutanen Auslosung einer Testreaktion bei Arzneimittelexanthemen. *Derm. Mschr., 168,* 402.
58. Bruynzeel, D.P., von Blomberg-van der Flier, M., Scheper, R.J., van Ketel, W.G. and de Haan, P. (1985): Penicillin allergy and the relevance of epicutaneous tests. *Dermatologica, 171,* 429–434.
59. Quirce, S., Parra, F., Lázaro, M., Gómez, M.I. and Cano, M.S. (1991): Generalized dermatitis due to oral nystatin. *Contact Dermatitis, 25,* 197–198.
60. Landwehr, A.J. and van Ketel, W.G. (1982): Delayed-type allergy to phenazone in a patient with erythema multiforme. *Contact Dermatitis, 8,* 283.
61. Lawrence, C.M. and Byrne. J.P.H. (1981): Eczematous eruption from oral diphenhydramine. *Contact Dermatitis, 7,* 276.
62. Merot, Y., Harms, M. and Saurat, J.-H. (1983): Photosensibilisation au carprofène (Imadyl®), un nouvel anti-inflammatoire non-stéroïdien. *Dermatologica, (Basel), 166,* 301.
63. De Shazo, R.D. and Stevenson, H.C. (1981): Generalized dermatitis to aminophylline. *Ann. Allergy, 46,* 152.
64. Valsecchi, R. and Cainelli, T. (1982): Penicillin allergy with positive skin test to cephalosporin alone. *Contact Dermatitis, 8,* 278.
65. Lang, P.G. Jr. (1983): Quinidine-induced photodermatitis confirmed by photopatch testing. *J. Am. Acad. Dermatol., 9,* 124.
66. Van Ketel, W.G. (1983): Allergy to carbimazole. *Contact Dermatitis, 9,* 161.
67. Rudzki, E., Grzywa, Z. and Maciejowska, E. (1976): Drug reaction with positive patch test to chloramphenicol. *Contact Dermatitis, 2,* 181.
66. White, I.R. (1983): Photopatch test in a hydrochlorothiazide drug eruption. *Contact Dermatitis, 9,* 237.
69. Van Ketel, W.G. (1983): An allergic eruption probably caused by ketoconazole. *Contact Dermatitis, 9,* 313.
70. Rudzki, E. and Dajek, Z. (1975): Drug eruption with positive patch test to phenol. *Contact Dermatitis, 1,* 322.
71. Maucher, O.M. and Fuchs, A. (1983): Kontakturtikaria im Epikutantest bei Pyrazolonallergie. Hautartz, 34, 383.
72. Van den Berg, W.H.H.W. and van Ketel, W.G. (1983): Fotosensibilisatie door Amantadine (Symmetrel®). *Nieuwsbr. Contactderm., 16,* 221.
73. Adams, R.M. and Fischer, T. (1990): Diagnostic patch testing. In: *Occupational Skin Disease, 2nd Edition.* Editor: R.M. Adams. W.B. Saunders Company, Philadelphia. Chapter 14, pp. 223–254.
74. Scheper, R.J. and von Blomberg, B.M.E. (1992): Cellular mechanisms in allergic contact dermatitis. In: *Textbook of Contact Dermatitis*. Editors: R.J.G. Rycroft et al. Springer, Heidelberg. Chapter 2, pp. 11–24.
75. Thestrup-Pedersen, K., Larsen, C.G. and Rønnevig, J. (1989): The immunology of contact dermatitis.

Contact Dermatitis, 20, 81–92.
76. Andersen, K.E., Benezra, C., Burrows, D. et al. (1987): Contact dermatitis, a review. *Contact Dermatitis, 16,* 55–78.
77. Keczkes, K., Basheer, A.M. and Wyatt, E.H. (1982): The persistence of allergic contact sensitivity: a 10-year follow-up in 100 patients. *Brit. J. Dermatol., 107,* 461.
78. Fregert, S. (1976): Respiratory symptoms with piperazine patch testing. *Contact Dermatitis, 2,* 61.
79. Maucher, O.M. and Fuchs. A. (1983): Kontakturtikaria im Epikutantest bei Pyrazolonallergie. *Hautarzt, 34,* 383.
80. Bruynzeel, D.P., van Ketel, W.G., Scheper, R.J. and von Blomberg-van der Flier, B.M.E. (1982): Delayed time course of irritation by sodium lauryl sulfate: observations on threshold reactions. *Contact Dermatitis, 8,* 236.
81. Angelini, G., Rantuccio, F. and Meneghini, C.L. (1975): Contact dermatitis in patients with leg ulcers. *Contact Dermatitis, 1,* 81.
82. Lawrence, C.M. and Smith, A.G. (1982): Ampliative medicament allergy: concomitant sensitivity to multiple medicaments including yellow soft paraffin, white soft paraffin, gentian violet and Span 20. *Contact Dermatitis, 8,* 240.
83. Bruynzeel, D.P. and Maibach, H.I. (1986): Excited skin syndrome (angry back). *Arch. Dermatol., 122,* 323–328.
84. Mathias, C.G.T. (1984): Dermographism and patch test reactions. *Contact Dermatitis, 10,* 110.
85. Dahl, M.V. and Jordan, W.P. Jr (1983): Topical steroids and patch tests. (Letter to the Editor). *Arch. Dermatol., 119,* 3.
86. Wong, G. and Maibach, H. (1982): Axillary lymphadenopathy possibly secondary to a positive patch test on the lower back. *Contact Dermatitis, 8,* 348.
87. Faure, M., Dambuyant. C., Chabeau, G. et al. (1981): Immune complex vasculitis and contact dermatitis to Frullania. *Contact Dermatitis, 7,* 320.
88. Bruynzeel, D.P., van Ketel, W.G., von Blomberg-van der Flier, M. and Scheper, R.J. (1983): Angry back or the excited skin syndrome. A prospective study. *J. Am. Acad. Dermatol., 8,* 392.
89. de Groot, A.C. and Frosch, P.J. (1992): Patch test concentrations and vehicles for testing contact allergens. In: *Textbook of Contact Dermatitis.* Editors: R.J.G. Rycroft et al. Springer, Heidelberg. Chapter 22, pp. 797–806.
90. Fisher, A. and Shapiro, A. (1956): Allergic eczematous contact dermatitis due to metallic nickel. *J. Am. Med. Assoc., 161,* 717.
91. Clark, R. A. and Rietschel, R. L. (1982): 0.1% Triamcinolone acetonide ointment and patch test responses. *Arch. Dermatol., 118,* 163.
92. Dahl, M.V. and Jordan, W.P. Jr. (1983): Topical steroids and patch tests. (Letter.) *Arch. Dermatol.,119,* 3.
93. Adams, R.M. (Ed.) (1990): *Occupational Skin Disease, 2nd Edition.* Saunders, Philadelphia.
94. Fisher, A.A. (Ed.) (1986): *Contact Dermatitis, 3rd Edition.* Lea and Febiger, Philadelphia.
95. Belsito, D.V. (1989): The immunologic basis of patch testing. *J. Am. Acad. Dermatol., 21,* 822–829.
96. Mathias, C.G.T., Caldwell, T.M. and Maibach, H.I. (1979): Contact dermatitis and gastrointestinal symptoms from hydroxyethylmethacrylate. *Brit. J. Dermatol., 100,* 447.
97. Andersen, K.E. (1986): Systemic symptoms related to patch tests with UV curable acrylic monomers. *Contact Dermatitis, 14,* 180.
98. Jirásek, L. and Kalensky, J. (1975): Kontaktní alergicky ekzém z krmnych smesi v zivocisné vyrobe. *Céskoslovenská Dermatologie, 50,* 217–225.
99. Maucher, O.M. and Fuchs, A. (1986): Der Hauttest zur Verifizierung der Pyrazolonallergie. *Allergologie, 9,* 305–314.
100. Ljunggren, B. and Bojs, G. (1991): A case of photosensitivity and contact allergy to systemic tricyclic drugs with unusual features. *Contact Dermatitis, 24,* 259–265.
101. Röhrborn, W. and Bräuninger, W. (1987): Thioridazine photoallergy. *Contact Dermatitis, 17,* 241.
102. Vaillant, L., Le Marchand, D., Grognard, C., Hocine, R. and Lorette, G. (1988): Photosensitivity to methyldopa. *Arch Dermatol., 124,* 326–328.
103. Przybilla, B., Ring, J., Galosi, A., Born, M. (1984): Photopatch test reactions to tiaprofenic acid. *Contact Dermatitis, 10,* 55–56.
104. Frosch, P.J. and Weickel, R. (1989): Photokontaktallergie durch Benzydamin (Tantum). *Hautarzt, 40,* 771–773.

105. Camarasa, J. and Serra-Baldrich, E. (1990): Tetrazepan allergy detected by patch test. *Contact Dermatitis, 22*, 246.
106. Goday, J., Aguirre, A. and Diaz-Perez, J.L. (1990): A positive patch test in a pyrazinamide drug eruption. *Contact Dermatitis, 22*, 181–182.
107. Pigatto, P.D., Morelli, M., Polenghi, M.M., Mozzanica, N. and Altomare, G.F. (1987): Phenobarbital-induced allergic dermatitis. *Contact Dermatitis, 16*, 279.
108. Cnudde, F., Leynadier, F. and Dry, J. (1990): Cutaneous reaction to captopril: value of patch tests. *Contact Dermatitis, 23*, 375–376.
109. Tomb, R.R., Lepoittevin, J.P., Espinassouze, F., Heid, E. and Foussereau, J. (1991): Systemic contact dermatitis from pseudoephedrine. *Contact Dermatitis, 24,* 89–93.
110. Mishimura, M. and Takano, Y. (1988): Systemic contact dermatitis medicamentosa occurring after intravesical dimethyl sulfoxide treatment for interstitial cystitis. *Arch Dermatol., 124*, 182–183.
111. Dooms-Goossens, A., Gidi de Alam, A., Degreef, H. and Kochayt, A. (1989): Local anesthetic intolerance due to metabisulfite. *Contact Dermatitis, 20*, 124–126.
112. De Groot, A.C. and Conemans, J. (1986): Allergic urticarial rash from codeine. *Contact Dermatitis, 14*, 209–214.
113. Rytter, M., Walther, Th., Süss, E. and Haustein, U.F. (1989): Allergische Reaktionen vom Sofort- und Spättyp nach Prednisolon-Medikation. *Dermatol. Mon. Schr., 175*, 44–48.
114. Voss, M. (1988): Eine Prednisolon-Allergie mit pustulösem Exanthem. *Dermatol. Mon. Schr., 174*, 221–225.
115. de Boer, E.M., van den Hoogenband, H.M. and van Ketel, W.G. (1984): Positive patch test reactions to injectable corticosteroids. *Contact Dermatitis, 11*, 261–262.
116. Cirne de Castro, J.L., Freitas, J.P., Menezes Brandao, F. and Themido, R. (1991): Sensitivity to thimerosal and photosensitivity to piroxicam. *Contact Dermatitis, 24*, 187–192.
117. Bruynzeel, D.P. and van Ketel, W.G. (1989): Patch testing in drug eruptions. *Seminars in Dermatology, 8*, 196–203.
118. Truchetet, F., Grosshans, E. and Brandenburger, M. (1987): Les tests cutanés dans l'allergie médicamenteuse endogène. *Ann. Derm. Venereol., 114*, 989–997.
119. de Groot, A.C. and Conemans, J. (1986): Allergic urticarial rash from oral codeine. *Contact Dermatitis, 14*, 209–214.
120. Peters, U. (1986): Delayed hypersensitivity to oral cimetidine. *Contact Dermatitis, 15*, 190–191.
121. Milligan, A. and Douglas, W.S. (1986): Contact dermatitis to cephalexin. *Contact Dermatitis, 15*, 91.
122. Keczkes, K. (1984): Does contact sensitivity last? *Int. J. Dermatol., 23*, 108–109.
123. Valsecchi, R., Rossi, A., Bigardi, A. and Pigatto, P.D. (1991): The loss of contact sensitization in man. *Contact Dermatitis, 24*, 183–186.
124. Nielsen, M. and Jørgensen, J. (1987): Persistence of contact sensitivity to ethylenediamine. *Contact Dermatitis, 16*, 275–276.
125. Rietschel, R.M. (1988): The case for patch test reading beyond day 2. *J. Am. Acad. Dermatol., 18*, 42–45.
126. Rietschel, R.L. (1985): Irritant and allergic responses as influenced by triamcinolone in patch test materials. *Arch Dermatol., 121*, 68–69.
127. Basketter, D.A. and Allenby, C.F. (1991): Studies of the quenching phenomenon in delayed contact hypersensitivity reactions. *Contact Dermatitis, 25*, 160–171.
128. Rycroft, R.J.G. (1986): False reactions to nonstandard patch tests. *Seminars in Dermatology, 5*, 225–230.
129. Alexander, S. (1988): Patch testing and menstruation. *Lancet, ii*, 751.
130. Edman, B. (1989): Seasonal influence on patch test results. *Contact Dermatitis, 20*, 226.
131. Ilchyshyn, A. (1985): False negative patch test response in coeliac disease. *Contact Dermatitis, 13*, 125–126.
132. Agathos, M. and Breit, R. (1989): Die Epicutantestung unter Berüchsichtigung falsch-positiver Reaktionen. *Allergologie, 12*, 1–6.
133. Aberer, W. (1988): Die 'falsch-positive' Epikutantest-Reaktion. *Dermatosen, 36*, 13–16.
134. Fischer, T. and Maibach, H.I. (1989): Easier patch testing with TRUE test. *J. Am. Acad. Dermatol., 20*, 447–453.
135. Foussereau, J. (1987): Les eczémas allergiques. Cosmétologiques, therapeutiques et vestimentaires. Masson, Paris.
136. Hannuksela, M. and Salo, H. (1986): The repeated open application test (ROAT). *Contact Dermatitis, 14*, 221–227.

3. Allergic contact dermatitis (general aspects)

137. Hannuksela, M. (1991): Sensitivity at various skin sites in the repeated open application test. *Am. J. Contact Dermatitis, 2*, 102–104.
138. Väänänen, A. and Hannuksela, M. (1986): Softisan — a new vehicle for patch testing. *Contact Dermatitis, 14*, 215–226.
139. Rietschel, R.L. (1992): The patch test as an exercise in cutaneous pharmacokinetics. Does compound allergy exist? *Arch. Dermatol., 128*, 678–679.

4. Unusual manifestations of allergic contact sensitivity

PURPURIC ALLERGIC CONTACT DERMATITIS

4.1 In some cases of allergic dermatitis the development of a definite purpuric component may be noted, even when laboratory studies, including blood count, bleeding time and clot retraction time, are normal. This phenomenon has been reported with contact allergic reactions to *p*-phenylenediamine (PPD) and the related compound *N*-isopropyl-*p*-phenylenediamine (IPPD) [28]. In these patients patch tests with PPD and IPPD [86] produced a similar purpuric reaction. Thioureas in boots have also been held responsible for purpuric allergic contact dermatitis [117]. Contact allergic purpura from industrial exposure to wool dust has been reported by Agarwal [38]. In this case nephritis was associated, which disappeared after strict avoidance of exposure to wool dust. Contact purpura to a positive patch test with *Frullania* has been documented; immune complex vasculitis was associated [58]. A purpuric vasculitis-like eruption (with the histopathologic picture of leukocytoclastic vasculitis [87]) has also been ascribed to contact allergy to balsam Peru in an antirheumatic ointment [44] and an ointment for dry skin [87]. A purpuric eruption caused by benzoyl peroxide for the treatment of acne has been observed [85]. A patch test to benzoyl peroxide was positive, and had the same vasculitis-like appearance. Histopathology showed leukocytoclastic vasculitis [85]. Purpura have also been observed in patients allergic to proflavine [121]. Petechial reactions following patch testing with cobalt are said to occur in 5% of all patients tested [25].

PIGMENTED CONTACT DERMATITIS

4.2 Riehl's melanosis is a non-itching pigmented dermatosis localized on the face and neck, and sometimes on other exposed areas. In Japan a series of patients has been reported presenting with a clinical picture similar to Riehl's melanosis, in some cases with pruritic lesions. These cases were considered to be 'pigmented cosmetic dermatitis' [30]. The skin manifestations of pigmented (cosmetic) contact dermatitis consist of diffuse or patchy brown hyperpigmentation on the cheeks and/or forehead, and the entire face may be involved. In severe cases, the pigmentation is sometimes black, purple, or blue-black. Occasionally, erythematous macules or papules, suggesting a mild contact dermatitis [88], are observed. This particular type of pigmented dermatitis could be related to contact allergy to coal tar dyes used in cosmetics, particularly to CI 15800 Brilliant Lake Red R (an azo-dye), and other 1-phenylazo-2-naphthol derivatives [11,12]. Fragrance materials were also involved, notably jasmin absolute, ylang-ylang oil (cananga oil), sandalwood oil, benzyl salicylate, benzyl alcohol, methoxycitronellal, β-santalol, geraniol, geranium oil, and patchouli oil [88]. The results of patch testing and of photopatch testing indicated that, as in most cases both the non-irradiated and irradiated patch tests were positive, the relevance of UV exposure was less than might have been expected. The number of patients with pigmented cosmetic dermatitis has decreased remarkably since 1978, when major cosmetic companies began to eliminate strong contact sensitizers from their products. The subject has been reviewed [88]. Pigmented cosmetic dermatitis may be caused by various cosmetic components and affects mostly women's faces; it is usually seen on mongoloids, not on Caucasians. Persistent secondary hyperpigmentation to contact dermatitis is often seen on mongoloids. It may be provoked by various contact allergens. All these reactions can be termed pigmented *contact* dermatitis. Pigmented *cosmetic* dermatitis is unique because of the affected sites, causation by cosmetic ingredients, and disappearance of the disfiguring pigmentation when contact with the offending allergens is avoided [88].

4.3 Pigmented contact dermatitis must be differentiated from phototoxic and photoallergic contact dermatitis.

Other causes of pigmented contact dermatitis have included:

- optical whiteners and textiles [9,19];
- chromium hydroxide used as a pigment in commercial toilet soap [42];
- occupational contact with azo dyes: Sudan I (CI 12055) (also in 'kumkum', i.e. coloured cosmetics used by Hindu women and applied as a round patch to the forehead [133]) and Vacanceine Red (CI 12175) [89];
- naphthol AS in clothes [90];
- airborne (occupational) contact with whitening dyes [91], formaldehyde [92], musk ambrette in incense [93] and possibly oak moss in a cosmetic cream [123];
- musk moskene in rouge [125].

FOLLICULAR CONTACT DERMATITIS

4.4 Sometimes, contact dermatitis may present as an itchy papular eruption. In such cases, the centre of the elementary papule is usually pierced by a hair; the skin between the papules remains normal. This form of follicular allergic contact dermatitis has been reported in cases of textile contact dermatitis due to formaldehyde. The eruption is presumably caused by the transfollicular absorption of formaldehyde [31]. Follicular contact dermatitis has also been reported in patients with contact allergy to homomenthyl salicylate (homosalate) [22].

This reaction should be differentiated from non-allergic pustular and papular reactions which may develop in patch tests with salts of metals (nickel, cobalt and, especially, copper) (§ 4.13).

ERYTHEMA MULTIFORME-LIKE ERUPTIONS

4.5 Erythema multiforme occasionally is a manifestation of allergic contact sensitivity. The lesions of erythema multiforme may present concurrently with those of the contact dermatitis, but erythema multiforme may also be the presenting and only sign of allergic contact sensitivity. The eruption, which may be bullous, commonly affects the face and extremities. In more severe cases, the lesions can become generalized. Oral lesions have been described. Patch tests with the causative allergens are strongly positive, and the development of the typical erythema multiforme "iris", "target" or "bull's-eye" lesions may result from patch testing. Biopsy specimens of clinical lesions (and sometimes of positive patch test reactions) usually reveal a picture consistent with erythema multiforme. The mechanism involved is not clear, though some authors suggest that the allergen is absorbed percutaneously and the eruption is caused by type III allergy according to Gell and Coombs [71]. Allergens which have been incriminated as causing erythema multiforme-like allergic contact dermatitis include [69,70,72,130]:

- 9-bromofluorene [20, 37]
- bufexamac [122,126]
- chloramphenicol [44]
- *p*-chlorbenzenesulfonylglycolic acid nitrile [21]
- clioquinol [44]
- deodorant [115]
- dimethoate [127]
- dinitrochlorobenzene (DNCB) [81]
- diphencyprone [79]
- econazole [41]
- epoxy resin [116]
- ethylenediamine [44,72]
- 5-fluorouracil [68]
- formaldehyde [52]
- *N*-hydroxyphthalimide [131]
- idoxuridine [151]
- isophoronediamine (epoxy hardener) [116]
- *N*-isopropyl-*p*-phenylenediamine [76]
- lauryl ether sulfate [132]
- lincomycin [73]
- mafenide acetate [67]
- mechlorethamine HCL [66]
- mercury [78]
- methyl parathion [128]
- neomycin [44]
- nickel [48,71]
- nickel and cobalt [49]
- perfume [51]
- *p*-phenylenediamine [115] in hair dye [75]
- a phenylsulfone-derivative [23]
- poison ivy [69]
- povidone-iodine [80]
- primula [7]
- proflavine hemisulfate [121]
- promethazine [44]
- pyrrolnitrin [44–46]
- scopolamine hydrobromide [6]
- sulfonamide [24,40,43,44,83]

- terpenes in Sloan's liniment [10]
- toxicodendron radicans (poison ivy) [53]
- trichloroethylene [82]
- trinitrotoluene [77]
- tropical woods [8,69].
- vitamin E [87]

Erythema multiforme may also be a complication of patch testing [130].

CONTACT URTICARIA (IMMEDIATE CONTACT REACTIONS)

4.6 Contact urticaria (synonym: immediate contact reactions) of immunological or non-immunological nature occurs from numerous sources. Immunological contact urticaria is usually due to an immediate-type hypersensitivity (Type I according to the classification of Gell and Coombs), but several case reports suggest that sometimes the delayed-type variety is also present. See Chapter 7 on contact urticaria.

LICHENOID ERUPTIONS

4.7 Allergic contact dermatitis has been reported to change after several weeks into a lichenoid eruption. This has been described in allergic contact sensitivity to substituted *p*-phenylenediamine derivatives used in the processing of colour films [14], and as a manifestation of contact sensitivity to *N*-isopropyl-*N'*-phenyl-*p*-phenylenediamine (IPPD), a rubber antioxidant [50]. Contact allergy to nickel has also been implicated as a cause of lichenoid dermatitis [64]. Both patch tests and oral provocation tests caused lichenoid papules to appear. Contact allergy to aminoglycoside antibiotics caused a lichenoid eruption. All positive patch tests had a lichenoid appearance [94]. A patient with pigmented dermatitis of the face caused by photoallergy to musk ambrette had histological features of a lichenoid reaction, both in clinical lesions and in the patch test [124]. Lichenoid eruptions in the mouth may be caused by allergy to metals in dental restoration materials, especially mercury amalgam (Chapter 13). Occupational lichenoid contact dermatitis from epoxy resin has been observed [129].

CONTACT GRANULOMA

4.8 Allergic contact granulomas (see also § 5.42)

Zirconium salts

Axillary granulomas characterized by lesions appearing as firm, shiny papules with a specific histological picture have been described after the use of zirconium salt containing deodorants and antiperspirants. Zirconium oxide or carbonate preparations have also been used in the treatment of Rhus dermatitis. Two types of skin reactions have been identified: one is a non-allergic foreign body inflammation healing spontaneously within a month. This type of reaction has been described in both sensitized and non-sensitized persons. The other reaction has only occurred in individuals sensitized to the zirconium salt. The epithelioid cell granulomas formed in these cases may persist for a year or longer [2].

Beryllium salts

Cutaneous contact with beryllium salts may cause the formation of a cutaneous epithelioid granuloma with positive patch test reactions [29]. Not only localized but also systemic granulomatous reactions have been reported.

Metals in tattoos

Delayed hypersensitivity reactions to mercury, chromium, manganese, cobalt or cadmium salts in tattoos may cause contact granulomata. Various histological patterns have been described (allergic and/or non-allergic) in tattoo reactions:
- a diffuse lymphohistiocytic infiltrate with an admixture of plasma cells and eosinophils [34,61]
- lichenoid reactions simulating lichen planus [36,62]
- granulomatous reactions [33,35]
- pseudolymphomatous reactions in areas containing mercury salts, chrome salts, and cobalt salts [32,98].

The histology of tattoo reactions has been reviewed by Goldstein [33]; *see also* § 5.42.

In jewellery

A female patient developed plaques under her metal jewellery. Histopathology was consistent with granuloma annulare. She proved to be allergic to nickel. After removal of the jewellery, the lesions disappeared within a few months [96]. Three patients developed benign lymphoplasia from hypersensitivity to gold in golden earrings [137].

4.9 Non-allergic contact granulomas have been caused by:

1. Chronic irritation, e.g. by glasses (granuloma fissuratum)
2. Oil, e.g. in cosmetics [1]
3. Talc [16]
4. Sodium stearate [3]
5. Zirconium salts
6. Metals in tattoos [3,35,95].
7. Corticosteroid powders (dubious report) [97]

FOCAL CONTACT SENSITIVITY

4.10 According to the basic immunological concept, in allergic contact sensitivity the entire skin is sensitized. Once sensitivity has developed, sensitized T-lymphocytes circulate through the skin, rendering all sites sensitive. In a patient treated for mycosis fungoides the entire skin surface was painted with topical nitrogen mustard (mechlorethamine hydrochloride 1/5000 aqueous). A remarkable focal contact sensitivity developed: the eczematous contact dermatitis was limited precisely to the area of clinically identifiable mycosis fungoides, whereas the uninvolved skin, though also painted with nitrogen mustard, showed no response whatsoever [27]. It is hypothesized that a malignant clone of T-cells had become specifically sensitized to nitrogen mustard. Thus sensitization would be restricted to the tumour sites.

TOXIC EPIDERMAL NECROLYSIS (LYELL)

4.11 *Monosulfiram (Sulfiram, tetraethylthiuram monosulfide)*

Monosulfiram is used in some antiscabietic preparations. A patient developed an extensive skin eruption diagnosed as toxic epidermal necrolysis of Lyell after application of a monosulfiram-containing lotion to her body below the neck as an antiscabietic treatment. According to her history she had developed a rubber dermatitis on her hands while working in a munition factory twenty-eight years earlier [18]. When the eruption had disappeared patch tests were performed. Positive reactions were found to the rubber chemical thiram disulfide and to the chemically related monosulfiram.

Perfume

A young adult female patient, on prolonged corticosteroid therapy for nephrotic syndrome, developed erythema multiforme with progression to toxic epidermal necrolysis and ultimately death following a double exposure to a locally applied unidentified perfume in spray cologne [51].

LYMPHOMATOID CONTACT DERMATITIS

4.12 Two conditions have been described under this name:

1. Orbaneja et al. [56] were the first to use the term 'lymphomatoid contact dermatitis'. They described 4 patients who had infiltrated plaque-like lesions of dermatitis mimicking histopathologically a cutaneous T-cell lymphoma. The condition was due to contact allergy from the striker surface of a matchbox and the special features were ascribed to the *prolonged* contact with the allergen. When contact with the source was avoided the lesions healed in a relatively short time. Similar cases have been observed from allergic contact dermatitis to ethylenediamine [57], phosphorus sesquisulphide [99], mercaptobenzothiazole [100] and azo dyes [101].
2. Ecker and Winkelmann [55] and Buechner and Winkelmann [54] use the term 'lymphomatoid contact dermatitis' to describe patients with a recurrent and progressive erythematous patchy dermatitis with temporary flares of generalized erythema (not unlike actinic reticuloid), in whom the histological findings consist of a distinct pattern of lymphocytic dermal reticulosis and chronic epithelial response. Although one or more positive patch test reactions to (unrelated) allergens were found in these patients a causal relationship

with the clinical picture has not been proven. and the eruption does *not* clear after avoidance of the chemicals producing positive patch tests. The authors argue that the similarity of these cases of lymphomatoid contact dermatitis both clinically and histologically with actinic reticuloid photosensitive dermatitis and airborne contact dermatitis indicates that these conditions represent a common transitional lymphoproliferative pre-malignant state. Lymphomatoid contact dermatitis is, according to these authors, considered to be a potential pre-Sézary state that can be recognized in the course and the histological pattern [55]. However, evolvement of such cases into cutaneous T-cell lymphoma has not (yet) been observed [101].

Alomar et al. [101] reviewed the literature and came to the following conclusions:

1. Two forms of lymphomatoid contact dermatitis (LCD) may be distinguished:
   - localized type: presenting as one or few infiltrated erythematous plaques resembling chronic eczema, and the
   - generalized type: characterized by an erythrodermic or generalized eruption in which transient circulating Sézary cells can be detected.
2. Allergens incriminated in these two types of LCD are as follows:
   localized
   - striker part of a box of matches (phosphorus sesquisulphide) [56,99]
   - mercaptobenzothiazole [100]
   - ethylenediamine [57]

   generalized
   - formaldehyde
   - glutaral
   - fig tree sawdust
   - phosphorus sesquisulphide
   - ragweed
   - potassium dichromate
   - tetramethylthiram
   - gold
   - azo dyes [101].
3. Diagnostic criteria of LCD should include:
   - a localized or generalized eruption in which the clinical history and physical examination suggests contact dermatitis;
   - mycosis fungoides-like histopathologic findings;
   - positive patch tests;
   - clearing of the lesions after corticosteroid therapy and total avoidance of the allergen.

PUSTULAR CONTACT DERMATITIS

4.13 Pustulogens are chemicals which cause sterile pustulation on topical application to the skin [103]. Pustular patch test reactions have been observed to metal compounds (nickel, chromate, mercury and arsenic), halogens (iodides, fluorides), croton oil [104] and sodium lauryl sulfate [105]. In a clinical setting, pustular eruptions as an expression of irritation have been caused by trichloroethylene [106] and hexafluorosilicate [105]. *Allergic* pustular contact dermatitis has been ascribed to nickel and nitrofurazone [107], and to rubber [134,135]. Rosacea(-like eruptions) have rarely been caused or worsened by contact allergic reactions: 5-fluorouracil [108], thimerosal in eyedrops [109], *p*-phenylenediamine in hair dye [109] and clindamycin [110].

MISCELLANEOUS UNUSUAL CUTANEOUS MANIFESTATIONS

4.14 – *Depigmented contact dermatitis* (airborne) from santalol and musk ambrette released from burning incense has been reported [111]. In principle, all allergens could induce post-inflammatory hypopigmentation, especially in pigmented individuals. Persistent vitiligo caused by the contact allergen diphencyprone used for the treatment of alopecia areata has been described several times [118–120].

– *Pellagra-like dermatitis* was ascribed to contact allergy to dithiocarbamate agricultural fungicide in one patient [112]. The report unfortunately lacks proper clinical description.

– *Urticarial papular and plaque eruptions.* Five patients had disseminated erythematous urticarial and plaque eruptions secondary to contact allergy to proflavine (4 cases) and permanent waving lotion (1 case). Some had 'iris-lesions', and the eruption clinically resembled erythema multiforme (§ 4.5). However, the histologic features of erythema multiforme were not present. The author assumes that many cases described as 'erythema multiforme-like contact dermatitis' should actually be included in this category which he called "urticarial papular and plaque eruptions" [113].

– *Small-plaque parapsoriasis.* A skin eruption typical of small-plaque parapsoriasis (syn: persistent superficial dermatitis) caused by contact allergy to cyanoacrylute glue was described in one patient [114].

– *Psoriasis-like contact dermatitis.* Rarely, contact allergic dermatitis may simulate psoriasis [136]. Of course, in psoriasis, contact allergy may worsen existing psoriasis (Koebner phenomenon).

ALLERGIC CONTACT DERMATITIS COMPLICATED BY EXTRACUTANEOUS SYMPTOMS

4.15 In extensive, severe or generalized allergic contact dermatitis non-specific constitutional symptoms may be observed:

– Headache, fever, anorexia, nausea and malaise have been reported in patients with severe allergic contact dermatitis from lauryl ether sulfate in a dish washing liquid containing an allergenic sulfone impurity [13].

In cases of limited dermatitis (e.g. limited to the hands) extracutaneous symptoms are rare:

– *Paraesthesia:* paraesthesia of the finger tips in the form of a burning sensation, tingling and slight numbness is a phenomenon described in cases of allergic contact dermatitis of the hands due to acrylic monomer. This type of paraesthesia accompanying an allergic contact dermatitis and persisting several weeks after the dermatitis had subsided, was reported in orthopaedic surgeons sensitized to methylmethacrylate bone cement [4].

– *Gastrointestinal symptoms:* in another case of allergic contact dermatitis of the hands due to hydroxyethylmethacrylate (in a laboratory technician), an association was found with nausea, diarrhoea and persistent paraesthesia of the finger tips. The gastrointestinal symptoms were reproduced by patch testing! Hydroxyethylmethacrylate was demonstrated to pass through vinyl gloves [15].

– *Respiratory symptoms:* a patient working in a factory where, among other substances, piperazine was processed, developed an eczema of the hands, arms, face and penis as well as respiratory symptoms. A patch test with 1% piperazine in water caused after about 17 hours itching of the piperazine patch test site and respiratory symptoms. The test was strongly positive after 48 hours. The respiratory symptoms disappeared after 5–6 hours [5]. In this case a sufficient amount of piperazine must have been absorbed from the patch test site in order to elicit the respiratory symptoms which, according to the author, probably were allergic (? Type 1 reaction). (Scratch, prick or intracutaneous tests are not mentioned.) Rhinitis has been associated with contact allergy to metals in dentures [65]. Patch tests with nickel and/or cobalt provoked the symptoms in some patients.

– *Fever:* four cases were reported in which treatment of psoriasis localized on the scalp with an ointment containing 3% 6-hydroxy-1,3-benzoxathiol-2-one resulted in a burning and itching erythema with vesiculation and edema, which extended in some cases to the face. In three cases body temperature was raised. Patch testing was impossible owing to the erythematous effect of this benzothiazole derivative on the skin [26].

– *Collapse:* a systemic reaction consisting of cyanosis and collapse after topical application of a mixture of 1% gentian violet (CI 42535) and 1% methyl green (CI 42590) on an ulcus cruris of a previously sensitized individual was described by Michel et al. [17].

– *Immune complex reaction: cutaneous vasculitis and nephritis:* a patient was patch-tested to *Frullania tamarisci* and *Frullania dilatata*. After 2 days a strong positive erythematous reaction was found. On the following day the two reactions were purpuric, and in the next 24–36 hours became bullous and necrotic. At the same time, a purpuric eruption with papulonodular lesions, lesions en cocarde and bullae with a tendency to necrose appeared on the lower limbs, on the pelvis and lower abdomen, and on the arms. Epistaxis accompanied the purpuric eruption. Histoimmunologic and immunologic findings were in favour of an immune complex reaction [58]. In a similar case [59], contact allergy to *Frullania* led to immune complex nephritis. Renal lesions accompanying poison oak dermatitis have been described previously [60]. Allergic contact purpura to wool dust was associated with nephritis in one case [38]; after strict avoidance of exposure to wool dust the nephritis disappeared.

– *Cataracts* occur in adults suffering from severe atopic dermatitis, especially of the face. A 34-year-old woman with mild atopic dermatitis has been described, who abruptly developed atopic cataracts in both eyes when she suffered from severe allergic cosmetic dermatitis of the face [102].

MISCELLANEOUS

4.16 – *Lymphangitis and lymphedema:* two cases have been described in which a recurrent allergic contact dermatitis of the hands led to lymphangitis and the development of a persistent lymphedema [47]. A similar observation was made by Worm et al. [63]. Recurrent bacterial infections may have been a contributory factor.

– *Permanent loss of finger nails:* a patient suffered a severe allergic reaction from sensitization to methylmethacrylate in a mixture of materials designed to make artificial nails. There was marked erythema, edema, and pain of the eponychial and paronychial tissues with persistent paraesthesia of the finger tips. Gradual destruction of the nail plates developed, and since no regrowth of the nails resumed in 6 years, the loss of the finger nails was considered to be permanent [39].

4.17 REFERENCES

1. Bergeron, J.R. and Stone, O.J. (1969): Multiple granulomas of the scalp of exogenous origin. *Cutis, 5,* 57.
2. Epstein, W.L., Skahen, J.R. and Krasnobrod, H. (1962): Granulomatous hypersensitivity to zirconium. Localization of allergen in tissue and its role in the formation of epitheloid cells. *J. Invest. Derm.*, 38, 223.
3. Fisher, A.A. (1973): *Contact Dermatitis.* Lea and Febiger, Philadelphia.
4. Fisher, A.A. (1979): Paresthesia of the fingers accompanying dermatitis due to methylmethacrylate bone cement. *Contact Dermatitis, 5,* 56.
5. Fregert, S. (1976): Respiratory symptoms with piperazine patch testing. *Contact Dermatitis, 2,* 61.
6. Guill, A., Goette, K., Knight, C.G., Peck, C.C. and Lupton, G.P. (1979): Erythema multiforme and urticaria. *Arch. Derm., 115,* 742.
7. Hjorth, N. (1966): Primula dermatitis. *Trans. St. John's Hosp. Derm. Soc. (Lond.), 52,* 207.
8. Holst, R., Kirby, J. and Magnusson, B. (1976): Sensitisation to tropical woods giving erythema multiforme-like eruptions. *Contact Dermatitis, 2,* 295.
9. Josephs, H. and Maibach, H.I. (1967): Contact dermatitis from Spandex brassieres. *J. Am. Med. Assoc., 201,* 880.
10. Kirby, D.J. and Darley, C.R. (1978): Erythema multiforme associated with a contact dermatitis to terpenes. *Contact Dermatitis, 4,* 238.
11. Kozuka, T., Tashiro, M., Sano, S., Fujimoto, K., Nakamura, Y., Hashimoto, S. and Nakaminami, G. (1979): Brilliant lake Red R as a cause of pigmented contact dermatitis. *Contact Dermatitis, 5,* 297.
12. Kozuka, T., Tashiro, M., Sano, S., Fujimoto, K., Nakamura, Y., Hashimoto, S. and Nakaminami, G. (1980): Pigmented contact dermatitis from azo-dyes. 1. Cross-sensitivity in humans. *Contact Dermatitis, 6,* 330.
13. Magnusson, B. and Gilje, O. (1973): Allergic contact dermatitis from a dishwashing liquid containing lauryl ether sulfate. *Acta Derm.-Venereol. (Stockh.), 53,* 136.
14. Mandel, E. H. (1960): Lichen planus-like eruptions caused by a color-film developer. *Arch. Dermatol., 81,* 516.
15. Mathias, C.G.T., Caldwell, T.M. and Maibach, H.I. (1979): Contact dermatitis and gastrointestinal symptoms from hydroxyethylmethacrylate. *Br. J. Dermatol., 100*, 447.
16. McCallum, D.I. and Hall, G.F.M. (1970): Umbilical granulomata with particular reference to talc granuloma. *Br. J. Dermatol., 83,* 151.
17. Michel, P.J., Buyer, R. and Delorme, G. (1958): Accidents géneraux (cyanose, collapsus cardiovasculaire) par sensibilisation à une solution aqueuse de violet de gentiane et vert de méthyle en applications locales. *Bull. Soc. Franç. Derm. Syph., 65,* 183.
18. Monckton Copeman, P.W. (1968): Toxic epidermal necrolysis caused by skin hypersensitivity to monosulfiram. *Br. Med. J., 1,* 623.
19. Osmundsen, B.J.D. (1970): Pigmented contact dermatitis. *Br. J. Dermatol., 83*, 296.
20. Powell, E.W. (1968): Skin reactions of 9-bromofluorene. *Br. J. Dermatol., 80,* 491.
21. Richter, G. and Scholz, H. (1970): Kontaktekzem und makulöses Exanthem bei *p*-Chlorbenzosulfonylglykolsäurenitril-Allergie. *Berufsdermatosen, 18,* 70.
22. Rietschel, R.L. and Lewis, Ch.W. (1978): Contact dermatitis to homomenthyl salicylate. *Arch. Dermatol., 114,* 442.
23. Roed-Petersen, J. (1975): Erythema multiforme as an expression of contact dermatitis. *Contact Dermatitis, 1,* 270.
24. Rubin, A. (1977): Ophthalmic sulfonamide-induced Stevens–Johnson syndrome. *Arch. Dermatol., 113,* 235.
25. Schmidt, H., Schultz Larsen, F., Øholm Larsen, P. and Søgaard, H. (1980): Petechial reaction following patch testing with cobalt. *Contact Dermatitis, 6,* 91.

26. Schoefinius, H.H. (1972): Kontaktdermatitis mit erhöhter Körpertemperatur unter Behandlung von Psoriasis vulgaris capillitii mit einem Benzoxathiol-Derivat. *Z. Haut- u. Geschlkr., 47,* 227.
27. Shelley, W.B. (1980): Focal contact sensitivity to nitrogen mustard in lesions of cutaneous T-cell lymphoma (mycosis fungoides). *Acta Derm.-Venereol. (Stockh.), 61,* 161.
28. Shmunes, E. (1978): Purpuric allergic contact dermatitis to paraphenylenediamine. *Contact Dermatitis, 4,* 225.
29. Sneddon, I.B. (1955): Berylliosis, a case report. *Br. Med. J., 1,* 1448.
30. Sugai, T., Takahashi, Y. and Takagi, T. (1977): Pigmented cosmetic dermatitis and coal tar dyes. *Contact Dermatitis, 3,* 249.
31. Uehara, M. (1978): Follicular contact dermatitis due to formaldehyde. *Dermatologica (Basel), 156,* 48.
32. Blumental, G., Okun, M.R. and Ponitch, J.A. (1982): Pseudolymphomatous reaction to tattoos. *J. Am. Acad. Dermatol., 6,* 485.
33. Goldstein, A. (1979): Histologic reactions to tattoos, *J. Derm. Surg. Oncol., 5,* 896.
34. Ravits, H.G. (1962): Allergic tattoo granuloma. *Arch. Dermatol., 86,* 287.
35. Verdich, J. (1981): Granulomatous reaction in a red tattoo. *Acta Derm.-Venereol. (Stockh.). 61,* 176.
36. Neild V.S. and Rhodes E.L. (1985): Tattoo reaction with generalized lichen planus. *Br. J. Dermatol., 113 (suppl. 29),* 76–77.
37. DeFeo, C.P. (1966): Erythema multiforme bullosum caused by 9-bromofluorene. *Arch. Dermatol., 94,* 545.
38. Agarwal, K. (1982): Contact allergic purpura to wool dust. *Contact Dermatitis, 8,* 281.
39. Fisher, A.A. (1980): Permanent loss of finger nails from sensitization and reaction to acrylic in a preparation designed to make artificial nails. *J. Derm. Surg. Oncol., 6,* 70.
40. Gottschalk, H.R. and Stone, O.J. (1976): Stevens–Johnson syndrome from ophthalmic sulfonamide. *Arch. Dermatol., 112,* 513.
41. Valsecchi, R., Tornaghi, A., Tribbia, G. and Cainelli, T. (1982): Contact dermatitis from econazole. *Contact Dermatitis, 8,* 422.
42. Mathias, T.C.G. (1982): Pigmented cosmetic dermatitis from contact allergy to a toilet soap containing chromium. *Contact Dermatitis, 8,* 29.
43. Goette, D.K. and Odom, R.B. (1980): Vaginal medications as a cause for varied widespread dermatitides. *Cutis, 26,* 406.
44. Meneghini, C.L. and Angelini, G. (1981): Secondary polymorphic eruptions in allergic contact dermatitis. *Dermatologica (Basel), 163,* 63.
45. Meneghini, C.L. and Angelini, G. (1982): Contact dermatitis from pyrrolnitrin. *Contact Dermatitis, 8,* 55.
46. Valsecchi, R., Foiadelli, L. and Cainelli, T. (1981): Contact dermatitis from pyrrolnitrin. *Contact Dermatitis, 7,* 340.
47. Lynde, C.W. and Mitchell, J.C. (1982): Unusual complication of allergic contact dermatitis of the hands: recurrent lymphangitis and persistent lymphoedema. *Contact Dermatitis, 8,* 279.
48. Calnan, C.D. (1956): Nickel dermatitis. *Br. J. Dermatol. 68,* 229.
49. Cook, L.J. (1982): Associated nickel and cobalt contact dermatitis presenting as erythema multiforme. *Contact Dermatitis, 8,* 280.
50. Ancona, A., Monroy, F. and Fernandez-Diez, J. (1982): Occupational dermatitis from IPPD in tyres. *Contact Dermatitis, 8,* 91.
51. Thompson, J.A. Jr. and Wansker, B.A. (1981): A case of contact dermatitis, erythema multiforme and toxic epidermal necrolysis. *J. Am. Acad. Dermatol., 5,* 666.
52. Nethercott, J.R., Albers, J., Guirguis, S. (1982): Erythema multiforme exudativum linked to the manufacture of printed circuit boards. *Contact Dermatitis, 8,* 314.
53. Mallory, S.B., Miller, O.F. and Tyler, W.B. (1982): *Toxicodendron radicans* dermatitis with black lacquer deposit on the skin. *J. Am. Acad. Dermatol., 6,* 363.
54. Buechner, S.A. and Winkelmann, R.K. (1983): Pre-Sézary erythroderma evolving to Sézary syndrome. *Arch. Dermatol., 119,* 285.
55. Ecker, R.I. and Winkelmann, R.K. (1981): Lymphomatoid contact dermatitis. *Contact Dermatitis. 7,* 84.
56. Orbaneja, J.G., Diez, L., Lozano, J.L.S. and Salazar, L.C. (1976): Lymphomatoid contact dermatitis: a syndrome produced by epicutaneous hypersensitivity with clinical features and a histopathologic picture similar to that of mycosis fungoides. *Contact Dermatitis, 2,* 139.
57. Wall, L.M. (1982): Lymphomatoid contact dermatitis due to ethylenediamine dihydrochloride. *Contact Dermatitis, 8,* 51.
58. Faure, M. Dambuyant, C., Chabeau, G. et al. (1981): Immune complex vasculitis and contact dermatitis

to Frullania. *Contact Dermatitis, 7,* 320.
59. Racadot, E. (1978): *Contribution à l'étude des syndromes néphrotiques allergiques. A propos d'un cas d'allergie à Frullania.* Thèse Médecine, Besançon.
60. Devich. K.B., Lee, J.C., Epstein, W.L. et al. (1975): Renal lesions accompanying poison oak dermatitis. *Clin. Nephrol., 3,* 106.
61. McGrouther, D.A., Downie, P.A. and Thompson, M.B. (1977): Reactions to red tattoos. *Br. J. Plast. Surg., 30,* 84.
62. Clarke, J. and Black, M.M. (1979): Lichenoid tattoo reactions. *Br. J. Dermatol., 100,* 451.
63. Worm, A.-M., Staberg, B. and Thomsen, K. (1983): Persistant oedema in allergic contact dermatitis. *Contact Dermatitis, 9.* 517.
64. Lombardi, P., Campolmi, P. and Sertoli, A. (1983): Lichenoid dermatitis caused by nickel salts? *Contact Dermatitis, 9,* 520.
65. Bork, K. (1978): Fließschnupfen durch Metallteile von Zahnprothesen. *Z. Hautkr. 53,* 814.
66. Brauwer, M.J., McEvoy, F.B., and Mitus, W.F. (1967): Hypersensitivity to nitrogen mustards in the form of erythema multiforme. *Arch. Intern. Med., 120,* 499.
67. Yaffee, M.S. and Dressler, D.P. (1969): Topical application of mafenide acetate. *Arch. Dermatol., 100,* 277.
68. Duvic, M. (1983): Erythema multiforme. *Dermatologic Clinics, 1,* 217.
69. Fisher, A.A. (1986): Erythema multiforme-like eruptions due to exotic woods and ordinary plants: Part I. *Cutis, 37,* 101–108.
70. Fisher, A.A. (1986): Erythema multiforme-like eruptions due to topical miscellaneous compounds: Part III. *Cutis, 37,* 262–264.
71. Friedman, S.J. and Perry, H.O. (1985): Erythema multiforme associated with contact dermatitis. *Contact Dermatitis, 12,* 21–23.
72. Fisher, A.A. (1986): Erythema multiforme-like eruptions due to topical medications: Part II. *Cutis, 37,* 158–161.
73. Conde-Salazar, L., Guimaraens, D., Romero, L., Gonzalez, M. and Yus, S. (1985): Erythema multiforme-like contact dermatitis from lincomycin. *Contact Dermatitis, 12,* 59–61.
74. Goh, C.L. (1987): Erythema multiforme-like and purpuric eruption due to contact allergy to proflavine. *Contact Dermatitis, 17,* 53–54.
75. Tosti, A., Bardazzi, F., Valeri, F. and Toni, F. (1987): Erythema multiforme with contact dermatitis to hair dyes. *Contact Dermatitis, 17,* 321–322.
76. Foussereau, J., Cavelier, C., Protois, J.C., Sanchez, M. and Heid, E. (1988): A case of erythema multiforme with allergy to isopropyl-*p*-phenylenediamine of rubber. *Contact Dermatitis, 18,* 183.
77. Goh, C.L. (1988): Erythema multiforme-like eruption from trinitrotoluene allergy. *Int. J. Dermatol., 27,* 650–651.
78. Sala, F., Crosti, C., Bencini, P.L., Perotta, E., Andreani, B., Greppi, F., Bertani, E. and Mansi, M. (1987): Esantema a tipo eritema polimorfo consequente all'applicazione topica prolungata di un unguento a base di mercurio metallico. *Chron. Dermatol., 18,* 937–943.
79. Perret, C.M., Steylen, P.M., Zaun, H., Happle, R. (1990): Erythema multiforme-like eruptions: a rare side effect of topical immunotherapy with diphenylcyclopropenone. *Dermatologica, 180,* 5–7.
80. Torinuki, W. (1990): Generalized erythema-multiforme-like eruption following allergic contact dermatitis. *Contact Dermatitis, 23,* 202–203.
81. Viraben, R., Labrousse, J.L. and Bazex, J. (1990): Erythema multiforme due to DNCB. *Contact Dermatitis, 22,* 179.
82. Phoon, W.H., Chan, M.O.Y. and Rajan, V.S. (1984): Stevens–Johnson syndrome associated with occupational exposure to trichloroethylene. *Contact Dermatitis, 10,* 270–276.
83. Genvert, G.J., Cohen, E.J. and Dunnenfield, E.D. (1985): Erythema multiforme after use of topical sulfacetamide. *Am. J. Opthalmol., 99,* 465–468.
84. Saperstein, H., Rapaport, M. and Rietschel, R.L. (1984): Topical Vitamin E as a cause of erythema multiforme-like eruptions. *Arch. Dermatol., 120,* 906–908.
85. van Joost, Th., van Ulsen, J., Vuzevski, D., Naafs, B. and Tank, B.H. (1990): Purpuric contact dermatitis to benzoyl peroxide. *J. Am. Acad. Dermatol., 22,* 359–361.
86. Roed-Peterson, J., Clemmensen, O.J., Menné, T. and Larsen, E. (1988): Purpuric contact dermatitis from black rubber chemicals. *Contact Dermatitis, 18,* 166–168.
87. Bruynzeel, D.P., van den Hoogenband, H.M. and Koedijk, F. (1984): Purpuric vasculitis-like eruption in a patient sensitive to balsam of Peru. *Contact Dermatitis, 11,* 207–209.

88. Nakayama, H., Matsuo, S., Hayakawa, K., Takhashi, K., Shigematsu, T. and Ota, S. (1984): Pigmented cosmetic dermatitis. *Int. J. Dermatol., 31*, 299–305.
89. Fujimoto, K., Hashimoto, S., Kozuka, T., Tashiro, M. and Sano, S. (1985): Occupational pigmented contact dermatitis from azo dyes. *Contact Dermatitis, 12*, 15–17.
90. Hayakawa, R., Matsunaga, K., Kojima, S., Kaniwa, M. and Nakamura, A. (1985): Naphthol AS as a cause of pigmented contact dermatitis. *Contact Dermatitis, 13*, 20–25.
91. Hayakawa, R., Kobayashi, M. and Matsunaga, K. (1981): 6 cases with occupational pigmented contact dermatitis. *Skin Research, 23,* 780–785.
92. Ukei, C., Oiwa, K., Matsunaga, K. and Hayakawa, R. (1983): Occupational contact dermatitis. *Skin Research, 23*, 368–376.
93. Hayakawa, R., Matsunaga, K. and Arima, Y. (1987): Airborne pigmented contact dermatitis due to musk ambrette in incense. *Contact Dermatitis, 16*, 96–98.
94. Lembo, G., Balato, N., Patruno, C., Pini, D. and Ayala, F. (1987): Lichenoid contact dermatitis due to aminoglycoside antibiotics. *Contact Dermatitis, 17*, 122–123.
95. Schwartz, R.A., Mathias, C.G.T., Miller, C.H., Rojas-Corona, R. and Lambert, W.C. (1987): Granulomatous reaction to purple tattoo pigment. *Contact Dermatitis, 16*, 198–202.
96. Stransky, L. (1987): Contact granuloma annulare. *Contact Dermatitis, 16*, 106.
97. Morelli, M., Fumagalli, M., Altomare, G.F. and Pigatto, P.D. (1988): Contact granuloma annulare. *Contact Dermatitis, 18*, 317–318.
98. Zinberg, M., Heilman, E. and Glickman, F. (1982): Cutaneous pseudolymphoma resulting from a tattoo. *J. Dermatol. Surg. Oncol., 8*, 955–958.
99. Ayala, F., Balato N., Nappa, P., de Rosa, G. and Lembo, G. (1987): Lymphomatoid contact dermatitis. *Contact Dermatitis, 17,* 311–313.
100. Fisher, A.A. (1987): Allergic contact dermatitis mimicking mycosis fungicides. *Cutis, 40*, 19–21.
101. Alomar, A., Pujol, R.M., Juneu, A. and Moreno, A. (1989): Lymphomatoid contact dermatitis. In: *Current Topics in Contact Dermatitis*. Editors: P.J. Frosch et al. Springer Verlag, Berlin, pp. 66–72.
102. Uehara, M. and Sato, T. (1986): Atopic cataract induced by severe allergic contact dermatitis on the face. *Dermatologica, 172,* 54–57.
103. Wahlberg, J.E. and Maibach, H.I. (1981): Sterile cutaneous pustules: a manifestation of primary irritancy? Identification of contact pustulogens. *J. Invest. Dermatol., 76*, 381–383.
104. Torinuki, W. and Tagami, H. (1988): Pustular irritant dermatitis due to croton oil. Evaluation of the role played by leukocytes and complement. *Acta Derm.-Venereol., 68*, 257–260.
105. Dooms-Goossens, A., Loncke, J., Michiels, J.L., De Greef, H. and Wahlberg, J. (1985): Pustular reactions to hexafluorosilicate in foam rubber. *Contact Dermatitis, 12*, 42–47.
106. Condé-Salazar, L., Guimaraens, D., Romero, L.V. and Sanchez Yus, E. (1983): Subcorneal pustular eruption and erythema from occupational exposure to trichloroethylene. *Contact Dermatitis, 9,* 235–237.
107. Burkhart, C.G. (1981): Pustular allergic contact dermatitis: a distinct clinical and pathological entitiy. *Cutis, 27*, 630–631, 638.
108. Sevadjian, C.M. (1985): Pustular contact hypersensitivity to fluorouracil with rosacea-like sequelae. *Arch. Dermatol., 121*, 240–242.
109. Bardazzi, F., Manuzzi, P., Riguzzi, G. and Veronesi, S. (1987): Contact dermatitis with rosacea. *Contact Dermatitis, 16*, 298.
110. de Kort, W.J.A. and de Groot, A.C. (1989): Lindamycin allergy presenting as rosacea. *Contact Dermatitis, 20*, 72–73.
111. Hayakawa, R., Matsunaga, K. and Arima, Y. (1987): Depigmented contact dermatitis due to incense. *Contact Dermatitis, 16,* 272–274.
112. Lisi, P. and Caraffini, S. (1985): Pellagroid dermatitis from mancozeb with vitiligo. *Contact Dermatitis, 13*, 124–125.
113. Goh, C.L. (1989): Urticarial papular and plaque eruptions. A noneczematous manifestation of allergic contact dermatitis. *Int. J. Dermatol., 28*, 172–176.
114. Shelley, E.D. and Shelley, W.B. (1984): Chronic dermatitis simulating small plaque parapsoriasis due to cyanoacrylate adhesive used on fingernails. *JAMA, 252*, 2455–2456.
115. Seidenari, S., Di Nardo, A., Motolese, A. and Pincelli, C. (1990): Erythema multiforme associated with contact sensitization. Report of 6 cases. *G. Ital. Dermatol. Venereol., 125*, 35–40.
116. Whitfield, M.J. and Rivers, J.K. (1991): Erythema multiforme after contact dermatitis in response to an epoxy sealant. *J. Am. Acad. Dermatol., 25*, 386–388.

4. Unusual manifestations of allergic contact sensitivity

117. Romaguera, C., Grimalt, F. and Vilaplana, J. (1989): Eczematous and purpuric allergic contact dermatitis from boots. *Contact Dermatitis, 21*, 269.
118. Duhra, P. and Foulds, I.S. (1990): Persistent vitiligo induced by diphencyprone. *Br. J. Dermatol., 123*, 415–416.
119. Hatzis, J., Gourgiotou, A. and Tosca, A. (1988): Vitiligo as a reaction to topical treatment with diphencyprone. *Dermatologica, 177*, 146–148.
120. MacDonald-Hull, S.P., Cotterill, J.A.C. and Norris, J.F.B. (1989): Vitiligo following diphencyprone dermatitis. *Br. J. Dermatol., 120*, 323.
121. Goh, C.L. (1987): Erythema multiforme-like and purpuric eruption due to contact allergy to proflavine. *Contact Dermatitis, 17*, 53–54.
122. Frosch, P.J. and Raulin, C. (1987): Kontaktallergie auf Bufexamac. *Hautarzt, 38*, 331–334.
123. Romaguera, C., Vilaplana, J. and Grimalt, F. (1991): Contact dermatitis from oak moss. *Contact Dermatitis, 24*, 224–225.
124. Parodi, G., Guarrera, M. and Rebora, A. (1987): Lichenoid photocontact dermatitis to musk ambrette. *Contact Dermatitis, 16*, 136–138.
125. Hayakawa, R., Hirose, O. and Arima, Y. (1991): Pigmented contact dermatitis due to musk moskene. *J. Dermatol. 18*, 420–424.
126. Poli, F., Pouget, F. and Revuz, J. (1991): Erytheme polymorphe après application de bufexamac (3 cas). *Ann. Dermatol. Venereol., 118*, 901–902.
127. Schena, B. and Barba, A. (1992): Erythema-multiforme-like contact dermatitis from dimethoate. *Contact Dermatitis, 27*, 116.
128. Bhargaua, R.U., Singh, V. and Soni, V. (1977): Erythema multiforme resulting from insecticide spray. *Arch. Dermatol., 113*, 686.
129. Lichter, M., Drury, D. and Remlinger, U. (1992): Lichenoid dermatitis caused by epoxy resin. *Contact Dermatitis, 26*, 275.
130. O'Donnell, B.F. and Tan, C.Y. (1992): Erythema multiforme reaction to patch testing. *Contact Dermatitis, 27*, 230–234.
131. Fregert, S., Gustafsson, K. and Trulsson, L. (1983): Contact allergy to *N*-hydroxyphthalimide. *Contact Dermatitis, 9*, 84–85.
132. Magnusson, B. and Gilje, O. (1973): Allergic contact dermatitis from a dish-washing liquid containing lauryl ether sulphate. *Acta. Derm. Venereol., 53*, 136–140.
133. Goh, C.L. and Kozuka, T. (1986): Pigmented contact dermatitis from "kumkum". *Clin. Exp. Dermatol., 11*, 603–606.
134. Pecegueiro, M. and Brandão, M. (1984): Contact plantar pustulosis. *Contact Dermatitis, 11*, 126–127.
135. Schoel, J. and Frosch, P.J. (1990): Allergisches Kontaktekzem durch Gummi-inhaltstoffe unter dem Bild einer Pustulosis Palmaris. *Dermatosen, 38*, 178–180.
136. Perno, P. and Lisi, P. (1990): Psoriasis-like contact dermatitis from a hair nitro dye. *Contact Dermatitis, 23*, 123–124.
137. Iwatsuki, K., Yamada, M., Takigawa, M., Inoue, K. and Matsumoto, K. (1987): Benign lymphoplasia of the earlobes induced by gold earrings: immunohistologic study on the cellular infiltrates. *J. Am. Acad. Dermatol., 16*, 83–88.

5. Allergic contact dermatitis from topical drugs

5.1 This chapter contains alphabetical tabulations of topical drugs and other topically applied substances that have caused contact allergy, as reported in the literature; for each drug one or more relevant references are provided. The drugs have been subdivided into several groups according to their clinical use and functional purposes. The last section in this chapter deals with contact allergy to drugs that are not usually applied topically but have accidentally come into contact with the skin, e.g. in medical and nursing personnel, or in the industry.

Patch test concentration and vehicle (see also Appendix)

5.2 For each drug the vehicle and concentration for patch testing is mentioned; usually this is the generally accepted concentration and vehicle, but sometimes it refers to the way the authors of the report mentioned have patch-tested the particular drug. Sources may be found in De Groot, A.C. (1994): *Patch Testing. Test Concentrations and Vehicles for 2800 Allergens, 3rd Edition*, Elsevier Science Publishers, Amsterdam.

5.3 Key to abbreviations

acet.	= acetone
alc.	= alcohol 70%
as is	= undiluted
BL	= butyrolactone
c.o.	= castor oil
comm. ointm. bas.	= commercial ointment basis
DEP	= diethyl phthalate
DMP	= dimethyl phthalate
euc.	= eucerin
glyc.	= glycerol
isopropyl alc.	= isopropyl alcohol
isopr. palm.	= isopropyl palmitate
MEK	= methyl ethyl ketone
m.o.	= mineral oil
o.o.	= olive oil
paraff. liq.	= paraffinum liquidum
pet.	= petrolatum
prop. glyc.	= propylene glycol

Estimated frequency of sensitization (EFS)

5.4 Estimated frequency of sensitization (EFS), based both on data from the literature and personal experience, is expressed as follows:
1: contact sensitization is common
2: contact sensitization may occur
3: contact sensitization is uncommon
4: contact sensitization is rare

Cross-reaction

5.5 Cross-reacting chemicals are listed, but only when such compounds have actually cross-reacted and *not* when they might be *expected* to do so on theoretical grounds.

PRESERVATIVES: ANTIMICROBIALS AND ANTIOXIDANTS

5.6 Cosmetic products and other topical preparations must be protected against deterioration caused by microbials (bacteria, yeasts, fungi) or by oxidation of lipid components (air oxygen). The microbial problem is solved by the addition of anti-microbials (preservatives). Usually a combination of two or more (even up to six) compounds is used for preservation.

Concentration levels of the preservatives vary widely. Most compounds (e.g. the paraben esters) are used at levels of 0.1 to 0.5%, but others are active at 0.0025% (25 p.p.m.) levels (e.g. organo-mercurials, methylisothiazolinones). Between these two extremes are the active levels of some important preservatives such as 2-bromo-2-nitropropane-1,3-diol (bronopol: 0.01–0.05%), quaternary ammonium compounds and chlorhexidine.

The antimicrobial level in deodorants is approximately 0.5%, which is higher than the level necessary for preservation. Antiseptic soaps and lotions contain the highest levels (ca. 2%). Cosmetics and other topical pharmaceuticals that do not contain water (salve, lipstick, baby oils and compact powders) do not need preservation.

The problem of oxidation of lipids which leads to rancidity, is solved by the addition of antioxidants. Chelating agents (e.g. EDTA, citric acid) will support antioxidant action by complexing trace heavy metal impurities in the product, which otherwise might catalyze the oxidation reaction.

Contact allergy from preservatives, though well known, must be considered infrequent when related to the widespread presence of these compounds in preparations handled by everyone. As these chemicals have a low sensitizing potential in the concentrations in which they are added to a product, sensitization after contact with *intact* skin, as in cosmetics, is infrequent; most reports of contact allergy to preservatives are from topical preparations used on eczematous or otherwise damaged skin.

Section 5.7 lists antioxidants, antimicrobials and preservatives that have caused contact allergy. An extensive listing of these compounds is given in § 30.5. For reviews of allergy to formaldehyde and formaldehyde donors, see [664]. For non-formaldehyde antimicrobials, see [745].

5.7 Contact allergy to preservatives: antimicrobials and antioxidants (see also [674–677])

Drug	Patch test conc. & vehicle (§ 5.2)	EFS (§ 5.4)	Cross-reactions (§ 5.5)	Comment	Ref.
alcohols					181 571
benzyl alcohol	5-10% pet.	4	patients hypersensitive to balsam Peru may cross-react to benzyl alcohol. Other primary alcohols(?)	Preservative in allergen extracts and solutions for injections, also used as solvent, in flavors and perfumes. *Cave:* irritant patch test reactions.	154 575
ethyl alcohol	10% aqua pure	4	other primary alcohols		444
isopropyl alcohol	10% aqua pure	4			245 283
aminacrine	0.1% pet.	4		Aminacrine is an acridine dye	465
ammonium sulfobituminate (ichthammol, ichthyol)	5% aqua	4	turpentine oil?	Ammonium sulfobituminate consists of sulfur (10%), ammonium sulfate (5–7%), hydrocarbons, nitrogenous bases, acids and derivatives of thiophene. The allergen is present in the water and the cyclohexane soluble fraction [80]. *Cave:* irritant patch test reactions with 5% aqua [537]	80 537
Ampholyt G®	0.1% sol.	3		Occupational allergy in hospital personnel. The active ingredients are: – 9-lauryl-3,6,9-triazanonanoic acid – 7-lauryl-1,4,7-triazaheptane – 6,9-dilauryl-3,6-triazanonanoic acid – 4,7-dilauryl-1,4,7-triaza-heptane The actual allergen is unknown	486
benzoic acid	5% pet.	3			661
BHA (butylated hydroxyanisole)	2% pet.	3		Antioxidant, primarily used in foods	156 163 351
BHT (butylated hydroxytoluene)	2% pet.	3		Antioxidant, primarily used in foods	119 163 351

(continued)

§ **5.7** *(continuation)*

Drug	Patch test conc. & vehicle (§ 5.2)	EFS (§ 5.4)	Cross-reactions (§ 5.5)	Comment	Ref.
bithionol	1% pet.	3	cross-reacts to halogenated salicylanilides	Usually photo-allergy (§ 6.5)	329
brilliant green	2% aqua	4	possibly to other triphenyl-methane dyes	*See also* under Triphenylmethane dyes	736
2-bromo-2-nitro-propane-1.3-diol (bronopol)	0.5% pet.	2		Formaldehyde donor Concomitant sensitization to formaldehyde is present in about 1/3 of patients. Review of formaldehyde (donors): *see* [664]	545 564 662
bromosalicylchlor-anilide	1% pet.	4			
chloroacetamide	0.2% pet.	2			125 258 404
chloramine-T	0.5% aqua	3		For industrial use, *see* [574]. For occupational allergy, *see* [737]	573 574
chlorbutanol	5% pet.	4			209
chlorhexidine (digluconate) (diacetate)	0.5 and 1% aqua	3		Chlorhexidine diacetate may be preferable for patch testing [279]. The 1% concentration is often irritant, so a lower concentration should be tested concomitantly. Other investigators have suggested to use chlorhexidine digluconate 1% in petrolatum and in water [456]. Patients with leg ulcers/stasis eczema are particularly at risk for developing contact sensitization to chlorhexidine [279,456]	279 456 477 478
dehydroacetic acid	0.1% and 1% pet.	4			744 811
diazolidinyl urea	2% aqua or pet.	2	to and from imidazolidinyl urea	Formaldehyde donor. Review of formaldehyde donors: *see* [664].	657 658 659
dibromopropa-midine	1-5% pet.	4			488
1,3-diiodo-2-hy-droxypropane	0.05% alc.	4			228 282

(continued)

§ **5.7** *(continuation)*

Drug	Patch test conc. & vehicle (§ 5.2)	EFS (§ 5.4)	Cross-reactions (§ 5.5)	Comment	Ref.
dipicolinic acid (2,6-pyridine dicarboxylic acid)	0.1% pet.	4		No controls performed, report probably reliable	669
DMDM hydantoin (dimethylol dimethyl hydantoin)	1-3% aqua	4	MDM hydantoin	All reactions have been caused by allergy to formaldehyde: (D)MDM hydantoin is a formaldehyde releaser. Review of formaldehyde (donors): *see* [664]	663
dodicin	1% aqua	4			409
eosin	1–2% alc or pet. 50% pet. (ICDRG)	4		The allergen is probably an (unidentified) impurity	741
ethacridine	1-2% pet.	2		Ethacridine is an acridine dye	359
ethylenediamine tetra-acetate (EDTA)	1% pet.	4	*not* to ethylenediamine hydrochloride [512,513]		266 341
fenticlor	1% pet.	4			129
formaldehyde	1% aqua	1		Formaldehyde donors: *see* [660]. Review of formaldehyde (donors): see [664]	115 384 780
Gallate esters (experimental sensitization: Ref. [810])					
lauryl gallate (dodecyl gallate)	0.1% pet.	3			671
octyl gallate				*See* index.	
propyl gallate	1% pet.	3		Contact allergy is usually caused from its presence in cosmetics and pharmaceutical preparations	62 109 779
glutaraldehyde	1% pet.	3	formaldehyde? [748]. Phthalic dicarboxaldehyde	Nasal and respiratory occupational problems: [288]. Occupational contact allergy *see* [748]	228 248 285 590
hexahydro-1,3,5-tris(2-hydroxyethyl) triazine	1% pet.	3			254 562 563
hexamidine	0.15% aqua	2			10 347

(continued)

§ **5.7** *(continuation)*

Drug	Patch test conc. & vehicle (§ 5.2)	EFS (§ 5.4)	Cross-reactions (§ 5.5)	Comment	Ref.
3-(hydroxyethyl)-5-methyl-8-(2-methyl-ethyl)-3,4-dihydro-2H-1,3-benzoxazine	0.01% alc	2		This is the allergen in Hirudoid® cream and is formed by reaction of the preservatives thymol and 1,3,5-trihydroxyethylhexa-hydrotriazine. Other allergens in Hirudoid cream are wool alcohols (including myristyl alcohol) [743]	740
imidazolidinyl urea (Germall 115®)	1% pet. or aqua	3	diazolidinyl urea	Formaldehyde donor. Review of formaldehyde (donors): *see* [664]	152 584 586 662
iodine, tincture of	0.5% aqua open test	2		Patch tests may show non-specific papulo-pustular reactions	293
iodoform	5% pet.	3		Use abandoned	242
isothiazolinones					
1,2-benzisothia-zolin-3-one	0.1% alc.	4			81
(5-chloro)-2-methyl-4-isothiazolin-3-one(Kathon CG)	100 ppm aqua	1	probably other isothiazolinones	Important cosmetic allergen; also in patients using 'moist toilet paper' [776]	441 555 672 673
4,5-dichloro-2-methyl-4-isothia-zolin-3-one	150 ppm alcohol	?	other isothiazolinones		360
mafenide hydro-chloride	10% pet.	2	other para-compounds		668
mercurial compounds			cross-reactions may occur between the metal, the organic and the inorganic mercurials [182,212]		182 212
ammoniated mercury	1% pet.	2	other mercurials	Inorganic mercurial compound, formerly used in the treatment of psoriasis and in skin lightening creams	138 212
merbromin (mercuro-chrome)	0.1-2% aqua	4	other mercurials	Organic mercurial compound	182 212

(continued)

§ **5.7** *(continuation)*

Drug	Patch test conc. & vehicle (§ 5.2)	EFS (§ 5.4)	Cross-reactions (§ 5.5)	Comment	Ref.
mercuric chloride	0.1% pet.	2	other mercurials	Inorganic mercurial compound. *Cave:* irritant patch test reactions	19 85
mercurous chloride	as is	3	other mercurials	Inorganic mercurial compound, formerly used for the treatment of syphilis and as a diuretic	183
p-chloro-mercuriphenol	0.067% pet.	4	phenylmercuric acetate		295
phenylmercuric acetate	0.01% aqua	3	other mercurials	Organic mercurical compound	315
phenylmercuric borate	0.01% aqua	3	other mercurials	Organic mercurial compound	315
phenylmercuric nitrate	0.01% aqua	3	other mercurials	Organic mercurial compound	315
thiomersal (merthiolate)	0.1% pet.	2	other mercurials	Organic mercurial compound. Also used as preservative in contact lens fluid causing many cases of allergic conjunctivitis [540]. *Cave:* irritant patch test reactions. Some patients are sensitized by the mercury, others by thiosalicylic acid. Contact allergy to thiosalicylic acid is associated with photosensitivity reactions to the non-steroidal antiinflammatory drug piroxicam [749]. Many cases of sensitization are caused by vaccination with thiomersal-preserved vaccines [750] and by hyposensitizing therapy for asthma and pollinosis [540]	166 212
methyldibromo-glutaronitrile (1,2-dibromo-2,4-dicyanobutane)	0.05% pet.	3			670 777 778
N-methylol chloro-accetamide	0.2% pet.	4	Chloroacetamide	Possibly formaldehyde donor	4 189
neutral red chloride	0.1% aqua	4			95 312
nitrofurazone	1% pet.	2	nitrofurantoin	Occupational airborne contact dermatitis *see* [739]	56 236
nordihydroguaia-retic acid (NDGA)	2% pet.	4		Antioxidant in topical preparations, formerly also used in foods	351

(continued)

§ **5.7** *(continuation)*

Drug	Patch test conc. & vehicle (§ 5.2)	EFS (§ 5.4)	Cross-reactions (§ 5.5)	Comment	Ref.
parabens					
esters of p-hydroxy-benzoic acid	15% pet.	3	between the various esters, benzocaine, 4-homosulfanilamide, *p*-phenylene-diamine and procaine	Parabens are also added to certain foods	280 297 325 381
– benzyl ester	3% pet.				
– butyl ester	3% pet.				
– ethyl ester	3% pet.				
– methyl ester	3% pet.				
– propyl ester	3% pet.				
phenolic compounds					
bismuth tribromophenol	as is	3			175 644
bromochlorophene	2%	4			564
p-chloro-*m*-cresol	1% pet.	3	*p*-chloro-*m*-xylenol		70 125 229 327
chloroxylenol	1% pet.	3	*p*-chloro-*m*-cresol dichloro-*m*-xylenol [815]	*Cave:* irritant patch test reactions with chloroxylenol 1% pet.	69 408
dichlorophene	1% pet.	3	hexachlorophene?	*Cave:* Irritant patch test reactions to dichlorophene 1% pet.	135 382 661
hexachlorophene	1% pet.	4	dichlorophene, bithionol and halogenated salicylanilides (usually *photo*-cross-reactions)		22 69 139 603
o-phenylphenol	1% pet.	3			530
phenoxyethanol	1% pet.	4			666
potassium sorbate	5% pet.	2	sorbic acid		587
povidone-iodine	10% pet. and comm. prep.	3	iodine	PVP-I solution has 10% bound iodine and 1% available iodine. Contact allergy to povidone iodine is sometimes associated with allergy to iodine [544,99]	24 520 544
proflavine dihydrochloride	0.1-1% pet.	3		Proflavine is an acridine dye	305
proflavine hemisulfate	1% pet.	2		Very commonly used in the tropics	654
propamidine	2% pet.	4			654
propylene oxide	0.1% alc.	4			245

(continued)

§ **5.7** *(continuation)*

Drug	Patch test conc. & vehicle (§ 5.2)	EFS (§ 5.4)	Cross-reactions (§ 5.5)	Comment	Ref.
quaternary ammonium compounds (may be tested 0.1% and 0.01% aqua) [180]				Irritant reactions with patch test concentrations of 0.1% occur frequently. Use test may be helpful in distinguishing allergic from irritant reactions [742]	
benzalkonium chloride	0.05–0.1% aqua	3	other quaternary ammonium compounds. e.g. hexamethonium bromide [534]	Benzalkonium chloride is a mixture of alkyl-dimethyl-benzyl-ammonium chlorides	3 162 533 534
benzethonium chloride	0.1% aqua	4	benzalkonium chloride		146
benzoxonium chloride	0.05% aqua	4	benzalkonium chloride		655
			domiphen bromide		656
cetalkonium chloride	0.1% aqua	4	benzalkonium chloride (?)		395
cetrimonium bromide (cetrimide)	0.1% aqua	3	benzalkonium chloride [533]		14 206 393
cetylpyridinium chloride	0.05% aqua	2			694
dequalinium chloride	0.01% aqua	4			175 368 460
domiphen bromide	0.1% aqua	4			72
lauryl pyridinum chloride	0.1% aqua	4			655
quaternium-15 (chloroallylhexaminium chloride)		2		Quaternium-15 is a formaldehyde releaser	110 584 585
quinoline derivatives					
chlorquinaldol	3% pet.	2	other quinoline derivatives	The frequency of sensitization decreases from Cl- via F- and Br- to the I-halogentated compounds. Cross reactions may be observed to – other halogenated quinoline derivatives – quinolines: aminoquinaldine, quinaldol, quinaldine, quinoline – isoquinolines: papaverine, eupaverine – chloroquine, amodiaquine	57 257 426 472 642

(continued)

§ **5.7** *(continuation)*

Drug	Patch test conc. & vehicle (§ 5.2)	EFS (§ 5.4)	Cross-reactions (§ 5.5)	Comment	Ref.
				– non-hydroxylated quinolines	
5-chloro-8-hydroxyquinoline	3% pet.	2	other quinoline derivatives		
clioquinol	3% pet.	2	other quinoline derivatives		
5,7-dibromo-8-hydroxyquinoline	3% pet.	2	other quinoline derivatives		
5,7-difluoro-8-hydroxyquinoline-p-hydroxymethylbenzoate	3% pet.	2	other quinoline derivatives		
8-hydroxyquinoline	3% pet.	2	other quinoline derivatives		
sodium benzoate	5% pet.	3			661
sodium hypochlorite	0.5% aqua	3			667
sodium metabisulfite	5% aqua	3			746 747
sodium sulfite	2-5% pet.	4			665
sorbic acid	2% pet.	2			59 107 539
sulfur	1-5% pet.	4			375
tetrachlorosalicylanilide	0.1% pet.	4			187
thymol (isopropyl *m*-cresol)	1% pet.	4	carvacrol rosemary		738
tocopherols	10%pet.	3		Patch testing with tocopherols may sensitize. *See* for patch testing also § 30.5.1	2 351 781
DL-α-tocopherol	10% pet.	3		For patch test sensitization, *see* [607]	
triclocarban	2% pet.	3	halogenated salicylanilides		287 811
triclosan (Irgasan DP 300®)	2% pet.	3			350 452 661 811

(continued)

§ **5.7** *(continuation)*

Drug	Patch test conc. & vehicle (§ 5.2)	EFS (§ 5.4)	Cross-reactions (§ 5.5)	Comment	Ref.
triphenyl-methane dyes (gentian violet, crystal violet, methyl violet, rosaniline, mala-chite green, brilliant green, chrysoidine and eosin)	2% aqua	3	other triphenyl-methane dyes		44 498
usnic acid	0.1% pet.	4			661
zinc pyrithione	1% pet.	4			661

CONTACT ALLERGY TO FRAGRANCE MATERIALS

5.8 Not only is fragrance the most important ingredient of perfumes and colognes, it is also a significant part of many other cosmetic products such as creams, lotions, powders, soaps, etc.

A perfume is a creative composition of fragrance materials. On opening a bottle, the most volatile components of the 'top note' will be smelled. After 5–20 minutes the 'heart' or the 'body' of the perfume is perceptible. With a good perfume this heart will last for 2–4 hours. What is left is the 'dry out', which will gradually disappear. There are distinct perfume materials that have a favorable influence on the perfume profile, tempering the top note, refinement and extension of the heart and strengthening the dry out. Such materials are called 'fixatives' and include balsam Peru, balsam Tolu, storax, benzoin, coumarin and musk.

The perfumer has approx. 200 fragrance materials of natural origin (e.g. essential oils) and approx. 3000 fragrance compounds, which are either isolates or derivatives of natural materials or synthetics. The most important fragrance materials are listed in § 30.7.

Perfumes contain approx. 12–20% of the so-called 'perfume compound'. It is expensive and actually too concentrated. The more diluted products (perfume lotion, perfume de toilette, eau de toilette, colognes) are therefore much more popular. There are no legally defined concentrations of the perfume compounds for these different products, but in general, colognes will contain 2–5%, perfume lotion and perfume de toilette 5–8% of the perfume compound. Most fragrance products are alcoholic solutions (70–96% ethanol), but perfume creams (sachets) and aerosols are also popular.

5.9 Typical **perfume formulas** are:

		Example:
Perfume:		
4–30%	water	water
70–96%	alcohol	ethanol
12–20%	perfume compound	perfume
Perfume aerosol:		
30%	propellant	chlorofluorocarhon 114
65%	alcohol	ethanol
5%	water	water
2–10%	perfume compound	perfume
Perfume sachet:		
70%	water	water
20%	lipid	glyceryl stearate, cetearyl alcohol
2%	surfactant: emulsifier	PEG-25 propylene glycol stearate
2–10%	perfume compound	perfume
0.2%	preservative	quaternium-15, methylparaben

IDENTIFICATION OF SENSITIZER

5.10 It is very difficult to establish the specific sensitizer in a perfume. Certain perfumes are both sensitizers and photosensitizers; others are solely photosensitizers. Therefore, patch tests with perfumes must be done, not only with the usual patch testing method but also with photopatch tests. Photosensitization is associated with a number of essential perfume oils, especially bergamot, lavender, cedar wood, neroli and petitgrain. Benzyl alcohol, a perfume solvent and gum benzoin as well as various balsams and other fixatives may be the actual sensitizers in perfumes [153].

A perfume ingredient which is a sensitizer may become hypoallergenic during the aging process of the perfume. In such cases patch tests with the aged perfume ingredient remain negative, whereas the tests with a freshly prepared solution will give a positive result. This explains for instance the fact that a patient with an allergic sensitivity to cinnamic aldehyde may tolerate an aged perfume containing cinnamic aldehyde, without acquiring a dermatitis [160].

Also, an allergenic perfume ingredient may become non-allergenic, owing to its neutralization by another ingredient of the perfume mixture, or to chemical interchanges between two or more components [35].

The phenomenon that a contact sensitizing substance no longer causes contact sensitization in combination with another compound has been coined as 'quenching effect' [328]. This has been observed in the human maximization test with the contact sensitizing aldehydes phenylacetaldehyde, citral aldehyde and cinnamic aldehyde. *See* § 3.13, item 8.

Although nowadays perfumes are considered to be the principal sensitizers in cosmetics [594], fragrance materials as possible sensitizing constituents of cosmetic products have been overlooked for many years. This may largely be explained by the concentrations of fragrances in cosmetics: these are often too low to elicit a positive patch test result when the cosmetic is tested 'as is', thus leading to false negative results.

It has been shown that contact allergy to certain well-known sensitizers such as balsam Peru, rosin (colophony) and wood tar is frequently associated with a perfume allergy. Therefore, contact allergy to these and/or other so-called 'markers' or 'indicators' of perfume allergy should alert the physician to the possibility of contact allergy to fragrance materials. These indicators are listed in § 5.11 [158].

More recently, a fragrance mixture has been introduced in the ICDRG standard series, which has facilitated testing for fragrance sensitivity. The fragrance mixture is a combination of the most common fragrance allergens. This mixture will in the future be modified as new fragrance allergens are defined. The fragrances in the mixture are shown in § 5.12.

The fragrance mixture detects possibly 70–80% of fragrance sensitivity, leaving 20–30% undetected [595]. In routine testing positive reactions to the fragrance mix have been noted in 6% [598], 8.2% [597], 18.7% [596], and 10.2% [683] of patients with contact dermatitis. Most positive reactions are to cinnamic aldehyde, hydroxycitronellal and isoeugenol, though data between various centres vary considerably [684]. One problem with the perfume mixture is that some false positive irritant reactions occur, especially with the Excited Skin Syndrome. Therefore, the patch test concentrations of the 8 individual fragrances in the mix have, in July 1984, been decreased from 2% to 1% each. Even then, positive reactions to the mix were observed in the absence of reactions to its ingredients. This was shown to be caused by the absence of sorbitan sesquioleate in the individual allergen preparations. Sorbitan sesquioleate is present in the mix as an emulsifier and appears to enhance the diagnostic power of the mix, probably by increasing the bioavailability of the ingredients. Some reactions to the mix have been caused by allergy to sorbitan sesquioleate itself [682]. Although at present this mixture is the most sensitive 'indicator' of perfume allergy, it has not rendered the other indicators obsolete [597].

5.11 Plant 'indicators' of perfume allergy

balsam Peru	25% pet.
rosin (colophony)	20% pet .
wood tar – pine 3%	
– beech 3%	
– juniper 3%	
– birch 3%	12% pet.
turpentine	10% o.o.
turpentine peroxides	0.3% pet.
sesquiterpene lactones (costus absolute)	1% pet.
lichen substances (atronin, oak moss)	1% pet.

5.12 Fragrance mixture (ICDRG)

	Before July 1984	After July 1984
cinnamic aldehyde	2% pet.	1% pet.
cinnamic alcohol	2% pet.	1% pet.
isoeugenol	2% pet.	1% pet.
oak moss	2% pet.	1% pet.
eugenol	2% pet.	1% pet.
geraniol	2% pet.	1% pet.
hydroxycitronellal	2% pet.	1% pet.
α-amylcinnamic aldehyde	2% pet.	1% pet.

5.13 A number of fragrance materials have been reported to cause contact allergy: these are listed in § 5.14. Many other ingredients will probably in future prove to be sensitizers and/or photosensitizers. Individual substances may be tested according to the recommendations of Fisher [153]. The relevant recommended patch test concentrations and vehicles are listed in § 5.15. (*See also* § 30.7 on fragrance materials.) Contact allergy to various fragrance materials is probably of great importance in the production of the state of persistent light reaction as seen in the photosensitivity dermatitis with actinic reticuloid; some of these allergens are also capable of involving photosensitivity mechanisms [592,593].

5.14 Contact allergy to fragrance materials

Substance	Patch test conc. & vehicle (§ 5.2)	EFS (§ 5.4)	Cross-reactions (§ 5.5)	Comment	Ref.
amyl cinnamate	32% pet.	4			290
α-amylcinnamic alcohol	2% pet.	2	α-amylcinnamic aldehyde	Commercial forms of α-amylcinnamic alcohol not infrequently contain α-amylcinnamic aldehyde	272 567
α-amylcinnamic aldehyde	2% pet.	3	α-amylcinnamic alcohol		567
anisylidene acetone	2% pet. (fresh)	4			681
atranorin	0.5% pet.	2		Present in oak moss perfumes	116 343
balsam Peru	25% pet.	1	benzoic acid, benzoin, benzyl alcohol, benzyl benzoate, cinnamates, cinnamic acid, cinnamic alcohol, cinnamon, essential oils, eugenol, orange peels, propolis, rosin (colophony), vanilla	*See also* under propolis (§ 5.41)	130 226 605 679 814

(continued)

§ **5.14** *(continuation)*

Substance	Patch test conc. & vehicle (§ 5.2)	EFS (§ 5.4)	Cross-reactions (§ 5.5)	Comment	Ref.
balsam Tolu	20% pet.	1	balsam Peru	Ingredients are listed by Mitchell [308]	226
benzaldehyde	5% pet.	1	balsam Peru		226
benzyl alcohol	5% pet.	4	*See* § 5.7		320 386
benzyl cinnamate	5% pet.	1	balsam Peru		226 681
benzylidene acetone	0.5% pet.	4			51 290 681
benzyl salicylate	1% pet.	3	balsam Peru, cananga oil, jasmin oil, ylang-ylang oil	Benzyl salicylate is a preservative. Also used as sunscreen (§ 29.19)	319 357
bergamot oil	5% pet.	4		Allergenic ingredients include α- and β-pinene and citral [812]	684 812
carvacrol	5% pet.	4			811
cananga oil	2% pet.	3			320
cinnamic alcohol	2% pet.	1	balsam Peru, cinnamic aldehyde	Consumer patch-test sensitization has been investigated [553]	271 319
cinnamic aldehyde (cinnamal)	1% pet.	1	balsam Peru, cinnamic alcohol, cinnamic acid [383]	Contact allergy from occupational exposure: *see* [483]. Pemphigoid-like allergic reaction to cinnamic aldehyde: Ref. [340]	326 385 605
cinnamon oil	2% pet.	4	balsam Peru, cinnamic aldehyde		77 751
cinnamyl benzoate	10% pet.	4			290
cinnamyl cinnamate	8% pet.	4			290
citral	2% pet. (fresh)	2		Citral is a mixture of geranial and neral. At higher temperatures citral may be a strong irritant (§ 2.4)	226 680 681
citronellal	2-4% pet.	2	hydroxycitronellal		272
citronella oil				*See* lemongrass oil	255
coniferyl alcohol	2% pet.	2	balsam Peru		226
costus absolute	1% pet.	3	plants containing sesquiterpene lactones	Principal allergens are sesquiterpene lactones, derived from *Saussurea lappa*, a Compositae plant. Perfume allergy indicator	306 310

(continued)

§ **5.14** *(continuation)*

Substance	Patch test conc. & vehicle (§ 5.2)	EFS (§ 5.4)	Cross-reactions (§ 5.5)	Comment	Ref.
coumarin	5% pet.	2	balsam Peru, vanilla, vanillin	Sensitization studies with various coumarins: Ref. [234]	434 681
cuminaldehyde	15% pet.	4			811
diethyl sebacate	20% alc.	3			376
dihydroabietyl alcohol	1% pet.	3	abietic acid, rosin (colophony)		124
dimethyl citracon-ate	12% pet.	4			681
dihydrocoumarin	5% pet.	2			290 681
eugenol	2% pet.	1	balsam Peru, isoeugenol		226
essential oils	2% pet.	3		For individual oils, *see* § 30.7 and § 39.2 Ref. [23]	
evernic acid	0.1% acet.	2		Present in oak moss perfumes	116 343
farnesol	4% pet.	2	balsam Peru		226
fumarprotocetraric acid	0.1% acet.	2		Present in oak moss perfumes	116 343
Galaxolide®	25% pet.	3			811
geranial	1-5% pet.	2	geranium, hydroxycitronellal, lavender oil, ylang-ylang oil		272 319
geraniol	2% pet.	2		Has caused patch-test sensitization	557 680
geranium oil	2% pet.	4			319
cis-3-hexenyl salicylate	3% pet.	4	*not* to benzyl salicylate, hexyl, methyl, and phenyl		475
hexylcinnamic aldehyde	2% pet.	4		Tested in a mixture: contact allergy not ascertained	811
hydroxycitronellal	2% pet.	1	citronellal, linalool [? 521]	Consumer patch-test sensitization has been investigated [554]	82 272
ionone	2% pet.	3			386
isoamyl salicylate	2% pet.	4			811
isoeugenol	1% pet.	1	balsam Peru, eugenol		226
jasmin oil	2% pet.	3			319

(continued)

§ **5.14** *(continuation)*

Substance	Patch test conc. & vehicle (§ 5.2)	EFS (§ 5.4)	Cross-reactions (§ 5.5)	Comment	Ref.
jasmin, synthetic	10% pet.	2			272 684
laurel oil	2% pet.	4			170
lavender oil	2% pet.	3			320
lemon oil	2% pet.	4	turpentine oil		255
lemon grass oil	2% pet.	3		Citral is the main constituent	298 751
lilial	1% pet.	4			557 811
linalool	30% pet.	3	hydroxycitronellal (?)	Caused facial psoriasis in the reported case	493
o-methoxycinnamic aldehyde	4% pet.	4			290
methoxycitronellal	1% pet.	3	hydroxycitronellal		320
methyl anisate	4% pet.	4			289 681
6-methyl coumarin	1% pet.	4			251
methyl heptine car-bonate	0.5% pet.	3	methyl octine carbonate		232 290 681
methyl octine car-bonate	1% MEK	4	methyl heptine carbonate	Occupational contact allergy in fragrance laboratory	232
γ-methylionone	10% pet.	4			572
musk ambrette	5% pet.	3	moskene		264
neral	1% pet.	4			681
nopyl acetate	25% pet.	4			811
oak moss	2% pet.	2		The main allergens are: atranorin, evernic acid, fumarprotocetraric acid, d-usnic acid.	343 487 609
orange oil	2% pet.	3			301
patchouli oil	2% pet.	4			319 782
phenylacetaldehyde (hyacinthin)	2% pet. (fresh)	1		Patch testing may sensitize	178
phenyl ethyl alcohol	5% pet.	4			811
peppermint oil	2% pet.	3			684
β-pinene	1% pet.	3			684
propylidene phthalide	2% pet.	4			681

(continued)

§ **5.14** *(continuation)*

Substance	Patch test conc. & vehicle (§ 5.2)	EFS (§ 5.4)	Cross-reactions (§ 5.5)	Comment	Ref.
rose oil Bulgaria	2% pet.	4		Geraniol is one of the allergenic ingredients [813]	319 813
rosin (colophony)	20% pet.	1	*See* § 5.10 and 5.11	Perfume allergy indicator	291
sandalwood oil	2% pet.	3			407 684
terpineol	5% pet.	3			684
usnic acid	0.1% pet.	3		Present in oak moss perfumes	343
ylang-ylang oil	2% pet.	1			320 823

Many other cosmetic (fragrance) materials will probably in future prove to be sensitizers and/or photosensitizers. Individual substances may be tested as follows (adapted from Fisher [153]):

5.15 Recommended patch test concentrations and vehicles for the screening of possible new sensitizers

Cosmetic ingredient	Patch test conc. & vehicle (§ 5.2)	Cosmetic ingredient	Patch test conc. & vehicle (§ 5.2)
p-anisaldehyde	1% pet.	cedartone V	as is
balm oil	1% pet.	trans-cinnamaldehyde	2% pet.
bay rum	as is	citracetal	10% DE
carnation oil	10% aqua	citron oil	1% pet.
coniferyl benzoate	1% pet (2% pet.: [180])	mirbane oil (nitrobenzene)	25% c.o. (10% o.o.: [180])
essential oils	1% alc. or 2% pet.	orange peel oil	1% alc. (2% pet.: [180])
gylan	as is	perfumes	as is (open and closed)
Hamamelis virg.	5% aqua	petitgrain oil	10% o.o.
4-hydroxy azobenzene carboxylic acid	2% pet.		
α-irisone	as is	sassafras oil	1% pet.
isoamyl salicylate	5% pet.	spice oil	5% pet. (*see also* § 5.39)
		terpineol extra	25% BL
		tetra-hydromuguol	as is
linalool oil	10% pet.	vanilla (alcoholic extract)	10% acet. (as is: [180])
linalyl acetate	1% pet.		
		verbena oil	1% pet.
menthanyl acetate	as is	versalide	10% pet.
mint oil	1% pet.	vetivert rectified	as is

LOCAL ANESTHETICS

5.16 Local anesthetics are widely used in topical preparations for their antipruritic and anesthetic properties, e.g. in the treatment of pruritus ani, hemorrhoids and, occasionally, pruritus vulvae. The efficacy however, is rather doubtful. Accidental contact with local anesthetics for injection may occur in medical and dental personnel. The allergenic potency of these drugs largely depends on their chemical structure.

The main groups of local anesthetics are the benzoic acid derivatives (esters of *p*-aminobenzoic acid, *m*-aminobenzoic acid and benzoic acid), the amide derivatives and the quinoline derivatives (see § 5.17). The esters of *p*-aminobenzoic acid frequently cause contact sensitization, whereas the aminoacyl amides, such as lidocaine, are less allergenic. Cross-sensitization is common, especially between the various benzoic acid derivatives; cross-reactivity with other para-compounds occasionally occurs. The most frequent sensitizers in Europe are benzocaine, tetracaine (amethocaine) and cinchocaine (dibucaine) [686]. A satisfactory 'caine-mix' for routine testing has not yet been developed [752].

The risk of developing a potentially serious anaphylactoid reaction upon injection of local anesthetics in patients with contact allergy to these drugs appears to be small [687] with possible exception of procaine.

Anesthetics for topical use that have caused contact allergy are listed in § 5.18.

5.17 Main classes of local anesthetics

A. BENZOIC ACID DERIVATIVES

***p*-Aminobenzoic acid esters:**
butacaine (butelline)
butethamine (monocaine)
butyl aminobenzoate (butamben, butesin)
ethyl aminobenzoate (benzocaine, anesthesin)
isobutyl *p*-aminobenzoate (cycloform)
naepaine (amylsine)
orthocaine (orthoform old & new)
procaine (novocaine)
propoxycaine (ravocaine)
risocaine (propaesin)
tetracaine (amethocaine, pantocaine)

Benzoic acid esters:
amylocaine (stovaine)
benoxinate hydrochloride (dorsacaine)
benzamine (β-eucaine)
cyclomethycaine (surfacaine, topocaine)
meprylcaine hydrochloride (oracaine)
metabutoxycaine (primacaine)
piperocaine (metycaine, neothesin)
propanocaine

***m*-Aminobenzoic acid esters:**
metabutethamine (unacaine)
proparacaine (alcaine)

B. ANILIDES OR AMIDE DERIVATIVES
bupivacaine (marcaine)
butanilicaine [687]
carticaine
lidocaine (lignocaine, xylocaine)
mepivacaine (carbocaine)
prilocaine (Citanest®)

C. QUINOLINE DERIVATIVES
dibucaine (cinchocaine, percaine, nupercaine)
dimethisoquin (quotane)

D. OTHER LOCAL ANESTHETICS
dyclonine hydrochloride
propanidid (intravenous compound)
propipocaine (falicaine)

5.18 Contact allergy to topical anesthetics

Drug	Patch test conc. & vehicle (§ 5.2)	EFS (§ 5.4)	Cross-reactions (§ 5.5)	Comment	Ref.
amylocaine hydrochloride	1% pet.	4			464
benzamine lactate	1% pet.	3			76
benzocaine (ethyl aminobenzoate)	5% pet.	1	para-compounds metabutethamine meprylcaine [516]		89 177 686
butacaine	5% pet.	3	procaine, benzocaine		270
butethamine	5% pet.	3	procaine, benzocaine		145
butyl aminobenzoate	5% pet.	3			440
dibucaine hydrochloride	5% pet.	2	clioquinol (?) *p*-phenylenediamine [687]		464 640 686
diperocaine	1% pet.	4			83
dyclonine hydrochloride	1% pet.	4	*not* to pramocaine		186
hydroxypolyethoxy-dodecane	5% pet.	3			80 216
lidocaine	2% pet.	3	bupivacaine prilocaine mepivacine dibucaine		525 640 641
mepivacaine	2% aqua	4	usually cross-reaction from lidocaine		685
orthoform, new	1% aqua/pet.	2	orthoform, old		270
orthoform, old	1% aqua/pet.	2	benzocaine, isobutyl PABA orthoform, new, risocaine		270
pramocaine	1% aqua	4			442 640
prilocaine	2% aqua	3	usually cross-reaction from lidocaine		685
procaine	1% pet.	2	para-compounds [687]		165 397
propanidid (intravenous anesthetic)	5% pet./aqua	4	balsam Peru cinnamon oil eugenol	Propanidid is a eugenol derivative	27 191 405
propanocaine	1% pet.	3			524
proparacaine hydro-chloride	2% aqua	4		Used in ophthalmology (§ 13.40)	26
propipocaine	1% pet.	2			39 377
quotane ointment (dimethisoquin hydrochloride)	as is	4			117
tetracaine	1% pet.	2	para-compounds [687]		111 252 464 686

VEHICLE CONSTITUENTS

5.19 The testing of vehicles as such is often fruitless because the concentrations of the various ingredients may be so low that epicutaneous tests on healthy skin remain negative. In addition, steroids in ointments may have a negative influence on test reactions. Classic ointment bases with petrolatum and mineral oils are usually harmless; cream bases contain at least preservatives and emulsifiers, but usually also antioxidants, lanolin or wool alcohols and perfumes as possible allergens (see the various relevant chapters). Synthetic vehicles containing polyethylene glycols, propylene glycol and/or fatty alcohols may also be sensitizers.

Those vehicle constituents that have caused contact allergy are listed in § 5.20.

5.20 Contact allergy to vehicle constituents

Vehicle constituent	Patch test conc. & vehicle (§ 5.2)	EFS (§ 5.4)	Cross-reactions (§ 5.5)	Comment	Ref.
acetone	10% o.o.	4		The patient had been deliberately sensitized to diphencyprone in acetone for treatment of alopecia areata.	757
Amerchol CAB®	pure	3	wool alcohols	Amerchol CAB® is a chemically modified lanolin preparation	783
Amerchol L101®	50% pet.	3	eucerin	Amerchol L101® is a chemically modified lanolin preparation	13
arachidis oil	pure	4			784
bismuth subnitrate	pure	4			759
butylene glycol	2–10% aqua	3	other glycols (hexylene, propylene)		755
carbowaxes	as is	4	other polyethylene glycols	Carbowaxes are solid polyethylene glycols	157
				see under polyethylene glycol	688
castor oil	pure	4		The offending chemical probably was ricinoleic acid (30% pet. and pure)	558 643
cera flava	pure	4		Possibly due to its allergenic ingredient propolis	754
ceteth-20	?	4		test concentration and vehicle not mentioned	689
cetyl alcohol	20% pet.	3	other higher fatty alcohols	Cetyl alcohol is an aliphatic alcohol. The actual allergens in commercial cetyl alcohol and cetylstearyl alcohol may be impurities [50] such as *n*-decyl alcohol and oleyl alcohol [753]	50 193 207

(continued)

§ **5.20** *(continuation)*

Vehicle constituent	Patch test conc. & vehicle (§ 5.2)	EFS (§ 5.4)	Cross-reactions (§ 5.5)	Comment	Ref.
chlorofluoromethane	pure	4	chemically related chlorofluoromethanes ethyl chloride (?)		437
n-decyl alcohol	5% pet.	4		Impurity in commercial cetyl and stearyl alcohol	753
decyl oleate	1% pet.	4		Emollient	781
dibutyl phthalate	5% pet.	3			74
diethyl sebacate	1% pet.	4			376
diisopropanolamine	1% pet.	4			697
diisopropyl sebacate	1–10% pet.	4			695
dimethyl sulfoxide	90% aqua	4		Histamine liberator	303
diphenylamine	1% pet.	4	*p*-phenylene-diamine (?)		79
emulgin RO/40®	0.1% and 1% pet.	4		Emulgin RO/40® is formed by the reaction of ethylene oxide and castor oil, producing a polyoxyethylene (Macrogol) ester	693
ethyl chloride	pure	4			756 816
ethylenediamine dihydrochloride	1% pet.	2	aminophylline (consists of 2/3 theophylline and 1/3 ethylenediamine), antazoline sulfate, ethylenediamine dihydroiodide, diethanolamine, diethylenetriamine, hexamethylene tetramine, ethylenediamine base, mepyramine maleate, piperazine, tetraethylenepentamine, triethylenetetramine		67 141 150 155 414 458 611
eucerin	as is	3	lanolin, wool alcohols	Eucerin is petrolatum with 6% wool alcohols	23
glycerin	1% aqua pure	4			208
glyceryl oleate	30% pet.	4			230
glyceryl stearate	30% pet.	3			209
hexantriol	5% aqua	4		Probably represents a cross-reaction after primary sensitization to stearyl alcohol and/or propylene glycol	333

(continued)

§ **5.20** *(continuation)*

Vehicle constituent	Patch test conc. & vehicle (§ 5.2)	EFS (§ 5.4)	Cross-reactions (§ 5.5)	Comment	Ref.
hexylene glycol	1-3-10-30% aqua	4	propylene glycol	Irritant when tested at 30%. Serial dilutions are advised to confirm allergy	655 691
hexyl laurate	30% pet.	4			696
hydroxypropyl cellulose	?% in alcohol or mineral oil	4			698
isopropyl alcohol	10% aqua pure	4			283
isopropyl myristate	5% pet.	4		Isopropyl myristate is a synthetic fatty alcohol	161
isopropyl palmitate	2% pet.	4			575
jojoba oil	20% o.o.	3		Lubricant, used in cosmetics	522
lanette N	20% pet.	2	lanolin, wool alcohols	Lanette N is a mixture of cetyl and stearyl alcohol (9 parts) and sodium cetyl stearyl acid ester (1 part). The actual allergen may be an impurity [50]	31 210
lanette O	20% pet.	2	wool alcohols	Lanette O is a mixture of cetyl and stearyl alcohol. The actual allergen may be an impurity [50]	31 492
lanette wax	30% paraff liq.	3	lanolin, wool alcohols	Lanette wax consists of cetyl and stearyl alcohol with 10% sulfated esters of fatty alcohols	210
lanolin	as is	3	other wool alcohols	Lanolin consists of a mixture of sterols (wool alcohols), fatty alcohols and fatty acids; for a discussion of its composition, see [374,541,542]. Removal of the wool alcohols reduces the risk of allergic reactions [92]. Lanolin is an uncommon sensitizer in the healthy population [543].	92 316 374 785
laureth-4	0.1–1% alc.	4	possibly wool alcohols	2 patients allergic also reacted to Amerchol L101, a lanolin derivative. Laureth-4 is a polyethylene glycol ether of lauryl alcohol	692
lauric acid dialkanolamide	1% pet.	4			209
lauryl dimethyl amine oxide	3.7% aqua	4		Foaming agent. *Cave:* irritant patch test reactions	317 538
myristamide DEA	1% pet.	4			209

(continued)

§ **5.20** *(continuation)*

Vehicle constituent	Patch test conc. & vehicle (§ 5.2)	EFS (§ 5.4)	Cross-reactions (§ 5.5)	Comment	Ref.
myristyl alcohol	20% pet.	3		*See* index	
nonoxynols	1–2% aqua	3	other nonoxynols, octoxynol 9	Nonoxynols are ethoxylated alkyl phenols or nonylphenyl ethers that conform in general to the formula $C_9H_{19}C_6H_4(OCH_2CH_2)_nOH$. Each nonoxynol name is followed by a number (n) that indicates the approximate number of ethylene oxide groups in the polyoxyethylene chain.	699
octyldodecanol	30% pet.	4			514
p-octylphenyl ethylene oxide	0.1% aqua	4			93
oleyl alcohol	pure and 30% pet.	3	stearyl alcohol	Allergenic impurity in commercial cetyl and stearyl alcohol [753]	84 151
olive oil	pure (freshly prepared)	3	*not* to other vegetable oils	The major constituents are: glycerides of oleic acid (85.5%), of palmitic acid (9.4%), of linoleic acid (4%), of stearic acid (2%), and of arachidic acid (0.9%). The exact allergen is unknown. Oleic acid has irritant properties and has been suspected as a sensitizer	201 536
pentaerythritol monooleate	10% o.o.	4			694
petrolatum (yellow, white)	pure	4		The sensitizing capacity of yellow and white petrolatum has been investigated [490], and some allergens have been identified [491]. For allergenicity prediction and pharmacopoieal requirements, *see* [599]	123 203 286
polyethylene glycol	pure	4	other polyethylene glycols	Polyethylene glycols are condensation products of ethylene glycol. The low molecular weight PEG's are liquid, PEG 1000-6000 are solid	157 688
polyethylene glycol stearate	pure	4			161
polyoxyethylene oxypropylene stearate (polysorbate 60)	20% pet.	3			210

(continued)

§ **5.20** *(continuation)*

Vehicle constituent	Patch test conc. & vehicle (§ 5.2)	EFS (§ 5.4)	Cross-reactions (§ 5.5)	Comment	Ref.
polyoxyethylene sorbitan monooleate (polysorbate 80)	10% pet.	4			13 210
polyoxyethylene sorbitan monopalmitate (polysorbate 40)	10% pet.	4			13 210
polyoxyethylene sorbitol lanolate	20% pet.	3			210
propylene glycol	2% pet.	3	other glycols (butylene, hexylene)	It is difficult to differentiate between toxic and allergic patch test reactions. In doubt patch tests should be repeated, and usage tests or oral provocation may be necessary for accurate diagnosis	159 211 755
sesame oil	as is sesamin 1% pet. sesamolin 1% pet.	3		Consists of triglycerides of oleic acid (48%), of linoleic acid (40%), and 10% of palmitic acid, stearic acid and arachoic acid; 2% is unsaponifiable and contains sesamolin and sesamin, which are the allergens	321 424
silicic acid	5% pet.	4		Silicic acid is colloidal silicon dioxide	760
sodium dioctyl sulfosuccinate	<1% aqua	3		Anionic surfactant	529
sodium lauryl sulfate	0.1% aqua	4		Well-known irritant, rare sensitizer. Certain batches of SLS solutions are preserved with formaldehyde [561]	337 561
soft paraffin				*See under* petrolatum	
sorbitan monolaurate	5% aqua	4			144 498
sorbitan monooleate	5% aqua	3			210 499
sorbitan monostearate	5% aqua	3			210
sorbitan sesquioleate	20% pet.	3	sorbitan monooleate and sorbitan monostearate		13 210
stearyl alcohol	30% pet.	4	oleyl alcohol, other higher fatty alcohols	Stearyl alcohol is an aliphatic alcohol	47 151 207 333

(continued)

§ **5.20** *(continuation)*

Vehicle constituent	Patch test conc. & vehicle (§ 5.2)	EFS (§ 5.4)	Cross-reactions (§ 5.5)	Comment	Ref.
TEA-oleyl hydrolyzed animal protein (oleyl polypeptide)	25% alcohol pure	3			12
thioglycerin	10% aqua	2	dimercaprol (BAL)		190
triethanolamine	2.5% pet.	2	ethylenediamine promethazine (?)		410 420 552 758
triethanolamine laurate	5% pet.	4			646
triethanolamine stearate	5% pet.	3			210
zinc oxide	10% pet.	4	zinc sulfate		423 784

ANTIBIOTICS AND CHEMOTHERAPEUTICS

5.21 Topical antibiotic-containing preparations have a variety of uses:
- treatment of primary bacterial skin infections
- eradication of pathogens from carrier sites
- lessening infection of granulating surfaces such as leg ulcers and burns
- in combination with topical corticosteroids for the treatment of (secondary infected) dermatitis.

Hazards of topical antibiotic administration

5.22 The main hazards in the use of topical antibiotics are:
- contact sensitivity (either immediate- or delayed-type)
- ecological shifts in the cutaneous microflora
- development of resistant strains of micro-organisms
- systemic effects (see Chapter 16)
- generalized reactions after oral or parenteral administration of antibiotics in previously sensitized individuals (see Chapter 17).

In this chapter only delayed-type hypersensitivity will be discussed. Some antibiotics are out of (topical) use because of their high sensitizing potential, such as penicillin and sulfonamides.

It must be stressed that the development of hypersensitivity to an antibiotic may greatly endanger the patient. Topical antibiotic preparations should therefore be used only on strict indications. Relatively 'safe' antibiotics for topical use are mupirocin, erythromycin, tetracycline, sodium fusidate and polymyxin. The reader is also referred to Chapters 16 and 17, on systemic side effects and systemic eczematous contact-type dermatitis medicamentosa, respectively. Those topical antibiotics that have caused contact allergic reactions are listed in § 5.23.

5.23 Contact allergy to antibiotics

Drug	Patch test conc. & vehicle (§ 5.2)	EFS (§ 5.4)	Cross-reactions (§ 5.5)	Comment	Ref.
amikacin	20% aqua	3	other aminoglycosides	Most if not all cases are cross-reactions after primary sensitization to neomycin	716
ampicillin	5% aqua	?		Occupational exposure in medical personnel	388
azidamfenicol	5% pet.	4	chloramphenicol	Chemically closely related to chloramphenicol	457
bacitracin	20% pet.	3	colistin, polymyxin	infrequent primary sensitizer; many reactions are concomitant reactions with neomycin [786]	45 435
cephalosporins	1–5% aqua	4	other cephalosporins	Accidental contact in a chemical analyst to the cephalosporins cephalothin, cephamandol and cephazolin	713
chloramphenicol	5% pet.	2	*p*-dinitrobenzene (?), dinitrochlorobenzene, *p*-nitrobenzoic acid	In one report chloramphenicol caused a drug eruption, patch tests were positive	140 262 364 390
chlorfenicone	1% pet.	4		Chloramphenicol derivative, used in pessaries	108
chlortetracycline	3% pet.	4	demethylchlortetra-cycline, tetracycline		73
clindamycin	1% aqua	3	lincomycin		104 489
colistin	comm. prep.	4		Accidental contact in pharmaceutical industry worker	719
dihydrostrepto-mycin	5% aqua 20% pet.	4	kanamycin, neomycin, streptomycin	Accidental contact	398
doxycycline	comm. prep.	4		Accidental contact in pharmaceutical industry worker	719
erythromycin	10 % pet.	4		Also immediate-type allergy reported [439]	439 501
framycetin	20% pet.	1	kanamycin (?), neomycin, paramomycin (?), streptomycin (?)	Framycetin consists of neomycin B (99%), neomycin C (1%) and neamine (0.2%)	90 336
gentamicin	20% pet.	1	kanamycin, neomycin,	Most reports are of cross-sensitivity to neomycin rather than of primary sensitization	32 284
hamycin	200,000 U/ml	3		Only listed; no details	761

(continued)

§ **5.23** *(continuation)*

Drug	Patch test conc. & vehicle (§ 5.2)	EFS (§ 5.4)	Cross-reactions (§ 5.5)	Comment	Ref.
4-4′-homo-sulfanilamide	5% pet.	2	related esters of *p*-aminobenzoic acid		23 25 447
kanamycin	sulfate, 20% pet.	4	other aminoglycosides	Rare primary sensitizer, usually cross-reaction from neomycin	718
kitasamycin	tartrate, powder pure and 4% aqua	4	not to other macrolide antibiotics	Airborn occupational contact allergy	379
lincomycin	1% aqua	4	clindamycin	Erythema multiforme-like dermatitis: [503]	503
mafenide	10% pet.	4			802
midecamicin	pure	4	not to other macrolides	Occupational airborne contact allergy	379
neomycin	20% pet.	1	ambutyrosin, amikacin [648], aminosydin, bacitracin, butirosin, cyclohexamide (?) [46], framycetin, gentamicin, kanamycin, paromomycin, ribostamycin, sisomicin, spectinomycin [516], *not* to streptomycin [648], tobramycin	Patch tests may become positive after 7 days only. Co-reacts with bacitracin. Sometimes contact allergy can only be detected with intradermal and usage tests. It has been suggested that short-term use (less than 1 week) on non-eczematous skin induces few allergic reactions [570]	136 167 334b 371 715 718 786
nitrofurazone	0.1–2% pet.	2	related nitrofuran derivatives		49 56 236
oxytetracycline	3% pet.	4	methacycline, tetracycline		52 313
paromomycin	sulfate , 20% pet.	4	other aminoglycosides	Rare primary sensitizer usually cross-reaction from neomycin	718
penicillin	10,000 IU/g pet. 100.000 IU/ml aqua	1	other pencillins	Occupational contact allergy in pharmaceutical workers, nurses and veterinary surgeons to penicillin, ampicillin, cloxacillin, carbenicillin, pivampicillin and pivmecillinam; [719,775,787]. Topical use largely abandoned	58 197 318 638
polymyxin B	3% pet.	3	bacitracin, polymyxin A		313 511

(continued)

§ **5.23** *(continuation)*

Drug	Patch test conc. & vehicle (§ 5.2)	EFS (§ 5.4)	Cross-reactions (§ 5.5)	Comment	Ref.
pristinamycin	5% pet.	4	virginiamycin	Factor IIa of pristinamycin and factor M of virginiamycin are identical	21
ribostamycin	25% aqua and pure	4	cross-reaction from neomycin	Erythoderma after systemic administration	714
rifampicin	comm. prep.	3		Occupational allergy in pharmaceutical industry workers	719
rifamycin	0.5–2.5% pet.	3			380
rolitetracycline	comm. prep.	4		Occupational contact allergy in pharmaceutical industry workers	718
sodium fusidate	2% pet.	3			118 503
streptomycin	5% aqua 1% pet.	3	dihydrostreptomycin, kanamycin, neomycin	Accidental contact in medical personnel	463 638
sulfonamide	5% pet.	1	chemically related diuretics, oral antidiabetics and sweetening agents, other sulfonamides and para-compounds		200 260 717
tobramycin	20% aqua	4	kanamycin, ribostamycin, sisomicin		715
tylosin tartrate	10% pet.	3		Occupational allergy in veterinary surgeons	719
tyrothricin	20% pet.	2			199
variotin P	10-50% pet.	4			204
virginiamycin	2-5% pet.	3	pristinamycin	*See also under* pristinamycin. For industrial contact, see [417]	48 269
xanthocillin	1% pet.	2			223

ANTIHISTAMINES

5.24 Primarily introduced as anti-allergic agents, antihistamines have also been found useful as tranquillizers, anticonvulsants, decongestants, local anesthetics and hypnotics. Most topical antihistamine preparations are used for their alleged antipruritic properties.

The nucleus of the typical antihistamine structure is a substituted ethylamine ($-CH_2CH_2N=$), which may comprise part of a straight chain or a ring structure, and is present in the histamine molecule as well. The main groups of compounds are (a) ethylenediamines (b) alkylamines, (c) ethanolamines, (d) piperazines and (e) phenothiazines (§ 5.27).

5.25 The antihistamines can readily sensitize the skin following topical application or occupational exposure, especially the ethylenediamine derivatives and the phenothiazines. Cross-sensitization occurs frequently, especially between chemically related antihistamines, or with other related drugs. Phototoxic and photoallergic reactions may be seen occasionally, especially in the phenothiazine group. In addition, the antihistamines or chemically related drugs may cause systemic eczematous contact-type dermatitis medicamentosa in previously sensitized individuals, when administered orally or parenterally (see Chapter 17).

5.26 Antihistamines for topical use include antazoline, bamipine, chlorcyclizine, (dex)chlorpheniramine maleate, diphenhydramine, doxylamine succinate, methapyrilene, phenindamine, pheniramine, promethazine, pyrilamine, thonzylamine and tripelennamine. Although the Committee on Drugs of the American Academy of Pediatrics [469] recommended "to discontinue the use of topical antihistamine preparations because their toxicity exceeds their limited benefit" and the American Medical Association came to the same conclusion [128] and convincing evidence for the usefullness of topical antihistamines has not been documented [301], topical antihistamine preparations are still widely used and are in many countries available 'over the counter', without prescription.

Antihistamines for topical use that have caused contact allergy are listed in § 5.28.

5.27 **Main classes of anthihistamines** (only some of these are used topically, see § 5.26)

Ethylenediamines
antazoline (phenazoline)
buclizine
chloropyramine
clemizole
methaphenilene
methapyrilene
pyrilamine (mepyramine)
thenyldiamine
thonzylamine
tripelennamine

Alkylamines
bamipine
brompheniramine maleate
chlorpheniramine maleate
dexbrompheniramine maleate
dexchlorpheniramine maleate
dimethindene maleate
mebhydroline
pheniramine

Ethanolamines
clemastine hydrogen fumarate
dimenhydrinate*
diphenhydramine
doxylamine
trimethobenzamide*

Piperazines
chlorcyclizine
cinnarizine
cyclizine*
hydroxyzine
meclizine (meclozine)

Phenothiazines
chlorpromazine*
N-hydroxyethyl promethazine chloride
isothipendyl hydrochloride
oxomemazine
perphenazine
promethazine hydrochloride
thiazinamium methylsulfate
trimeprazine tartrate
methylpromazine

Miscellaneous
cyproheptadine
deptropine citrate
diphenylpyraline
phenindamine tartrate

* Antiemetics.

5.28 Contact allergy to topical antihistamines

Drug	Patch test conc. & vehicle (§ 5.2)	EFS (§ 5.4)	Cross-reactions (§ 5.5)	Comment	Ref.
antazoline	1% pet.	2	ethylenediamine and its derivatives		148 394
brompheniramine	pure (?)			The reaction represented a cross-reaction to other pyridine derivatives	579
chlorcyclizine	1% pet.	4			15
chlorpheniramine maleate	5% pet.	4			431 645
chlorphenoxamine	1.5% pet./aqua	3			438
chlorpromazine	0.1% pet.	2	phenothiazines	Accidental contact in medical personnel	399
dexchlorpheni-ramine maleate	1% aqua	4	possibly to mepyramine, diphenhydramine; definitely to pheniramine, chlorpheniramine and brompheniramine maleate [807]		496
diphenhydramine hydrochloride	1% pet.	2	antazoline, dimenhydrinate [148]		112 301 481
doxylamine succinate	?	?		No case reports	148
isothipendyl	1% pet.	4	*not* to phenothiazine derivatives	Structurally similar to phenothiazine	600
methapyrilene	2% pet.	3			281
perphenazine	2% pet.	3			645
phenindamine tartrate	5% pet.	2			134
phenothiazine antihistamines		2	other phenothiazine derivatives		588
promazine	2% pet.	3			645
promethazine hydrochloride	2% pet.	1	ethylenediamine and its derivatives, para-compounds, phenothiazines, triethanolamine (?)		148 399
pyrilamine maleate	2% pet.	3			112
tripelennamine	2% pet.	2	antazoline, ethylene-diamine-derived antihista-mines [148], phenothiazines, promethazine, sulfapyridine		148 301 400

ANTIMYCOTICS

5.29 Antifungal drugs are becoming more important as the incidence of fungal infections increases. This increase is largely iatrogenic; large-scale employment of broad-spectrum antibiotics, and the increasing use of immunosuppressive therapeutics in patients with malignancies, autoimmune diseases and organ transplants disturb the ecological balance and lead to a rising incidence of fungal diseases. Also, the use of hormonal contraceptives predisposes to candidal infections of the vagina. In addition the recent AIDS epidemic resulted in an increase of local and systemic fungal infections.

Therefore, new antifungal drugs are being developed nearly every year. Recently introduced antimycotics, which may be used both systemically and topically, are the *imidazoles*. These include: bifonazole, clotimazole, croconazole, econazole, enilconazole, isoconazole, ketoconazole, miconazole, oxiconazole, sulconazole and tioconazole [406]. These imidazoles are being used extensively nowadays for topical treatment, because of their high antifungal activity and lack of side effects; contact allergy to the imidazoles appears to be infrequent. Cross-reactions have been observed between the various imidazoles, but the exact pattern of cross-reactivity has not yet been elucidated because of (i): the small number of patients sensitized, (ii): the unavailability of certain imidazoles and (iii): technical difficulties with patch testing (testing the antifungals in petrolatum may result in false-negative reactions). Bifonazole, clotrimazole and possibly ketoconazole may usually be considered safe for patients allergic to other imidazoles [791], although cross-reactions have sometimes been observed [804]. Testing the imidazoles in MEK (methyl ethyl ketone) may be preferable to petrolatum [342]. In animal experiments, croconazole was shown to be a strong sensitizer and bifonazole to be a moderate sensitizer. The other imidazoles were found to be weak sensitizers [790]. Topical antimycotics that have caused contact allergy are listed in § 5.30.

5.30 Contact allergy to antimycotics

Drug	Patch test conc. & vehicle (§ 5.2)	EFS (§ 5.4)	Cross-reactions (§ 5.5)	Comment	Ref.
benzoic acid	5% pet.	3			20
5-bromo-4′-chlorosalicylanilide	1% pet.	2	other halogenated salicylanilides (usually photo-cross reactions)	*only* photosensitizer (§ 6.5)	66
buclosamide	5% pet.	2	halogenated salicylanilides, sulfonamides, sulfonamide-anti diabetics and diuretics (usually photo-cross-reactions)	*only* photosensitizer (§ 6.5)	68 249
candicidin	0.05% pet.	4			106

(continued)

§ **5.30** *(continuation)*

Drug	Patch test conc. & vehicle (§ 5.2)	EFS (§ 5.4)	Cross-reactions (§ 5.5)	Comment	Ref.
Castellani's solution	as is	3	hexyl resorcinol		294
chlordantoin	1% pet.	4			218
chlormidazole	1% pet.	3			233
chlorphenesin	1% pet.	4			61
clophenoxyde	1% ethyl acetate	4	ω-chloroacetophenone		168
clotrimazole	1% MEK or alc.	4	not to other imidazoles (econazole, miconazole,)	Imidazole. *See* § 5.29	352 354
croconazole	1% pet.	3	other imidazoles	Imidazole. *See* § 5.29	348
cyclopyroxolamine	1% pet.	4			817
dibenzthione	1% acet. 3% pet.	3	possibly antihypertensive drugs derived from triazines, hydrochlorthiazide		40 275
3,5-dichloro-4-fluoro-thiocarbanilide	1% isopropyl alc.	3			426
econazole	1% alc.	3		Imidazole. *See* § 5.29	370 500
enilconazole	2% pet.	4	other imidazoles	Enilconazole is a fungicide for veterinary use. Imidazole. *See* § 5.29	476
etisazole	1% pet.	4		Veterinary fungicide. Accidental contact. Imidazole. *See* § 5.29	113 429
haloprogin	1% pet.	4			358
hexetidine	0.1% pet.	4		Quaternary ammonium compound	526
isoconazole	2% alc. or MEK	3		Imidazole. *See* § 5.29	370 515
ketoconazole	1% pet.	4	possibly to bifonazole, miconazole, sulconazole	Imidazole. Generalized rash after oral keto-conazole [296]. See § 5.29	296 804
mesulfen	5% pet.	3			96 433 502
methyl captan	2% aqua, 5% lan-vas	4			401

(continued)

§ **5.30** *(continuation)*

Drug	Patch test conc. & vehicle (§ 5.2)	EFS (§ 5.4)	Cross-reactions (§ 5.5)	Comment	Ref.
metronidazole	2% pet.	4	cross-reaction from tioconazole	Imidazole. *See* § 5.29	790
miconazole nitrate	2% alc. or MEK	3	other imidazoles	Imidazole. *See* § 5.29	370 450 497
mycanodin	1–2% ?	4		Mycanodin is a combination of 3-(2-oxychlorophenyl)-pyrazole and bamipine	65
naftifine hydrochloride	1% pet.	3		Allylamine, not chemically related to the imidazoles	649 650 762
nifuratel	1% acet.	4		Also used for the treatment of trichomoniasis. Connubial contact dermatitis, *see* [763]	479
nifuroxime	?	4			1
nystatin	100,000–300,000 U/g PEG-400	3			101 172
oxiconazole	1% alc. or MEK	4	other imidazoles	Imidazole. *See* § 5.29	196 370
pecilocin	1% pet.	3			323
phenylmercuric borate	0.1% pet.	2	other mercurials		467
pyrrolnitrin	1% pet.	2	possibly dinitrochlorbenzene		299 353 560
sodium thiosulfate	20% aqua	3		No details provided; only listed	761
sulconazole nitrate	1% pet.	4	other imidazoles	Imidazole. *See* § 5.29	473 788
tioconazole	1% pet.	4	other imidazoles	Imidazole. *See* § 5.29	121 789
tolciclate	1% pet.	4			651
tolnaftate	0.01–1% pet.	4			195 652
undecylenic acid	2–5% pet.	4	zinc undecylenate		194
zinc undecylenate	20% talc	4	undecylenic acid		194

CORTICOSTEROIDS

5.31 Contact dermatitis to topical corticosteroid preparations used to be considered an uncommon event. However, cases of contact sensitivity are being reported with increasing frequency [623] and routine testing yields prevalence rates of sensitization of 2.9% [708] and even more [709,710] in patients suspected of allergic contact dermatitis. Contact allergy to ingredients of topical corticosteroid preparations should be considered in cases of long-standing therapy-resistant dermatitis, or exacerbation of dermatitis after topical corticosteroid therapy. Oral or parenteral administration of corticosteroids in sensitized individuals may lead to systemic contact dermatitis (Chapter 17).

5.32 Hypersensitivity to commercial corticosteroid preparations may be caused by the corticosteroid itself, by one or more other ingredients of the preparation (preservatives, vehicles), or both. Ingredients in corticosteroid ointment or cream bases which have been identified as sensitizers (by their presence in corticosteroid preparations) include:

- benzyl alcohol [634]
- cetearyl alcohol (cetylstearyl alcohol) [621]
- cetyl alcohol [619]
- *p*-chloro-*m*-cresol [327]
- citric acid [621]
- disodium edetate [341,621]
- ethylenediamine hydrochloride [635]
- glyceryl oleate [627]
- isopropyl myristate [621]
- isopropyl palmitate [634]
- lanolin [619]
- PEG cetyl ether [621]
- PEG stearate [621]
- parabens [459,637]
- phenol [78]
- polysorbate 60 [636]
- propyl gallate [621]
- propylene glycol [327,459]
- pyridoxine hydrochloride
- ricinus oil [621]
- silicone fluid [621]
- sodium benzoate [621]
- sodium citrate [621]
- sodium lauryl sulfate [7,78]
- sorbic acid
- sorbitol [621]
- stearyl alcohol [47]
- vaselinum album [621]

5.33 Patch testing

There still remains much discussion about the patch testing conditions for corticosteroids [711]. In general, higher concentrations than the use concentrations in the commercial products are required, although the anti-inflammatory properties may cause false-negative reactions. The main problems are, however, the solubility of the corticosteroids in the vehicles and insufficient bioavailability. Ethanol 94% seems to be suitable for most corticosteroids, although degradation reactions may occur. With a mixture of 45% alcohol, 45% isopropanol and 10% propylene glycol more positive reactions are observed, but there can be contact sensitivity to propylene glycol. Xerogel formulations may hold promise [793]. Suitable 'markers' for corticosteroid allergy are tixocortol pivalate [712,805] and budesonide [708], both 1% in petrolatum. These steroids should routinely be tested. Hydrocortisone 17-butyrate, also considered to be a useful marker for corticosteroid allergy [620,709], was found to have no advantages over budesonide and to be superfluous when budesonide is routinely tested [708], although the reverse situation has also been found [805]. Corticosteroids tend to become positive only after a considerable period of time and patch test readings should be performed not only at day 2 and 3 but preferably also 6 or 7 days after application. Intradermal testing may sometimes be necessary, either to detect sensitivity [610,795] or to exclude false positive patch test reactions [796]. Most corticosteroid allergic patients suffer from long-standing dermatitis: hand eczema, foot eczema and eczema caused by chronic venous insufficiency (often with leg ulcers). Multiple sensitivities are the rule rather than the exception [708]. A suggested series of corticosteroids for patch testing with a suitable test concentration and vehicle is provided [708] in Table 5.34.

Table 5.34. Test concentrations and vehicles for corticosteroids [708]

Alclomethasone dipropionate	1% pet.	Hydrocortisone	2% alc.
Amcinonide	1% epi.	Hydrocortisone acetate	1% epi.
Beclomethasone dipropionate	5% pet.	Hydrocortisone-17-butyrate	1% alc.
Budesonide	1% pet.	Hydrocortisone-21-butyrate	2% epi.
Clobetasone butyrate	1% epi.	Isofluprednone acetate	5% pet.
Clobetasol propionate	1% alc.	Medrysone	1% alc.
Cloprednol	2% alc.	Methylprednisolone acetate	1% alc.
Cortisone acetate	1% epi.	Meprednisone	1% alc.
Desonide	1% epi.	Momethasone furoate	1% alc.
Dexamethasone	1% epi.	Prednisolone	1% epi.
Dexamethasone sodium phosphate	1% epi.	Prednisolone caproate	1% epi.
Dichlorisone acetate	1% epi.	Prednisolone metasulfobenzoate	1% epi.
Diflorasone diacetate	1% epi.	Prednicarbate	1% alc.
Fludrocortisone acetate	1% epi.	Prednisone	1% alc.
Fluocinonide	1% pet.	Triamcinolone acetonide	1% alc.
Fluocortin butyl ester	1% alc.	Tixocortol pivalate	1% pet.
Fluorometholone	1% pet.	Triamcinolone	1% alc.
		Triamcinolone diacetate	1% alc.

alc. = alcohol; epi. = 45% ethanol (alcohol), 10% propylene glycol, 45% isopropanol.
pet. = petrolatum.

5.35 Cross-reactions between corticosteroids occur frequently. This makes the choice of an appropriate steroid in allergic patients difficult. Relevant to cross-reactivity, 4 groups of corticosteroids have been defined [707]. Patients allergic to a particular corticosteroid tend to cross-react to other steroids in the same group, but not to other groups; this provides some help to the prescribing physician (Table 5.35). Possible cross sensitivity between hydrocortisone and 17-α-OH-progesterone may play an etiological role in autoimmune progesterone dermatitis [794].

Table 5.35. Cross-reaction pattern of corticosteroids

Group A	Group B
Cloprednol	Amcinonide
Cortisone	Budesonide
Cortisone acetate	Desonide
Fludrocortisone	Fluocinolone acetonide
Hydrocortisone	Fluocinonide
Hydrocortisone acetate	Halcinonide
Methylprednisolone acetate	Triamcinolone acetonide
Prednisolone	Triamcinolone alcohol
Prednisolone acetate	
Prednisone	
Tixocortol pivalate	
Group C	**Group D**
Betamethasone	Alclometasone dipropionate
Betamethasone sodium phosphate	Betamethasone dipropionate
Dexamethasone	Betamethasone valerate
Dexamethasone sodium phosphate	Clobetasol-17-propionate
Fluocortolone	Fluocortolone caproate
	Fluocortolone pivalate
	Fluprednidene acetate
	Hydrocortisone-17-butyrate
	Hydrocortisone-17-valerate

Reported contact allergy to corticosteroids [792,708]

5.36 Topical steroids that have caused contact allergy are listed in § 5.36. Other local and systemic side effects are discussed in Chapters 14 and 16.

Contact allergy to topical corticosteroids (reviews: Ref. [178,623,631]

Corticosteroid	Ref.
alclomethasone dipropionate	105,708
amcinonide	5,102,627,708
beclomethasone dipropionate	63,708
betamethasone	78
betamethasone 21-(dihydrogen phosphate) disodium salt	78

(continued)

§ **5.36** *(continuation)*

Corticosteroid	Ref.
betamethasone dipropionate	63
betamethasone sodium phosphate	63
betamethasone valerate	629,630,633,765
budesonide	132,205,708
chlorprednisone acetate	448
clobetasol 17-propionate	443,628,708
clobetasone butyrate	619,708
clocortolone pivalate	765
cloprednol	708
cortisone	471
cortisone acetate	708
desonide	132,622,708
desoximetasone	613
dexamethasone	78,708
dexamethasone 21-(dihydrogen phosphate) disodium salt	78
dexamethasone sodium phosphate	708
dichlorisone acetate	708
diflorasone diacetate	708
diflucortolone-21-valerate	60,613
fludrocortisone acetate	708
fluocinolone acetonide	471,611,630
fluocinonide	611,622,708
fluocortin butylester	416,708
fluocortolone	302,625,765
fluocortolone caproate	302
fluocortolone monohydrate	60,613
fluocortolone pivalate	302
fluorometholone	708
fluperolone acetonide	471
flurandrenolide	30
halcinonide	622
hydrocortisone	471,610,616,617,626,708,818
hydrocortisone acetate	708
hydrocortisone alcohol	617
hydrocortisone butyrate	620,624,632,708
hydrocortisone-17-butyrate	620,624,632,708
hydrocortisone-21-butyrate	708
hydrocortisone butyrate propionate	633
hydrocortisone 21-diol acetate	615
hydrocortisone phosphate	468
hydrocortisone sodium phosphate	633,764
hydrocortisone sodium succinate	63,764
hydrocortisone succinate	626,764
hydrocortisone valerate	622
isofluprednone acetate	708
medrysone	708
methylprednisolone	459,471,708

(continued)

§ **5.36** *(continuation)*

Corticosteroid	Ref.
methylprednisolone acetate	708
momethasone furoate	708
paramethasone acetate	633
prednicarbate	428,627,708,765,766
prednisolone	459,471,616,617,626,622,708
prednisolone 21-trimethylacetate	462
prednisolone butylacetate	633
prednisolone caproate	708
prednisolone hemisuccinate	468
prednisolone metasulfobenzoate	708
prednisone	616
tixocortol pivalate	614,615,708
triamcinolone	621
triamcinolone acetonide	622,624,634,708
triamcinolone diacetate	

DRUGS USED IN THE TREATMENT OF PSORIASIS, ACNE, ECZEMA AND PRURITUS

5.37 Contact allergy to drugs used in psoriasis, acne, eczema and pruritus treatment

Drug	Patch test conc. & vehicle (§ 5.2)	EFS (§ 5.4)	Cross-reactions (§ 5.5)	Comment	Ref.
6-aminonicotinamide	1% dimethyl sulfoxide open test	4		Rarely used	470
ammonium sulfobituminate			*See* § 5.7		
antihistamines, topical			*See* §§ 5.24–5.28		
benzoyl peroxide	1% pet.	2		The main indications for BP are acne and leg ulcers. When used for leg ulcers contact sensitization is very frequent [546,550], but when used for acne, adverse effects are usually of irritant nature [548]. Usage tests may be indicated	276 546 548 550

(continued)

§ **5.37** *(continuation)*

Drug	Patch test conc. & vehicle (§ 5.2)	EFS (§ 5.4)	Cross-reactions (§ 5.5)	Comment	Ref.
chrysarobin	0.03% pet.	4		No contact allergy reported	149
corticosteroids			*See* § 5.31–5.36		
crotamiton	10% aqua 1% MEK	3		Also used as scabicide	43 425
dithranol	0.02% acet. or pet.	3			120 797
ethyl lactate	1% pet.	4			274
menthol	1–2% pet.	4			86 684
8-methoxypsoralen (methoxsalen)	0.1% alc.	4	trimethylpsoralen	Exacerbation after oral 8-methoxypsoralen administration [568]	367 568
nitrofurylamino-thiadazoles	1% pet.	4	related compounds		176
phenol	0.5–1% aqua	4	cresols, hydroquinone (?), resorcinol		20 591
polidocanol	5% pet 0.5% aqua [235]	3		Also used for ulcus cruris therapy	235
resorcinol	2% pet.	3	hexylresorcinol, hydroquinone, hydroxyhydroquin-one, meta dihydroxy-benzenes, orcinol, phenol, pyrocatechol, pyrogallol, resorcinol acetate, resorcinol monobenzoate [806]		256 294
salicylic acid	2% pet.	4			366
sulfur	1–5% pet.	4			375 461
tar, coal	5% pet.	3	wood tars (?) [402]		361 402
tar, wood (pine, beech, juniper, birch)	4×3% pet.	1	balsams, essential oils, perfumes, rosin and woods (?)	Perfume allergy indicator	357
tioxolone	0.05–0.5% alc.	3			451
tretinoin	0.005% alc.	4			277 365

PLANT-DERIVED SUBSTANCES IN TOPICAL DRUGS

5.38 Contact allergy to plant-derived substances in topical drugs and cosmetics

Drug	Patch test conc. & vehicle (§ 5.2)	EFS (§ 5.4)	Cross-reactions (§ 5.5)	Comment	Ref.
abietic acid	5% pet.	3			339 453
aloe extract	aloe leaf jelly	4			825 826
arnica tincture	20% pet.	2		The main suspected allergens are helenalin and its methacryl acid ester (sesquiterpene lactones)	217 363 556
balsam Peru				See § 5.14	
balsam Tolu				*See* § 5.14	
beeswax	30% pet.	2	balsam Peru	Contains vanillin and cinnamic acid	332
belladonna plaster	pure, atropine 1% pet.	4		Belladonna plaster contains belladonna alkaloids (derived from Atropa belladonna): atropine, scopolamine. Systemic symptoms from its use may occur: headache, dizziness, blurred vision	547
benzoin tincture	2-10% pet. 10% alc.	3	balsam Peru, benzyl alcohol, benzyl cinnamate, eugenol, α-pinene, storax, vanilla	Benzoin tincture is 10% benzoin in alcohol: benzoin contains; benzoic acids, cinnamic acids, vanillin and coniferyl benzoate	103 147 233
bergamot oil	2% pet.	4		Contains 5-methoxypsoralen	213
Centelase®	1% pet. (powder)	4		Centelase® contains the triterpenic fraction of the plant Centella Asiatica (umbelliferae). This fraction consists of asiaticoside, asiatic acid and madecassic acid	531
centella asiatica	extract 2% alc.	4		Synonym: Indian pennywort (umbelliferae)	824
chamomile oil	25% o.o.	3		The allergen is presumably a sesquiterpene lactone called desacetyl matricarin	36 556 559
coumarin				*See* § 5.14	
esculin	1% pet.	4			94

(continued)

§ **5.38** *(continuation)*

Drug	Patch test conc. & vehicle (§ 5.2)	EFS (§ 5.4)	Cross-reactions (§ 5.5)	Comment	Ref.
gums (karaya, acacia and tragacanth)	– gum: as is – tragacanth: 0.1% aqua	4			323 506 507
henna (lawsonia)	10 mg henna powder in 100 ml aqua, ether and alcohol	4		Used for hair colouring. The patient reacted to the active ingredient 2-hydroxy-1,4-naphthoquinone (lawsone)	331
karaya powder	karaya seal ring	4		Used in a drainable polyethylene bag at colostomy sites	88
linseed	as is, raw and cooked	4		Folk medicine, used for hidradenitis axillaris	64
niaouli oil	1% alc.	3	thyme oil	Constituent of biogaze (§ 5.41). The main allergen is limonene	238
rosin (colophony)	20% pet.	1	abietic acid, abietic alcohol, balsam Peru, dehydroabietic acid, dextropimaric acid, dihydroabietic acid, levopimaric acid, maleopimaric acid, methylabietate, neoabietic acid, palustric acid, tetrahydroabietic acid	Rosin (colophony) is a solidified product derived from the balsams (gum rosin) of coniferous trees. Three types of rosin (gum rosin, wood rosin and tall oil rosin) are distinguished depending on the mode of recovery. Abietic acid is the main resin acid in most colophony types (50–80%). The main allergens appear to be oxidation products of abietic acid and dehydroabietic acid [701, 705]. Pure abietic itself is not allergenic [704], though some authors consider it to be a major allergen in unmodified colophony [700]. Derivatives of colophony with specific properties can be prepared by hydration, dehydration, disproportionation, dimerisation, polymerisation and the formation of esters, alcohols, ethers, adducts and other compounds [700]. Hydrogenation reduces the allergenicity of colophony [702]. Maleic acid modification, however, forms a new very potent allergen: maleopimaric acid [703]. This allergen may also be present after esterification, unless this process is carried to completion [703]. Modified colophony products are usually stronger sensitizers than unmodified colophony [706]	173 566 602

(continued)

§ **5.38** *(continuation)*

Drug	Patch test conc. & vehicle (§ 5.2)	EFS (§ 5.4)	Cross-reactions (§ 5.5)	Comment	Ref.
storax	2% pet.	2	benzoin, balsam Peru		309
tar (wood and coal)				*See* § 5.37	
tea tree oil	pure	3		The allergen was eucalyptol. Systemic contact dermatitis from ingestion with honey	828
terpineol	5% pet.	3		In e.g. thyme oil and niaouli oil	244
thuja occidentalis	commercial extract	4	concomitant reaction to abietol, cedar wood oil, rosin, pine resin, and turpentine of larch	Allergen not identified	827
thyme oil	1–5% alc.	3	niaouli oil	Constituent of biogaze (§ 5.41). The main allergen is limonene	238
turpentine, vegetable	– turpentine peroxide 0.3% o.o. – α-pinene 15% pet. – dipentene 2% pet.	2		*Cave:* irritant patch test reactions. Contact allergy to turpentine has become infrequent as turpentine oil in paints has been replaced by white spirit	335 604

Other plant-derived substances and their test concentrations are provided in § 5.39. *See also* §§ 5.8–5.15 on contact allergy to fragrance materials, and § 30.7 on fragance materials.

5.39 Plant-derived substances and patch testing dilutions (adapted from Fregert [180])

Substance	Patch test conc. & vehicle (§ 5.2)	Comment
alantolactone	0.1% pet.	Patch testing may sensitize
balsam of pine	20% pet.	
balsam of spruce	20% pet.	
dammar resin	20% alc./pet.	
fruits (orange, citrus peels)	as is	*Cave*: irritant patch test reactions
mirbane oil	10% o.o.	
pentadecyl-catechol	0.1% pet.	Patch testing may sensitize
α-pinene	15% pet.	
plant, leaf, flower, pollen, bulb	as is	*Cave:* irritant patch test reactions

(continued)

§ **5.39** *(continuation)*

Substance	Patch test conc. & vehicle (§ 5.2)	Comment
pyrethrum	2% pet.	
spice	as is	
spice oils	5% alc. (*see also* § 5.15)	
storax, oil of	2% pet.	
tobacco	as is	
vanilla	as is	
Venice turpentine (larch turpentine)	20% pet.	
wood, exotic	dry sawdust	*Cave:* irritant patch test reactions
wood, pine and spruce	balsams of pine and spruce	

ANTIPARASITIC DRUGS

5.40 Contact allergy to antiparasitic drugs

Drug	Patch test conc. & vehicle (§ 5.2)	EFS (§ 5.4)	Cross-reactions (§ 5.5)	Comment	Ref.
acetarsol	1% pet.	4		Also present in several toothpastes and mouthwashes (?)	346
benzyl benzoate	5% pet.	3	balsam Peru, balsam Tolu		226 502
crotamiton	5% pet.	3		Also used as antipruritic drug	42
DDT	1% pet.	4		May produce chloracne and possibly porphyria	37
lindane	1% pet.	4			38
malathion	1% alc. (open test) 0.5% pet. 1% aqua [180]	4			304
mesulfen	5% pet.	3			502
monosulfram	1% pet.	4	disulfiram, tetramethylthiuram disulfide		314

MISCELLANEOUS DRUGS

5.41 Contact allergy to miscellaneous topical drugs

Drug	Use	Patch test conc. & vehicle (§ 5.2)	EFS (§ 5.4)	Cross-reactions (§ 5.5)	Comment	Ref.
acyclovir	antiviral drug	5% aqua/prop. glyc.	3		Oral acyclovir resulted in drug rash [809]	169
aluminium acetate	used in eardrops	1% and 5% aqua	4			820
3-(amino-methyl)-pyri-dine/pyridyl salicylate	analgesic	1% aqua	3		Para-compounds	731 767
benzarone	anti-hemorrhoidal drug	pure and 2% pet.	4			202
benzydamine hydrochloride	non-steroidal anti-inflamma-tory drug	5% aqua or pet.	4			53
biogaze	wound treatment	as is	2		The main allergen is limonene in thyme oil and niaouli oil	238 523
boric acid	in topical remedies	5% glyc. 3% aqua	4			20
bufexamac	anti- inflamma-tory drug	5% pet.	2			300 601
buphenine	β-sympathico-mimetic drug used as vasodilator	1% alc. and pure	4			198
butoxyethyl nicotinate	vasodilator	2.5% pet.	4	3-(aminomethyl)-pyri-dine, benzyl nicotinate		527
camphor	folk medicine, decubitus prevention	10% pet.	4			28
capsicum	antirheumatic drug	0.5% pet.	4			300
carmustine (BCNU)	topical cytostatic drug for mycosis fungoides	1% aqua (?)	1			608
chloral hydrate	counterirritant, hypnotic	1-5% aqua	4			734
chlorambucil	cytostatic drug	pure 2.5% pet.	4		Drug was admin-istered systemically. No controls used with patch testing	259

(continued)

§ **5.41** *(continuation)*

Drug	Use	Patch test conc. & vehicle (§ 5.2)	EFS (§ 5.4)	Cross-reactions (§ 5.5)	Comment	Ref.
cinnoxicam	non-steroidal anti-inflammatory drug	?	4	?	Only listed; no details provided. Syn: piroxicam	808
clonidine	anti-hypertensive in trans- dermal therapeutic system	9% pet.	1		Oral clonidine is usually well-tolerated in allergic individuals [770]	768 769
collagenase A	treatment of leg ulcers	1.2 mg/g pet.	4			55
dexpanthenol	wound treatment	5% pet.	3			240
dianobol cream	wound treatment	pure	4			391
diclofenac	non-steroidal anti-inflamma-tory drug	2.5% pet.	4	not to other NSAID's	Urticaria after systemic administration	799
diethylstil-bestrol	hormone	1% pet.	4	balsam Peru, benz-estrol, benzylester of *p*-hydroxybenzoic acid, *p*-benzylphenol, bisphenol-A, dienestrol, hexestrol, monobenzone, storax,		185
dihydroxy-acetone	tanning agent	10% aqua	4			215
diisopropoxy-phosphoryl fluoride (DPF)	cholinesterase inhibitor	0.1% o.o	4	related chemicals		184
diphencyprone (diphenylcyclo-propenone)	treatment of alopecia areata	0.1% acet.	1		Diphencyprone 2% in acetone is used for (deliberate) sensitization	482
enoxolone	anti-inflamma-tory drug	10% pet.	4			802
estradiol benzoate	hormone	0.01% MEK	4	balsam Peru, resorcinol monobenzoate	Contact allergy to estradiol transdermal therapeutic systems is caused by the adhesive and hydroxypropyl cell-ulose, not by estradiol itself [768,769,771]	278
etofenamate	antirheumatic drug	2% pet.	3	possibly to flufenamic acid		430 726

(continued)

§ **5.41** *(continuation)*

Drug	Use	Patch test conc. & vehicle (§ 5.2)	EFS (§ 5.4)	Cross-reactions (§ 5.5)	Comment	Ref.
fepradinol	anti-inflammatory drug	1% aqua	4	not to other NSAIDs		803
5-fluorouracil	cytostatic drug	5% pet.	2		Sometimes patch test are negative, but scratch tests positive. *Cave:* irritant patch test reactions	137 519 569
gelatin	in adhesives	pure	4			506
glycol salicylate	treatment of sports injuries	1% pet.	4			733
heparine	treatment of phlebitis	comm. prep.	3	other heparines		378 819
hydroquinone	bleaching agent	2% pet.	4	monobenzone		732 800
ibuprofen	non-steroidal anti-inflammatory drug	5% pet.	4			722
ibuproxam	non-steroidal anti-inflammatory drug	5% pet.	3	ketoprofen		721
idoxuridine	antiviral drug	1% pet.	3	brominated and chlorinated pyrimidine analogs, trifluorthymidine		11 580 821
5-iodo-2′-deoxycytidine	antiviral drug	5% pet.	3	idoxuridine		821
imidazoline chlorhydrate	α-adrenergic sympathicomimetic	0.1% pet.	4	oximetazoline chlorhydrate		505
indomethacin	non-steroidal anti-inflammatory drug	5% pet.	4			724
4-isopropylcatechol	bleaching agent	5% pet.	4			122
ketoprofen	non-steroidal anti-inflammatory drug	5% pet.	2	ibuproxam		419 422
mechlorethamine hydrochloride	cytostatic drug	0.02% aqua (open test)	1	mechlorethamine homologs [445]		576 639
mephenesin	muscle relaxant	5% pet.	3			733

(continued)

§ **5.41** *(continuation)*

Drug	Use	Patch test conc. & vehicle (§ 5.2)	EFS (§ 5.4)	Cross-reactions (§ 5.5)	Comment	Ref.
methyl nicotinate	vasodilatant	1% pet.	4			733
methyl salicylate	counter-irritant	2% pet.	3	sodium salicylate		224
minoxidil	treatment of alopecia androgenetica	2% in 70% alc. and 10% propylene glycol	2			18 425
monobenzone (monobenzyl-ether of hydro-quinone)	depigmenting agent	1% pet.	2	bisphenol A, diethyl-stilbestrol (?), *p*-hydroxybenzoic acid ester,	Dermatitis may be restricted to pigmented areas in vitiligo patients [127]	41 127 732
mustard oil	folk medicine	0.1% pet.	4		Also causes toxic reactions. Contains allylisothiocyanate	192
nicotine	in transdermal therapeutic system for smoking withdrawal	commercial product			Nicotine was not tested separately	773
nitroglycerin	coronary vasodilator	2% pet.	3		Contact dermatitis in transdermal therapeutic systems: [220,768,769]	372 589
oxyphenbuta-zone	anti-inflamma-tory drug	1% pet.	2	phenylbutazone, pheprazone, suxibuzone		263 725
palmitoyl collagenic acid	treatment of keloids	1-10% pet.			Palmitoyl collagenic acid is a lipoaminoacid obtained from a condensation reaction between palmitic acid and a collagen hydrolyzate	735
pellidol	wound treatment	2% pet.	2	other azo-dyes, para-compounds		396
phenylbutazone	anti-inflamma-tory drug	1-5% pet.	3		*See under* pyrazinobutazone	418
piroxicam	non-steroidal anti-inflamma-tory drug	1% pet.	4		Contact allergy not proven	801
potassium iodide	formerly used for diagnosing dermatitis herpetiformis	30% pet.	4			8

(continued)

§ **5.41** *(continuation)*

Drug	Use	Patch test conc. & vehicle (§ 5.2)	EFS (§ 5.4)	Cross-reactions (§ 5.5)	Comment	Ref.
propolis	folk medicine, in cosmetics	10% pet.	2	Pseudo-cross-reactions to balsam Peru and Tolu. Common constituents are: benzoic acid, benzyl alcohol, benzyl benzoate, benzyl cinnamate, benzyl ferulate, farnesol, benzyl isoferulate, caffeic acid, cinnamic alcohol cinnamic acid, coniferyl benzoate, nerolidol, and vanillin. (Pseudo) cross-reactions to essential oils, cera flava.	Sensitization also occurs during beeswax modelling and in beekeepers. Review: [728]. The main allergen in propolis is 'LB-1' which consists of 3-methyl-2-butenyl caffeate (54%), 3-methyl-3-butenyl caffeate (28%), 2-methyl- 2-butenyl caffeate (4%), phenylethyl caffeate (8%), caffeic acid (1%) and benzyl caffeate (1%) [729]. Poplar bud constituents are probably responsible for propolis allergy [730]. Sensitization studies with ingredients of propolis, *see* [798]	565 729
pyrazinobutazone	non-steroidal anti-inflammatory drug	pyrazinobutazone 5% pet. piperazine hexahydrate 5% aqua. phenylbutazone 1-5% pet.	4	Salt of piperazine and phenylbutazone. Oral provocation positive		726
ruscus aculeatus	vasoconstrictor, treatment of hemorrhoids	1% alcohol	4			578
scopolamine	prevention of motion sickness in transdermal therapeutic system	1% aqua or pet.	2	not to atropine		768 769 772
Solcoseryl®	wound treatment	comm. prep.	4			289
sulfadiazine silver (Flammazine®)	treatment of burns	silver nitrate 1%?	4		Contact allergic reactions to sulfadiazine silver cream are not rare and usually caused by cetyl alcohol or propylene glycol	365

(continued)

§ **5.41** *(continuation)*

Drug	Use	Patch test conc. & vehicle (§ 5.2)	EFS (§ 5.4)	Cross-reactions (§ 5.5)	Comment	Ref.
tannic acid	adstringent	0.25% aqua	4			273
tattoos					For fuller data, *see* § 5.42	392
tetrachlordeca-oxide	treatment of leg ulcers	comm. prep. pure	4			829
thiosinamine	skin massage	0.05% alc.	3		Also used in photography	413
tiger balm	folk medicine	as is	3	balsam Peru		226
transdermal therapeutic systems					See under clonidine, estradiol, nitroglycerin and scopolamine	768 769
triaziquone	cytostatic drug	0.05% euc.	4			219
triethanolamine polypeptide oleate conden-sate	cerumenolytic drug	1% pet.	3			265
trioxyethylrutin	treatment of venous disorders	2% pet.	4			13
tromantadine	antiviral drug	1% pet.	1	amantadine [495]	Contact allergy to the commercial ointment is nearly always caused by the active ingredient tromantadine [474]	142 338
vitamin K_1 (phy-tonadione)	vitamin	commercial preparation	3	not to vitamin K_3	Allergy caused by subcutaneous injection	720

PIGMENTS USED IN TATTOOS

5.42 Contact allergy to tattoos [392]

Colour	Pigment	Patch testing	Comment	Ref.
blue	– cobalt blue – indigo	cobalt chloride 2% pet.	Contact allergy to cobalt caused granulomatous skin reactions	356
green	– trivalent chromic oxide – chromic hydrate – hydrated chromium sesquioxide	potassium dichromate 0.5% pet.	No primary sensitization to the pigment. Usually preceeded by cement eczema	71

(continued)

§ **5.42** *(continuation)*

Colour	Pigment	Patch testing	Comment	Ref.
red	– mercuric sulfide (cinnabar)	0.1% pet. (?)	Contact allergy has caused lichenoid and granulomatous reactions; these reactions also occur without mercury sensitivity (§ 4.8 and 4.9)	412 466
yellow	– cadmium sulfide – ochre – curcuma yellow		Only phototoxic reactions described from cadmium sulfide (§ 6.5)	
purple	– manganese	manganese oxide pure		322 392

ACCIDENTAL CONTACTANTS

5.43 Contact allergy to accidental contactants

Drug	Use	Patch test conc. & vehicle (§ 5.2)	Cross-reactions (§ 5.5)	Comment	Ref.
alprenolol	β-adrenergic blocking agent	0.1–10% aqua	metroprolol		133
p-aminosalicylic acid	tuberculostatic drug	3% pet.			421
aminophylline	smooth muscle relaxant	2.5% pet.	ethylenediamine hydrochloride	Aminophylline consists of theophylline and ethylenediamine	17
anileridine	narcotic	anileridine injection undiluted			131
apomorphine	treatment of alcoholism	0.01–0.1 and 1% aqua	morphine	Has also caused rhinitis and respiratory symptoms in the reported cases	114
benzidine	organic intermediate	1% pet. or MEK [180]	other p-amino compounds		16 521
1,4-bis-chloromethyl-benzene		?		Possibly related to bis-(4-chlorophenyl)-methylchloride	241

(continued)

§ **5.43** *(continuation)*

Drug	Use	Patch test conc. & vehicle (§ 5.2)	Cross-reactions (§ 5.5)	Comment	Ref.
bis-(4-chlorophenyl)-methylchloride	DDT substitute	1% chloroform		For other chlorinated methyl derivatives *see* [241]	34
bromocholine bromide	antihypertensive drug	pure			373
butyl acetate	in penicillin preparation	5% o.o.			349
carbimazole	thiourea antithyroid drug	10% pet.			822
carbocromen	coronary vasodilator	0.8% aqua			239
p-chlorobenzene-sulfonylglycolic acid nitrile	synthesis of benzodiazepines	0.01% acet.		Controls may react to 0.01% and 0.1%	449
chloroquine diphos-phate	antimalarial drug	5% aqua	mepacrine		221
chloroquine sulfate	antimalarial drug	1% pet.			510
chlorpromazine	sedative	0.1% pet.	diethazine hydrochloride, ethopropazine hydrochloride, promethazine hydrochloride, thiazinamium		345 387
chlorprothixene	tranquillizer	1% aqua	chlorpromazine derivatives		267
codeine	analgesic	1% ethanol	paracompounds ?	Also occupational rhinitis, sinusitis, bronchitis and conjunctivitis. Concomitant reactions to other opium alkaloids (notably morphine)	480
cycloheximide	fungicide	1% pet.	possibly cross-reacting to primary sensitization to neomycin		46
dibenzyline	α-adrenergic receptor blocking agent	1% aqua			307
diethylaminoethyl-chloride hydroioide	cleaning of syringes	0.1% aqua			253

(continued)

§ **5.43** *(continuation)*

Drug	Use	Patch test conc. & vehicle (§ 5.2)	Cross-reactions (§ 5.5)	Comment	Ref.
dimercaprol	chelating agent	<5% pet.			100
emetine hydrochloride	antiparasitic drug	3% alc.			389
ethambutol	antituberculosis drug	1% aqua	2,2′-(ethylenediimino)-di-1-propanol		455
ethoxyquin	antioxidant in animal feed	0.5% aqua or pet.			485
etisazole	antifungal drug	2% pet.		Used in veterinary medicine	429
famotidine	H_2-receptor antagonist	0.1% aqua			508
furazolidone	antibiotic in animal feed	2% in PEG-400	nitrofurazone		362
hydrazines	various	1% pet.	dihydralazine, hydralazine, hydralazine sulfate, isoniazid, β-phenylethyl-hydrazine, phenylhydrazine	May cause toxic reactions	188 411 432 579
hydroquinone	antioxidant	1% pet.			246
isoamylether of phenylaminoacetate	antispasmodic	5% aqua			164
isoniazid	antituberculosis drug	2% aqua			455
meclofenoxate	improves cerebral uptake of oxygen and glucose	2.5% ?			171
2-[4(5)-methyl-5(4)-imidazolyl-methyl-thio]-C13	H_2-antagonist	0.1% and 1% aqueous and ethanol solution			87
morphine	analgesic	1% aqua		Histamine releaser, urticariogenic. *See also under* codeine	126 480
nicotinic acid	vitamin	1% aqua	possibly other pyridine derivatives	In the reported case, the reaction to nicotinic acid was a cross-reaction to other pyridine derivatives	579

(continued)

§ **5.43** *(continuation)*

Drug	Use	Patch test conc. & vehicle (§ 5.2)	Cross-reactions (§ 5.5)	Comment	Ref.
omeprazole	treatment of peptic ulcer	0.1–1% pet. or alcohol			
oxprenolol hydrochloride	antihypertensive drug	1% pet.	possibly to or from propranolol hydrochloride		362
penethamate hydroiodide	antibiotic	25% o.o.	benzyl penicillin		227 231
phenolphthalein	in laxatives	0.5% alc.			403
phenoxybenzamine	α-adrenergic receptor blocking agent	1% aqua	related haloalkylamines		9 311
phenylephrine hydrochloride	mydriatic agent in eye drops	5% aqua		Unreliable report	774
piperazine	anthelmintic	1% pet.	*N,N′*-dimethyl-piperazine, ethylenediamine hydrochloride, *N*-methyl-piperazine, methyl-2-piperazine	Patch testing may have caused respiratory symptoms	75 179 504
propranolol hydrochloride	β-adrenergic receptor blocking agent	1% pet.	possibly to or from oxprenolol hydrochloride		307 362
quinidine sulfate	antiarrhythmic	1% aqua			143 454
quinine sulfate	antipyretic; antimalarial drug, in beverages (tonic)	1% pet.	clioquinol (?)		174
ranitidine (base and chlorhydrate)	H_2 histamine receptor antagonist	5% pet.	ranitidine chlorhydrate (1% pet.)		647
spiramycin	antibiotic in veterinary medicine	10% aqua or pet.	tylosin (?)		231 446
spironolactone	antihypertensive drug	1% alc.			268
streptomycin	antibiotic	1% pet.			577
tetraethylthiuram disulfide (disulfiram)	therapy for alcoholism	0.25% pet.	thiram and related compounds		250

(continued)

§ **5.43** *(continuation)*

Drug	Use	Patch test conc. & vehicle (§ 5.2)	Cross-reactions (§ 5.5)	Comment	Ref.
tetramisole hydrochloride	veterinary anthelmintic	1% (?)	levamisole (1%?)		509
tribromoethanol	anaesthetic	1% aqua			29
tropicamide	mydriatic agent in eyedrops	1% ?		Unreliable report	774
tylosin	antibiotic	5% pet.	spiramycin		231 446 484 494
vincamine tartrate	used for cerebral circulatory disturbance	1% aqua			427
vitamin B_1	vitamin	10% pet.	co-carboxylase		225
vitamin K_1	antidote to anticoagulants	0.1% pet or aqua			222
vitamin K_3 sodium bisulfite	vitamin	0.1% aqua/pet.	vitamin K_4		355
vitamin K_4	vitamin	0.1% pet.	vitamin K_3		247

5.44 REFERENCES

1. Aaronson, C.M. (1969): Generalised urticaria from sensitivity to nifuroxime. *J. Am. Med. Assoc., 210, 557.*
2. Aeling, J.L., Panagotacos, P.J. and Andreozzi, R.J. (1973): Allergic contact dermatitis to vitamin E in aerosol deodorant. *Arch. Derm., 108,* 579.
3. Afzelius, H., and Thulin, H. (1979): Allergic reactions to benzalkonium chloride. *Contact Dermatitis, 5,* 60.
4. Ägren, S., Dahlquist, J., Fregert, S. and Person, K. (1980): Allergic contact dermatitis from the preservative N-methylol-chloracetamide. *Contact Dermatitis, 6,* 302.
5. Hayakawa, R., Matsunaga, K., Suzuki, M., Ogino, Y., Arisu, K., Arima, Y. and Hirose, O. (1990): Allergic contact dermatitis due to amcinoide. *Contact Dermatitis, 23,* 49–50.
6. Alani, S.D. and Alani, M.D. (1976): Allergic contact dermatitis and conjunctivitis from epinephrine. *Contact Dermatitis, 2,* 147.
7. Eubanks, S.W. and Patterson, J.W. (1984): Dermatitis from sodium lauryl sulfate in hydrocortisone cream. *Contact Dermatitis, 11,* 250–251.
8. Alcon, D.N. (1947): Sensitivity to iodides and bromides in dermatoses other than dermatitis herpetiformis. *J. Invest. Dermatol., 8,* 287.
9. Alexander, S. and Spector, R.G. (1975): Phenoxybenzamine. *Contact Dermatitis, 1,* 59.
10. Dooms-Goossens, A., Vandaele, M., Bedert, R. and Marien, K. (1989): Hexamidine isethionate: a sensitizer in topical pharmaceutical products and cosmetics. *Contact Dermatitis, 21,* 270.
11. Amon, R.B., Lis, A.W. and Hanifin, J.M. (1975): Allergic contact dermatitis caused by idoxuridine: pattern of cross-reactivity with other pyrimidine analogues. *Arch. Dermatol., 111,* 1581.

12. Balato, N., Lembo, G., Patruno, C. and Ayala, F. (1989): Allergic contact dermatitis from Cerumenex® in a child. *Contact Dermatitis, 21,* 348–349.
13. Tosti, A., Guerra, L., Morelli, R. and Bardazzi, F. (1990): Prevalence and sources of sensitization to emulsifiers: a clinical study. *Contact Dermatitis, 23,* 68–72.
14. Pecegueiro, M. (1990): Allergic contact dermatitis to cetrimide after preoperative skin preparation. *Ninth Int. Symp. on Contact Dermatitis,* p. 90. Stockholm.
15. Ayres III, S. and Ayres Jr., S. (1954): Contact dermatitis from chlorcyclizine hydrochloride. *Arch. Dermatol. Syph., 69,* 502.
16. Baer, R.L. (1945): Benzidine as cause of occupational dermatitis in a physician. *J. Am. Med. Assoc., 129,* 442.
17. Baer, R.L., Cohen, H.J. and Neideroff, A.H. (1959): Allergic eczematous sensitivity to aminophyllin. *Arch. Dermatol. 81,* 647.
18. Veraldi, S., Benelli, C. and Pigatto, P.D. (1992): Occupational allergic contact dermatitis from minoxidil. *Contact Dermatitis, 26,* 211–212.
19. Baer, R.L., Ramsey. D.L. and Biondi, E. (1973): The most common contact allergens. *Arch. Dermatol., 108,* 74.
20. Baer, R.L., Serri, F. and Weissenbach-Vidal, Chr. (1955): Studies on allergic sensitization to certain topical therapeutic agents. *Arch. Dermatol. Syph., 71,* 19.
21. Baes, H. (1974): Allergic contact dermatitis to virginiamycin. *Dermatologica (Basel), 149,* 231.
22. Baker, H., Ive. F.A. and Lloyd, M.J. (1969): Primary irritant dermatitis of the scrotum due to hexachlorophene. *Arch. Dermatol., 99,* 693.
23. Bandmann, H.J. (1967): Kontaktekzem und Ekzematogene. *Münch. med. Wschr., 109,* 1572.
24. Van Ketel, W.G. and Van den Berg, W.H.H.W. (1990): Sensitization to povidone iodine. *Dermatol. Clinics, 8,* 107–109.
25. Bandmann, H.J. and Breit, R. (1973): The mafenide story. *Br. J. Dermatol., 89,* 219.
26. Bandmann, H.J., Breit. R. and Mutzeck, E. (1974): Allergic contact dermatitis from Proxymetacaine. *Contact Dermatitis Newsl., 15,* 451.
27. Bandmann, H.J. and Doenicke, A. (1971): Allergisches Kontaktekzem durch Propanidid bei einem Anesthesisten. *Berufsdermatosen, 19,* 160.
28. Bandmann, H.J. and Dohn, W. (1967): *Die Epikutantestung,* p.170. Bergmann, Munich.
29. Bandmann, H.J. and Dohn, W. (1967): *Die Epikutantestung,* p.288. Bergmann, Munich.
30. Hausen, B.M. and Kulenhamp, D. (1985): Kontaktallergie auf Fludroxycortid und Cetylalkohol. *Dermatosen, 33,* 27–28.
31. Bandmann, H.J. and Keilig, W. (1980): Lanette O — another test substance for lower leg series. *Contact Dermatitis, 6,* 227.
32. Bandmann, H.J. and Mutzeck, E. (1973): Contact allergy to gentamycin sulfate. *Contact Dermatitis Newsl., 13,* 371.
33. Bandmann, M. (1967): *Zur monovalenten Kontaktallergie gegen Eucerinum anhydricum.* Thesis, Munich.
34. Bang-Pedersen, N., Thormann, J. and Senning, A. (1980): Occupational contact allergy to bis-4(4-chlorophenyl)-methylchloride. *Contact Dermatitis, 6,* 56.
35. Bedoukian, P.Z. (1952): Aspects of aging in perfumes. *Am. Perfumer Essent. Oil Rev., 22,* 263.
36. Beetz, D., Cramer, H.J. and Mehlhorn, H.Ch. (1971): Zur Häufigkeit der epidermalen Allergie gegenüber Kamille in Kamillenhaltigen Arzneimitteln und Kosmetika. *Derm. Mschr., 157,* 505.
37. Behrbohm, P. (1962): Über allergische Krankheit durch DDT und HCH. *Allergie u. Asthma, 8,* 237.
38. Behrbohm, P. and Brandt, B. (1960): Allergisches Kontaktekzem durch technische und gereinigte Hexachlorcyclohexanpräparate bei der Anwendung im Pflanzenschutz und in der Schädlingsbekämpfung. *Berufsdermatosen, 8,* 95.
39. Behrbohm, P. and Lenzner, M. (1975): Sensitivity to falicain (propoxypiperocainhydrochloride). *Contact Dermatitis, 1,* 187.
40. Behrbohm, P. and Zschunke, E. (1965): Allergisches Ekzem durch das Antimykotikum 'Afungin' (Dibenzthion). *Derm. Wschr., 151,* 1447.
41. Bentley-Phillips, B. and Bayler, M.A.H. (1975): Cutaneous reactions to topical application of hydroquinone. *S. Afr. Med. J., 49,* 1391.
42. Baptista, A. and Barros,A. (1992): Contact dermatitis from crotamiton. *Contact Dermatitis, 27,* 59.
43. Hausen, B.M. and Kresken, J. (1988): The sensitizing capacity of crotamiton. *Contact Dermatits, 18,* 298–299.
44. Bielicky, T. and Novak, M. (1969): Contact group sensitisation to triphenylmethane dyes. *Arch. Dermatol., 100,* 540.

45. Katz, B.E. and Fisher, A.A. (1987): Bacitracin; a unique topical antibiotic sensitizer. *J. Am. Acad. Dermatol., 17,* 1016–1024.
46. Black, H. (1971): Allergy to cycloheximide (Actidione). *Contact Dermatitis Newsl., 10,* 243.
47. Black, H. (1975): Contact dermatitis from stearyl alcohol in Metosyn (fluocinonide) cream. *Contact Dermatitis, 1,* 125.
48. Bleumink, E. and Nater, J.P. (1972): Allergic contact dermatitis to virginiamycin. *Dermatologica (Basel), 144,* 253.
49. Bleumink, E., Te Lintum, J.C.A. and Nater, J.P. (1974): Kontaktallergie durch Nitrofurazon (furacin) and Nifurprazin (Carofur). *Hautarzt, 25,* 403.
50. Hannuksela, M. (1988): Skin contact allergy to emulsifiers. *Int. J. Cosm. Sc., 10,* 9–14.
51. Bloom, D. (1940): Eczema venenatum (perfume). *Arch. Dermatol., 42,* 968.
52. Bojs, G. and Möller, H. (1974): Eczematous contact allergy to oxytetracycline with cross-sensitivity to other tetracyclines. *Berufsdermatosen, 22,* 202.
53. Vincenzi, C., Cameli, N., Tardio, M. and Piraccini, B.M. (1990): Contact and photocontact dermatitis due to benzydamine hydrochloride. *Contact Dermatitis, 23,* 125–126.
54. Yoshikawa, K., Watanabe, K. and Mizuno, N. (1985): Contact allergy to hydrocortisone 17-butyrate and pyridoxine hydrochloride. *Contact Dermatitis, 12,* 55–56.
55. Braun, W.P.H. (1975): Contact allergy to collagenase mixture (IRUXOL). *Contact Dermatitis, 1,* 241 .
56. Braun, W. and Schütz, R. (1968): Kontaktallergie gegen Nitrofurazon (Furacin). *Dtsch. Med. Wschr., 93,* 1524.
57. Breit, R. and Bandmann, H.J. (1973): The wide world of antimycotics. *Brit. J. Dermatol., 89,* 657.
58. Brown, E.A. (1948): Reactions to penicillin. A review of the literature 1943–1948. *Ann. Allergy, 6,* 723.
59. Brown, R. (1979) Another case of sorbic acid sensitivity. *Contact Dermatitis, 5*, 268.
60. Junghans, C. (1985): Allergische Kontaktdermatitis gegen drei verschiedene topische Corticosteroide. *Derm. U. Kosmet., 26*, 92–95.
61. Burns, D.A. (1986): Allergic contact sensitivity to chlorphenesin. *Contact Dermatitis, 14,* 246.
62. Kraus, A.L., Stotts, J., Altringer, L.A. and Allgood, G.S. (1990): Allergic contact dermatitis from propyl gallate; dose response comparison using various application methods. *Contact Dermatitis, 22,* 132–136.
63. Akaeda, T., Shoji, H., Taniguichi, Y., Nishijima, S., Komura, J. and Asada, Y. (1988): A case of allergic contact dermatitis to topical corticosteroids: betamethasone sodium phosphate, dipropionate and valerate. *J. Kansai. Med. Univ., 40 (suppl.),* 60–64.
64. Burckhardt, W. and Hellerström, S. (1932): Sensibilisierung gegen Leinsamen. *Acta Derm.-venereol. (Stockh.), 13,* 712.
65. Burckhardt. W., Mahler, F. and Schwarz-Speck, M. (1968): Photoallergische Ekzeme durch Mycanodin. *Dermatologica (Basel), 137,* 208.
66. Burry, J.N. (1967): Photoallergies to fenticlor and multifungin. *Arch. Derm., 95,* 287.
67. Balato, N., Cusano, F., Lembo, G. and Ayala, F. (1986): Ethylenediamine dermatitis. *Contact Dermatitis, 15,* 263–265.
68. Burry, J.N. and Hunter G.A. (1970): Photocontact dermatitis from Jadit. *Brit. J. Dermatol., 82,* 224.
69. Myatt, A.E. and Beck, M.H. (1985): Contact sensitivity to parachlorometaxylenol (POMX). *Clin. exp. Dermatol., 10,* 491–494.
70. Burry, J.N. Kirk, J. Reid, J.G. and Turner, T. (1975): Chlorocresol sensitivity. *Contact Dermatitis, 1,* 41 .
71. Cairns. R.J. and Calnan. C.D. (1962): Green tattoo reactions associated with cement dermatitis. *Br. J. Dermatol., 74,* 288.
72. Calnan. C.D. (1962): Contact dermatitis from drugs. *Proc. Roy. Soc. Med., 55,* 39.
73. Calnan, C.D. (1967): Chlortetracycline sensitivity. *Contact Dermatitis Newsl., 1,* 16.
74. Wilkinson, S.M. and Beck, M.H. (1992): Allergic contact dermatitis from dibutyl phthalate, propyl gallate and hydrocortisone in Timodine®. *Contact Dermatitis, 27,* 197.
75. Calnan, C.D. (1975): Occupational piperazine dermatitis. *Contact Dermatitis, 1,* 126.
76. Calnan. C.D. (1975): Sensitivity to benzamine lactate. *Contact Dermatitis, 1,* 56.
77. Calnan, C.D. (1976): Cinnamon dermatitis from an ointment. *Contact Dermatitis, 2,* 167.
78. Maucher, O.M., Faber, M., Knipper, H., Kirchner, S. and Schöpf, E. (1987): Kortikoidallergie. *Hautarzt, 38,* 577–582.
79. Calnan. C.D. (1978): Diphenylamine. *Contact Dermatitis, 4,* 301.
80. Schwale, M. and Frosch, P.J. (1983): Kontaktallergie auf Ammoniumbituminosulfonat. *Dermatosen., 31,* 183–186.

5. Allergic contact dermatitis from topical drugs

81. Freeman, S. (1984): Allergic contact dermatitis due to 1,2-benzisothiazolin-3-one in gum arabic. *Contact Dermatitis, 11,* 146–149.
82. Calnan. C.D. (1979): Unusual hydroxycitronellal perfume dermatitis. *Contact Dermatitis, 5,* 123.
83. Calnan. C.D. (1980): Allergy to the local anaesthetic diperodon. *Contact Dermatitis, 6,* 367.
84. Calnan. C.D. and Sarkany, L. (1960): Sensitivity to oleyl alcohol. *Trans. St. John's Hosp. Derm. Soc. (Lond.,) 44,* 47.
85. Osawa, J., Kitamura, K., Ikezawa, Z. and Nakajima, H. (1991): A probable role for vaccines containing thimerosal in thimerosal hypersensitivity. *Contact Dermatitis, 24,* 178–182.
86. Camarasa, G. and Alomar, A. (1978): Mentholdermatitis from cigarettes. *Contact Dermatitis, 4,* 169.
87. Camarasa, G. and Alomar, A. (1980): Contact dermatitis to an H2-antagonist. *Contact Dermatitis, 6, 152.*
88. Camarasa, J.M.G. and Alomar, A. (1980): Contact dermatitis from Karaya seal ring. Contact Dermatitis 6, 139.
89. Caro. J. (1978): Contact allergy/photoallergy to glyceryl PABA and benzocaine. *Contact Dermatitis, 4.* 381.
90. Carruthers, J.A. and Cronin, E. (1976): Incidence of neomycin and framycetin sensitivity. *Contact Dermatitis, 2,* 269.
91. Motley, R.J. and Reynolds, A.J. (1988): Contact allergy to 2,4-dichlorophenylethyl imidazole derivatives. *Contact Dermatitis, 19,* 381–382.
92. Edman, B. and Möller, H. (1989): Testing a purified lanolin preparation by a randomized procedure. *Contact Dermatitis, 20,* 287–290.
93. Comaish, J.S. (1970): Reaction to Triton X 45. *Contact Dermatitis Newsl., 7,* 167.
94. Comaish, J.S. and Kersey, P.J. (1980): Contact dermatitis to extract of horse chestnut (esculin). *Contact Dermatitis, 6, 150.*
95. Conant M. and Maibach, H.I. (1974): Allergic contact dermatitis due to neutral red. *Arch. Dermatol., 109,* 735.
96. Connor. B.L. (1973): Mesulphen in tineafax ointment. *Contact Dermatitis Newsl., 14,* 417.
97. Bunney, M.H. (1972): Contact dermatitis due to betamethasone-17-valerate (Betnovate). *Contact Dermatitis Newsl., 12,* 318.
98. Dupont, C. (1972): Sensitivity to Fentichlor. *Contact Dermatitis Newsl., 12,* 327.
99. Böckers, M. and Bork, K. (1986): Kontakt dermatitis durch PVP-Jod. *Deutsche Med. Wschr., 111,* 1110–1112.
100. Cornbleet, T. (1947): Skin sensitization to B.A.L. *J. invest. Dermatol., 9,* 281.
101. Coskey, R.J. (1971): Contact Dermatitis due to nystatin. *Arch. Dermatol., 103,* 228.
102. Dunkel, F.G., Elsner, P., Pevny, I., Röger, J. and Burg, G. (1990): Amcinonide-induced contact dermatitis, possibly due to the ketal structure. *Am. J. Contact Dermatitis, 1,* 246–249.
103. James, W.D., White, S.W. and Yanklowitz, B. (1984): Allergic contact dermatitis to compound tincture of benzoin. *J. Am. Acad. Dermatol., 11,* 847–850.
104. de Kort, W.J.A. and de Groot, A.C. (1989): Clindamycin allergy presenting as rosacea. *Contact Dermatitis, 20,* 72–73.
105. Kabasawa, Y. and Kanzaki, T. (1990): Allergic contact dermatitis from alclometasone dipropionate. *Contact Dermatitis, 23,* 374–375.
106. Council on Drugs (1966): A new agent for the treatment of candidal vaginitis: Candicidin (Candeptin). *J. Am. Med. Assoc., 196,* 1144.
107. Coyle, H.E., Miller, E. and Chapman, R.S. (1981): Sorbic acid sensitivity from unguentum Merck *Contact Dermatitis. 7,* 56.
108. Cronin, E. (1969) Genetris pessaries. *Contact Dermatitis Newsl., 6,* 134.
109. Heine, A. (1988): Contact dermatitis from propyl gallate. *Contact Dermatitis, 18,* 313–314.
110. Parker, L.U. (1990): A five-year study of contact allergy to quaternium-15. *Am. J. Contact Dermatitis, 1,* 144.
111. Cronin, E. (1980): Medicaments. In: *Contact Dermatitis,* p. 198. Churchill Livingstone, Edinburgh.
112. Cronin, E. (1980): *Contact Dermatitis,* p. 236. Churchill Livingstone, Edinburgh.
113. Dahlquist, I. (1977): Contact dermatitis to a veterinary fungicide. *Contact Dermatitis, 3,* 277.
114. Dahlquist, I. (1977): Allergic reactions to apomorphine. *Contact Dermatitis, 3.* 349.
115. Dahlquist, I. and Fregert, S. (1978): Formaldehyde releasers. *Contact Dermatitis, 4,* 173.
116. Dahlquist, I. and Fregert S. (1980): Contact allergy to atranorin in Lichens and perfumes. *Contact Dermatitis 6,* 111.
117. Daly, J.F. (1952): Contact dermatitis due to 'Quotane'. *Arch. Dermatol. Syph., 66.* 393.

118. Baptista, A. and Barros, M.A. (1990): Contact dermatitis from sodium fusidate. *Contact Dermatitis, 23,* 186–187.
119. Bardazzi, F., Misciali, C., Borello, P. and Capobianco, C. (1988): Contact dermatitis due to antioxidants. *Contact Dermatitis, 19,* 385–386.
120. Romaguera, C., Grimalt, F. and Vilaplana, J. (1990): Acute contact dermatitis by dithranol. *Am. J. Contact Dermatitis, 1,* 186–188.
121. Jones, S.K. and Kennedy, C.T.C. (1990): Contact dermatitis from tioconazole. *Contact Dermatitis, 22,* 122–123.
122. Dong Gil Byun, Young Hoe Kim, Yang Ja Park and Soon Bok Lee (1975): Treatment of hyperpigmented disease with 4-isopropyl catechol (Korean). *Kor. J. Dermatol., 13, 5.*
123. Dooms-Goossens, A. and Degreef, H. (1980): Sensitization to yellow petrolatum used as a vehicle for patch testing. Contact Dermatitis, 6, 146.
124. Dooms-Goossens, A., Degreef, H. and Luytens, E. (1979): Dihydroabietyl alcohol (Abitol), a sensitizer in mascara. *Contact Dermatitis, 5,* 350.
125. Dooms-Goossens, A., Degreef, H., Van Hee, J., Kerkhofs L. and Chrispeels, M.T. (1981): Chlorocresol and chloracetamide, allergens in medications, glues and cosmetics. *Contact Dermatitis, 7, 51.*
126. Dore. S.E. and Prosser Thomas, E.W. (1944): Contact dermatitis in a morphine factory. Br. J. Dermatol., 56, 177.
127. Nordlund, J.J., Forget, B., Kirkwood, J., Lerner, A.B. (1985): Dermatitis produced by applications of monobenzone in patients with active vitiligo. *Arch. Dermatol., 121,* 1141–1143.
128. Drug Evaluations (1971): *Antihistamines,* pp. 367–368. American Medical Association, Chicago, IL.
129. Dupont, C. (1972): Sensitivity to Fentichlor. *Contact Dermatitis Newsl., 12,* 327.
130. Ebner, H. (1974): Perubalsam und Parfums. Untersuchungen über allergologische Beziehungen zwischen diescn Substanzen. *Hautarzt, 25,* 123.
131. Ecker, R.J. (1980): Contact dermatitis to anileridine. *Contact Dermatitis, 6,* 495.
132. Piraccini, B.M., Bardazzi, F., Morelli, R., Tosti, A. (1991): Contact dermatitis due to budesonide. *Contact Dermatitis, 24,* 54–55.
133. Ekenval, L. and Forsbeck, M. (1978): Contact eczema produced by a β-adrenergic blocking agent (alprenolol). *Contact Dermatitis, 4,* 190.
134. Ellis, F.A. and Bundick, W.R. (1949): Reactions to the local use of thephorin. *J. Invest. Dermatol., 13,* 25.
135. Epstein, E. (1966): Dichlorophene allergy. *Ann. Allergy, 24,* 437.
136. Epstein, E. (1980): Contact dermatitis to neomycin with false negative patch tests: Allergy established by intradermal and usage tests. *Contact Dermatitis, 6,* 219.
137. Epstein, E. (1980): Contact dermatitis to 5-fluorouracil with false negative patch tests. *Contact Dermatitis, 6,* 220.
138. Aberer, W., Gerstner, G., Pehamberger, H. (1990): Ammoniated mercury ointment: outdated but still in use. *Contact Dermatitis, 23,* 168–171.
139. Epstein, J.H., Wuepper, K.D. and Maibach, H.I. (1968): Photocontact dermatitis to halogenated salicylanilides and related compounds. *Arch. Dermatol., 97,* 236.
140. Eriksen, K. (1978): Cross allergy between paranitro-compounds with special reference to DNCB and chloramphenicol. *Contact Dermatitis, 4,* 29.
141. Hogan, D.J. (1990): Allergic contact dermatitis to ethylenediamine, a continuing problem. *Dermatologic Clinics, 8,* 133–136.
142. Hausen, B.M., Schulz, R. (1986): Vergleichende Untersuchungen über das Sensibilisierungsvermögen angewandter Herpes-Simplex Therapeutika. *Dermatosen, 34,* 163–170.
143. Fernström, A.T.B. (1965): Occupational quinidine contact dermatitis, a concept apparently not yet described. *Acta derm.-venereol. (Stockh.), 45,* 129.
144. Finn, O.A. and Forsyth, A. (1975): Contact dermatitis due to sorbitan monolaurate. *Contact Dermatitis, 1,* 318.
145. Fisher, A.A. (1965): Paraphenylene diamine, one of the 'BIG FIVE' in allergic contact dermatitis. *Cutis, 1,* 171.
146. Fisher. A.A. (1973): Allergic reactions to feminine hygiene sprays. *Arch. Dermatol., 108,* 801.
147. Fisher. A.A. (1973): *Contact Dermatitis, 2nd Edition*, p. 59. Lea and Febiger, Philadelphia.
148. Fisher, A.A. (1973): *Contact Dermatitis, 2nd Edition,* pp. 295–297. Lea and Febiger, Philadelphia.
149. Fisher, A.A. (1973): *Contact Dermatitis, 2nd Edition*, p. 371. Lea and Febiger, Philadelphia.

150. Nielsen, M., Jørgensen, J. (1987); Persistence of contact sensitivity to ethylenediamine. *Contact Dermatitis, 16,* 275–276.
151. Fisher, A.A. (1974): Contact dermatitis from stearyl alcohol and propylene glycol. *Arch. Dermatol., 110,* 636.
152. van Neer, P.A.F.A., van der Kley, A.M.J. (1991): Imidazolidinyl urea (Germall 115) should be patch tested in water. *Contact Dermatitis, 24,* 302.
153. Fisher, A.A. (1975): Patch testing with perfume ingredients. *Contact Dermatitis, 1,* 166.
154. Shmunes, E. (1984): Allergic dermatitis to benzyl alcohol in an injectable solution. *Arch. Dermatol., 120,* 1200–1201.
155. Fisher, A.A. (1986): Cross reactions between ethylenediamine base in merthiolate tincture with ethylenediamine HCL. *Contact Dermatitis, 14,* 181–182.
156. Fisher, A.A. (1975): Contact dermatitis due to food additives. *Cutis, 16,* 961.
157. Fisher, A.A. (1978): Immediate and delayed allergic contact reactions to polyethylene glycol. *Contact Dermatitis, 4,* 135.
158. Fisher, A.A. (1980): Perfume dermatitis, part 1. *Cutis, 26,* 458.
159. Catanzaro, J.M., Smith, J.G. (1991): Propylene glycol dermatitis. *J. Am. Acad. Dermatol., 24,* 90–95.
160. Fisher, A.A. and Dooms-Goossens, A. (1976): The effect of perfume 'aging' on the allergenicity of individual perfume ingredients. *Contact Dermatitis 2,* 155.
161. Fisher, A.A., Pascher, F. and Kanof, F.N.B. (1971): Allergic contact dermatitis due to ingredients of vehicles. *Arch. Dermatol., 104,* 286.
162. Fisher, A.A. and Stillman, M.A. (1972): Allergic contact sensitivity to benzalkoniumchloride (BAK). Cutaneous, ophthalmic and general medical implications. *Arch. Dermatol., 106.* 169.
163. White, I.R., Lovell, C.R., Cronin, E. (1984): Antioxidants in cosmetics. *Contact Dermatitis, 11,* 265–267.
164. Folesky, H.J. and Zschunke. E. (1962): Allergisches Ekzem durch Phenylaminoessigsaure Isoamylester (Aklonin). *Berufsdermatosen. 10.* 337.
165. Förstrom, L., Hannuksela, M., Idanpään-Heikkilä, J. and Salo, O.P. (1977): Hypersensitivity reactions to Gerovital. *Dermatologica (Basel) 154,* 367.
166. Lachapelle, J.M., Chabeau, G., Ducombs, G. et al. (1988): Enquête multicentrique rélative a la fréquence des tests épicutanés positifs au mercure et au thiomersal. *Ann. Dermatol. Venereol, 115,* 793–796.
167. Macdonald, R.M., Beck, M. (1983): Neomycin: a review with particular reference to dermatological usage. *Clin. exp. Dermatol., 8,* 249–258.
168. Foussereau, J. and Benezra, Cl. (1970): *Les Eczémas Allergiques Professionnels,* p. 61. Masson et Cie., Paris.
169. Vincenzi, C., Peluso, A.M., Cameli, N., Tosti, A. (1992): Allergic contact dermatitis caused by acyclovir. *Am. J. Contact Dermatitis, 3,* 105–107.
170. Foussereau, J., Benezra, C. and Ourisson, G. (1967): Contact dermatitis from Laurel. *Trans. St. John's Hosp. Med. Soc. (Lond.), 53,* 141.
171. Foussereau, J. and Lantz, J.P. (1972): Allergy to meclofenoxate. *Contact Dermatitis Newsl., 12,* 321.
172. De Groot, A.C., Conemans, J.M.H. (1990): Nystatin allergy. Petrolatum is not the optimal vehicle for patch testing. *Dermatologic Clinics, 8,* 153–155.
173. Foussereau, J., Schlewer, G., Chabeau, G. and Reimeringer, A. (1980): Étude allergologique d'intolèrances à la colophane. *Dermatosen, 28,* 14.
174. Frain Bell, W., Johnson, B.E., Gardiner, J.M. and Zaynoun, S. (1975): A study of persistent light reaction in quindoxin and quinine photosensitivity. *Brit. J. Dermatol., 93,* suppl. 11, 21.
175. Fräki. J.E., Peltonen, L. and Hopsu-Havu, V.K. (1979): Allergy to various components of topical preparations in stasis dermatitis and leg ulcers. *Contact Dermatitis, 5,* 97.
176. Fregert. S. (1968): Cross-sensitization among nitrofurylaminothiadazoles. *Acta derm.-venereol. (Stockh.), 48,* 106.
177. Fregert, S. et al (1969): Epidemiology of contact dermatitis. *Trans. St. John's Hosp. Derm. Soc. (Lond.),55,* 17.
178. Fregert, S. (1970): Sensitization to phenylacetaldehyde. *Dermatologica (Basel), 141,* 11.
179. Fregert, S. (1976): Respiratory symptoms with piperazine patch testing. *Contact Dermatitis, 2,* 61.
180. Fregert, S. (1981): *Manual of Contact Dermatitis,* 2nd Edition. Munksgaard, Copenhagen.
181. Fregert, S., Groth, O., Gruvberger, B., Magnusson, B., Mobacken, H. and Rorsman, H. (1971): Hypersensitivity to secondary alcohols. *Acta derm.-venereol. (Stockh.), 51,* 271.
182. Bardazzi, F., Vassilopoulou, A., Valenti, R., Paganini, P., Morelli, R. (1990): Mercurochrome-induced allergic contact dermatitis. *Contact Dermatitis, 23,* 381–382.

183. Fregert, S. and Hjorth, N. (1979): In: *Textbook of Dermatology,* 3rd Edition, p. 476. Editors: A. Rook, D.S. Wilkinson and F.J.G. Ebling. Blackwell Scientific Publications, Oxford.
184. Fregert, S. and Möller, H. (1962): Hypersensitivity to the cholinesterase inhibitor di-iso-propoxyphosphorylfluoride. *J. invest. Dermatol., 38,* 371.
185. Fregert. S. and Rorsman, H. (1962): Hypersensitivity to diethylstilbestrol with cross-sensitization to benzestrol. *Acta derm.-venereol. (Stockh.), 42,* 290.
186. Purcell, S.M., Dixon, S.L. (1985): Allergic contact dermatitis to dyclonine hydrochloride simulating extensive herpes simplex labialis. *J. Am. Acad. Dermatol., 12,* 231–234.
187. Frenk. E. (1962): Akute Putzmittelekzeme der Hände durch Tetrachlorsalicylanilid. *Dermatologica (Basel), 124,* 433.
188. Frost. J. and Hjorth, N. (1959): Contact dermatitis from hydrazine hydrochloride in soldering flux. *Acta derm.-venereol. (Stockh.), 39,* 82.
189. Farli, M., Ginanneschi, M., Francalanci, S., Martinelli, C., Sertoli, A. (1987): Occupational contact dermatitis to N-methylol-chloracetamide. *Contact Dermatitis, 17,* 182–184.
190. Gasser, E. (1953): Coiffeur-Ekzem, verursacht durch Thioglycerin enthaltende Kaltdauerwellenwasser. Inaugural Diss. Zürich.
191. Gastelain, P.Y and Piriou, A. (1980): Contact dermatitis due to propanidid in an anesthesist. *Contact Dermatitis, 6,* 360.
192. Gaul. L.E. (1964): Contact dermatitis from synthetic Oil of Mustard (allylisothiocyanate). *Arch. Dermatol., 90,* 158.
193. Gaul, L.E. (1969): Dermatitis from cetyl and stearyl alcohols. *Arch. Dermatol., 99,* 593.
194. Gelfarb, M. and Leiden, M. (1960): Allergic eczematous contact dermatitis. *Arch. Dermatol., 82,* 642.
195. Gellin, G.A., Maibach, H.I. and Wachs, G.N. (1972): Contact allergy to tolnaftate. *Arch. Dermatol. 106,* 715.
196. Raulin, C., Frosch, P.J. (1987): Contact allergy to oxiconazole. *Contact Dermatitis, 16,* 39–40.
197. Girard, J.P. (1978): Recurrent angioneurotic oedema and contact dermatitis due to penicillin. *Contact Dermatitis. 4,* 309.
198. Alomar, A. (1984): Buphenine sensitivity. *Contact Dermatitis, 11,* 315.
199. Goldman. L., Feldman, M.D. and Altemeier, W.A. (1948): Contact dermatitis from topical tyrothricin and associated with polyvalent hypersensitivity to various antibiotics. *J. invest. Dermatol., 11,* 243.
200. Rudzki, E., Rebandél, P. (1987); Primary sensitivity to sulphonamide and secondary sensitization to aromatic amines. *Contact Dermatitis, 17,* 49.
201. Hackel, H., Elsner, P., Burg, G. (1991): Sensitization to olive oil. *Am. J. Contact Dermatitis, 2,* 50–51.
202. Pevny, I. (1984): Benzaron allergy. *Contact Dermatitis, 11,* 122.
203. Grimalt, F. and Romaguera, C. (1978): Sensitivity to petrolatum. *Contact Dermatitis, 4,* 377.
204. Groen, J., Bleumink, E. and Nater, J.P. (1973): Variotin sensitivity. *Contact Dermatitis Newsl., 15,* 456.
205. Hayakawa, R., Matsunaga, K., Suziki, M., et al. (1991): Allergic contact dermatitis due to budesonide. *Contact Dermatitis, 24,* 136–137.
206. Haidar, Z. (1978): An adverse reaction to a topical antiseptic (cetrimide). *Br. J. Oral Surg., 16,* 86.
207. Hannuksela, M. (1979): Frequent contact allergy to higher fatty alcohols. *IV International Symposion on Contact Dermatitis.* San Francisco, March 29–31, 1979.
208. Hannuksela, M. and Forström, L. (1976): Contact hypersensitivity to glycerol. *Contact Dermatitis, 2,* 291.
209. Hannuksela. M., Kousa. M. and Pirilä, V. (1976): Allergy ingredients of vehicles. *Contact Dermatitis, 2,* 105.
210. Hannuksela, M., Kousa, M. and Pirilä, V. (1976): Contact sensitivity to emulsifiers. *Contact Dermatitis, 2,* 201.
211. Frosch, P.J., Pekar, U., Enzmann, H. (1990): Contact allergy to propylene glycol. Do we use the appropriate test concentration? *Derm. Clinics, 8,* 111–113.
212. von Mayenburg, J. (1989): Quecksilber als Allergen. *Allergologie, 12,* 235–242.
213. Harber, C.L., Harris, H., Leder, M. and Baer, R.L. (1964): Berloque dermatitis. *Arch Dermatol., 90,* 572.
214. Hardie. R.A., Savin, J.A., White, D.A. and Pumford, S. (1978): Quinine dermatitis: investigation in a factory outbreak. *Contact Dermatitis, 4,* 121.
215. Morren, M., Dooms-Goossens, A., Heidbuchel, M., Sente, F., Damas, M.C. (1991): Contact allergy to dihydroxyacetone. *Contact Dermatitis, 25,* 326–327.
216. Hartung, J. and Rudolph, P.O. (1970): Epidermale Allergie gegen Hydroxypolyaethoxydodekan. *Z. Haut. u. Geschl.kr. 45,* 547.

5. Allergic contact dermatitis from topical drugs

217. Hausen, B.M. (1978): Identification of allergens in Arnica Montana. *Contact Dermatitis, 4,* 308.
218. Helander, I., Hollmén, A. and Hopsu-Havu, V.K. (1979): Allergic contact dermatitis to chlordantoin. *Contact Dermatitis, 5,* 54.
219. Helm, F.and Klein, E. (1965): Effects of allergic contact dermatitis on basal cell epitheliomas. *Arch. Dermatol., 91,* 142.
220. di Landro, A., Valsecchi, R., Cainelli, T. (1989): Contact dermatitis from Nitroderm. *Contact Dermatitis, 21,* 115–116.
221. Herrmann, W.P. and Schulz, K.H. (1965): Allergisches Kontaktekzem durch Resochin. *Dermatologica (Basel), 130,* 216.
222. Heydenreich, G. (1977): A further case of adverse skin reaction from vitamin K1. *Br. J. Dermatol., 97,* 697.
223. Heyer, A. (1961): Sensitisation to xanthocillin in salve. *Acta derm.-venereol. (Stockh.), 41,* 201.
224. Hindson, C. (1977): Contact eczema from methyl salicylate reproduced by oral aspirin (acetylsalicylic acid). *Contact dermatitis, 3,* 348.
225. Hjorth, N. (1958): Contact dermatitis from vitamin B (thiamine). *J. invest. Dermatol., 30,* 261.
226. Hjorth, N. (1961): Eczematous allergy to balsams, allied perfumes and flavouring agents. *Acta derm.-venereol. (Stockh.), 41,* suppl. 46.
227. Hjorth, N. (1967): Occupational dermatitis among veterinary surgeons caused by penethamate. *Berufsdermatosen, 15,* 163.
228. Hjorth, N. (1972): Contact dermatitis from 1,3-diiodo-2-hydroxypropane. *Contact dermatitis Newsl., 12,* 322.
229. Andersen, K.E., Carlsen, L., Egsgaard, H., Larsen, E. (1985): Contact sensitivity and bioavailability of chlorocresol. *Contact Dermatitis, 13,* 246–251.
230. Hjorth, N. and Trolle-Lassen, C. (1963): Skin reactions to ointment bases. *Trans. St. John's Hosp. derm. Soc. (Lond.), 49,* 127.
231. Hjorth, N. and Weissmann, K. (1973): Occupational dermatitis among veterinary surgeons caused by spiramycin, tylosin and penethamate. *Acta derm.-venereol. (Stockh.), 53,* 229.
232. English, J.S.C., Rycroft, R.J.G. (1988): Allergic contact dematitis from methyl heptine and methyl octine carbonates. *Contact Dermatitis, 18,* 174–175.
233. Hoffman, Th.E. and Adams R.M. (1978): Contact dermatitis to grease paint make up. *Contact Dermatitis, 4,* 379.
234. Hausen, B.M., Schmieder, M. (1986): The sensitizing capacity of coumarins (I). *Contact Dermatitis, 15,* 157–163.
235. Frosch, P.J. and Schulze-Dirks, A. (1989): Kontaktallergie durch Polidocanol (Thesit). *Hautartz, 40,* 146–149.
236. Ancona, A. (1985): Allergic contact dermatitis to nitrofurazone. *Contact Dermatitis, 13,* 35.
237. Hunziker, N. (1961). Reaction eczémateuses aux dérivés de l'oxyquinaléine. *Dermatologica (Basel), 122,* 26.
238. Huriez, C. and Martin, P. (1974): Conséquences pratiques des recherches d'isolement et d'identification chimiques des allergènes végétaux. In: *Actualités allergologiques,* pp. 83–87. Expansion Scientifique. Paris.
239. Huriez, Cl., Martin, P., Bétourné, M. and Martin, H.J. (1974): Sensitivity to carbocromène. *Contact Dermatitis Newsl., 15,* 429.
240. Schulze-Dirks, A., Frosch, P.J. (1988): Kontaktallergie auf Dexpanthenol. *Hautarzt, 39,* 375–377.
241. Ippen. H. and Liebeskind, H. (1978): Kontaktekzem durch 1,4-Bis-chlormethylbenzol. *Dermatosen, 26,* 97.
242. Jadassohn, J. (1896): Verhandlungen der Deutschen Dermatologischen Gesellschaft. Bericht über die Verhandlung des V. Kongresses. *Arch. Dermatol. Syph. (Berl.). 34,* 103.
243. Jannasch, G. (1962): Beitrag zur Kontaktallergie durch moderne Antibiotika. Z. *Haut-u. Geschl.kr., 33,* 158.
244. Jelen, G., Schlewer, G., Chabeau, G. and Foussereau, J. (1979): Eczemas due to plant allergens in manufactured products. *Acta derm.-venereol. (Stockh.), 59,* suppl. 85, 91.
245. Jensen, O. (1981): Contact allergy to propylene oxide and isopropyl alcohol in a skin disinfectant swab. *Contact Dermatitis, 7,* 148.
246. Jirásek, L. and Kalensky, J. (1975): Kontaktni alergicky ekzém z krmnych smesi v zivocisne vyrobe. *Cz. Derm., 50,* 217.

247. Jirásek, L. and Schwank, R. (1965): Berufskontaktekzem durch Vitamin K. *Hautarzt, 16,* 351.
248. Zemtsov, A. (1992): Evaluation of antigenic determinant in glutaraldehyde contact dermatitis by patch testing with chemically related substances. *Am. J. Contact Dermatitis, 3,* 138–141.
249. Jung. E.G. and Schwarz, K. (1965): Photoallergy from 'Jadit' with photocrossreactions to derivatives of sulfanilamide. *Int. Arch. Allergy, 27,* 313.
250. Kaalund-Jörgensen, O. (1949): Eczem efter ekstern pävirkning of Antabus. *Ugeskr. Laeg., 31/3,* 373.
251. Kaidbey, K.H. and Kligman, A.M. (1978): Photocontact allergy to 6-methyl coumarin. *Contact Dermatitis, 4,* 277.
252. Kalveram, K., Günnewig, W., Wehling, K. and Forck, G. (1978): Tetracaine allergy: cross-reactions with para compounds? *Contact Dermatitis, 4,* 376.
253. Kärcher, K.H. (1957): Zur pathogenese der lokalen Sensibilisierung durch Penicillinester. (Pulmo 500). *Derm. Wschr., 136,* 1071.
254. Keczkes, K. and Brown, P.M. (1976): Hexahydro-1,3,5,tris(2-hydroxyethyl)triazine, a new bactericidal agent as a cause of allergic contact dermatitis. *Contact Dermatitis, 2,* 92.
255. Keil, H. (1947): Contact dermatitis due to oil of citronella. *J. invest. Dermatol. 8,* 327.
256. Keil, H. (1962): Group reactions in contact dermatitis due to resorcinol. *Arch. Dermatol., 86, 212.*
257. Hutzler, D., Pevny, I. (1988): Allergien gegen 8-Hydroxychinolin-Derivate. Dermatosen, 36, 86–90.
258. Klaschka, F. (1975): Contact allergy to chloracetamide. *Contact Dermatitis, 1,* 265.
259. Knisley, R.E., Settipane, G.A. and Albala, M.M. (1971): Unusual reaction to chlorambucil in a patient with chronic Iymphatic leukaemia. *Arch. Dermatol., 104,* 77.
260. Kooy, R. and van Vloten, Th.J. (1952): Epidermal sensitization due to sulphonamide drugs. *Dermatologica (Basel), 104,* 151.
261. Kounis, N.G. (1976): Untoward reaction to corticosteroids: intolerance to hydrocortisone. *Ann. Allergy, 36,* 203.
262. van Joost, Th., Dikland, W., Stolz, E., Prens, E. (1986): Sensitization to chloramphenicol; a persistent problem. *Contact Dermatitis, 14,* 176–178.
263. Camelli, N., Vincenzi, C., Morelli, R., Bardazzi, F., Tardio, M. (1991): Contact allergy to oxyphenbutazone. *Contact Dermatis, 24,* 75–76.
264. Wojnarowska, F., Calnan, C.D. (1986): Contact and photocontact allergy to musk ambrette. *Br. J. Dermatol., 114,* 667–675.
265. Kroon, S. (1981): Contact dermatitis from oleyl polypeptide in Xerumenex® eardrops. *Contact Dermatitis, 7,* 271.
266. Kruyswijk, M.R.J. and Polak, B.C.P. (1980): Contactallergie na toepassing van oogdruppels en oogzalven. *Ned. T. Geneesk., 124,* 1449.
267. Kull, E. and Schwarz-Speck, K. (1961): Gruppenspezifische Ekzemreaktion bei Largactilsensibilisierung. *Dermatologica (Basel), 122,* 263.
268. Klijn, J. (1984): Contact dermatitis from spironolactone. *Contact Dermatitis, 10,* 105.
269. Lachapelle, J.M. and Lamy, F. (1973): On allergic contact dermatitis to virginiamycin. *Dermatologica (Basel), 146,* 320.
270. Lane, C.G. and Luikart II, R. (1951): Dermatitis from local anaesthetics. *J. Am. Med. Assoc., 146,* 717.
271. Larsen, W.G. (1975): Contact dermatitis due to a perfume. *Contact Dermatitis, 1,* 142.
272. Larsen, W.G. (1977): Perfume dermatitis. *Arch. Dermatol., 113,* 625.
273. Lewis, G.M. (1944): Dermatitis venenata due to tannins. *Arch. Dermatol. Syph., 50,* 138.
274. Marot, L. and Grosshans, E. (1987): Allergic contact dermatitis to ethyl lactate. *Contact Dermatitis, 17,* 45–46.
275. Lidén, S. and Göransson, K. (1975): Contact allergy to dibenzthion. *Contact Dermatitis, 1,* 258.
276. Morelli, R., Lanzarini, M., Vincenzi, C. and Reggiani, M. (1989): Contact dermatitis due to benzoyl peroxide. *Contact Dermatitis, 20,* 238–239.
277. Tosti, A., Guerra, L., Morelli, R. and Piraccini, M. (1992): Contact dermatitis due to topical retinoic acid. *Contact Dermatitis, 26,* 276.
278. Ljunggren, B. (1981): Contact dermatitis to estradiol benzoate. *Contact Dermatitis, 7,* 141.
279. Knudsen, B.B. and Avnstorp, C. (1991): Chlorhexidine gluconate and acetate in patch testing. *Contact Dermatitis, 24,* 45–49.
280. Lorenzetti, O.J. and Wernet, T.C. (1977): Topical parabens: benefit and risks. *Dermatologica (Basel), 154,* 244.
281. Loveman, A.B. and Fliegelman, M.T. (1951): Local cutaneous sensitivity to methapyrilene. *Arch. Dermatol. Syph., 63,* 250.

282. Löwenfeld, W. (1928): Überempfindlichkeit gegen lodthion mit gleichzeitiger urtikarieller Reaktion. *Derm. Wschr. 78,* 502.
283. Ludwig, E. and Hausen, B.M. (1977): Sensitivity to isopropyl alcohol. *Contact Dermatitis. 3,* 240.
284. Lynfield, Y.L. (1970): Allergic contact sensitization to gentamycin. *N.Y. St. J. Med., 70,* 2235.
285. Hansen, E.M. and Menné, T. (1990): Glutaraldehyde: patch test, vehicle and concentration. *Contact Dermatitis, 23,* 369.
286. Maibach, H.I. (1978): Chronic dermatitis and hyperpigmentation from petrolatum. *Contact Dermatitis 4,* 62.
287. Maibach, H.I. et al. (1978): Triclocarban: evaluation of contact dermatitis potential in man. *Contact Dermatitis, 4,* 283.
288. Ballantyne, B., Berman, B. (1984): Dermal sensitizing potential of glutaraldehyde: a review and recent observations. *J. Toxicol.- Cut. Ocular Toxicol., 3,* 251–262.
289. Malten, K.E. (1977): Sensitization to solcoseryl and methyl anisate (fragrance ingredient). *Contact Dermatitis, 3,* 219.
290. Malten, K.E. (1979): Four bakers showing positive patch tests to a number of fragrance materials, which can also be used as flavors. *Acta derm.-venereol. (Stockh), Suppl. 85,* 117.
291. Malten, K.E. Nater, J.P. and van Ketel, W.G. (1976): *Patch testing guidelines.* Dekker en van de Vegt, Nijmegen, Holland.
292. Mansell, P.W.A., Litwin, M.S., Ichinose, H. and Krementz, E.T. (1975): Delayed hypersensitivity to 5-fluorouracil following topical chemotherapy of cutaneous cancers. *Cancer Res. 35,* 1288.
293. Marcussen, P.V. (1962): Variations in the incidence of contact hypersensitivities. *Trans. St. John's Hosp. Derm. Soc. (Lond.) 48,* 40.
294. Serrano, G., Fortea, J.M., Millan, F., Botella, R. and Latasa, J.M. (1992): Contact allergy to resorcinol in acne medications: report of three cases. *J. Am. Acad. Dermatol., 26,* 502–504.
295. Mathias, C.G.I., Maibach, H.I. and Chappler, R.R. (1981): Contact dermatitis to parachloromercuriphenol. *Contact Dermatitis 7,* 117.
296. Verschueren, G.L.A., Bruynzeel, D.P. (1992): Hypersensitivity to ketoconazole. *Contact Dermatitis, 26,* 47–48.
297. Maucher. O.M. (1974): Beitrag zur Kreuz- oder Kopplungsallergie auf Parahydroxy-benzoe-säureester. *Berufsdermatosen, 22,* 183.
298. Mendelsohn, H.V. (1946): Lemon grass oil. *Arch. Dermatol. 53,* 94.
299. Meneghini, C.L. and Angelini, G. (1975): Contact dermatitis from pyrrolnitrin (an antimycotic agent). *Contact Dermatitis 1,* 288.
300. Perret, C.M., Happle, R. (1989): Contact allergy to bufexamac. *Contact Dermatitis, 20,* 307–308.
301. De Groot, A.C. (1993): Topical antihistamines — what use are they? *Drugs and Therapeutics Bulletin.* In press.
302. Menné, T. and Andersen, K.E. (1977): Allergic contact dermatitis from fluocortolone, fluocortolone pivalate and fluocortolone caproate. *Contact Dermatitis, 3,* 337.
303. Merck Index (1976): An encyclopedia of chemicals and drugs. Ninth edition. Merck and Co., Inc. Rahway, N.J., U.S.A.
304. Milby. T.H. and Epstein, W.L. (1964): Allergic contact sensitivity to malathion. *Arch. environm. Hlth, 9,* 434.
305. Mitchell, J.C. (1972): Contact dermatitis from proflavine dihydrochloride. *Arch. Dermatol., 106,* 924.
306. Mitchell, J.C. (1974): Contact sensitivity to costusroot oil, an ingredient of some perfumes. *Arch. Dermatol., 109,* 572.
307. Mitchell, J.C. (1974): Allergic contact dermatitis from alpha- and beta-adrenergic receptor blocking agents (Dibenzyline and propranolol). *Contact Dermatitis Newsl., 16,* 488.
308. Mitchell. J.C. (1975): Contact hypersensitivity to some perfume materials. *Contact Dermatitis, 1,* 196.
309. Mitchell, J.C. and Dupuis, G. (1972): Allergic contact dermatitis from storax (styrax). *Contact Dermatitis Newsl., 11,* 274.
310. Mitchell, J.C. and Epstein, W.L. (1974): Contact hypersensitivity to a perfume material, Costus Absolute. *Arch. Dermatol., 110,* 871.
311. Mitchell, J.C. and Maibach, H.I. (1975): Allergic contact dermatitis from phenoxybenzamine hydrochloride. *Contact Dermatitis 1,* 363.
312. Mitchell, J.C. and Stewart, W.D. (1973): Allergic contact dermatitis from neutral red applied for herpes simplex. *Arch. Dermatol., 108,* 689.

313. Möller, H. (1976): Eczematous contact allergy to oxytetracycline and polymyxin B. *Contact Dermatitis, 2,* 289.
314. Monkton Copeman, P.W. (1968): Toxic epidermal necrolysis caused by skin hypersensitivity to monosulfiram. *Brit. Med. J., i,* 623.
315. Morris. G.E. (1960): Dermatoses from phenylmercuric salts. *Arch. Environm. Health, 1,* 53.
316. Mortensen, T. (1979): Allergy to lanolin. *Contact Dermatitis, 5,* 137.
317. Muston, H.L., Boss. J.M. and Summerly. R. (1977): Dermatitis from Ammonyx LO, constituent of surgical scrub. *Contact Dermatitis, 3,* 347.
318. Nagreh, D.S. (1976): Contact dermatitis from proprietary preparations in Malaysia. *Int. J. Dermatol., 15,* 34.
319. Nakayama, H., Hanaoka, H. and Oshiro, A. (1974): *Allergen Controlled System (ACS),* p. 42. Kanehara Shappan, Tokyo.
320. Nakayama, H., Harada, R. and Toda, M. (1976): Pigmented cosmetic dermatitis. *Int. J. Dermatol., 15,* 673.
321. Hayakawa, R., Matsunaga, K., Suzuki, M., et al. (1987): Is sesamol present in sesame oil? *Contact Dermatitis, 17,* 133–135.
322. Nguyen, L.Q. and Allen, H.B. (1979): Reactions to manganese and cadmium in tattoos. *Cutis, 23,* 71.
323. Nilsson, D.C. (1960): Sources of allergenic gums. *Ann. Allergy, 18,* 518.
324. Norgaard, O. (1977): Pecilocinum-Allergie. *Hautarzt, 25,* 35.
325. North American Contact Dermatitis Group (1973): Epidemiology of contact dermatitis in North America: 1972. *Arch. Dermatol., 108,* 573.
326. Ogier. M. and Duverneuil, G. (1977): Dermitis allergiques à l'aldehyde cinnamique. *Arch. Mal. prof. Med. Trav. Secur. soc., 38,* 835.
327. Oleffe, J.A., Blondeel. A. and De Coninck, A. (1979): Allergy to chlorocresol and propylene glycol in a steroid cream. *Contact Dermatitis, 5,* 53.
328. Opdyke. D. (1976): Inhibition of sensitization induced by certain aldehydes. *Food Cosm. Toxic., 14,* 197.
329. O'Quinn. S.E., Kennedy, B.C. and Isbell, K.H. (1967): Contact photodermatitis due to bithionol and related compounds. *J. Am. Med. Assoc., 199,* 89.
330. Pankok, E. (1964): Uatrogene Kontaktallergie gegen Antimykotika. *Arch. klin. exp. Derm., 219, 555.*
331. Gupta, B.N., Mathur, A.U., Agarwal, C. and Singh, A. (1986): Contact sensitivity to henna. *Contact Dermatitis, 15,* 303–304.
332. Petersen, H.O. (1977): Hypersensitivity to propolis. *Contact Dermatitis. 3,* 278.
333. Pevny. I. and Uhlich, M. (1975): Allergie gegen Bestandteile medizinischer und kosmetischer Externa. *Hautartz, 26,* 252.
334a. Pirilä, V., Kilpiö, O., Olkkonen, A., Pirilä, L. and Siltanen, E. (1969): On the chemical nature of the eczematogens in oil of turpentine. V. *Dermatologica (Basel), 139,* 183.
334b. Pirilä, V. and Kajama. H. (1962): Über Neomycinallergie mit besonderer Berücksichtigung der sich anschlieszenden Gruppenallergie. *Hautartz, 13,* 261.
335. Pirilä. V., Kilpiö, O., Olkkonen, A., Pirilä, L. and Siltanen, E. (1969): On the chemical nature of the eczematogens in oil of turpentine. V. *Dermatologica (Basel), 139,* 183.
336. Pirilä. V. and Rouhunkoski, S. (1959): On sensitisation to neomycin and bacitracin. *Acta derm.-venereol. (Stockh.), 39,* 470.
337. Prater, E., Göring. H.D. and Schubert, H. (1978): Sodium lauryl sulfate in contact allergy. *Contact Dermatitis, 4,* 242.
338. Patruno, C., Auricchio, L., Mozzillo, R. and Brunetti, B. (1990): Allergic contact dermatitis due to tromantadine hydrochloride. *Contact Dermatitis, 22,* 187.
339. Rapaport, M.J. (1980): Sensitization to Abitol. *Contact Dermatitis, 6,* 137.
340. Goh, C.L. and Ng, S.K. (1988): Bullous contact allergy from cinnamon. *Dermatosen, 36,* 186–187.
341. De Groot, A.C. (1986): Contact allergy to EDTA in a topical corticosteroid preparation. *Contact Dermatitis, 15,* 250–252.
342. Perret, C.M. and Happle, R. (1988): Contact allergy to miconazole. *Contact Dermatitis, 19,* 75.
343. Gonçalo, S., Cabral, F. and Gonçalo, M. (1988): Contact sensitivity to oak moss. *Contact Dermatitis, 19,* 355–357.
344. Rietschel, R.L. (1978): Photocontact dermatitis to hydrocortisone. *Contact Dermatitis, 4,* 334.
345. Rives, H. (1956): *Contribution à l'étude des dermatoses profesionnelles provoquées par la chlorpromazine.* Thesis. Lyon.

346. Robin, J. (1978): Contact dermatitis to acetarsol. *Contact Dermatitis, 4,* 309.
347. Revuz, J., Poli, F., Wechsler, J. and Dubertret, L. (1984): Dermite de contact a l'hexamidine. *Ann. Dermatol. Venereol, 111,* 805–810.
348. Shono, M., Hayashi, K. and Sugimoto, R. (1989): Allergic contact dermatitis from croconazole hydrochloride. *Contact Dermatitis, 21,* 225–227.
349. Roed-Petersen, J. (1980): Allergic contact dermatitis from butylacetate. *Contact Dermatitis, 6,* 55.
350. Veronesi, S., de Padova, P., Vanni, D. and Melino, M. (1986): Contact dermatitis to triclosan. *Contact Dermatitis, 15,* 257–258.
351. Flyvholm, M.A. and Menné, T. (1990): Sensitizing risk of butylated hydroxytoluene based on exposure and effect data. *Contact Dermatitis, 23,* 341–345.
352. Raulin, C.H. and Frosch, P.J. (1987): Kontaktallergie auf Clotrimazol und Azidamfenicol. *Dermatosen., 35,* 64–66.
353. Romaguera, C. and Grimalt. F. (1980): Five cases of contact dermatitis from pyrrolnitrin. *Contact Dermatitis, 6,* 352.
354. Balato, N., Lembo, G., Nappa, P. et al. (1985): Contact dermatitis from clotrimazole. *Contact Dermatitis, 12,* 110.
355. Dinu, A., Brandão, M. and Faria, A. (1988): Occupational contact dermatitis from vitamin K3 sodium bisulphite. *Contact Dermatitis, 18,* 170–171.
356. Rorsman, H., Brehmer-Andersson, E., Dahlquist, I., Ehinger, B., Jacobsson, S., Lindt, F. and Rorsman, G. (1969): Tattoo granuloma and uveitis. *Lancet, 2,* 27.
357. Rothenborg, H.W. and Hjorth. N. (1968): Allergy to perfumes from toilet soaps and detergents in patients with dermatitis. *Arch. Dermatol., 97,* 417.
358. Rudolph, R.I. (1975): Allergic contact dermatitis caused by haloprogin. *Arch. Dermatol., 111,* 1487.
359. Rudzki, E. and Baranowska, A. (1974): Contact sensitivity in stasis dermatitis. *Dermatologica (Basel), 148,* 353.
360. Bruze, M., Dahlquist, I. and Gruvberger, B. (1989): Contact allergy to dichlorinated methylisothiazolinone. *Contact Dermatitis, 20,* 219–220.
361. Gonçalo, S., Sousa, I. and Moreno, A. (1984): Contact dermatitis to coal tar. *Contact Dermatitis, 10,* 57–58.
362. Rebandel, P. and Rudzki, E. (1990): Dermatitis caused by epichlorohydrin, oxprenolol hydrochloride and propranolol hydrochloride. *Contact Dermatitis, 23,* 199.
363. Rudzki. E. and Grzywa, Z. (1977): Dermatitis from arnica montana. *Contact Dermatitis, 3,* 281.
364. Kubo, Y., Nonaka, S. and Yoshida, H. (1987): Contact sensitivity to chloramphenicol. *Contact Dermatitis, 17,* 245–247.
365. Fraser-Moodie, A. (1992): Sensitivity to silver in a patient treated with silver sulphadiazine (Flamazine). *Burns, 18,* 74–77.
366. Goh, C.L. and Ng, S.K. (1986): Contact allergy to salicylic acid. *Contact Dermatitis, 14,* 114.
367. Takashima, A., Yamamoto, K., Kimura, S., Takakuwa, Y. and Mizuno, N. (1991): Allergic contact and photocontact dermatitis due to psoralens in patients with psoriasis treated with topical puva. *Br. J. Dermatol., 124,* 47–42.
368. Salo. O.P. and Pirilä, V. (1968): Sensitisation to topical Dequaline. *Contact Dermatitis Newsl., 4,* 66.
369. de Groot, A.C. and Conemans, J.M.H. (1990): Contact allergy to furazolidone. *Contact Dermatitis, 22,* 202–205.
370. Raulin, C. and Frosch, P. (1988): Contact allergy to imidazole antimycotics. *Contact Dermatitis, 18,* 76–80.
371. Samsoën, M., Metz, R., Melchior, E. and Foussereau, J. (1980): Cross-sensitivity between aminoside antibiotics. *Contact Dermatitis, 6,* 141.
372. Sausker. W.F. and Frederick, F.D. (1978): Allergic contact dermatitis secondary to topical nitroglycerin. *J. Am. Med. Assoc., 239,* 1743.
373. Saynisch. F. (1957): Allergische Dermatosen durch beruflichen Kontakt mit Bromcholinbromid und Nitrosomethylharnstoff. *Berufsdermatosen, 5,* 197.
374. Schlossman. M.L. and McCarthy, J.P. (1979): Lanolin and -derivatives chemistry: relationship to allergic contact dermatitis. *Contact Dermatitis, 5,* 65.
375. Schneider, H.G. (1978): Schwefel-allergie. *Hautarzt, 29,* 340.
376. Kabasawa, Y. and Kanzaki, T. (1990): Allergic contact dermatitis from ethyl sebacate. *Contact Dermatitis, 22,* 226.
377. Scholz. A. and von Richter, G. (1977): Zur Allergie gegen Falikain (Propipokainhydrochlorid). *Derm. Mschr., 163,* 966.

378. Valsecchi, R., Rozzoni, M. and Cainelli, T. (1992): Allergy to subcutaneous heparin. *Contact Dermatitis, 26,* 129–130.
379. Dooms-Goossens, A., Bedert, R., Degreef, H. and Vandaele, M. (1990): Airborne allergic contact dermatitis from kitasamysin and midecamycin. *Contact Dermatitis, 23,* 118–119.
380. Guerra, L., Adamo, F., Venturo, N. and Tardio, M. (1991): Contact dermatitis due to rifamycin. *Contact Dermatitis, 25,* 328.
381. Menné, T. and Hjorth, N. (1988): Routine patch testing with paraben esters. *Contact Dermatitis, 19,* 189–191.
382. Schorr, W.F. (1970): Dichlorophene (G-4) allergy. *Arch Dermatol., 102,* 515.
383. Weibel, H., Hansen, J. and Andersen, K.E. (1989): Cross-sensitization pattern in guinea pigs between cinnamaldehyde, cinnamyl alcohol and cinnamic acid. *Acta. Derm. Venereol., 69,* 302–307.
384. Schorr, W.F. (1971): Formaldehyde in shampoo and toiletries. *Contact Dermatitis Newsl., 9,* 220.
385. Speight, E.L. and Lawrence, C.M. (1990): Cinnamic aldehyde 2% pet. is irritant on patch testing. *Contact Dermatitis, 23,* 379–380.
386. Schultheiss, E. (1957): Überempfindlichkeit gegenüber Ionon und Benzylalkohol. *Derm. Mschr., 135,* 629.
387. Schulz, K.H. and Herrmann, W.P. (1955): Allergische Kontaktdermatitis durch Megaphen. *Hautartz, 6,* 542.
388. Schülz, K.H., Schöpf, E. and Wex, O. (1970): Allergische Berufsekzeme durch Ampicillin. *Berufsdermatosen, 18, 132.*
389. Schwank, R. and Jirásek, L. (1952): Skin sensitization due to emetine. *Cs. Derm., 27,* 50.
390. Schwank, R. and Jirásek, L. (1963): Kontaktallergie gegen Chloramphenicol mit besonderer Berücksichtigung der Gruppensensibilisierung. *Hautartz, 14,* 24.
391. Schwarz, K. and Storck, H. (1966): Ekzematöse Sensibilisierung auf Methandrostenolon in Salbenform. *Dermatologica (Basel) 132,* 73.
392. Geier, J., Fuchs, Th. and Ippen, H. (1989): Tätowierungen. *Dermatosen., 37,* 4–12.
393. Sharvill, D. (1965): Reaction to chlorhexidine and cetrimide. *Lancet, i,* 771.
394. Sherman, W.B. and Cooke, R.A. (1950): Dermatitis following the use of pyribenzamine and antistine. *J. Allergy, 21,* 63.
395. Shmunes, E. and Levy. E.J. (1972): Quaternary ammonium compound dermatitis from a deodorant. *Arch. Dermatol., 105,* 91.
396. Sidi, E. and Arouette, J. (1959): Hautallergien durch Azofarbstoffe. *Hautarzt, 10,* 193.
397. Sidi, E. and Dobkevitch-Morrill, S. (1951): The injection and ingestion test in cross-sensitization to the para-group. *J. invest. Dermatol. 15,* 165.
398. Sidi, E., Gervais, A. and Gervais, P. (1962): Les sensibilisations cutanées dans la groupe Streptomycine–neomycine–framycetine. *Acta allerg. (Kbh.), 17,* 529.
399. Sidi, E., Hincky, M. and Gervais, A. (1955): Allergic sensitization and photosensitization to phenergan-cream. *J. invest. Dermatol., 24,* 345.
400. Sidi, E., Melki, G. and Longueville, R. (1952): Dermatitis aux pomades antihistaminiques. *Acta allerg. (Kbh.), 5,* 292.
401. Simeray, M.A. (1966): Action d'un fongicide agricole (orthocide) dans 250 cas de pityriasis versicolor. *Bull. Soc. franc Derm. Syph., 73,* 337.
402. Cusano, F., Capozzi, M. and Errico, G. (1992): Allergic contact dermatitis from coal tar. *Contact Dermatitis, 27,* 51–52.
403. Skinner, L.C. (1949): Contact dermatitis due to phenolphthaleine. *Arch. Dermatol. Syph., 59,* 338.
404. Smeenk, G. and Prins, F.J. (1972): Allergic contact eczema due to chloracetamide. *Dermatologica (Basel), 144,* 108.
405. Sneddon, I.B. and Glew, R.C. (1973): Contact dermatitis due to propanidid in an anesthesist. *Practitioner, 211,* 321.
406. Baes, H. (1991): Contact sensitivity to miconazole with ortho-chloro cross-sensitivity to other imidazoles. *Contact Dermatitis, 24,* 89–93.
407. Starke, J.C. (1967): Photoallergy to Sandalwood Oil. *Arch. Dermatol., 96,* 62.
408. Storrs, F. (1975): Para-chloro-meta-xylenol allergic contact dermatitis in seven individuals. *Contact Dermatitis, 1,* 211.
409. Suhonen, R. (1980): Contact allergy to dodecyl-di-(aminoethyl)glycine (Desimex i). *Contact Dermatitis, 6,* 290.
410. Suurmond, D. (1966): Patch test reactions to phenergancream, promethazine and triethanolamine. *Dermatologica (Basel), l33,* 503.

411. Suzuki, Y. and Ohkido, Y. (1979): Contact dermatitis from hydrazine. *Contact Dermatitis, 5,* 113.
412. Taaffe, A., Knight, A.G. and Marks, R. (1978): Lichenoid tattoo hypersensitivity. *Br. Med. J., 1,* 616.
413. Tarnick, M. (1976): Hautsensibilisierungen gegen Thiosinamin (Aminosin®, Allylthiokarbamid). *Derm. Mschr., 162,* 905.
414. Tas, J. and Weissberg, D. (1958): Allergy to aminophylline. *Acta allerg. (Kbh.), 12,* 39.
415. Meding, B. (1986): Contact allergy to omeprazole. *Contact Dermatitis, 15,* 36.
416. Martinez-Falero, A.A., Gutierrez, M.J.C., Salvador, J.Z. and Diaz-Perez, J.L. (1990): Allergic contact dermatitis from fluocortin butyl. *Contact Dermatitis, 22,* 241–242.
417. Tennstedt, D., Dumont-Fruytier, M. and Lachapelle, J.M. (1978): Occupational allergic contact dermatitis to virginiamycin, an antibiotic used as a food-additive for pigs and poultry. *Contact Dermititis, 4,* 133.
418. Thormann, J. and Kaaber, K. (1978): Contact sensitivity to phenylbutazone ointment (Butazolidine). *Contact Dermatitis, 4,* 235.
419. Tosti, A., Gaddoni, G., Valeri, F. and Bardazzi, F. (1990): Contact allergy to ketoprofen: report of 7 cases. *Contact Dermatitis, 23,* 112–113.
420. Scheuer, B. (1983): Kontaktallergie auf Triäthanolamin. *Hautarzt, 34,* 126–133.
421. Tzanck, A., Sidi, E. and Herbault (1950): Un cas d'intolerance à l'acide para-amino-salicylique. *Bull. Soc. franc. Derm. Syph., 57,* 504.
422. Mozzanica, N. and Pigatto, P.D. (1990): Contact and photocontact allergy to ketoprofen: clinical and experimental study. *Contact Dermatitis, 23,* 336–340.
423. Van der Meer, B.J. (1957): Een geval van contactallergie voor koper en zink. *Ned. T. Geneesk., 101,* 2166.
424. Kubo, Y., Nonaka, S. and Yoshida, H. (1986): Contact sensitivity to unsaponifiable substances in sesame oil. *Contact Dermatitis, 15,* 215–217.
425. Whitmore, S.E. (1992): The importance of proper vehicle selection in the detection of minoxidil sensitivity. *Arch. Dermatol., 128,* 653–656.
426. Van Hecke, E. (1969): Contact allergy to the topical antimycotic Fluoro-4-dichloro-3′-5′-thiocarbanilid. *Dermatologica (Basel), 138,* 480.
427. Van Hecke, E. (1981): Contact sensitivity to vincamine tartrate. *Contact Dermatitis, 7.* 53.
428. Dunkel, F.G., Elsner, P. and Burg, G. (1991): Allergic contact dermatitis from prednicarbate. *Contact Dermatitis, 24,* 59–60.
429. VanHee, J., Ceuterick, A., Dooms, M. and Dooms-Goossens, A. (1980): Etisazole: an animal antifungal agent with skin sensitizing properties in man. *Contact Dermatitis, 6,* 443.
430. Götze, A., Teikemeier, G. and Goerz, G. (1992): Contact dermatitis from etofenamate. *Contact Dermatitis, 26,* 209.
431. Tosti, A., Bardazzi, F. and Piancastelli, E. (1990): Contact dermatitis due to chlorpheniramine maleate in eyedrops. *Contact Dermatitis, 22,* 55.
432. Van Ketel, W.G. (1964): Contact dermatitis from a hydrazine-derivative in a stain remover. Cross sensitization to Apresoline and Isoniazid. *Acta Derm.-Venereol. (Stockh.), 44,* 49.
433. Van Ketel, W.G. (1967): Allergic dermatitis caused by Tineafax ointment. *Dermatologica (Basel), 135,* 121.
434. Van Ketel, W.G. (1973): Allergy to cumarin and cumarin-derivatives. *Contact Dermatitis Newsl., 13,* 355.
435. Held, J.L., Kalb, R.E., Ruszkowski, A.M. and deLeo, V. (1987): Allergic contact dermatitis from bacitracin. *J. Am. Acad. Dermatol., 17,* 592–594.
436. Pevny, I. and Hutzler, D. (1988): Gruppenallergien bzw. Merfachreaktionen bei Patienten mit Allergie gegen Hydroxychinolin-derivate. *Dermatosen, 36,* 91–98.
437. Van Ketel, W.G. (1976): Allergic contact dermatitis from propellants in deodorant sprays in combination with allergy to ethylchloride. *Contact Dermatitis, 2,* 115.
438. Van Ketel, W.G. (1976): Sensitivity to chlorphenoxamine hydrochloride. *Contact Dermatitis, 2,* 121.
439. Van Ketel, W.G. (1976): Immediate- and delayed-type allergy to erythromycin. *Contact Dermatitis, 2,* 363.
440. Van Ketel, W.G. (1978): Allergic contact dermatitis from butylaminobenzoate. *Contact Dermatitis, 4,* 55.
441. Menné, T., Frosch, P.J., Veien, N.K. et al. (1991): Contact sensitization to 5-chloro-2-methyl-4-isothiazolin-3-one and 2-methyl-4-isothiazolin-3-one (MCI/MI). *Contact Dermatitis, 24,* 334–341.
442. Van Ketel, W.G. (1981): Allergy to pramoxine (pramocaine). *Contact Dermatitis, 7,* 49.
443. Cox, N.H. (1988): Contact allergy to clobetasol propionate. *Arch. Dermatol., 124,* 911–913.
444. Melli, M.C., Giogini, S. and Sertoli, A. (1986): Sensitization from contact with ethyl alcohol. *Contact Dermatitis, 14,* 315.

445. Van Scott, E.J. and Yu, R.F. (1974): Antimitotic, antigenic and structural relationships of nitrogen mustard and its homologues. *J. invest. Dermatol., 62,* 378.
446. Veien, N.K., Hattel, T., Justesen, O. and Norholm, A. (1980): Occupational contact dermatitis due to spiramycin and/or tylosin among farmers. *Contact Dermatitis, 6,* 410.
447. Velasco, J.E. and Africk, J.A. (1971): Contact dermatitis to mafenide acetate. *Arch. Dermatol., 103,* 61 .
448. Vermeulen, C.W. and Malten, K.E. (1963): Contacteczeem door 6-alpha-chloorprednison en neomycine. *Ned. T. Geneesk., 107,* 548.
449. Von Richter, G. and Scholz, A. (1970): Kontaktekzem und makulöses Exanthem bei p-Chlorbenzolsulfonyl-glykolsäurenitril-Allergie. *Berufsdermatosen, 18,* 70.
450. Wade, T.R., Jones, H.E. and Artis, W.A. (1979): Irritant and allergic reactions to topically applied Micatin cream. *Contact Dermatitis, 5,* 168.
451. Näher, H. and Frosch, P.J. (1987): Contact dermatitis to thioxolone. *Contact Dermatitis, 17,* 250–251.
452. Steinkjer, B. and Braathen, L.R. (1988): Contact dermatitis from triclosan (Irgasan DP 300). *Contact Dermatitis, 18,* 243–244.
453. Wahlberg, J.E. (1978): Abietic acid and colophony. *Contact Dermatitis, 4,* 55.
454. Wahlberg, J.E. and Boman, A. (1981): Contact sensitivity to quinidine sulfate from occupational exposure. *Contact Dermatitis, 7,* 27.
455. Holdiness, M.R. (1986): Contact dermatitis to antituberculosis drugs. *Contact Dermatitis, 15,* 282–288.
456. Lasthein Andersen, B. and Brandrup, F. (1985): Contact dermatitis from chlorhexidine. *Contact Dermatitis, 13,* 307–309.
457. Raulin, Ch. and Frosch, P.J. (1987): Kontaktallergie auf Clotrimazol und Azidamfenicol. *Dermatosen, 35,* 64–66.
458. White, M.I. (1978): Contact dermatitis from ethylenediamine. *Contact Dermatitis, 4,* 291.
459. Rytler, M., Walther, Th., Süss, E. and Haustein, U.F. (1989): Allergische Reaktionen vom Sofort- und Spättyp nach Prednisolon-Medikation. *Dermatol. Mon. Schr., 175,* 44–48.
460. Wilkinson, D.S. (1970): Durch Dequalinium hervorgerufene Hautnekrosen. *Hautarzt, 21,* 114.
461. Wilkinson, D.S. (1975): Sulphur sensitivity. *Contact Dermatitis, 1,* 58.
462. Schmoll, M. and Hausen, B.M. (1988): Allergic contact dermatitis due to prednisolon-21-trimethyl-acetate. *Z. Hautkr., 63,* 311–313.
463. Wilson, H.T.H. (1958): Streptomycin dermatitis in nurses. *Brit. Med. J., i,* 1378.
464. Wilson, H.T.H. (1966): Dermatitis from anaesthetic ointments. *Practitioner, 197,* 673.
465. Wilson, H.T.H. (1971): Dermatitis from an acridine dye. *Contact Dermatitis Newsl., 9,* 212.
466. Winkelmann, R.K. and Harris, R.B. (1979): Lichenoid delayed hypersensitivity reactions in tattoos. *J. cutan. Path., 6,* 59.
467. Wortmann, F. (1972): Erfahrungen mit dem neuen Antimykotikum Exomycol. *Mykosen, 15,* 295.
468. Fernandez de Corres, L., Bernaola, G., Urrutia, I. and Munoz, D. (1990): Allergic dermatitis from systemic treatment with corticosteroids. *Contact Dermatitis, 22,* 104–106.
469. Yaffe, J., Bierman, W., Cann, M. et al. (1973): Antihistamines in topical preparations. *Pediatrics, 51,* 299.
470. Zackheim, H.S. (1975): Treatment of psoriasis with 6-nicotinamide. *Arch Dermatol., 111,* 880.
471. Zina, G. and Bonu, G. (1967): Contact sensitivity to corticosteroids. *Contact Dermatitis Newsl., 2,* 26.
472. Soesman-Van Waadenoyen Kernekamp, A. and Van Ketel, W.G. (1980): Persistence of patch test reactions to clioquinol (vioform) and cross-sensitization. *Contact Dermatitis, 6,* 455.
473. Tamiya, Y., Matsumura, E. and Sasaki, E. et al. (1989): Allergic contact dermatits due to sulconazole nitrate, streptomycin sulphate and prednisolone valerate acetate. *Skin Research, 31 (suppl.),* 206–211.
474. Schneider, K.W. (1982): Tromantadin-Kontaktallergien. *Therapiewoche, 32,* 5691.
475. Van Ketel, W.G. (1983): Sensitization to cis-3-hexenyl salicylate. *Contact Dermatitis, 9,* 154.
476. Van Heeke, E. and De Vos, L. (1983): Contact sensitivity to enilconazole. *Contact Dermatitis, 9,* 144.
477. Bechgaard, E., Ploug, E. and Hjorth, N. (1985): Contact sensitivity to chlorhexidine? *Contact Dermatitis, 13,* 53–55.
478. Reynolds, N.J. and Harman, R.R.M. (1990): Allergic contact dermatitis from chlorhexidine diacetate in a skin swab. *Contact Dermatitis, 22,* 103–104.
479. Valsecchi, R., Imberti, L. and Cainelli, T. (1990): Nifuratel contact dermatitis. *Contact Dermatitis, 23,* 187.
480. Condé-Salazar, L., Guimaraens, D., Gonzales, M. and Fuente, C. (1991): Occuptational allergic contact dermatitis from opium alkaloids. *Contact Dermatitis, 25,* 202–203.
481. Coskey. R.J. (1983): Contact dermatitis caused by diphenhydramine hydrochloride. *J. Am. Acad. Dermatol., 8,* 204.

5. Allergic contact dermatitis from topical drugs

482. Happle, R., Hausen, B.M. and Wiesner-Menzel, L. (1983): Diphencyprone in the treatment of alopecia areata. *Acta Derm.-venereol (Stockh.) 63,* 49.
483. Nethercott, J.R., Pilger, C., O'Blenis, L. and Roy, A.M. (1983): Contact dermatitis due to cinnamic aldehyde induced in a deodorant manufacturing process. *Contact Dermatitis, 9,* 241.
484. Jung, H.-D. (1983): Beruflich bedingte Kontaktekzeme durch Tylosin (Tylan®). *Derm. Mschr., 169,* 235.
485. Savini, C., Morelli, R., Piancastelli, E. and Restani, S. (1989): Contact dermatitis due to ethoxyquin. *Contact Dermatitis, 21,* 342–343.
486. Foussereau, J., Samsoen, M. and Hecht, M.Th. (1983): Occupational dermatitis to Ampholyt G in hospital personnel. *Contact Dermatitis, 9,* 233.
487. Fregert, S. and Dahlquist, I. (1983): Patch testing with oak moss extract. *Contact Dermatitis, 9,* 227.
488. Lützow-Holm, C. and Rønnevig, J.R. (1988): Allergic contact dermatitis from dibrompropamidine cream. *Contact Dermatitis, 18,* 100–101.
489. Yokoyama, R., Mizuno, E., Takeuchi, M., Abe, M. and Ueda, H. (1991): Contact dermatitis due to clindamycin. *Contact Dermatitis, 25,* 125.
490. Dooms-Goossens, A. and Degreef, H. (1983): Contact allergy to petrolatums. (I). Sensitizing capacity of different brands of yellow and white petrolatums. *Contact Dermatitis, 9,* 175.
491. Dooms-Goossens, A. and Degreef, H. (1983): Contact allergy to petrolatums. (II). Attempts to identify the nature of the allergens. *Contact Dermatitis, 9,* 247.
492. Keilig, W. (1983): Kontaktallergie auf Cetylstearylalkohol (Lanette O) als therapeutisches Problem bei Stauungsdermatitis und Ulcus cruris. *Dermatosen, 31,* 50.
493. De Groot, A.C. and Liem, D.H. (1983): Facial psoriasis caused by contact allergy to linalool and hydroxycitronellal in an after-shave. *Contact Dermatitis, 9,* 230.
494. Verbov, J. (1983): Tylosin dermatitis. *Contact Dermatitis, 9,* 325.
495. Przybilla, B. (1983): Allergic contact dermatitis to tromantadine. *J. Am. Acad. Dermatol., 9,* 165–166.
496. Cusano, F., Capozzi, M. and Errico, G. (1989): Contact dermatitis from dexchlorpheniramine. *Contact Dermatitis, 21,* 340.
497. Van Hecke, E. and Van Brabant, S. (1981): Contact sensitivity to imidazole derivatives. *Contact Dermatitis, 7,* 348.
498. Lawrence, C.M. and Smith, A.G. (1982): Ampliative medicament allergy: concomitant sensitivity to multiple medicaments including yellow soft paraffin, white soft paraffin, gentian violet and Span 20. *Contact Dermatitis, 8,* 240.
499. Austad, J. (1982): Allergic contact dermatitis to sorbitan monooleate (Span 80). *Contact Dermatitis, 8,* 426.
500. Valsecchi, R., Tornaghi, A., Tribbia, G. and Cainelli, T. (1982): Contact dermatitis from econazole. *Contact Dermatitis, 8,* 422.
501. Lombardi, P., Campolmo, P., Spallanzani, P. and Sertoli, A. (1982): Delayed hypersensitivity to erythromycin. *Contact Dermatitis, 8,* 416.
502. Meneghini, C.L., Vena, G.A. and Angelini, G. (1982): Contact dermatitis to scabicides. *Contact Dermatitis, 8,* 285.
503. Condé-Salazar, L., Guimaraens, D., Romero, L., Gonzalez, M. and Yus, S. (1985): Erythema multiforme-like contact dermatitis from lincomycin. *Contact Dermatitis, 12,* 59–60.
504. Menezes Brandào, F. and Foussereau, J. (1982): Contact dermatitis to phenylbutazone–piperazine suppositories (Carudol®) and piperazine–gel (Carudol®). *Contact Dermatitis. 8,* 264.
505. Romaguera, C. and Grimalt, F. (1982): Contact dermatitis from nasal sprays and amyl nitrite. *Contact Dermatitis, 8,* 266.
506. Hardie, R.A., Benton, E.C. and Hunter, J.A.A. (1982): Adverse reactions to paste bandages. *Clin exp. Dermatol., 7,* 135.
507. Nilsson, D.C. (1960): Sources of allergic gums. *Ann. Allergy, 18,* 518.
508. Monteseirin, J. and Conde, J. (1990): Contact eczema from famotidine. *Contact Dermatitis, 22,* 290.
509. Pambor, M. and Hein, K. (1982): Tetramisolhaltiges Anthelminthikum (Nilverm®) als berufliches Ekzematogen in der Viehwirtschaft. *Derm. Mschr., 168.* 314.
510. Kellet, J.K. and Beck, M.H. (1984): Contact sensitivity to chloroquine sulphate. *Contact Dermatitis, 13,* 47.
511. Grandinetti, P.J. and Fowler, J.F. (1990): Simultaneous contact allergy to neomycin, bacitracin and polymyxin. *J. Am. Acad. Dermatol., 23,* 646–647.
512. Fisher, A.A. (1980): The antihistamines. *J. Am. Acad. Dermatol., 3,* 303.

513. Fisher, A.A. (1981): Contact dermatitis: Questions and answers. Part 1. *Cutis, 28,* 610.
514. Tucker, W.F.G. (1983): Contact dermatitis to Eutanol G. *Contact Dermatitis, 9,* 88.
515. Frenzel, U.H. and Gutekunst, A. (1983): Contact dermatitis to isoconazole nitrate. *Contact Dermatitis, 9,* 74.
516. Fisher, A.A. (1982): Topical medicaments which are common sensitizers. *Ann. Allergy, 49,* 97.
517. McGeorge, B.C.L. and Steele, M.C. (1991): Allergic contact dermatitis of the nipple from Roman chamomile ointment. *Contact Dermatitis, 24,* 139–140.
518. Trancik, R.J. and Maibach, H.I. (1982): Propylene glycol: irritation or sensitization? *Contact Dermititis, 8,* 185.
519. Tennstedt, D. and Lachapelle, J.M. (1987): Allergic contact dermatitis to 5-fluorouacil. *Contact Dermatitis, 16,* 279–280.
520. Tosti, A., Vincenzi, C., Bardazzi, F. and Mariani, R. (1990): Allergic contact dermatitis due to povidine–iodine. *Contact Dermatitis, 23,* 197–198.
521. Grimalt, F. and Romaguera, C. (1981): Cutaneous sensitivity to benzidine. *Dermatosen, 29,* 95.
522. Scott, M.J. and Scott, M.J. Jr. (1982): Jojoba oil (Letter to the Editor). *J. Am. Acad. Dermatol., 6.* 545.
523. Le Roy, R., Grosshans, E. and Foussereau, J. (1981): Recherche d'allergie de contact dans 100 cas d'ulcère de jambe. *Dermatosen, 29.* 168.
524. Foussereau, J. (1986): Contact dermatitis from propanocaine. *Contact Dermatitis, 15,* 40.
525. Black, R.J., Dawson, T.A.J. and Strang, W.C. (1990): Contact sensitivity to lignocaine and prilocaine. *Contact Dermatitis, 23,* 117–118.
526. Merk, H., Ebert, L. and Goerz, G. (1982): Allergic contact dermatitis due to the fungicide hexetidine. *Contact Dermatitis, 8,* 216.
527. Audicana, M., Schmidt, R. and Fernandez de Corres, L. (1990): Allergic contact dermatitis from nicotinic acid esters. *Contact Dermatitis, 22,* 60–61.
528. Meneghini, C.L. and Angelini, G. (1982): Contact dermatitis from pyrrolnitrin. *Contact Dermatitis, 8,* 55.
529. Staniforth, P. and Lovell, C.R. (1981): Contact dermatitis related to constituent of an orthopaedic wool. *Brit. Med. J., 283,* 1297.
530. Adams, R.M. (1981): Allergic contact dermatitis due to o-phenylphenol. *Contact Dermatitis, 7,* 332.
531. Santucci, B., Picardo, N. and Cristaudo, A. (1985): Contact dermatitis due to Centelase®. *Contact Dermatitis, 13,* 39.
532. Valsecchi, R., Foiadelli, L. and Cainelli, T. (1981): Contact dermatitis from pyrrolnitrin. *Contact Dermatitis, 7,* 340.
533. Lovell, C.R. and Staniforth, P. (1981): Contact allergy to benzalkonium chloride in plaster of Paris. *Contact Dermatitis, 7,* 343.
534. Fisher, A.A. (1987): Allergic contact dermatitis and conjunctivitis from benzalkonium chloride. *Cutis, 39,* 381–383.
535. Van Hecke, E. and Van Brabandt, S. (1981): Contact sensitivity to imidazole derivatives. *Contact Dermatitis, 7,* 348.
536. Malmkvist Padoan, S., Pettersson, A. and Svensson, A. (1990): Olive oil as a cause of allergy in patients with venous eczema and occupationally. *Contact Dermatitis, 23,* 73–76.
537. Lawrence, C.M. and Smith, A.G. (1981): Ichthammol sensitivity. *Contact Dermatitis, 7,* 335.
538. Roberts, D.L., Summerly, R. and Byrne, J.P.H. (1981): Contact dermatitis due to the constituents of Hibiscrub. *Contact Dermatitis, 7,* 326.
539. Göransson, K. and Lidén, S. (1981): Contact allergy to sorbic acid and Unguentum Merck. *Contact Dermatitis, 7,* 277.
540. Tosti, A., Guerra, L. and Bardazzi, F. (1989): Hyposensitizing therapy with standard antigenic extracts: and important source of thimerosal sensitization. *Contact Dermatitis, 20,* 173–176.
541. Motiuk, K. (1979): Wool wax acids. A review. *J. Am. Oil Chem. Soc., 56,* 91.
542. Motiuk, K. (1979): Wool wax alcohols. A review. *J. Am. Oil Chem. Soc., 56,* 651.
543. Kligman, A.M. (1983): Lanolin allergy: crisis or comedy. *Contact Dermatitis, 9,* 99.
544. Kunze, J., Kaiser, H.J. and Petres, J. (1983): Relevanz einer Jodallergie bei handelsüblichen Polyvidon-Jod-Zubereitungen. Z. *Hautkr., 58,* 255.
545. Storrs, F.J. and Bell, D.E. (1983): Allergic contact dermatitis to 2-bromo-2-nitropropane-1,3-diol in a hydrophilic ointment. *J. Am. Acad. Dermatol., 8,* 157.
546. Bandmann, H.J. and Agathos, M. (1985): Die posttherapeutische Benzoylperoxidkontaktallergie bei Ulcus-cruris-Patienten. *Hautarzt, 36,* 670–674.

547. Haustein, U.F., Tegetmeyer, L. and Ziegler, V. (1985): Allergic and irritant potential of benzoyl peroxide. *Contact Dermatitis, 13,* 252–257.
548. Williams, H.C. and du Vivier, A. (1990): Belladona plaster — not as bella as it seems. *Contact Dermatitis, 23,* 119–120.
549. Nater, J.P. and De Groot, A.C. (1984): Drugs used on the skin and cosmetics. In: *Side Effects of Drugs, Annual 8, Chapter 15,* pp. 151–152. Editor M.N.G. Dukes. Elsevier, Amsterdam.
550. Jensen, O., Petersen, S.H. and Vesterager, L. (1980): Contact sensitization to benzoyl peroxide following topical treatment of chronic leg ulcers. *Contact Dermatitis, 6,* 179.
551. Pecegueiro, M., Brandão, M., Pinto, J. and Conçalo, S. (1987): Contact dermatitis to hirudoid cream. *Contact Dermatitis, 17,* 290–293.
552. Scheuer, B. (1983): Kontaktallergie durch Triäthanolamin. *Hautarzt, 34,* 126.
553. Steltenkamp, R.J., Booman, K.A., Dorsky, J. et al. (1980): Cinnamic alcohol: A survey of consumer patch-test sensitization. *Food Cosmet. Toxicol., 18,* 419.
554. Steltenkamp, R.J., Booman, K.A., Dorsky, J. et al. (1980): Hydroxycitronellal: A survey of consumer patch test sensitization. *Food Cosmet. Toxicol., 18,* 407.
555. De Groot, A.C. and Weyland, J.W. (1988): Kathon CG. A review. *J. Am. Acad. Dermatol., 18,* 350–358.
556. Bruynzeel, D.P., van Ketel, W.G., Young, E., van Joost, Th. and Smeenk, G. (1992): Contact sensitization by alternative topical medicaments containing plant extracts. *Contact Dermatitis, 27,* 278–279.
557. Larsen, W.G. (1983): Allergic contact dermatitis to the fragrance material lilial. *Contact Dermatitis, 9,* 158.
558. Lodi, A., Leuchi, S., Mancini, L., Chiarelli, G. and Crosti, C. (1992): Allergy to castor oil and colophony in a wart remover. *Contact Dermatitis, 26,* 266–267.
559. Van Ketel, W.G. (1982): Allergy to Matricaria chamomilla. *Contact Dermatitis, 8,* 143.
560. Balato, N., Lembo, G., Cusano, F. and Ayala, F. (1983): Contact dermatitis from pyrrolinitrin. *Contact Dermatitis, 9,* 238.
561. Fisher, A.A. (1981): Dermatitis due to the presence of formaldehyde in certain sodium lauryl sulfate (SLS) solutions. *Cutis, 27,* 360.
562. Rycrort, R. (1978): Is Grotan BK a contact sensitizer? *Brit. J. Dermatol., 99,* 346.
563. Dahl, M.G.C. (1981): Patch test concentrations of Grotan BK (letter). *Brit. J. Dermatol., 104,* 607.
564. Frosch, P.J., White, I.R. and Rycroft, R.J.G. et al. (1990): Contact allergy to bronopol. *Contact Dermatitis, 22,* 24–26.
565. Machácková, J. (1988): The incidence of allergy to propolis in 605 consecutive patients patch tested in Prague. *Contact Dermatitis, 18,* 210–212.
566. Hausen, B.M., Kuhlwein, A. and Schulz, K.H. (1982): Kolophonium-Allergie. Part 1 and 2. *Dermatosen Beruf Umw., 30,* 107 and 145.
567. Guin, J.D. and Hamey, P. (1983): Sensitivity to α-amylcinnamic aldehyde and α-amylcinnamic alcohol. *J. Am. Acad. Dermatol., 8,* 76.
568. Möller, H. (1990): Contact and photocontact allergy to psoralens. *Photodermatol. Photoimmunol. Photomed., 7,* 43–44.
569. Epstein, E. (1985): Fluorouracil paste treatment of thin basal cell carcinomas. *Arch. Dermatol., 121,* 207–213.
570. MacDonald, R.H. and Beck, M. (1983): Neomycin: a review with particular reference to dermatological usage. *Clin. exp. Dermatol., 8,* 249.
571. Fisher, A.A. (1983): Topically applied alcohol as a cause of contact dermatitis. *Cutis, 31,* 588.
572. Bernaola, G., Escayol, P., Fernández, E. and Fernández de Corrés, L. (1989): Contact dermatitis from methylionone fragrance. *Contact Dermatitis, 21,* 71–72.
573. Osmundsen, P. (1978): Contact dermatitis due to sodium hypochlorite. *Contact Dermatitis, 4,* 177.
574. Dooms-Goossens, A., Gevers, D., Mertens, A. and Van der Heyden, D. (1983); Allergic contact urticaria due to chloramine. *Contact Dermatitis, 9,* 319.
575. Lazzarini, S. (1982): Contact allergy to benzyl alcohol and isopropyl palmitate, ingredients of topical corticosteroid. *Contact Dermatitis, 8.* 349.
576. Vega, F.A., Halprin, K.M., Taylor, J.R. et al. (1982): Failure of periodic ultraviolet radiation treatments to prevent sensitization to nitrogen mustard: a case report. *Brit. J. Dermatol., 106,* 361.
577. Levene, G.M. and Withers, A.F.D. (1969): Anaphylaxis to streptomycin and hyposensitization (parasensitization). *Trans. St. John's Hosp. Derm. Soc., 55,* 184–188.
578. Landa, N., Aguirre, A., Goday, J., Ratón, J.A. and Diaz-Pérez, J.L. (1990): Allergic contact dermatitis from

a vasoconstrictor cream. *Contact Dermatitis, 22,* 290–291.
579. Pevny, I. and Peter, G. (1983): Allergisches Kontaktekzem auf Pyridin- und Hydrazinderivate. *Dermatosen Beruf Umw., 31,* 78.
580. Senff, H., Engelmann, L., Kunze, J. and Hausen, B.M. (1990): Allergic contact dermatitis from idoxuridine. *Contact Dermatitis, 23,* 43–45.
581. Gattefosse, R.M. (1950): *Formulaire de Parfumerie et de Cosmetologie.* Girardot & Cie, Paris.
582. Neumann, H. (1983): Allergische und toxische Nebenwirkungen von Ethylendiamin. *Allergologie, 6,* 27.
583. Frosch, P.J. and Weickel, R. (1987): Kontaktallergie auf das Konservierungsmittel Bronopol. *Hautarzt, 38,* 267–270.
584. Fisher, A.A. (1980): Cosmetic dermatitis, Part. II. Reactions to some commonly used preservatives. *Cutis, 26,* 136.
585. Jordan, W.P., Sherman, W.T. and King, S.E. (1979): Threshold responses in formaldehyde-sensitive subjects. *J. Am. Acad. Dermatol., 1,* 44.
586. Mandy, S.H. (1974): Contact dermatitis to substituted imidazolidinyl urea, a common preservative in cosmetics. *Arch. Dermatol., 110,* 463.
587. Fisher, A.A. (1980): Cutaneous reactions to sorbic acid and potassium sorbate. *Cutis, 25,* 350, 352, 423.
588. Fisher, A.A. (1982): Contact dermatitis from topical medicaments. *Semin. Dermatol., 1,* 49.
589. Chandraratna, P.A.N. and O'Dell, R.E. (1979): Allergic reactions to nitroglycerin ointment: Report of five cases. *Curr. ther. Res., 25,* 481.
590. Di Prima, T., de Pasquale, R. and Nigro, M. (1988): Contact dermatitis from glutaraldehyde. *Contact Dermatitis, 19,* 219–220.
591. Pecegueiro, M. (1992): Contact dermatitis due to resorcinol in a radiotherapy dye. *Contact Dermatitis, 26,* 273.
592. Addo, H.A., Ferguson, J., Johnson, B.E. and Frain-Bell, W. (1982): The relationship between exposure to fragrance materials and persistent light reaction in the photosensitivity dermatitis with actinic reticuloid syndrome. *Brit. J. Dermatol., 107,* 261.
593. Frain-Bell, W. (1982): Photosensitivity dermatitis and actinic reticuloid. *Semin. Derm., 1,* 161.
594. Eiermann, H.J., Larsen, W., Maibach, H.I. et al. (1982): Prospective study of cosmetic reactions: 1977–1980. *J. Am. Acad. Dermatol., 6.* 909.
595. Larsen, W.G. (1985): Perfume dermatitis. *J. Am. Acad. Dermatol., 12,* 1–9.
596. Lynde, C.W. and Mitchell, J.C. (1982): Patch testing with balsam of Peru and fragrance mix. *Contact Dermatitis, 8,* 274.
597. Veien, N.K., Hattel. T., Justesen. O. and Norholm, A. (1982): Patch testing with perfume mixture. *Acta Derm-venereol. (Stockh.), 62,* 341.
598. Calnan, C.D., Cronin, E. and Rycroft, R.J.G. (1980): Allergy to perfume ingredients. *Contact Dermatitis, 6,* 500.
599. Dooms-Goossens, A. and Dooms, M. (1983): Contact allergy to petrolatums (III). Allergenicity prediction and pharmacopoeial requirements. *Contact Dermatitis, 9,* 352.
600. Tokashima, A. and Yoshikawa, K. (1983): Contact allergy to isothipendyl. *Contact Dermatitis, 9,* 429.
601. Frosch, P.J. and Raulin, C. (1987): Kontaktallergie auf Bufexamac. *Hautarzt, 38,* 331–334.
602. Karlberg, A.-T., Boman, A. and Wahlberg, J.E. (1980): Allergenic potential of abietic acid, colophony and pine resin-HA. *Contact Dermatitis, 6,* 481.
603. Romaguera, C. and Grimalt, F. (1980): Statistical and comparative study of 4600 patients tested in Barcelona (1973–1977). *Contact Dermatitis, 6,* 309.
604. Cronin, E. (1979): Oil of turpentine — a disappearing allergen. *Contact Dermatitis, 5,* 308.
605. Collins, F.W. and Mitchell, J.C. (1975): Aroma chemicals. Reference sources for perfume and flavour ingredients with special reference to cinnamic aldehyde. *Contact Dermatitis, 1,* 43.
606. Sugai, T. and Higashi, J. (1975): Hypersensitivity to hydrogenated lanolin. *Contact Dermatits, 1,* 146.
607. Roed-Petersen, J. and Hjorth, N. (1975): Patch test sensitization from, d,l-alpha-tocopherol (vitamin E). *Contact Dermatitis, 1,* 391.
608. Zackheim, H.S., Epstein, E.H. Jr. and Crain, W.R. (1990): Topical carmustine (BCNU) for cutaneous T cell lymphoma. A 15-year experience in 143 patients. *J. Am. Acad. Dermatol., 22,* 802–810.
609. Thune, P., Solberg, Y., McFadden, N. et al. (1982): Perfume allergy due to oak moss and other lichens. *Contact Dermatitis 8,* 396.
610. Wilkinson, S.M., Cartwright, P.H. and English, J.S.C. (1991): Hydrocortisone; an important cutaneous allergen. *Lancet, 337,* 761–762.

5. Allergic contact dermatitis from topical drugs

611. Feldman, S.B., Sexton, F.M., Buzas, J. and Marks, J.G. (1988): Allergic contact dermatitis from topical steroids. *Contact Dermatitis, 19,* 226–228.
612. Bruning, P.F., Meyer, W.J. and Migeon, C.J. (1979): Glucocorticoid receptor in cultured human skin fibroblasts. *J. Steroid Bioch., 10,* 587.
613. Junghans, C., Kuhlwein, A. and Hausen, B.M. (1986): Mehrfachsensibilisierung gegen topisch angewandte Kortikosteroide. *Dermatosen, 34,* 68–70.
614. Dooms-Goossens, A., Andersen, K.E. and Burrows, D. et al. (1989): A survey of the results of patch tests with tixocortol pivalate. *Contact Dermatitis, 20,* 158.
615. Foussereau, J. and Jelen, G. (1986): Tixocortol pivalate — an allergen closely related to hydrocortisone. *Contact Dermatitis, 15,* 37–38.
616. Church, R. (1960): Sensitivity to hydrocortisone acetate ointment. *Br. J. Dermatol., 72,* 341.
617. Comaish, S. (1969): A case of hypersensitivity to corticosteroids. *Br. J. Dermatol., 81,* 919.
618. Coskey, R.J. (1965): Contact dermatitis due to topical hydrocortisone and prednisone. *Michigan Med., 64,* 669.
619. Dooms-Goossens, A., Degreef, H., Parijs, M. and Kerkhofs, L. (1979): A retrospective study of patch test results from 163 patients with stasis dermatitis or leg ulcers. *Dermatologica (Basel), 159,* 93.
620. Reitamo, S., Lauerma, A.I. and Förström, L. (1989): Detection of contact hypersensitivity to topical corticosteroids with hydrocortisone-17-butyrate. *Contact Dermatitis, 21,* 159–165.
621. Rafanelli, L. (1984): Azione dei corticosteroidi topici. *Chronica Dermatologica, 15*, 73–80.
622. Esser, B. (1983): Beitrag zur Kortisonallergie. Z. *Hautkr., 58,* 29.
623. Guin, J.D. (1984): Contact sensitivity to topical corticosteroids. *J. Am. Acad. Dermatol., 10,* 773–778.
624. Förstrom, L., Lassus, A., Salde, L. and Niemi, K.-M. (1982): Allergic contact eczema from topical corticosteroids. *Contact Dermatitis, 8,* 128.
625. Van Ketel, W.G. (1974): Allergy to Ultralan preparations. *Contact Dermatitis Newsl., 15,* 427.
626. Kooij, R. (1959): Hypersensitivity to hydrocortisone. *Br. J. Dermatol., 71,* 392.
627. Hopf, G. and Mathias, B. (1989): Glukokortikoid-Externa und Kontaktdermatitis. *Münch. Med. Wschr., 131,* 595–599.
628. Kuhlwein, A., Hausen, B.M. and Hoting, E. (1983): Kontaktallergie durch halogenierte Kortikosteroide. *Z. Hautkr., 58,* 796.
629. Malten, K.E. (1973): Betnelan V® lotion contact sensitivity. *Contact Dermatitis Newsl. 13,* 360.
630. Pasricha, J.S. and Gupta, R. (1983): Contact sensitivity to betamethasone 17-valerate and fluocinolone acetonide. *Contact Dermatitis, 9.* 330.
631. Uter, W. (1990): Allergische Reaktionen auf Glukokortikoide. *Dermatosen, 38,* 75–90.
632. Soesman-Van Waadenoijen Kernekamp, A. and Van Ketel, W.G. (1979): Contact allergy to hydrocortisone-17-butyrate. *Contact Dermatitis, 5,* 268.
633. Sasaki, E. (1990): Corticosteroid sensitivity and cross-sensitivity. *Contact Dermatitis, 23,* 306–315.
634. Lazzarini, S. (1983): Contact allergy to benzyl alcohol and isopropyl palmitate, ingredients of topical corticosteroid. *Contact Dermatitis, 8,* 349.
635. Fisher, A.A. (1983): Allergic reactions to topical corticosteroids or their vehicles. *Cutis, 32,* 122.
636. Maibach, H.I. and Conant, M. (1977): Contact urticaria to a corticosteroid cream: polysorbate 60. *Contact Dermatitis, 3,* 350.
637. Fisher, A.A. (1982): Cortaid cream dermatitis and the 'paraben paradox'. *J. Am. Acad. Dermatol., 6,* 116.
638. Fisher, A.A. (1983): Allergic contact dermatitis to penicillin and streptomycin. *Cutis, 32,* 314.
639. Thestrup-Pedersen, K., Christiansen, J.V. and Zachariae, H. (1982): Precautions for personnel applying topical nitrogen mustard to patients with mycosis fungoides. *Dermatologica (Basel), 165,* 108.
640. Van Ketel, W.G. (1983): Contact allergy to different antihaemorrhoidal anaesthetics. *Contact Dermatitis, 9,* 512.
641. Nurse, D.S. and Rosner, S.A. (1983): Contact dermatitis due to lignocaine. *Contact Dermatitis, 9.* 513.
642. Myatt, A.E. and Beck, M.H. (1983): Contact sensitivity to chlorquinaldol. *Contact Dermatitis, 9,* 523.
643. Sai, S. (1983): Lipstick dermatitis caused by ricinoleic acid. *Contact Dermatitis, 9,* 524.
644. Wereide, K., Thune, P. and Hanstad, I. (1983): Contact allergy to xeroform in leg ulcer patients. *Contact Dermatitis, 9,* 525.
645. Angelini, G., Vena, G.A. and Meneghini, C.L. (1985): Allergic contact dermatitis to some medicaments. *Contact Dermatitis, 12,* 263–269.
646. Lindemayr, H. and Drobil, M. Unterschenkelekzem und Kontaktallergie. *Hautarzt, 36,* 227–231.

647. Romaguera, C., Grimalt, F. and Vilaplana, J. (1988): Epidemic of occupational contact dermatitis from ranitidine. *Contact Dermatitis, 18,* 177–178.
648. Jerez, J., Rodriguez, F., Jiménez, J. and Martin-Gil, D. (1987): Cross-reactions between aminoside antibiotics. *Contact Dermatitis, 17,* 325.
649. Senff, H., Tholen, S., Stider, W. et al. (1989): Allergic contact dermatitis to naftifine. Report of two cases. *Dermatologica, 178,* 107–108.
650. Hoting, E., Küchmeister, B. and Hausen, B.M. (1987): Kontaktallergie auf das Antimykotikum Naftifin. *Dermatosen, 35,* 124–127.
651. Veraldi, S. and Schianchi-Veraldi, R. (1991): Allergic contact dermatitis from tolciclate. *Contact Dermatitis, 24,* 315.
652. Lang, E. and Goos, M. (1985): Combined allergy to tolnaftate and nystatin. *Contact Dermatitis, 12,* 182.
653. Buckley, D.B. (1986): Allergic contact dermatitis to bromsalicylchloranilide. *Contact Dermatitis, 14,* 319.
654. Goh, C.L. (1986): Contact sensitivity to proflavine. *Int. J. Dermatol., 25,* 449–451.
655. Bruynzeel, D.P., de Groot, A.C. and Weyland, J.W. (1987): Contact dermatitis to lauryl pyridinium chloride and benzoxonium chloride. *Contact Dermatitis, 17,* 41–42.
656. de Groot, A.C., Conemans, J. and Liem, D.H. (1984): Contact allergy to benzoxonium chloride (Bradophen). *Contact Dermatitis, 11,* 324.
657. de Groot, A.C., Bruynzeel, D.P., Jagtman, B.A. and Weyland, J.W. (1988): Contact allergy to diazolidinyl urea (Germall II®). *Contact Dermatitis, 18,* 202–205.
658. Perret, C.M. and Happle, R. (1989): Contact sensitivity to diazolidinyl urea (Germall II). In: *Current Topics in Contact Dermatitis*, Editors: P.J. Frosch et al. pp. 92–94. Springer Verlag, Berlin.
659. Tosti, A., Restani, S. and Lanzarini, M. (1990): Contact sensitization to diazolidinyl urea: report of 3 cases. *Contact Dermatitis, 22,* 127–128.
660. Fiedler, H.P. (1983): Formaldehyd-Formaldehyd-Abspalter. *Dermatosen, 31,* 187–189.
661. Meynadier, J.M., Meynadier J., Colmas, A. et al. (1982): Allergie aux conservateurs. *Ann. Derm. Venereol, 109,* 1017–1027.
662. Ford, G.P. and Beck, M.H. (1986): Reactions to quaternium 15, bronopol and Germall 115 in a standard series. *Contact Dermatitis, 14,* 271–274.
663. de Groot, A.C., van Joost, Th., Bos, J.D. et al. (1988): Patch test reactivity to DMDM hydantoin. Relationship to formaldehyde allergy. *Contact Dermatitis, 18,* 197–201.
664. Fransway, A.F. (1991): The problem of preservation in the 1990s: I. Statement of the problem. Solution(s) of the industry and the current use of formaldehyde and formaldehyde-releasing biocides. *Am. J. Contact Dermatitis, 2,* 6–23.
665. Vissers-Croughs, K.J.M., van der Kley, A.M.J., Vulto, A.G. and Hulsmans, R.F.H.J. (1988): Allergic contact dermatitis from sodium sulfite. *Contact Dermatitis, 18,* 252–253.
666. Lovell, C.R., White, I.R. and Boyle, J. (1984): Contact dermatitis from phenoxyethanol in aqueous cream BP. *Contact Dermatitis, 11,* 187.
667. Hostynek, J.J., Patrick, E., Younger, B. and Maibach, H.I. (1989): Hypochlorite sensitivity in man. *Contact Dermatitis, 20,* 32–37.
668. Breit, R. and Seifert, P. (1989): Mafenide — still an allergen of importance? In: *Current Topics in Contact Dermatitis*. Editors: P.J. Frosch et al. pp. 222–225. Springer Verlag, Berlin.
669. Hums, R. (1988): Dipicolinsäure — ein Allergen? *Dermatol. Mon. Schr., 174,* 333–338.
670. de Groot, A.C., Bruynzeel, D.P., Coenraads, P.J. et al. (1991): Frequency of allergic reactions to methyldibromoglutaronitrite (1,2-dibromo-2,4-dicyanobutane) in the Netherlands. *Contact Dermatitis, 25,* 260–261.
671. van der Meeren, H.L.M. (1987): Dodecyl gallate, permitted in food, is a strong sensitizer. *Contact Dermatitis, 16,* 260–262.
672. de Groot, A.C. and Herxheimer, A. (1989): Isothiazolinone preservative; cause of a continuing epidemic of contact dermatitis. *Lancet, i,* 314–316.
673. de Groot, A.C. (1990): Methylisothiazolinone/methyl-chloroisothiazolinone (Kathon CG) allergy: an updated review. *Am. J. Contact Dermatitis, 1,* 151–156.
674. de Groot, A.C., Weyland, J.W., Bos, J.D. and Jagtman, B.A. (1986): Contact allergy to preservatives (I). *Contact Dermatitis, 14,* 120–122.
675. de Groot, A.C., Bos, J.D., Jagtman, B.A. et al. (1986): Contact allergy to preservatives (II). *Contact Dermatitis, 15,* 218–222.

676. Bajaj, A.K. and Gupta, S.C. (1986): Contact hypersensitivity to topical antibacterial agents. *Int. J. Dermatol., 25,* 103–105.
677. Ford-Jones, E.L. (1989): Topical antiseptics. *Clinics in Dermatology, 7,* 142–155.
678. Romaguera, C., Grimalt, F. and Vilaplana, J. (1986): Geraniol dermatitis. *Contact Dermatitis, 14,* 185–186.
679. Fisher, A.A. (1990): Perfume dermatitis in children sensitized to balsam of Peru in topical agents. *Cutis, 45,* 21–22.
680. Cardullo, A.C., Ruszkowski, A.M. and deLeo, V.A. (1989): Allergic contact dermatitis resulting from sensitivity to citrus peel, geraniol and citral. *J. Am. Acad. Dermatol., 21,* 395–397.
681. Malten, K.E., van Ketel, W.G., Nater, J.P. and Liem, D.H. (1984): Reactions in selected patients to 22 fragrance materials. *Contact Dermatitis, 11,* 1–10.
682. Enders, F., Przybilla, B. and Ring, J. (1991): Patch testing with fragrance mix and its constituents: discrepancies are largely due to the presence or absence of sorbitan sesquioleate. *Contact Dermatitis, 24,* 238–239.
683. Malanin, G. and Ohela, K. (1989): Allergic reactions to fragrance-mix and its components. *Contact Dermatitis, 21,* 62.
684. Santucci, B., Cristaudo, A., Cannistrad, C. and Picardo, M. (1987): Contact dermatitis to fragrances. *Contact Dermatitis, 16,* 93–95.
685. Curley, R.K., Macfarlane, A.W. and King, C.M. (1986): Contact sensitivity to the amide anesthetics lidocaine, prilocaine and mepivacaine. *Arch. Dermatol., 122,* 924–926.
686. Beck, M.H. and Holden, A. (1988): Benzocaine — an unsatisfactory indicator of topical local anaesthetic sensitization for the U.K. *Br. J. Dermatol., 118,* 91–94.
687. Ruzicka, T., Gerstmeier, M., Przybilla, B. and Ring, J. (1987): Allergy to local anaesthetics: comparison of patch test with prick and intradermal test result. *J. Am. Acad. Dermatol., 16,* 1202–1208. (Also published in *Z. Hautkr. (1987), 62,* 455–460.)
688. Bajaj, A.K., Gupta, S.C., Chatterjee, A.K. and Singh, K.G. (1990): Contact sensitivity to polyethylene glycols. *Contact Dermatitis, 22,* 291–292.
689. Wölbling, R.H. and Rapprich, K. (1985): Zur Verträglichkeit von Lomaherpan® Creme bei der Behandlung des Herpes simplex. *Therapiewoche, 35,* 4057–4058.
690. Daly, B.M. (1987): Bactroban allergy due to polyethylene glycol. *Contact Dermatitis, 17,* 48–49.
691. Kinnunen, T. and Hannuksela, M. (1989): Skin reactions to hexylene glycol. *Contact Dermatitis, 21,* 154–158.
692. Svensson, A. (1988): Allergic contact dermatitis to laureth-4. *Contact Dermatitis, 18,* 113–114.
693. Jones, S.K. and Kennedy, C.T.C. (1988): Contact dermatitis from Emulgin RO/40, an emulsifier in Hioxyl cream. *Contact Dermatitis, 18,* 108–110.
694. Dastychová, E. and Zahejsky, J. (1990): Investigation of undesirable effects of the protective ointment Indulona A/85 in subjects with eczema. *Ceskoslovenská Dermatologie, 65,* 47–50.
695. Dooms-Goossens, A., de Veylder, H., de Boulle, K. and Maertens, M. (1986): Allergic contact dermatitis due to diisopropyl sebacate. *Contact Dermatitis, 15,* 192.
696. Hausen, B.M. and Overbeck, M. (1989): Kontaktallergie auf Hexyllaurat. *Akt. Dermatol., 15,* 328–329.
697. Fujimoto, K., Hashimoto, S., Kuzuka, T. and Yoshikawa, K. (1989): Contact dermatitis due to diisopropanolamine. *Contact Dermatitis, 21,* 56.
698. Schwartz, B.K. and Clendenning, W.E. (1988): Allergic contact dermatitis from hydroxypropyl cellulose in a transdermal estradiol patch. *Contact Dermatitis, 18,* 106–107.
699. Dooms-Goossens, A., Deveylder, H., Gidi de Alam, A., Lachapelle, J.M., Tennstedt, D. and Degreef, H. (1989): Contact sensitivity to nonoxynols as a cause of intolerance to antiseptic preparations. *J. Am. Acad. Dermatol., 21,* 723–727.
700. Hausen, B.M., Krueger, A., Mohnert, J., Hahn, H. and König, W.A. (1989): Contact allergy due to colophony (III). Sensitizing potency of resin acids and some related products. *Contact Dermatitis, 20,* 41–50.
701. Karlberg, A.-T. (1988): Contact allergy to colophony. Chemical identification of allergens, sensitization experiments and clinical experiences. *Acta. Derm. Venereol, suppl. 139,* 1–43.
702. Karlberg, A.-T., Boman, A. and Nilsson, L.G. (1988): Hydrogenation reduces the allergenicity of colophony (rosin). *Contact Dermatitis, 19,* 22–29.
703. Karlberg, A.-T., Gäfuert, E., Hagelthorn, G. and Nilsson, J.L.G. (1990): Maleopimaric acid — a potent sensitizer in modified rosin. *Contact Dermatitis, 22,* 193–201.

704. Karlberg, A.-T., Bergstedt, E., Boman, A. et al. (1985): Is abietic acid the allergenic component of colophony? *Contact Dermatitis, 13,* 209–215.
705. Karlberg, A.-T., Boman, A., Hacksell, U., Jacobsson, S. and Nilsson, J.L.G. (1988): Contact allergy to dehydroabietic acid derivatives isolated from Portuguese colophony. *Contact Dermatitis, 19,* 166–174.
706. Hausen, B.M. and Mohnert, J. (1989): Contact allergy due to colophony (V). Patch test results with different types of colophony and modified colophony products. *Contact Dermatitis, 20,* 295–301.
707. Coopman, S., Degreef, H. and Dooms-Goossens, A. (1989): Identification of cross-reaction patterns in allergic contact dermatitis from topical corticosteroids. *Br. J. Dermatol., 121,* 27–32.
708. Dooms-Goossens, A. and Morren, M. (1992): Results of routine patch testing with corticosteroid series in 2073 patients. *Contact Dermatitis, 26,* 182–191.
709. Lauerma, A.I. (1991): Screening for corticosteroid contact sensitivity. Comparison of tixocortol pivalate, hydrocortisone-17-butyrate and hydrocortisone. *Contact Dermatitis, 24,* 123–130.
710. Wilkinson, S.M., Cartwright, P.A. and English, J.S.C. (1991): Hydrocortisone: and important cutaneous allergen. *Lancet, 337,* 761–762.
711. Dooms-Goossens, A. (1990): Contact dermatitis to topical corticosteroids: diagnostic problems. In: Menné, T., Maibach, H.I., Eds: Exogenous dermatoses: environmental dermatitis. Boca Raton: *CRC Press,* 299–310.
712. Dooms-Goossens, A., Degreef, H.J., Marien, K.J. and Coopman, S.A. (1989): Contact allergy to corticosteroids: A frequently missed diagnosis? *J. Am. Acad. Dermatol., 21,* 538–543.
713. Condé-Salazar, L., Guimaraens, D., Romero, L.V. and Gonzalez, M.A. (1986): Occuptational dermatitis from cephalosporins. *Contact Dermatitis, 14,* 70–71.
714. Puig, L.L., Abadias, M. and Alomar, A. (1989): Erythroderma due to ribostamycin. *Contact Dermatitis, 21,* 79–82.
715. Menéndez Ramos, F., Martin, R.L., Olivo, Z., Bris, J.D. and Luque, V. (1990): Allergic contact dermatitis from tobramycin. *Contact Dermatitis, 22,* 305–306.
716. Rudzki, E., Zakrzewski, Z., Rebandel, P., Grzywa, Z. and Hudymowicz, W. (1989): Sensitivity to amikacin. *Contact Dermatitis, 20,* 391.
717. Degreef, H. and Dooms-Goossens, A. (1985): Patch testing with silver sulfadiazine cream. *Contact Dermatitis, 12,* 33–37.
718. Rudzki, E., Zakrzewski, Z., Rebandel, P., Grzywa, Z. and Hudymowicz, W. (1988): Cross reactions between aminoglycoside antibiotics. *Contact Dermatitis, 18,* 314–316.
719. Rudzki, E. and Rebandel, P. (1984): Contact sensitivity to antibiotics. *Contact Dermatitis, 11,* 41–42.
720. Finkelstein, H., Champion, M.C. and Adam, J.E. (1987): Cutaneous hypersensitivity to vitamin K1 injection. *J. Am. Acad. Dermatol., 16,* 540–545.
721. Molinini, R. (1991): Contact allergy to Ibuproxam. *Contact Dermatitis, 24,* 302–303.
722. Veronesi, S., de Padova, M.P., Bardazzi, F. and Melino, M. (1986): Contact dermatitis to ibuprofen. *Contact Dermatitis, 15,* 103–104.
723. Kubo, K., Shirai, K., Akaeda, T. and Oguchi, M. (1988): Contact dermatitis from ibuprofen piconol. *Contact Dermatitis, 18,* 188–189.
724. Beller, U. and Kaufmann, R. (1987): Contact dermatitis to indomethacin. *Contact Dermatitis, 17,* 121–122.
725. Figueiredo, A., Gonçalo, S. and Freitas, J.D. (1985): Contact sensitivity to pyrazolone compounds. *Contact Dermatitis, 13,* 271.
726. Bris, J.M.D., Montanes, M.A., Candela, M.S. and Diez, A.G. (1992): Contact sensitivity to pyrazinobutazone (Carudol) with positive oral provocation test. *Contact Dermatitis, 26,* 355–356.
727. Schuler, T.M. and Frosch, P.J. (1988): Kontaktallergie auf Propolis (Bienen-Kittharz). *Hautarzt, 39,* 139–142.
728. Hausen, B.M., Wollenweber, E., Senff, H. and Post, B. (1987): Propolis allergy. (I). Origin, properties, usage and literature review. *Contact Dermatitis, 17,* 163–170.
729. Hausen, B.M. and Wollenweber, E. (1988): Propolis allergy. (III). Sensitization studies with minor constituents. *Contact Dermatitis, 19,* 296–303.
730. Ginanneschi, M., Acciai, M.C., Bracci, S. and Sertoli, A. (1991): Studies on propolis components — synthesis and haptenic activity of 1,1-dimethyl allyl ester of caffeic acid and of its *o*-methyl derivatives. A qualitative approach to structure activity relationship. *Am. J. Contact Dermatitis, 2,* 60–64.
731. Schmidt, R.J. and Fernández de Corrés, L. (1987): Allergic contact dermatitis from proprietary topical analgesic sprays containing 3-(aminomethyl)-pyridylsalicylate. *Dermatologica, 174,* 272–279.

732. van Ketel, W.G. (1984): Sensitization to hydroquinone and the monobenzyl ether of hydroquinone. *Contact Dermatitis, 10,* 253.
733. Degreef, H., Bonamie, A., van der Heyden, D. and Dooms-Goossens, A. (1984): Mephenesin contact dermatitis with erythema multiforme features. *Contact Dermatitis, 10,* 220–223.
734. de Groot, A.C. and Conemans, J. (1987): Chloral hydrate. The contact allergen that fell asleep. *Contact Dermatitis, 16,* 229–231.
735. Bordalo, O. and Brandão, F.M. (1991): Contact allergy to palmitoyl collagenic acid in an anti-keloid cream. *Contact Dermatitis, 24,* 316–317.
736. Shehade, S.A. and Foulds, I.S. (1986): Allergic contact dermatitis to Brilliant Green. *Contact Dermatitis, 14,* 186–187.
737. Lombardi, P., Gola, M., Acciai, M.C. and Sertoli, A. (1989): Unusual occuptational allergic contact dermatitis in a nurse. *Contact Dermatitis, 20,* 302–303.
738. Fisher, A.A. (1989): Allergic contact dermatitis due to thymol in Listerine® for treatment of paronychia. *Cutis, 43,* 531–532.
739. Lo, J.S., Taylor, J.S. and Oriba, H. (1990): Occupational allergic contact dermatitis to airborne nitrofurazone. *Dermatologic Clinics, 8,* 165–168.
740. Smeenk G., Kerckhoffs, H.P.M. and Schreurs, P.H.M. (1987): Contact allergy to a reaction product in Hirudoid® cream: an example of compound allergy. *Br. J. Dermatol., 116,* 223–231.
741. Tomb, R.R. (1991): Allergic contact dermatitis from eosin. *Contact Dermatitis, 24,* 27–29.
742. Klein, G.F., Sepp, N. and Fritsch, P. (1991): Allergic reactions to benzalkonium chloride? Do the use test. *Contact Dermatitis, 25,* 269–270.
743. Pecegueiro, M., Brandão, M., Pinto, J. and Conçalo, S. (1987): Contact dermatitis to Hirudoid® cream. *Contact Dermatitis, 17,* 290–293.
744. Dejobert, Y., Martin, P., Thomas, P. and Bergoend, H. (1991): Contact dermatitis from topical leech extract. *Contact Dermatitis, 24,* 366–367.
745. Fransway, A.F. (1991): The problem of preservation in the 1990s: II. Agents with preservative function independent of formaldehyde release. *Am. J. Contact Dermatitis, 2,* 145–174.
746. Fisher, A.A. (1989): Reactions to injectable local anaesthetics part IV: reactions to sulfites in local anaesthetics. *Cutis, 44,* 283–284.
747. Fisher, A.A. (1989): Reactions to sulfites in foods: delayed eczematous and immediate urticarial, anaphylactoid and asthmatic reactions. Part III. *Cutis, 44,* 187–188.
748. Nethercott, J.R. and Holness, D.L. and Page, E. (1988): Occupational contact dermatitis due to glutaraldehyde in health care workers. *Contact Dermatitis, 18,* 193–196.
749. Serrano, G., Bonillo, J., Aliaga, A. et al. (1990): Piroxicam induced photosensitivity and contact sensitivity to thiosalicylic acid. *J. Am. Acad. Dermatol., 23,* 479–483.
750. Aberer, W., Reiter, E., Ziegler, V. and Gailhofer, G. (1991): The importance of including thimerosal and increasingly frequent allergen in Europe, in standard screening series for allergic contact dermatitis. *Am. J. Contact Dermatitis, 2,* 110–112.
751. Rudzki, E. and Grzywa, Z. (1985): The value of a mixture of cassia and citronella oils for detection of hypersensitivity to essential oils. *Dermatosen, 33,* 59–62.
752. Wilkinson, J.D., Andersen, K.E., Lahti, A., Rycroft, R.J.G., Shaw, S. and White, I.R. (1990): Preliminary patch testing with 25% and 15% 'caine'-mixes. *Contact Dermatitis, 20,* 244–245.
753. Ishiguro, N. and Kawashima, M. (1991): Contact dermatitis from impurities in alcohol. *Contact Dermatitis, 25,* 257.
754. Panneck, W.B. (1990): Kontaktallergie auf Unguentum leniens. *Allergologie, 13,* 183–184.
755. Fan, W., Kinnunen, T., Niinimäki, A. and Hannuksela, M. (1991): Skin reactions to glycols used in dermatological and cosmetic vehicles. *Am. J. Contact Dermatitis, 2,* 181–183.
756. Aberer, W. and Zonzits, E. (1989): Allergy to ethyl chloride does occur and might frequently be misdiagnosed. *Contact Dermatitis, 21,* 352–353.
757. Tosti, A., Bardazzi, F. and Ghetti, P. (1988): Unusual complication of sensitizing therapy for alopecia areata. *Contact Dermatitis, 18,* 322.
758. Jones, S.K. and Kennedy, C.T. (1988): Contact dermatitis from triethanolamine in E45 cream. *Contact Dermatitis, 19,* 230.
759. Goh, C.L. (1989): Contact sensitivity to topical medicaments. *Int. J. Dermatol., 28,* 25–28.
760. Mitchell, D.M., Ganpule, M.T. and Beck, M.H. (1987): Contact sensitivity to silicic acid in Unguentum Merck. *Contact Dermatitis, 16,* 178.

761. Mahaur, B.S., Sharma, V.K., Kumar, B. and Kaur, S. (1987): Prevalence of contact hypersensitivity to common antiseptics, antibacterials and antifungals in normal persons. *Indian J. Dermatol. Venereol. Leprol., 53,* 269–272.
762. Mehringer, A., Hartmann, A.A., Pevny, I. and Burg, G. (1990): Fünf Fälle einer Kontaktallergie durch Naftifin (Exoderil®). *Akt. Dermatol., 16,* 193–195. (letter: p. 326)
763. Diprima, T.M., de Pasquale, R. and Nigro, M.A. (1990): Connubial contact dermatitis from nifuratel. *Contact Dermatitis, 22,* 117–118.
764. Wilkinson, S.M. and English, J.S.C. (1991): Hydrocortisone sensitivity. An investigation into the nature of the allergen. *Contact Dermatitis, 25,* 178–181.
765. Dunkel, F.G., Elsner, P. and Burg, G. (1991): Contact allergies to topical corticosteroids: 10 cases of contact dermatitis. *Contact Dermatitis, 25,* 97–103.
766. Senff, H., Kunz, R., Köllner, A. and Kunze, J. (1991): Allergische Kontaktdermatitis gegen Prednicarbat. *Hautarzt, 42,* 53–55.
767. Camarasa, J.G. (1990): Analgesic spray contact dermatitis. *Dermatologic Clinics, 8,* 137–138.
768. Hogan, D.J. and Maibach, H.I. (1990): Adverse reactions to transdermal dermatologic drug delivery systems. *J. Am. Acad. Dermatol., 22,* 811–814.
769. Holdiness, M.R. (1989): A review of contact dermatitis associated with transdermal therapeutic systems. *Contact Dermatitis, 20,* 3–9.
770. Maibach, H.I. (1987): Oral substitution in patients sensitized by transdermal clonidine treatment. *Contact Dermatitis, 16,* 1–8.
771. McBurney, E.I., Noel, S.B. and Collins, J.H. (1989): Contact dermatitis to transdermal estradiol system. *J. Am. Acad. Dermatol., 20,* 508–510.
772. Gordon, C.R., Shupak, A, Doweck, I. and Spitzer, O. (1989): Allergic contact dermatitis caused by transdermal hyoscine. *Brit. Med. J., 298,* 1220–1221.
773. Eichelberg, D., Stolze, P., Block, M. and Buchkremer, G. (1989): Contact allergies induced by TTS-treatment. *Meth. Find. Exp. Clin. Pharmacol, 11,* 223–225.
774. Okamoto, H. and Kawai, S. (1991): Allergic contact sensitivity to mydriatic agents on a nurse's fingers. *Cutis, 47,* 357–358.
775. Pecegueiro, M. (1990): Occupational contact dermatitis from penicillin. *Contact Dermatitis, 23,* 190–191.
776. Lucker, G.P.H., Hulsmans, R.F.H.J., van der Kley, A.M.J. and van de Staak, W.J.B.M. (1992): Evaluation of the frequency of contact allergic reactions to Kathon CG in the Maastricht area — 1987–1990. *Dermatology, 184,* 90–93.
777. Fuchs, Th., Enders, F., Przybilla, B. et al. (1991): Contact allergy to Euxyl K400. *Dermatosen, 39,* 151–153.
778. Torres, V. and Soares, A.P. (1992): Contact allergy to dibromodicyanobutane in a cosmetic cream. *Contact Dermatitis, 27,* 114–115.
779. Marston, S. (1992): Propyl gallate on liposomes. *Contact Dermatitis, 27,* 74–76.
780. Fylvholm, M.A. and Menné, T. (1992): Allergic contact dermatitis from formaldehyde. *Contact Dermatitis, 27,* 27–36.
781. Garcia-Bravo, B. and Mozo, P. (1992): Generalized contact dermatitis from vitamin E. *Contact Dermatitis, 26,* 280.
782. Hausen, B.M. and Kunze, B. (1991): Kontaktallergie auf Patchouli-Öl. *Akt. Dermatol., 17,* 199–202.
783. Bojs, G., Bruze, M. and Svensson, A. (1992): Contact allergy to the lanolin derivative Amerchol CAB. *Am. J. Contact Dermatitis, 3,* 83–85.
784. Lohfink, H.D. (1992): Langzeitbeobachtungen bei Unterschenkelekzem — Patienten mit Allergie gegen Salbengrundlagen und Kosmetika. *Phlebologie, 21,* 31–34.
785. Carmichael, A.J., Foulds, I.S. and Bransbury, D.S. (1991): Loss of lanolin patch test positivity. *Br. J. Dermatol., 125,* 573–576.
786. Gette, M.T., Marks, J.G. and Maloney, M.E. (1992): Frequency of postoperative allergic contact dermatitis to topical antibiotics. *Arch. Dermatol., 128,* 365–367.
787. Møller, N.E. and von Würden, U. (1992): Hypersensitivity to semisynthetic penicillins and cross reactivity with penicillin. *Contact Dermatitis, 26,* 351–352.
788. Machet, L., Vaillant, L., Muller, C., Cochelin, N. and Lorette, G. (1992): Contact dermatitis and cross sensitivity from sulconazole nitrate. *Contact Dermatitis, 26,* 352–353.
789. Stubbs, S., Heikkilä, H., Reitamo, S. and Förström, L. (1992): Contact allergy to tioconazole. *Contact Dermatitis, 26,* 155–158.

5. Allergic contact dermatitis from topical drugs

790. Hausen, B.M. and Angel, M. (1992): Studies on the sensitizing capacity of imidazole and triazole derivatives Part II. *Am. J. Contact Dermatitis, 3,* 95–101.
791. Hausen, B.M., Heesch, B. and Kiel, U. (1990): Studies on the sensitizing capacity of imidazole derivatives. *Am. J. Contact Dermatitis, 1,* 25–33.
792. Lauerma, A.I. (1992): Contact hypersensitivity to glucorticosteroids. *Am. J. Contact Dermatitis, 3,* 112–132.
793. Dooms-Goossens, A., Pauwels, M., Bourda, A., Degreef, H. and Kinget, R. (1992): Patch testing with corticosteroids in xerogel formulations. *Contact Dermatitis, 26,* 206.
794. Schoenmakers, A., Vermorken, A., Degreef, H. and Dooms-Goossens, A. (1992): Corticosteroid or steroid allergy? *Contact Dermatitis, 26,* 159–162.
795. Wilkinson, S.M. and English, J.S.C. (1992): Patch tests are poor detectors of corticosteroid allergy. *Contact Dermatitis, 26,* 67–68.
796. Wilkinson, S.M., Heagerty, A.H.M. and English, J.S.C. (1992): A prospective study into the value of patch and intradermal tests in identifying topical corticosteroid allergy. *Br. J. Dermatol., 127,* 22–25.
797. Di Landro, A., Valsecchi, R. and Cainelli, T. (1992): Contact allergy to dithranol. *Contact Dermatitis, 26,* 49–50.
798. Hausen, B.M., Evers, P., Stüwe, H.T., König, W.A. and Wollenweber, E. (1992): Propolis allergy (IV). *Contact Dermatitis, 26,* 34–44.
799. Schiavino, D., Papa, G., Nucera, E. et al. (1992): Delayed allergy to diclofenac. *Contact Dermatitis, 26,* 357–358.
800. Pasricha, J.S. and Parmar, K.A. (1991): Contact dermatitis due to hydroquinone. *Indian J. Dermatol. Venereol. Leprol., 57,* 194.
801. Green, C. and Lowe, J.G. (1992): Contact allergy to piroxicam gel. *Contact Dermatitis, 27,* 261–262.
802. Fernández, J.C., Gamboa, P., Jáuregui, I., González, G. and Antépara, I. (1992): Concomitant sensitization to enoxolone and mafenide in a topical medicament. *Contact Dermatitis, 27,* 262.
803. Izu, R., Aguirre, A., Irazabal, B., Goday, J. and Diaz-Perez, J.L. (1992): Allergic contact dermatitis from fepradinol. *Contact Dermatitis, 27,* 266–267.
804. Santucci, B., Cannistraci, C., Cristaudo, A. and Picardo, M. (1992): Contact dermatitis from ketoconazole cream. *Contact Dermatitis, 27,* 274–275.
805. Burden, A.D. and Beck, M.H. (1992): Contact hypersensitivity to topical corticosteroids. *Br. J. Dermatol., 127,* 497–500.
806. Nakagawa, M., Kawai, K. and Kawai, K. (1992): Cross sensitivity between resorcinol monobenzoate and phenyl salicylate. *Contact Dermatitis, 27,* 199–200.
807. Santacci, B., Cannistraci, C., Cristaudo, A. and Picardo, M. (1992): Contact dermatitis from topical alkylamines. *Contact Dermatitis, 27,* 200–201.
808. Pigatto, P.D., Mozzanica, N., Legori, A. et al. (1992): Topical NSAID allergic contact dermatitis. Italian Experience. *Abstract Book 1st Congress European Society of Contact Dermatitis, Brussels,* page 24.
809. Tennstedt, D. and Lachapelle, J.M. (1992): Patch testing and oral challenge with acyclovir. *Abstract Book 1st Congress European Society of Contact Dermatitis, Brussels,* page 26.
810. Hausen, B.M. and Beyer, W. (1992): The sensitizing capacity of the antioxidants propyl, octyl and dodecyl gallate and some related gallic acid esters. *Contact Dermatitis, 26,* 253–258.
811. de Groot, A.C., Liem, D.H., Nater, J.P. and van Ketel, W.G. (1985): Patch tests with fragrance materials and preservatives. *Contact Dermatitis, 12,* 87–92.
812. Zacher, K.D. and Ippen, H. (1984): Kontaktekzem durch Bergamottöl. *Dermatosen, 32,* 95–97.
813. Vilaplana, J., Romaguera, C. and Grimalt, F. (1991): Contact dermatitis from geraniol in Bulgarian rose oil. *Contact Dermatitis, 24,* 301.
814. Oxholm, A., Heidenheim, M., Larsen, E., Batsberg, W. and Menné, T. (1990): Extraction and patch testing of methylcinnamate, a newly recognised fraction of Balsam of Peru. *Am. J. Contact Dermatitis, 1,* 43–46.
815. Ranchoff, R.E., Steck, W.D., Taylor, J.S. and Evey, P. (1986): Electrocardiograph electrode and hand dermatitis from parachlorometaxylenol. *J. Am. Acad. Dermatol., 15,* 348–350.
816. Aberer, W. (1991): Local anaesthetics with ethyl chloride freezing: problems despite proper application. *Br. J. Dermatol., 124,* 113.
817. Goitre, M., Bedello, P.G., Cane, D. et al. (1986): Contact dermatitis due to cyclopyroxolamine. *Contact Dermatitis, 15,* 94–95.
818. Wilkinson, S.M. and English, J.S.C. (1992): Hydrocortisone sensitivity: clinical features of fifty-nine cases. *J. Am. Acad. Dermatol., 27,* 683–687.

819. Bircher, A.J., Flückiger, R. and Buchner, S.A. (1990): Eczematous infiltrated plaques to subcutaneous heparin: a type IV allergic reaction. *Br. J. Dermatol., 123,* 507–514.
820. O'Driscoll, J.B.O., Beck, M.B., Kesseler, M.E. and Ford, G. (1991): Contact sensitivity to aluminium acetate eardrops. *Contact Dermatitis, 24,* 156–157.
821. Foussereau, J. and Tomb, R.R. (1987): Cross-allergy between 5-iodo-2′-deoxycytidine and idoxuridine. *J. Am. Acad. Dermatol., 17,* 145–147.
822. Goh, C.L. and Ng, S.K. (1985): Photallergic contact dermatitis to carbimazole. *Contact Dermatitis, 12,* 58–59.
823. Sugawara, M., Nakayawa, H. and Watanabe, S. (1990): Contact hypersensitivity to ylang-ylang oil. *Contact Dermatitis, 23,* 248–249.
824. Izu, R., Aguirre, A., Gil, N. and Díaz-Pérez, J.L. (1992): Allergic contact dermatitis from a cream containing centella asatica extract. *Contact Dermatitis, 26,* 192.
825. Klein, A.D. and Penneys, N.S. (1988): Aloe vera. *J. Am. Acad. Dermatol., 18,* 714–720.
826. Kwahck, H., Lee, H.S. and Hann, S.K. (1991): A case of allergic contact dermatitis to Aloe Vera. *Kor. J. Dermatol., 29,* 518–521.
827. Grimm, I. (1991): Kontaktallergie auf einen Thuja-occidentalis-Extrakt. *Allergologie, 14,* 272–274.
828. de Groot, A.C. and Weyland, J.W. (1992): Systemic contact dermatitis from tea tree oil. *Contact Dermatitis, 27,* 279–280.
829. Schallreuter, K.U. and Gupta, M.A. (1987): Allergic contact dermatitis from tetrachlordecaoxide (Oxoferin®). *Contact Dermatitis, 17,* 253–254.

6. Phototoxic and photoallergic contact dermatitis

6.1 Photosensitivity is the term used to describe abnormal or adverse cutaneous reactions to light energy. The broad spectrum of clinical photosensitivity reactions has been classified as follows [24]:

Classification of Photosensitivity Diseases [24]

Type	Disease
Genetic and metabolic	Xeroderma pigmentosum
	Erythropoietic protoporphyria
	Erythropoietic porphyria
	Erythropoietic coproporphyria
	Porphyria cutanea tarda
	Albinism
	Pellagra
	Kwashiorkor
	Hartnup disease
Phototoxic and photoimmunologic	Phototoxic
	Internal (drugs)
	External (drugs, plants, fruits)
	Photoallergic
	Solar urticaria (immediate hypersensitivity)
	"Drug" photoallergy (delayed hypersensitivity)
	Langerhans' cell alteration (delayed hypersensitivity depression)
Degenerative and neoplastic	Actinic keratosis
	Squamous-cell carcinoma
	Malignant melanoma
	Basal-cell epithelioma
Idiopathic	Polymorphous light eruption
	Hydroa aestivale
	Hydroa vacciniforme
	Actinic reticuloid
	Actinic prurigo

(continued)

§ **6.1** *(continuation)*

Type	Disease
Photoaggravated	Discoid lupus erythematosus Systemic lupus erythematosus Dermatomyositis Herpes simplex Darier's disease Bloom's disease Acne vulgaris Atopic dermatitis Disseminated superficial actinic porokeratoses Hartnup disease Lichen planus actinicus Pellagra Pemphigus foliaceus Transient acantholytic dermatosis

Drug-induced photosensitivity refers to adverse cutaneous responses which follow the combined or successive exposure to certain chemicals (photosensitizers) and light. A subdivision can be made into phototoxic and photoallergic reactions. Phototoxicity is the common response which will occur in everybody if enough light energy of the proper wave lengths and, in the case of a photosensitized system, enough of the photosensitizer, is present in the skin. Thus, phototoxicity can be likened to a primary irritant response [91]. Photoallergy can be defined as an acquired altered photoreactivity dependent on an antigen-antibody or cell-mediated hypersensitivity state.

6.2 Adverse responses due to the presence of a photosensitizer

The photosensitizers comprise:
A. Endogenous photosensitizers; which play a role in some of the porphyrias.
B. Exogenous photosensitizers; which are subdivided into:
 1. *Topical photosensitizers* (see § 6.5).
 2. *Systemic photosensitizers*. Well-known systemic photosensitizers are sulfonamides, sulfonylurea derivatives, chlorothiazides, phenothiazines, tetracyclines, griseofulvin, nalidixic acid and furocoumarins (see also Chapter 18 on Photochemotherapy). Recently, several NSAIDs (non-steroidal anti-inflammatory drugs) such as piroxicam, naproxen and carprofen and quinolone antibiotics (e.g. ciprofloxacin, enoxacin, norfloxacin, ofloxacin) have been responsible for many cases of photosensitivity. Drugs that have caused photosensitivity reactions are listed in Table 6.2, together with the mechanism responsible (phototoxic and/or photoallergic), if elucidated. It must be stressed, however, that there is often uncertainty and sometimes controversy about the mechanisms involved.

Table 6.2. Systemic photosensitizers [25,74,93,97–99,144,145]

Drug Name	Mechanism	
Psychopharmaca, hypnotics, antiepileptics		
Amitriptyline	PA ?	
Barbiturates	PA ?	
Carbamazepine	PA	[158]
Chlordiazepoxide	PA	
Chlorprothixene	PA	
Clomipramine	PA	[147]
Desipramine	?	
Diazepam	?	
Dothiepin	?	
Haloperidol	?	
Imipramine	PA	
Maprotiline	?	
Meprobamate	?	
Methylphenidate	?	
Nortriptyline	PA	
Phenothiazines	PT & PA	
– Chlorpromazine		
– Levopromazine		
– Perazine		
– Promazine		
– Promethazine		
– Prothipendyl		
– Thiopropazate		
– Thioridazine		[150]
– Triflupromazine		
– Trimeprazine		
Phenytoine	PA ?	
Protriptyline	PT	
Pyritinol	PA	
Trimethadione	PA ?	
Antihistamines		
Cimetidine	?	
Cyproheptadine	?	
Dimenhydrinate	?	
Diphenhydramine	PA	
Phenothiazines	see above	
Terfenadine	PA	
Triprolidine	?	
Antiphlogistics		
Azapropazone	PT	
Benoxaprofen	PT	
Carprofen	PT & PA	[124]
Diclofenac	PT & PA	[124]

(continued)

§ **6.2** *(continuation)*

Drug Name	Mechanism	
Diflunisal	?	
Fenclofenac	?	
Gold salts	PA ?	
Ibuprofen	?	
Ketoprofen	PT & PA	[124]
Mefenamic acid	?	
Naproxen	?	
Oxaprozin	PT	
Oxyphenbutazone	?	
Phenylbutazone	?	
Piroxicam	PT & PA	[124]
Salicylates	PT & PA	[124]
Sulindac	PT	
Tenoxicam	PT	
Tiaprofenic acid	PT & PA	[124]
Antidiabetics		
Carbutamide	PA	
Chlorpropamide	PA ?	
Glibenclamide	PA ?	
Tolbutamide	PA	
Cardiovascular drugs		
Amiodarone	PT	
Atenolol	?	
Captopril	PA	
Diltiazem	?	
Disopyramide	?	
Fenofibrate	?	[149]
Labetalol	?	
Methyldopa	PA	
Nifedipine	?	
Oxprenolol	?	
Propranolol	?	
Quinidine	PA & PT	[151]
Quinine	PA & PT	[151]
Reserpine	?	
Diuretics		
Amiloride	?	
Bendrofluazine	PT	
Chlorothiazide	PA & PT	
Chlorthalidon	PA ?	
Cyclopenthiazode	?	
Diazoxide	?	
Furosemide	PT	
Hydrochlorothiazide	PA & PT	

(continued)

§ **6.2** *(continuation)*

Drug Name	Mechanism	
Quinethazone	PA ?	
Triamterene	PA ?	
Xipamide	PA ?	
Dermatological drugs		
Etretinate	PT	
Isotretinoin	PT ?	
5-Methoxypsoralen	PT	
8-Methoxypsoralen	PT & PA	
Trimethylpsoralen	PT	
Antibiotics		
Chloramphenicol	PA ?	
Chlortetracycline	PT	
Cinoxacin	PT	[160]
Ciprofloxacin	PT	[155]
Cotrimoxazol	?	
Demethylchlortetracycline	PT, PA ?	
Doxycycline	PT	
Enoxacin	PT & PA	[153]
Griseofulvin	PA ? & PT	
Ketoconazole	?	
Lamefloxacin	PA	[152]
Methacycline	PT	
Minocycline	PT	
Nalidixic acid	PT	
Norfloxacin	PT	[154]
Ofloxacin	PT	
Oxytetracycline	PT	
Pefloxacin	PT	
Penicillin	PA ?	
Salazosulfapyridine	PA	
Sulfonamides	PA & PT	
Tetracycline	PT	
Antituberculosis and antiprotozoal drugs		
Amodiaquin	PT	
p-Aminosalicylic acid	PA ?	
Chloroquine	PA	
Clofazimine	PT	
Dapsone	PA	
Hydroxychloroquine	PT	
Isoniazid	PT	
Mepracine	PT ?	
Pyrazinamide	?	
Pyrimethamine	PA	
Quinine	PA	

(continued)

§ **6.2** *(continuation)*

Drug Name	Mechanism
Streptomycin	?
Thiambutosine	PT
Trimethoprim	PT
Cytostatic drugs	
Azathioprine	?
Cyclophosphamide	?
Dacarbazine	PT
5-Fluorouracil	PT & PA
Methotrexate	PT
Procarbazine	?
Triethylenemelamine	PA ?
Vinblastine	PT
Miscellaneous drugs	
Amantadine	PA
Diethylstilbestrol	?
Moquizone	?
Oral Contraceptive	?

PA = Photoallergic
PT = Phototoxic
? = Mechanism unknown.

6.3 Many articles have reviewed drug-induced photosensitivity:
- photosensitivity from systemic drugs [25,50,99]
- photosensitivity from topical and systemic drugs [29,74,98]
- photoallergy from topical and systemic drugs [46,97]
- photosensitivity from topical drugs [94]
- phototoxicity from topical drugs [96]
- photocontact allergy to sunscreens [165,166]

PHOTOSENSITIVITY DUE TO TOPICAL PHOTOSENSITIZERS (PHOTOCONTACT DERMATITIS)

6.4 Photosensitivity due to topical photosensitizers may be phototoxic, photoallergic, or a combination of both. It is not always easy to determine whether a particular photosensitivity reaction is phototoxic or photoallergic in nature; a combination of both types of reactions frequently occurs. In § 3.7 some characteristics of phototoxic and photoallergic types of reactions are given that may help to differentiate these conditions. Photopatch testing has not completely been standardized [92,94,140–143]. A test tray for topical photoallergens is presented in § 6.6.

The most serious consequence of photocontact-allergy is the development of persistent photosensitivity in a small group of patients, despite strict avoidance of further exposure to the photosensitizer. For this group of patients the term '*persistent light reactors*' has been coined [28,94].

A comprehensive list of topical photosensitizers in provided in § 6.5.

6.5 Topical photosensitizers [140–142,161]

Drug	Use	Type of reaction	Comment	Ref.
6-acetoxy-2,4-dimethyl-m-dioxane	preservative	photoallergic	*See also under* dimethoxane	110
p-aminobenzoic acid (derivatives) (PABA)	sunscreens	photoallergic phototoxic		39 52 78 108
amyl (= pentyl) dimethyl PABA	sunscreen	photoallergic		108 141
balsam Peru	fragrance	phototoxic		90
benzocaine	local anaesthetic	photoallergic		17 22 42 108
benzydamine	analgesic and antipyretic drug	photoallergic	Photoallergic dermatitis after oral intake: Ref. [117]	20 116
β-carotene	sunscreen	photoallergic	Photocontact allergy not proven	10
bithionol	antiseptic	photoallergic phototoxic	Has photo-cross-reacted with halogenated salicylanilides and hexachlorophene. Has caused persistent light reactions	9 40 57
blankophores (optical whiteners)	in soaps,detergents and cosmetics	photoallergic		14
brilliant lake red R (DC-Red 31, CI 15800)	coal tar dye in cosmetics	photoallergic		70
5-bromo-4′-chlorsalicy-lanilide	antiseptic	photoallergic phototoxic	Has photo-cross-reacted with other halogenated salicylanilides. Has caused persistent light reactions	8 36
buclosamide	antifungal drug	phototoxic photoallergic	Has cross reacted with sulfanilamide antidiabetics and diuretics. Has caused 'localized persistent light reactions'	12 56
butyl methoxydi-benzoylmethane	sunscreen	photoallergic	photocross-reactivity to and from 4-isopropyldibenzoylmethane	139
cadmium sulfide	yellow tattoo pigment	phototoxic	Has produced papular and nodular lesions in tattoos	6
chlorhexidine	antiseptic	photoallergic		75
chloromercapto-dicarboximide	antiseborrhoeic agent	photoallergic		23
chloro-2-phenyl-phenol	antiseptic	photoallergic		1

(continued)

§ **6.5** *(continuation)*

Drug	Use	Type of reaction	Comment	Ref.
chlorpromazine hydrochloride	sedative	photoallergic phototoxic	Occupational contact in medical and nursing professionals, in industry and in veterinary medicine	13 17 95
chlorprothixene	tranquillizer	photoallergic	Accidental contact in a nurse who was allergic to chlorpromazine	49
cinnamates	sunscreens, fragrances	photoallergic		33
cinnamic aldehyde	fragrance	photoallergic		86
cinoxate	sunscreen	photoallergic		72
coal tar (and derivatives including acridine, anthracene, benzpyrene, fluoranthene, phenanthrene)	psoriasis and eczema therapy, cosmetics	phototoxic photoallergic	Has caused persistent light reaction: photocontact urticaria [90]. Vegetable and bituminous tars are *not* phototoxic	4 19 43 79 100
colophony	resin	phototoxic		140
coumarin (derivatives)			See 6-methyl coumarin	
desoximethasone	topical corticosteroid	uncertain	Diagnosis made per exclusionem. The steroid itself was not tested	134
dibenzthione	antifungal drug	photoallergic	Has photo-cross-reacted with hydrochlorthiazide	5
dibromsalan	antiseptic	photoallergic	Has photo-cross-reacted with other halogenated salicylanilides, hexachlorophene, dichlorophene and carbanilides	26 35 54
dichlorophene	antiseptic	photoallergic		141
dibucaine HCl	local anaesthetic	photoallergic	photocross sensitivity from benzocaine	38 108
digalloyl trioleate	sunscreen	photoallergic	Digalloyl trioleate is a mixture of tannic acid derivatives	66
dimethoxane	preservative (in sunscreen)	photoallergic		86
dimethoxydibenzoylmethane	sunscreen	photoallergic		106 107
diphenydramine	topical antihistamine	photoallergic		21 37
dyes e.g.: methylene blue fluorescein eosin rose bengal acridine orange acriflavin neutral red	various	phototoxic		16 55

(continued)

§ **6.5** *(continuation)*

Drug	Use	Type of reaction	Comment	Ref.
erythrocine-AL (FDC-Red 3, CI 45430)	coal tar dye in cosmetics	photoallergic		70
essential oils: bergamot oil cedar oil citron oil lavender oil lime oil neroli oil petitgrain oil sandalwood oil	perfumes	phototoxic	Sandalwood oil has caused persistent light reaction	34 69 81
2-ethoxyethyl-*p*-methoxycinnamate	sunscreen	photoallergic phototoxic		18 89 107 108 109
ethylenediamine	stabilizer in steroid cream	photoallergic	Dubious report	157
fenticlor	antifungal drug	photoallergic phototoxic	Has photo-cross-reacted with bithionol and hexachlorophene. Has caused persistent light reactions. Photoallergic contact dermatitis from occupational exposure: Ref. [133]	8 9 62
fluorescein	diagnostic dye used in ophthalmology	photoallergic	photo provocation with intravenous injection of fluorescein was positive	132
fluorouracil	cytostatic drug	phototoxic(?)	Accelerates inflammatory processes	67
formaldehyde	preservative	uncertain	Immediate sunburn-like reaction in the test situation	87
furocoumarins	cosmetics containing plant extracts, essential oils, colognes, direct contact with many plants (Umbelliferae, Rutaceae)	phototoxic photoallergic (?)	Have caused postinflammatory hyperpigmentation (berloque dermatitis). Plants containing furocoumarins may cause dermatitis bullosa striata pratensis	60
glyceryl PABA	sunscreen	photoallergic	In the reported cases often also a positive reaction to benzocaine. During the manufacture of glyceryl-*p*-aminobenzoate benzocaine is produced. Sometimes impurities may be the actual cause of alleged glyceryl PABA photosensitivity [112]	17 27 108 112

(continued)

§ **6.5** *(continuation)*

Drug	Use	Type of reaction	Comment	Ref.
hexachlorophene	antiseptic	photoallergic phototoxic	Rare primary photosensitizer: more often photo-cross-reacts with other compounds e.g. halogenated phenols. Has caused persistent light reaction [131]	53 57 131
homosalate (homo-menthyl salicylate)	sunscreen	photoallergic		141
hydrocortisone	corticosteroid	photoallergic		65
isoamyl-*p*-*N,N*-dimethyl-aminobenzoate	sunscreen	phototoxic		78 44
isoamyl-*p*- methoxy cinnamate	sunscreen	photoallergic	Photocross sensitivity to and from octyl methoxycinnamate	86 139
isobutyl PABA	sunscreen	photoallergic		146
isopropyl dibenzoyl-methane	sunscreen	photoallergic phototoxic		103 104 105 106 107 139 159
ketoprofen	non-steroidal anti-inflammatory drug (NSAID)	photoallergic	Photocross reactions to tiaprofenic acid, ibuproxam, flubiprofen and fenofibrate	120 125 138
lithol Red-CA (DC Red 11, CI 15630)	coal tar dye in cosmetics	photoallergic		70
4-methylbenzylidene camphor	sunscreen	photoallergic phototoxic		104 139
8-methoxypsoralen	PUVA therapy	phototoxic photoallergic	Photocross-reactions to 3-carbethoxypsoralen. Also primary photosensitization to trimethylangelicin and 3-carbethoxypsoralen [31]	31 163
6-methyl coumarin	fragrance	photoallergic phototoxic	Has photo-cross-reacted with 7-methyl coumarin, coumarin, 7-methoxycoumarin	45 47
mexenone (benzo-phenone-10)	sunscreen	photoallergic	Has photo-cross-reacted with oxybenzone (benzophenone 3)	10 63
minoxidil	treatment of baldness	photoallergic		162

(continued)

§ **6.5** *(continuation)*

Drug	Use	Type of reaction	Comment	Ref.
musk ambrette	perfumes	photoallergic phototoxic	Has caused persistent light reactions [158]. Photo-cross-reactions to musk xylene and musk moskene, but not to musk ketone and tibetene: Refs [64,84]. Lichenoid photocontact dermatitis: Ref. [126]. PUVA treatment of persistent light reactor: Ref. [48]. Analysis of musk ambrette and other nitromusks: Ref. [32]. Other nitromusks have a low or no photosensitizing potential [128]	11 32 82 83 85
mycanodin	antifungal drug	photoallergic		7
oak moss	fragrance	photoallergic	Photocontact allergy to the ingredient evernic acid	101 135
octyl dimethyl PABA	sunscreen	photoallergic	Possible cross-sensitivity to isobutyl PABA	102 108 139
octyl methoxycinnamate	sunscreen	photoallergic	Photocross-sensitivity to and from isoamyl methoxycinnamate	139
oxybenzone (benzophenone-3)	sunscreen	photoallergic phototoxic		88 108 111 113 114 139
permanent orange (DC Orange 17, CI 12075)	coal tar dye in cosmetics	photoallergic		70
phenylbenzimidazole sulfonic acid	sunscreen	photoallergic		86 110 139
2-phenyl-5-methyl-benzoxazol (witisol)	sunscreen	photoallergic		139
p-phenylenediamine	various	photoallergic	Possible photocross-reaction from PABA [108]. Possible photo-cross-reaction to or from local anaesthetics [129]	76 108
piroxicam	non-steroidal anti-inflammatory drug (NSAID)	photoallergic? phototoxic?	*Systemic* photosensitivity to piroxicam: Ref. [119]. Most patients photoallergic to piroxicam either from systemic or topical administration are contact allergic to thiosalicylic acid and thiomersal [118,136]. Persistent light reactions: Ref. [119]	118

(continued)

§ **6.5** *(continuation)*

Drug	Use	Type of reaction	Comment	Ref.
procaine HCl	local anaesthetic	photoallergic	Photo cross-sensitivity from benzocaine	108
promethazine hydrochloride	(topical) antihistamine	photoallergic phototoxic	Oral use in sensitized individuals may provoke photosensitivity. Has caused persistent light reactions	56 61 68 73
quinine sulfate	antimalarial drug	photoallergic	Accidental contact. Has caused persistent light reactions	41
sulfanilamide	chemotherapeutic	photoallergic phototoxic	Has (photo)-cross-reacted with other para-compounds. Has caused persistent light reactions	3
sulizobenzone (benzophenone-4)	sunscreen	photoallergic		141
tetrachlorsalicylanilide	antiseptic	photoallergic phototoxic	Has photo-cross-reacted with other halogenated salicylanilides, hexachlorophene. Has caused persistent light reactions	15 77
thiocolchicoside	topical analgesic	photoallergic		164
tiaprofenic acid	non-steroidal anti-inflammatory drug (NSAID)	phototoxic photoallergic	Photo-cross-sensitivity to flurbiprofen [122]. Exacerbation by oral ketoproten [122]. Photosensitivity after oral administration of tiaprofenic acid: Refs. [123,124]. Photopatch test sensitization: Ref. [137]	121 122 140
toluidine red (Pigment Red 3, CI 12120)	coal tar dye in cosmetics	photoallergic		70
tribromsalan	antiseptic	phototoxic photoallergic	Has photo-cross-reacted with other halogenated salicylanilides, triclocarban, hexachlorophene and fenticlor	35 58 59
triclocarban	antiseptic	phototoxic photoallergic	Has photo-cross-reacted with halogenated salicylanilides. Rare primary photosensitizer	2 30 51
triclosan	antiseptic	phototoxic photoallergic		140 141
zinc pyrithione	dandruff therapy	photoallergic (?)	May lead to photosensitive eczema and actinic reticuloid syndrome	80

6.6 Several test trays of (topical) photosensitisers have been suggested. A survey is presented in the following table.

Photopatch Test Substances

Photosensitizer	Ref. [140]	[141]	[142]	[143]
Antiseptic substances				
Bithionol	1.0%	1.0%	1.0%	
Bromochlorosalicylanilide	1.0%			
Buclosamide	5.0%			
Chlorhexidine gluconate			0.5%	
Dichlorophene		1.0%		
Diphenylphenol		2.0%		
Fenticlor	1.0%	1.0%	1.0%	
Hexachlorophene	1.0%	1.0%	1.0%	
Tetrachlorosalicylanilide	0.1%	1.0%	0.1%	
Tribromosalicylanilide	1.0%	1.0%	1.0%	
Triclocarbon		1.0%	1.0%	
Triclosan	2.0%		2.0%	
Therapeutic agents				
Benzocaine				2.0%
Carprofen	5.0%			
Chlorpromazine	0.1%	1.0%	0.1%	0.1%
Chlorthiazide	1.0%			
Diphenhydramine chloride			1%	
Furosemide	1.0%			
Promethazine	1.0%	2.0%	1.0%	1.0%
Quinidine	1.0%			
Quinine		1.0%		
Sulfanilamide	5.0%			
Tiaprofenic acid	5.0%			
Tolbutamide	5.0%			
Cosmetic ingredients				
6-Methylcoumarin	1.0%	5.0%	1% alc	
Musk ambrette	5.0%	5% alc	1.0%	5.0%
Musk mix	5.0%			
Oil of bergamot		5.0%		
Perfume mix	8.0%		6.0%	
Plants (-derivatives)				
Balsam of Peru	25.0%		25.0%	
Chrysanthemum oleoresin		10% alc		
Colophony	20.0%			
Compositae mix	6.5%			
Lichen mixture			16.0%	
Ragweed		?		
Wood tars	3.0%		20.0%	

(continued)

§ **6.6** *(continuation)*

Photosensitizer	Ref. [140]	[141]	[142]	[143]
Sunscreens				
p-Aminobenzoic acid (PABA)	5.0%	10% alc	5% alc	2.0%
Amyl dimethyl PABA		5.0%		
Benzophenone		5.0%		
Butyl methoxydibenzoylmethane				2.0%
Cinnamate		5.0%		
2-Ethoxyethyl-*p*-methoxycinnamate				2.0%
Homosalate		2.0%		
4-Isopropyl dibenzoylmethane	5.0%			2.0%
Methylbenzylidene camphor	5.0%			2.0%
Mexenone				2.0%
Octyl dimethyl PABA				2.0%
Octyl methoxycinnamate				2.0%
Oxybenzone	2.0%			2.0%
Sulisobenzone		10.0%		
Miscellaneous				
Cyclamate	1.25%			
Saccharin	0.40%			
Thiourea	0.1%		0.01% aqua	

Test vehicle is petroleum unless otherwise indicated.
When no test concentration is given in any column, this indicates that that particular substance is no part of the photopatch test tray of the referenced group of investigators.

One should bear in mind that photocontact dermatitis to several of these compounds is exceptional (e.g. hexachlorophene), whilst others are well-known photosensitizers and therefore hardly used any more; several are prohibited in some countries (e.g. several halogenated salicylanilides).

6.7 REFERENCES

1. Adams, R.M. (1972): Photoallergic contact dermatitis to chloro-2-phenylphenol. *Arch. Dermatol., 106,* 711.
2. Agren-Jonsson, S. and Magnusson, B. (1976): Sensitisation to propantheline bromide, trichlorocarbanilide and propylene glycol in an antiperspirant. *Contact Dermatitis, 2,* 79.
3. Aokï, K. and Saito, T. (1974): Studies on the mechanism of photosensitivity caused by sulfa drugs. In: *Sunlight and Man, Normal and Abnormal Photobiologic Responses. Ch. 27, p.* 431. University of Tokyo Press, Tokyo.
4. Barefoot, S.W. (1979): Report of a persistent light eruption due to pitch. *Cutis, 24,* 395.
5. Behrbohm, P. and Zschunke, E. (1965): Allergisches Ekzem durch das Antimykotikum 'Afungin' (Dibenzthion). *Derm. Wschr., 151,* 1447.
6. Björnberg, A. (1963): Reactions to light in yellow tattoos from cadmium sulfide. *Arch. Dermatol., 88,* 267.
7. Burckhardt, W., Mahler, F. and Schwarz-Speck, M. (1968): Photoallergische Ekzeme durch Mycanodin. *Dermatologica (Basel), 137,* 208.
8. Burry, J.N. (1967): Photoallergies to fentichlor and multifungin. *Arch. Dermatol., 95,* 287.
9. Burry, J.N. (1968): Cross sensitivity between fentichlor and bithionol. *Arch. Dermatol., 97,* 497.
10. Burry, J.N. (1980): Photoallergies from benzophenones and beta carotene in sunscreens. *Contact Dermatitis, 6,* 211.

11. Serrano, G., Aliaga, A., de la Cuadra, J., Planells, I., Lorente, M. and Bonillo, J. (1986): Photosensitivity to musk ambrette in Spain. *Photodermatol., 3,* 186–188.
12. Burry, J.N. and Hunter, G.A. (1970): Photocontact dermatitis from Jadit. *Br. J. Dermatol., 82,* 224.
13. Calnan, C.D. (1958): Studies in contact dermatitis. V. Photosensitivity from chlorpromazine. *Trans. St. John's Hosp. derm. Soc. (Lond.), 41,* 26.
14. Calnan, C.D. (1973): Hazards of optic bleaches. *Trans. St. John's Hosp. derm. Soc. (Lond.), 59,* 275.
15. Calnan, C.D., Harman, R.R.M. and Wells, G.C. (1961): Photodermatitis from soaps. *Br. med. J., ii,* 1266.
16. Calnan, C.D. and Sarkany, J. (1957): Studies in Contact Dermatitis. II. Lipstick cheilitis. *Trans. St. John's Hosp. derm. Soc. (Lond.), 39,* 28.
17. Caro, I. (1978): Contact allergy/photoallergy to glycerol PABA and benzocaine. *Contact Dermatitis, 4,* 381.
18. Cronin, E. (1980): Photosensitisers. In: *Contact Dermatitis* p. 454. Churchill Livingstone, Edinburgh.
19. Crow, K.D., Alexander, E., Buck, W.H.L., Johnson, B.E., Magnus, I.A. and Porter, A.D. (1961): Photosensitivity due to pitch. *Br. J. Dermatol., 73,* 220.
20. Vincenzi, C., Cameli, N., Tardio, M. and Piraccini, B.M. (1990): Contact and photocontact dermatitis due to benzydamine hydrochloride. *Contact Dermatitis, 23,* 125–126.
21. Emmett, E.A. (1974): Diphenhydramine Photoallergy. *Arch. Dermatol., 110,* 249.
22. Epstein, S. (1965): Photocontact dermatitis from benzocain. *Arch. Dermatol., 92,* 591.
23. Epstein, S. (1968): Photoallergic contact dermatitis: report of a case due to Dangard. *Cutis, 4,* 856.
24. Harber, L.C. and Whitman, G.B. (1986): Photosensitivity. Classification. *Dermatologic Clinics, 4,* 167–169.
25. Ljunggren, B. and Bjellerup, M. (1986): Systemic drug photosensitivity. *Photodermatology, 3,* 26–35.
26. Epstein, J.H., Wuepper, K.D. and Maibach, H.I. (1968): Photocontact dermatitis to halogenated salicylanilides and related compounds. *Arch. Dermatol., 97,* 236.
27. Fisher, A.A. (1977): The presence of benzocaine in sunscreens containing glyceryl PABA (Escalol 106). *Arch. Dermatol., 113,* 1299.
28. Burry, J.N. (1984): Persistent light reactions. *Contact Dermatitis, 10,* 170–173.
29. Johnson, B.E. and Ferguson, J. (1990): Drug and chemical photosensitivity. *Semin. Dermatol., 9,* 39–46.
30. Freeman, R.G. and Knox, J.M. (1968): The action spectrum of photocontact dermatitis. *Arch. Dermatol., 97,* 130.
31. Takashima, A., Yamamoto, K., Kimura, S., Takahuwa, Y. and Mizuno, N. (1991): Allergic contact and photocontact dermatitis due to psoralens in patients with psoriasis treated with topical PUVA. *Br. J. Dermatol., 124,* 27–32.
32. Goh, C.L. and Kwok, S.F. (1986): A simple method of qualitative analysis for musk ambrette, musk ketone and musk xylene in cologne. *Contact Dermatitis, 14,* 53–56.
33. Goodmann, T.F. (1970): Photodermatitis from a sunscreening agent (letter). *Arch. Dermatol., 102,* 563.
34. Harber, C.L., Harris. H., Leder, M. and Baer, R.L. (1964): Berloque dermatitis. *Arch. Dermatol., 90,* 505.
35. Harber, L.C., Targovnik, S.E. and Baer, R.L. (1967): Contact photosensitivity patterns to halogenated salicylanilides. *Arch. Dermatol., 96,* 646.
36. Herman, P.S. and Sams, W.M. (1972): *Soap Photodermatitis. Photosensitivity to Halogenated Salicylanilides.* Charles C. Thomas, Springfield, III.
37. Horio, T. (1976): Allergic and photoallergic dermatitis from diphenhydramine. *Arch. Dermatol., 112,* 1124.
38. Horio, T. (1980): Photosensitivity reactions to dibucaine. *Arch. Dermatol., 115,* 973.
39. Horio, T. and Hituchi, T. (1978): Photocontact dermatitis from p-aminobenzoic acid. *Dermatologica (Basel). 156,* 124.
40. Jillson, O.F. and Baughman, R.D. (1963): Contact photodermatitis from bithionol. *Arch. Dermatol., 88,* 409.
41. Johnson, B.E., Zaynoun, S., Gardiner, J.M. and Frain-Bell, W. (1975): A study of persistent light reaction in quindoxin and quinine photosensitivity. *Br. J. Dermatol., 93,* suppl. 11, 21.
42. Kaidbey, K.H. and Allen, H. (1981): Photocontact allergy to benzocaine. *Arch. Dermatol., 117,* 77.
43. Kaidbey, K.H. and Kligman, A.M. (1977): Clinical and histological study of coal tar phototoxicity in humans. *Arch. Dermatol., 113,* 592.
44. Kaidbey, K.H. and Kligman, A.M. (1978): Phototoxicity to a sunscreen ingredient. Padimate A. *Arch. Dermatol., 114,* 547.
45. Kaidbey, K.H. and Kligman, A.M. (1978): Photocontact allergy to 6-methylcoumarin. *Contact Dermititis, 4,* 277.
46. Elmets, C.A. (1986): Drug-induced photoallergy. *Dermatol Clinics, 4,* 231–241.

47. Kaidbey, K.H. and Kligman, A.M. (1981): Photosensitization by coumarin derivatives. *Arch. Dermatol., 117,* 258.
48. Lindberg, L., Larkö, O. and Roupe, G. (1986): Successful PUVA-treatment for musk ambrette-induced persistent light reaction. *Photodermatol., 3,* 111–112.
49. Kull, E. and Schwarz-Speck, K. (1961): Gruppenspezifische Ekzemreaktionen bei Largactilsensibilisierung. *Dermatologica (Basel), 122,* 263.
50. Drug induced cutaneous photosensitivity. Drug therapy 1990: June: 44,51,52,54,57.
51. Maibach, H. et al. (1978): Triclocarban. Evaluation of contact dermatitis potential in man. *Contact Dermatitis, 4,* 283.
52. Marmelzat, J. and Rapaport, M.J. (1980): Photodermatitis with PABA. *Contact Dermatitis, 6,* 230.
53. Masuda, T. et al. (1971): Photocontact dermatitis due to bithionol, TBS, diaphene and hexachlorophene. *Jpn. J. Dermatol., 81,* 238.
54. Molloy, J.F. and Mayer, J.A. (1966): Photodermatitis from dibromosalicylanilide. *Arch. Dermatol., 93,* 331.
55. Morikawa, F., Fukuda, M., Naganuma, M. and Nakayama, Y. (1976): Phototoxic reactions to xanthine dyes induced by visible light. *J. Derm. (Tokyo), 3,* 59.
56. Nagreh, D.S. (1975): Photodermatitis study of the condition in Kuantan, Malaysia. *Contact Dermatitis, 1,* 27.
57. O'Quinn, S.E., Kennedy, C.B. and Isbell, K.H. (1967): Contact photodermatitis from bithionol and related compounds. *J. Am. Med. Assoc., 199,* 125.
58. Osmundsen, P.E. (1968): Contact photodermatitis due to tribromsalicylanilide. *Br. J. Dermatol., 80,* 228.
59. Osmundsen, P.E. (1970): Contact photodermatitis due to tribromsalicylanilide (cross reaction pattern). *Dermatologica (Basel), 140,* 65.
60. Pathak, M.A. (1974): Phytophotodermatitis. In: *Sunlight and Man,* p. 502. University of Tokyo Prcss, Tokyo.
61. Prisco, D.J., Soto, J.M. and Herrera, E. (1968): Phenergan sensitivity. *Contact Dermatitis Newsl., 4,* 63.
62. Ramsay, C.A. (1979): Skin responses to ultraviolet radiation in contact photodermatitis due to fentichlor. *J. invest. Dermatol., 48,* 255.
63. Ramsay, D.L., Cohen, H.J. and Baer, R.L. (1972): Allergic reactions to benzophenones. *Arch. Derm, 105,* 906.
64. Cronin, E. (1984): Photosensitivity to musk ambrette. *Contact Dermatitis, 11,* 88–92.
65. Rietschel, R.L. (1978): Photocontact dermatitis to hydrocortisone. *Contact Dermatitis, 4,* 334.
66. Sams, W.M. (1956): Contact photodermatitis. *Arch. Dermatol., 73,* 142.
67. Sams, W.M. (1968): Untoward response with topical fluorouracil. *Arch. Dermatol., 97,* 14.
68. Sidi, E., Hincky, M. and Gervais, A. (1955): Allergic sensitisation and photosensitization to phenergan cream. *J. invest. Dermatol., 24,* 345.
69. Starke, J.C. (1967): Photoallergy to sandalwood oil. *Arch. Dermatol., 96,* 62.
70. Sugai, T., Takahashi, Y. and Tagaki, T. (1977): Pigmented cosmetic dermatitis and coal tar dyes. *Contact Dermatitis, 3,* 249.
71. Sulser, H., Schwarz, K. and Schwarz, M. (1963): Über Kreuzreaktionen bei experimenteller photoallergischer Chlorpromazinsensibilisierung. *Dermatologica (Basel), 127,* 108.
72. Thompson, G., Maibach, H. and Epstein, J. (1977): Allergic contact dermatitis from sunscreen preparations complicating photodermatitis. *Arch. Dermatol., 113,* 1252.
73. Tzanck, A., Sidi, E., Mazalton, and Kohen, (1951): Sur deux cas de dermite au phenergan avec photosensibilisation. *Bull. Soc. franc. Derm. Syph., 58,* 433.
74. Epstein, J.H. and Wintroub, B.U. (1985): Photosensitivity due to drugs. *Drugs, 30,* 42–57.
75. Wahlberg, J.E. and Wennersten, G. (1971): Hypersensitivity and photosensitivity to chlorhexidine. *Dermatologica, (Basel), 143,* 376.
76. Wasserman, G.A. and Haberman, H.F. (1975): Photosensitivity: results of investigation in 250 patients. *Canad. med. Ass. J., 113,* 1055.
77. Wilkinson, D.S. (1962): Further experiences with halogenated salicylanilides. *Br. J. Dermatol., 74,* 295.
78. Willis, J. and Kligman, A.M. (1970): Aminobenzoic acid and its esters. *Arch. Dermatol., 102,* 405.
79. Wiskemann, A. and Hoyer, H. (1971): Zur Phototoxizität von Teerpräparaten. *Hautarzt, 22,* 257.
80. Yates, V.M. and Finn, O.A. (1980): Contact allergic sensitivity to zinc pyrithione followed by the photosensitivity dermatitis and actinic reticuloid syndrome. *Contact Dermatitis, 6,* 349.
81. Zaynoun, S.T., Johnson, B.E. and Frain-Bell, W. (1977): A study of oil of bergamot and its importance as a phototoxic agent. *Contact Dermatitis, 3,* 225.

6. Phototoxic and photoallergic contact dermatitis

82. Ducombs, G., Abbadie, D. and Maleville, J. (1986): Persistent light reaction from musk ambrette. *Contact Dermatitis, 14,* 129–130.
83. Sánchez-Pedreño, P., García-Bravo, B., Rodriguez-Pichardo, A. and Camacho, F. (1989): Different clinical presentations in photosensitivity to musk ambrette. *Photodermatol., 6,* 103–105.
84. Galosi, A. and Plewig, G. (1982): Photoallergisches Ekzem durch Ambrette Moschus. *Hautarzt, 33,* 589.
85. Ramsay, C.A. (1984): Transient and persistent photosensitivity due to musk ambrette. Clinical and photobiological studies. *Br. J. Dermatol., 111,* 423–429.
86. Fagerlund, V.-L., Kalimo, K. and Jansén, C. (1983): Photocontact allergy from sunscreens. *Duodecim, 99,* 146.
87. Shelley, W.B. (1982): Immediate sunburn-like reaction in a patient with formaldehyde photosensitivity. *Arch. Dermatol., 118,* 117.
88. Holzle, E. and Plewig, G. (1982): Photoallergische Kontaktdermatitis durch benzophenonhaltige Sonnenschutzpräparate. *Hautarzt, 33,* 391.
89. Davies, M.G., Hawk, J.L.M. and Rycroft, R.J.G. (1982): Acute photosensitivity from the sunscreen 2-ethoxyethyl-p-methoxycinnamate. *Contact Dermatitis, 8,* 190.
90. Kroon, S. (1983): Standard photopatch testing with Waxtar, para-aminobenzoic acid, potassium dichromate and balsam of Peru. *Contact Dermatitis, 9,* 5.
91. Lowe, N.J. (1986): Cutaneous phototoxicity reactions. *Br. J. Dermatol., 115,* (suppl. 31): 86–92.
92. Przybilla, B. (1987): Phototestungen bei Lichtdermatosen. *Hautarzt, 38,* 23–28.
93. Schauder, S. and Ippen, H. (1988): Photosensitivität. In: *Manuale Allergologicum V* (Eds: E. Fuchs and K.H. Schulz), Chapter 15. Dustri Verlag, Deisenhoven.
94. Wennersten, G., Thune, P., Jansén, C.T. and Brodthagen, H. (1986): Photocontact dermatitis: current status with emphasis on allergic contact photosensitivity occurrence, allergens and practical phototesting. *Semin. Dermatol., 5,* 277–289.
95. Ertle, T. (1982): Beruflich bedingte Kontakt und Photokontaktallergie bei einem Landwirt durch Chlorpromazin. *Dermatosen Beruf Umw., 30,* 120.
96. Maibach, H.I. and Marzulli, F.N. (1986): Photoirritation (phototoxicity) from topical agents. *Dermatologic Clinics, 4,* 217–222.
97. Pevny, I. and Lurz, Ch. (1985): Photoallergische Dermatitis. *Allergologie, 8,* 128–138.
98. Hawk, J.L.M. (1984): Photosensitizing agents used in the United Kingdom. *Clin. Exp. Dermatol., 9,* 300–302.
99. Rosen, C. (1989): Photo-induced drug eruptions. *Semin. Dermatol., 8,* 149–157.
100. Diette, K.M., Gange, R.W. and Stern, R.S. et al (1983): Coal tar phototoxicity: Kinetics and exposure parameters. *J. invest. Dermatol., 81,* 347.
101. Fernández de Corres, L., Munoz, D., Leaniz-Barrutia, I. and Corrales, J.L. (1983): Photocontact dermatitis from oak moss. *Contact Dermatitis, 9,* 528.
102. Weller, P. and Freeman, S. (1984): Photocontact allergy to octyldimethyl PABA. *Aust. J. Dermatol., 25,* 73–76.
103. Haussman, A. and Kleinhans, D. (1986): Allergisches Kontaktekzem durch UV-Strahlenfilter in Sonnenschutzcremes — Zwei Fallbeobachtungen. *Z. Hautkr., 61,* 1654–1656.
104. Schauder, S. and Ippen, H. (1988): Photoallergisches und allergisches Kontaktekzem durch Dibenzoylmethan-Verbindungen und andere Lichtschutzfilter. *Hautarzt, 39,* 435–440.
105. English, J.S.C., White, I.R. and Cronin, E. (1987): Sensitivity to sunscreens. *Contact Dermatitis, 17,* 159–162.
106. Schauder, S. and Ippen, H. (1986): Photoallergic and allergic contact dermatitis from dibenzoylmethane. *Photodermatology, 3,* 140–147.
107. English, J.S.C., White, I.R. and Cronin, E. (1987): Sensitivity to sunscreens. *Contact Dermatitis, 17,* 159–162.
108. Thune, P. (1984): Contact and photocontact allergy to sunscreens. *Photodermatol., 1,* 5–9.
109. Murphy, G.M. and White, I.R. (1987): Photoallergic contact dermatitis to 2-ethoxyethyl-p-methoxycinnamate. *Contact Dermatitis, 16,* 296.
110. Kalimo, K., Fagerlund, V.-L. and Jansen, C.T. (1984): Concomitant photocontact allergy to a benzophenone derivative and a sunscreen preservative, 6-acetoxy-2,4,-dimethyl-m-dioxane. *Photodermatol., 1,* 315–317.
111. Lenique, P., Machet, L., Vaillant, L. et al. (1992): Contact and photocontact allergy to oxybenzone. *Contact Dermaititis, 26,* 177–181.

112. Bruze, M., Gruvberger, B. and Thune, P. (1988): Contact and photocontact allergy to glyceryl para-aminobenzoate. *Photodermatol., 5,* 162–165.
113. Marguery, M.C. and Bazex, J. (1989): Photoallergic contact dermatitis due to 2-hydroxy-4-methoxybenzophenone (oxybenzone): report of four cases. *Br. J. Dermatol., 121,* suppl. 34, 59–60.
114. Green, C., Norris, P.G. and Hawk, J.L.M. (1991): Photoallergic contact dermatitis from oxybenzone aggravating polymorphic light eruption. *Contact Dermatitis, 24,* 62–63.
115. Gudmundsen, K.J., Murphy, G.M., O'Sullivan, D., Powell, F.C. and O'Loughlin, S. (1991): Polymorphic light eruption with contact and photocontact allergy. *Br. J. Dermatol., 124,* 379–382.
116. Motley, R.J. and Reynolds, A.J. (1988): Photodermatitis from benzydamine cream. *Contact Dermatitis, 19,* 66.
117. Frosch, P.J. and Weickel, R. (1989): Photokontaktallergie durch Benzydamin (Tantum). *Hautarzt, 40,* 471–473.
118. Serrano, G., Bonillo, J., Aliaga, A., Cuadra, J, Pujol, C., Pelufoc, Cervera, P. and Miranda, M.A. (1990): Piroxicam-induced photosensitivity and contact sensitivity to thiosalicylic acid. *J. Am. Acad. Dermatol., 23,* 479–483.
119. Serrano, G., Fortea, J.M., Latasa, J.M. et al. (1992): Oxicam-induced photosensitivity. *J. Am. Acad. Dermatol., 26,* 545–548.
120. Serrano, G., Fortea, J.M., Latasa, J.M. et al. (1992): Photosensitivity induced by fibric acid derivatives and its relation to photocontact dermatitis to ketoprofen. *J. Am. Acad. Dermatol., 27,* 204–208.
121. Neumann, R.A., Knobler, R.M. and Lindemayr, H. (1989): Tiaprofenic acid induced photosensitivity. *Contact Dermatitis, 20,* 270–273.
122. Valsecchi, R., Di Landro, A., Pigatto, P. and Cainelli, T. (1989): Tiaprofenic acid photodermatitis. *Contact Dermatitis, 21,* 345–346.
123. Galosi, A., Przybilla, B., Ring, J. and Dorn, M. (1984): Systemische Photoprovokation mit Surgam. *Allergologie, 7,* 143–144.
124. Przybilla, B., Ring, J., Schwab, U., Galosi, A., Dorn, M. and Braun-Falco, O. (1987): Photosensibilisierende Eigenschaften nichtsteroidaler Antirheumatika im Photopatch Test. *Hautarzt, 38,* 18–25.
125. Cusano, F. and Capozzi, M. (1992): Photocontact dermatitis from ketoprofen with cross-reactivity to ibuproxam. *Contact Dermatitis, 27,* 50–51.
126. Parodi, G., Guarrera, M. and Rebora, A. (1987): Lichenoid photocontact dermatitis to musk ambrette. *Contact Dermatitis, 16,* 136–138.
127. Leroy, D. and Dompmartin, A. (1989): Connubial photosensitivity to musk ambrette. *Photodermatol., 6,* 137–139.
128. Parker, R.D., Buehler, E.V. and Newmann, E.A. (1986): Phototoxicity, photoallergy and contact sensitization of nitro musk perfume raw materials. *Contact Dermatitis, 14,* 103–109.
129. LeVine, M. (1984): Idiopathic photodermatitis with a positive paraphenylene-diamine photopatch test. *Arch. Dermatol., 120,* 1488–1490.
130. Möller, H. (1990): Contact and photocontact allergy to psoralens. *Am. J. Contact Dermatitis, 1,* 254.
131. Kalb, R.E. (1991): Persistent light reaction to hexachlorophene. *J. Am. Acad. Dermatol., 24,* 333–334.
132. Hochsattel, R., Gall, H., Weber, L. and Hauffmann, R. (1990): Photoallergic reaction to fluorescein. *Contact Dermatitis, 22,* 42–44.
133. Norris, P.G., Hawk, J.L.M. and White, I.R. (1988): Photoallergic contact dermatitis from fenticlor. *Contact Dermatitis, 18,* 318–319.
134. Stierstorfer, M.B. and Baughman, R.D. (1988): Photosensitivity to desoximetasone emollient cream. *Arch. Dermatol., 124,* 1870–1871.
135. Fernández de Corres, L. (1986): Photosensitivity to oak moss. *Contact Dermatitis, 15,* 118.
136. Cirne de Castro, J.L., Freitas, J.P., Menezes Brandao, F. and Themido, R. (1991): Sensitivity to thimerosal and photosensitivity to piroxicam. *Contact Dermatitis, 24,* 187–192.
137. Przybilla, B., Ring, J., Galosi, A. and Dorn, M. (1984): Photopatch test reactions to tiaprofenic acid. *Contact Dermatitis, 10,* 55–56.
138. Mozzanica, N. and di Pigatto, P.D. (1990): Contact and photocontact allergy to ketoprofen: Clinical and experimental study. *Contact Dermatitis, 23,* 336–340.
139. Schauder, S. (1991): Kontaktekzem durch Lichtfilterhaltige Lichtschutzmittel und Kosmetika. *Akt. Dermatol., 17,* 47–57.
140. Hölze, E., Neumann, N., Hausen, B., Przybilla, B., Schauder, S., Hönigsmann, H., Bircher, A. and Plewig, G. (1991): Photopatch testing: The 5-year experience of the German, Austrian and Swiss Photopatch Test

Group. *J. Am. Acad. Dermatol., 25,* 59–68. (Partly) also published in: Allergologie 1989: 13–20 and Aktuelle Dermatologie 1991: 17: 117–123.

141. Menz, J., Muller, S.A. and Connolly, S.M. (1988): Photopatch testing: A six-year experience. *J. Am. Acad. Dermatol., 18,* 1044–1047.
142. Thune, P., Jansen, C., Wennersten, G., Rystedt, I., Brodthagen, H. and McFadden, N. (1988): The Scandinavian multicenter photopatch study 1980–1985: final report. *Photodermatol., 5,* 261–269.
143. White, I.R. (1992): Photoallergens and photosensitivity: Current Problems. In: R.J.G. Rycroft et al. (Editors), *Textbook of Contact Dermatitis*, Chapters 2–4, pp. 75–88. Springer, Heidelberg.
144. Bruinsma, W. (1990): *A Guide to Drug Eruptions. Fifth edition.* Free University, Amsterdam.
145. *Side Effects of Drugs, Annuals 12–15* (Editors: M.N.G. Dukes, L. Beeley and J.K. Aronson). Amsterdam. Elsevier Science Publishers, 1988–1991.
146. Jeanmougin, M. (1986): Determination du povoir photosensibilisant d'un médicament par la méthode des photopatch tests. *Nouv. Dermatol., 5,* (suppl. 3): 204–208.
147. Ljunggren, B. and Bojs, G. (1991): A case of photosensitivity and contact allergy to systemic tricyclic drugs, with unusual features. *Contact Dermatitis, 24,* 259–265.
148. Terui, T. and Tagami, H. (1989): Eczematous drug eruption from carbamazepine: co-existence of contact and photocontact sensitivity. *Contact Dermatitis, 20,* 260–264.
149. Merino, V., Llamas, R. and Iglesias, L. (1990): Phototoxic reaction to fenofibrate. *Contact Dermatitis, 23,* 284.
150. Röhrborn, W. and Bräuninger, W. (1987): Thioridazine photoallergy. *Contact Dermatitis, 17,* 241.
151. Ljunggren, B., Hindsen, M. and Isaksson, M. (1992): Systemic quinine photosensitivity with photoepicutaneous cross-reactivity to quinidine. *Contact Dermatitis, 26,* 1–4.
152. Kurumaji, Y. and Shono, M. (1992): Scarified photopatch testing in lomefloxacin photosensitivity. *Contact Dermatitis, 26,* 5–10.
153. Kawabe, Y., Mizuno, N. and Sahakibara, S. (1989): Photoallergic reaction caused by enoxacin. *Photodermatology, 6,* 57–69.
154. Shelley, E.D. and Shelley, W.B. (1988): The subcorneal pustular drug eruption: an example induced by norfloxacin. *Cutis, 42,* 24–27.
155. Nederost, S.T., Dijkstra, J.W.E. and Handel, D.W. (1989): Drug-induced photosensitivity reaction. *Arch. Dermatol., 125,* 433.
156. Highet, A. (1986): Bullous eruption associated with cinoxacin and long wave ultraviolet A light. *Br. med. J., 292,* 732.
157. Burry, J.N. (1986): Photocontact dermatitis from ethylenediamine. *Contact Dermatitis, 15,* 305–306.
158. Megahed, M., Hölzle, E. and Plewig, G. (1991): Persistent light reaction associated with photoallergic contact dermatitis to musk ambrette and allergic contact dermatitis to fragrance mix. *Dermatologica, 182,* 199–202.
159. Jacobi, H. and Pinzer, B. (1990): Photoallergisches Kontaktekzem durch 4-Isopropyldibenzoylmethan. *Dermatol Mon. Schr., 176,* 669–672.
160. Gudmundsen, K.J., Murphy, G.M., O'Sullivan, D., Powell, F.C. and O'Loughlin, S.O. (1991): Polymorphic light eruption with contact and photocontact allergy. *Br. J. Dermatol., 124,* 379–382.
161. Dromgoole, S.H. and Maibach, H.I. (1990): Sunscreening agent intolerance: Contact and photocontact sensitization and contact urticaria. *J. Am. Acad. Dermatol., 20,* 1068–1078.
162. Tosti, A., Guerra, L. and Bardazzi, F. (1991): Contact dermatitis caused by topical minoxidil: case reports and review of the literature. *Am. J. Contact Dermatitis, 2,* 56–59.
163. Möller, H. (1990): Contact and photocontact allergy to psoralens. Photodermatol. Photoimmunol. *Photomed., 7,* 43–44.
164. Foti, C., Vena, G.A. and Angelini, G. (1992): Photocontact allergy due to thiocolchicoside. *Contact Dermatitis, 27,* 201–202.
165. Freeman, S. and Frederiksen, P. (1990): Sunscreen allergy. *Am. J. Contact Dermatitis, 1,* 240–243.
166. Dromgoole, S.H. and Maibach, H.I. (1990): Sunscreening agent intolerance: contact and photocontact sensitization and contact urticaria. *J. Am. Acad. Dermatol., 22,* 1068–1078.

7. The contact urticaria syndrome

7.1 Contact urticaria denotes a wheal-and-flare response after cutaneous exposure to certain agents; usually the reaction is elicited within 30–60 minutes, but delayed-onset urticaria (up to 6 hours) may infrequently occur, possibly through slower percutaneous penetration. The broad spectrum of clinical manifestations described justifies the term 'the contact urticaria syndrome'. The subject has been thoroughly reviewed [52–54,72,76]; a monograph on non-immunologic contact urticaria has been published [27]. A recent frequently used synonym for contact urticaria is 'immediate contact reactions' [52,72].

7.2 On the basis of the action mechanisms involved, contact urticaria may be subdivided into three types [30,36,72], which are characterized as follows:

Type A: Non-immunologic contact urticaria
- The response may be evoked in many or nearly all exposed individuals.
- Contact with the incriminated chemical induces release of histamine and other vasoactive substances, without involving immunologic processes.
- Passive transfer is not possible.
- This type of contact urticaria occurs frequently.

Type B: Immunologic contact urticaria
- The response may be evoked in previously sensitized individuals only.
- Immunologic mechanisms are involved in releasing histamine and other vasoactive substances.
- Passive transfer is possible.
- This type of contact urticaria occurs less frequently.

Type C: Uncertain mechanism contact urticaria
- The mechanisms involved are not clarified: neither an immunologic nor a nonspecific direct release of mediators has been proven.

7.3 On a clinical basis, the following division has been suggested [52]:

Cutaneous reactions only

Stage 1: Localized urticaria;
dermatitis/dermatosis;
non-specific symptoms (e.g. itching, tingling and burning).
Stage 2: Generalized urticaria.

Extracutaneous reactions:

Stage 3: Bronchial asthma;
rhinoconjunctivitis;
otolaryngeal;
gastrointestinal.
Stage 4: Anaphylactoid reactions.

7.4 Contact urticaria may be elicited by contact with various foods, plants, animal products, physical influences, textiles, cosmetics and industrial contactants [36,52–54]. Sometimes a positive delayed test-response may develop subsequent to the initial wheal-and-flare reaction. For patients exhibiting combined reactions in the test situation the term 'contact dermatitis of immediate and delayed type' has been proposed [52]. For test procedures to evaluate the immediate-type responses the reader is referred to the review articles on the subject [52–54]. To identify substances which may cause non-immunologic contact urticaria, the NICU-test was developed [77]. This test showed the following chemicals (not included in Table 7.5) to be urticariogens: acetaldehyde, ethyl nicotinate, histamine, methyl salicylate and octylamine. Erythema *alone* is not a reliable sign of contact urticaria. This would disqualify α-amylcinnamic alcohol, anisyl alcohol, benzyl alcohol, bronopol, coumarin, geraniol, imidazolidinyl urea and Kathon CG, which have been proposed as contact urticariogens [97]. Any strong irritant can induce whealing under the right conditions, which should be appreciated when studying cases of suspected non-immunologic contact urticaria [77].

Table 7.5 lists chemicals used in dermatology and cosmetology, which have caused contact urticaria. In many reported cases the authors believe the contact urticaria to be of immunologic origin, but substantial evidence for this is often lacking. Therefore, the mechanism of action for a particular drug is only then listed as 'immunologic' (type B) if passive transfer has been successful or if specific antibodies have been demonstrated.

7.5 Contact urticaria caused by topical drugs

Drug	Use	Mechanism involved	Comment	Ref.
acetylsalicylic acid	analgesic	immunologic (?)	Only listed; no references	36 52
aminophenazone	antipyretic analgesic	uncertain	Generalized urticaria upon patch testing. Also delayed-type allergy. Caused also anaphylactic shock. Has cross-reacted to propyphenazone and metamizole [62]	7 20 62

(continued)

§ **7.5** *(continuation)*

Drug	Use	Mechanism involved	Comment	Ref.
ammonium persulfate	in hair bleaches	uncertain	Scratch tests in an atopic patient have caused a mild asthmatic attack. May induce urticarial responses to scratch tests in controls. Negative in the NICU-test [77]. Anaphylaxis has occurred	5 12
ampicillin	antibiotic	uncertain	A patch test evoked the urticarial reaction	38
amyl alcohol	solvent	immunologic	The reported patient also reacted to butyl alcohol, ethyl alcohol and propyl alcohol	41
arsphenamine	formerly used for treating syphilis	uncertain		46
bacitracin	antibiotic	immunologic	Anaphylactic reaction [43]. Also delayed type allergy [87]. Specific reagins were demonstrated. Negative in the NICU-test [77]	43 87 111
balsam Peru	various	non-immunologic	The % of positive reactions depends upon the test concentration. A concentration of 12.5% yields the largest number [13]. Also positive reactions to cinnamic aldehyde, cinnamic acid, benzoic acid and benzaldehyde in some cases. Sometimes also delayed-type allergy. Positive in the NICU-test [77]. Anaphylactic symptoms with patch testing recorded [52]	13 48 64
benzaldehyde		non-immunologic	*See under* balsam Peru	
benzocaine	local anesthetic	uncertain	Scratch tests positive. Also anaphylactic reaction. Also delayed-type hypersensitivity. Negative in the NICU-test [77]	24
benzoic acid		non-immunologic immunologic [52]	*See also under* balsam Peru. Benzoic acid in food has caused perioral contact urticaria. Positive in the NICU-test [77]. *See under* denatonium benzoate. Quenching by eugenol: Ref. [118]	63
benzoyl peroxide	acne therapy	uncertain		59
bithionol	antiseptic in soap		*Photo*contact urticaria. Also delayed type photoallergy in the 2 reported cases	106

(continued)

§ **7.5** *(continuation)*

Drug	Use	Mechanism involved	Comment	Ref.
butyl alcohol		non-immunologic	*See under* amyl alcohol. Negative in the NICU-test [77]	
butylated hydroxyanisole (BHA)	antioxidant	uncertain	Also delayed-type hypersensitivity in the reported case	42
butylated hydroxytoluene (BHT)	antioxidant	uncertain	Also delayed-type hypersensitivity in the reported case	42
camphor	rubefacient	probably non-immunologic		48
capsicain	counter-irritant	non-immunologic	Only listed: no references	52
caraway seed oil	in toothpastes	uncertain	Also caused 'sub-shock'	22
cephalosporins	antibiotics	uncertain	Also sneezing, watery nasal discharge, lacrimation and difficulty of breathing in the reported case	50
cetyl alcohol	vehicle constituent	uncertain	Both urticarial response and delayed type hypersensitivity in the reported case with concomitant reactions to stearyl alcohol	16
chloramine-T	disinfectant	immunologic	Specific IgE antibodies demonstrated. Also dyspnea and rhinitis in the reported case	57
chloramphenicol	antibiotic	uncertain	Has caused a 'sub-shock'	26
chlorhexidine digluconate	antiseptic	immunologic	Most cases are caused by application to the mucous membranes. Passive transfer tests have been positive [78]. Severe anafylactic reactions have been observed [79]. Also delayed type allergy [80]	78 79 80 81
p-chloro-*m*-cresol	disinfectant	uncertain	Also delayed type allergy in the reported case	90
chlorproethazine	analgesic	non-immunologic	*Photo*contact urticaria. Also delayed phototoxicity	126
chlorpromazine	sedative	?	Only listed: no references	36
	sedative	immunologic	*Photo*contact urticaria. Also delayed type (photo) allergy in the reported case	104
	sedative	uncertain	*Photo*contact urticaria. Also delayed type photoallergy in the reported case	105

(continued)

§ **7.5** *(continuation)*

Drug	Use	Mechanism involved	Comment	Ref.
cinnamic acid		non-immunologic	*See under* balsam Peru. Positive in the NICU-test [77]	
cinnamic aldehyde (cinnamal)	flavoring agent	non-immunologic	Some controls were positive on patch testing. Was shown to release histamine from human leukocytes. Quenching by eugenol: Ref. [118]. Positive in the NICU-test [77]	35
cinnamon oil		non-immunologic	*See also under* sorbic acid. In patients with urticaria displaying contact urtication to patch tests with cinnamon oil, oral provocation induced urticaria. Cinnamon oil consists mainly of cinnamic aldehyde [98]	64 98
clioquinol	antimicrobial	uncertain		51 119
clobetasol-17-propionate	corticosteroid	uncertain		61
denatonium benzoate	denaturant in alcoholic preparations	uncertain	Also asthmatic symptoms in the reported patient	3
diethyl toluamide (DEET)	insect repellent	immonologic	Passive transfer demonstrated. Negative in the NICU-test [77]	30 58
1,3-diiodo-2-hydroxypropane	antiseptic	uncertain	Also delayed type hypersensitivity in the reported case	28
dimethyl sulfoxide (DMSO)	solvent	non-immunologic	Concentrations below 20% only cause erythema. Positive in the NICU-test [77]	25 33
dinitrochlorobenzene (DNCB)	contact allergen for treatment of alopecia areata	uncertain		83
diphenycyclone	contact allergen for treatment of alopecia areata	uncertain		114
disodium cromoglycate	topical mast cell stabilizer	uncertain	No controls performed	99
Emulgade F®	emulsifier	uncertain	Emulgade F contains cetearyl alcohol, PEG-40 castor oil and sodium cetearyl sulfate	100
estrogen cream	topical hormone preparation	uncertain		8

(continued)

§ **7.5** *(continuation)*

Drug	Use	Mechanism involved	Comment	Ref.
ethyl alcohol	antiseptic	immunologic	Passive transfer only after scratching. The patient reported also reacted to amyl alcohol, butyl alcohol and propyl alcohol. In another patient [67] who displayed erythema 20 minutes after cutaneous contact with ethyl alcohol, a generalized eruption developed after drinking alcoholic beverages. Anaphylaxis from drinking alcohol may be caused by immediate-type allergy to the alcohol metabolite acetic acid [82]. Flushes from drinking alcohol by Orientals may be caused by genetically determined slow aldehyde reductase and subsequent accumulation of acetaldehyde (which causes non-immunologic contact urticaria, Ref. [77]) [96]. Late phase reaction after 10 hours, Ref. [123]	41 67
ethylenediamine	stabilizer	uncertain	Contact urticarial response upon patch testing in a patient with urticaria	64
ethyl vanillin	flavoring agent	uncertain		44
eugenol	fragrance/flavor	uncertain, probably nonimmunologic	Contact urticarial response upon patch testing in patients with urticaria. Also delayed-type allergy in some cases. Oral provocation caused urticaria. Quenching of reactions caused by benzoic acid, cinnamic aldehyde and sorbic acid: Ref. [118]	64
formaldehyde	preservative	uncertain	The reaction was provoked by contact with gaseous formaldehyde [65]. Asthma from occupational exposure caused by type-I allergy to formaldehyde: Ref. [110]. Contact urticaria and pulmonary dysfunction from a patch test with formaldehyde: Ref. [121]. Positive in the NICU-test [77]	65
gentamicin	antibiotic	immunologic		52
gentian violet	antiseptic	uncertain		14
henna	hair dye	uncertain	Also sneezing, wheezing and throat complaints in the reported case [9]. Prick tests were positive. The allergen was *not* 2-hydroxy-1,4-naphthoquinone [91]	9

(continued)

§ **7.5** *(continuation)*

Drug	Use	Mechanism involved	Comment	Ref.
hexamidine isethionate	disinfectant	uncertain	The reaction was caused by a scarification	122
hexantriol	vehicle constituent	uncertain		47
p-hydroxybenzoic acid	preservative	uncertain		60
iodine	antiseptic	non-immunologic	Only listed: no references	52
isopropyl alcohol	antiseptic	uncertain		68
isopropyl dibenzoyl-methane	sunscreen	uncertain	*photo*contact urticaria	120
lanolin alcohol	vehicle constituent	uncertain		51
lemon perfume constituents	perfume	non-immunologic		70
levomepromazine	sedative	uncertain		109
lidocaine	local anesthetic	uncertain		113
lindane	antiparasitic drug	?	Industrial contactant, also induces asthma. Only listed: no references	36
mechlorethamine hydrochloride	cytostatic drug	uncertain	Has also caused anaphylaxis and dyspnea	10 17 18 75
menthol	antipruritic	uncertain		37
merbromin (mercuro-chrome)	antiseptic	immunologic	Passive transfer test positive, also to merthiolate (thimerosal)	86
metamizole	analgesic	uncertain	Contact urticarial reaction upon patch testing in patients with anaphylaxis after oral administration. Cross-reactions occur between pyrazolone derivatives	62
methyl green	antiseptic	uncertain		14
mezlocillin	antibiotic	uncertain	No cross-reaction to penicillin	116
monoamylamine	antifungal drug	uncertain		49
neomycin	antibiotic	uncertain	Also delayed-type hypersensitivity to neomycin in the reported case, with cross-reaction to paromomycin and kanamycin [32]. Anaphylaxis after open test [32]	32 103
nicotinyl alcohol	vasodilator	uncertain		32

(continued)

§ **7.5** *(continuation)*

Drug	Use	Mechanism involved	Comment	Ref.
nitrofuroxime	antifungal drug	uncertain	Also delayed-type hypersensitivity in the reported case	1
papain	enzyme in contact lens cleaning solution	uncertain		85
parabens	preservatives	immunologic and non-immunologic	Passive transfer demonstrated	21 64
penicillin	antibiotic	uncertain	Anaphylaxis after oral administration and testing [52]	32 60
peppermint oil	flavor in toothpaste	uncertain		101
phenol	antipruritic	non-immunologic		4
phenylbutazone	analgesic	uncertain	Cross-reaction to propyphenazone in a patient with anaphylaxis after oral propyphenazone. Also delayed type hypersensitivity to phenylbutazone in the reported case	62
p-phenylenediamine	in hair preparations	uncertain	Also difficulty in breathing. Also delayed type allergy [92]. The oxidation product *N'N'*-bis-(4-aminophenyl)-2,5-diamino- 1,4-quinonediimine caused immunologic contact urticaria with anaphylaxis in one patient [93]	6 92
phenylmercuric compounds	antiseptics	immunologic	Inhalation produced asthma. Passive transfer demonstrated	31
o-phenylphenate	preservative	immunologic	passive transfer positive	95
polyethyleneglycol 400 (PEG-400)	vehicle constituent	uncertain		11
polysorbate 60	vehicle constituent	uncertain	Only urticarial response when patch-tested on the forehead	29
pristinamycin	antibiotic	uncertain	Also delayed-type hypersensitivity in the reported patient	2
promethazine hydrochloride	antihistamine	uncertain		20
propipocaine	local anesthetic	uncertain	Anaphylactic shock	112
propyl alcohol	solvent	immunologic	The patient reported also reacted to amyl alcohol, ethyl alcohol and butyl alcohol. Negative in the NICU-test [77]	41

(continued)

§ **7.5** *(continuation)*

Drug	Use	Mechanism involved	Comment	Ref.
propylene glycol	vehicle constituent	uncertain		55
propyphenbutazone	analgesic	uncertain	Contact urticarial reaction upon patch testing in patients with anaphylaxis after oral propyphenbutazone. Cross-reactions between pyrazolone derivatives	62
pyrazolone derivatives	analgesics	uncertain	Contact urticarial reactions upon patch testing in patients with anaphylaxis after oral administration. *See under* aminophenazone, propyphenbutazone, metamizole and phenylbutazone	62
resorcinol	acne therapy	non-immunologic	Only listed: no references	52
rouge	cosmetic	uncertain	The patient had a delayed-type reaction to γ-methylionone, a perfume ingredient of the cosmetic. The relevance of this finding remained uncertain. The contact urticarial reaction was limited to the face	56
rifamycin	topical antibiotic	immunologic	Cross-reaction to rifampicin [108]. Anaphylactic shock [125]	108 125
salicylic acid	keratolytic drug	uncertain		36
sodium benzoate	preservative	non-immunologic	*See also under* denatonium benzoate. Negative in the NICU-test [77]. Airborne contact urticaria: Ref. [88]	3
sodium sulfite	preservative	uncertain	anaphylaxis and asthma	
sorbic acid	preservative	non-immunologic and immunologic (?) [40]	Sorbic acid in food has caused perioral contact urticaria [63]. Quenching by eugenol: Ref. [118]. Positive in the NICU-test [77]	15 40
sorbitan laurate	emulsifier	uncertain	Also delayed type allergy in the reported case	94
squaric acid dibutyl ester	contact allergen for treatment of alopecia areata	uncertain		115
stearyl alcohol	vehicle constituent	uncertain	Also delayed type hypersensitivity in the reported case, with concomitant reaction to cetyl alcohol	16
streptomycin	antibiotic	uncertain	*See also under* neomycin. Rhinitis and conjunctivitis after open test	32 45

(continued)

§ **7.5** *(continuation)*

Drug	Use	Mechanism involved	Comment	Ref.
sulfur	antiseborrheic drug	uncertain		60
sulisobenzone (benzophenone-4)	sunscreen	uncertain	Also delayed type hypersensitivity in the reported patient	39
terpinyl acetate	fragrance	uncertain	Terpinyl acetate was a fragrance ingredient in spray starch	74
tetracycline	antibiotic	uncertain	Also asthma in the reported case. Generalized urticaria upon patch-testing	73
thiomersal	preservative	immunologic	only listed: no references	72
thurfyl nicotinate	rubefacient	non-immunologic	Histamine releaser. Positive in the NICU test [77]	34
α-tocopherol (vitamin E)	antioxidant	uncertain		23
tropicamide	anticholinergic ophthalmic preparation	uncertain		19
virginiamycin	antibiotic	immunologic		52
wheat bran	in baths	immunologic	The patient was an atopic infant whose eczema improved on a gluten-free diet	71

7.6 Cosmetics that have caused contact urticaria include:

- bath oil [102]
- casein-containing diaper rash ointment [107]
- deodorant [48]
- fixation fluid for permanent wave [51]
- hair bleach (*see* § 7.5 *under* ammonium persulfate)
- hair conditioner [117]
- hair dye [92, 93]
- hair spray [69]
- henna [91]
- nail varnish [69]
- perfumes [44,69,70]
- permanent wave fluid [51]
- rouge (*see* § 7.5)
- shampoo [40], egg-containing [89]
- toothpaste [40] (*see* § 7.5 *under* sorbic acid)

7.7 REFERENCES

1. Aaronson, C.M. (1969): Generalized urticaria from sensitivity to nifuroxime. *J. Am. Med. Assoc., 210, 557.*
2. Baes, H. (1974): Allergic contact dermatitis to virginiamycin. Dermatologica (Basel), 149, 231.
3. Björkner, B. (1980): Contact urticaria and asthma from denatonium benzoate (Bitrex®). *Contact Dermatitis, 6,* 466.
4. Björkner, A. (1968): *Skin reactions to primary irritants in patients with hand eczema.* O. Isacson Tryckeri, Gothenburg.
5. Brubaker, M.M. (1972): Urticarial reaction to ammonium persulphate. *Arch. Dermatol., 106,* 413.
6. Temesvari, E. (1984): Contact urticaria from paraphenylenediamine. *Contact Dermatitis, 11,* 125.
7. Camarasa, J.M.G., Alomar, A. and Perez, M. (1978): Contact urticaria and anaphylaxis from aminophenazone. *Contact Dermatitis, 4,* 243.
8. Cole, H., Marmelzat, W. and Walker, A. (1948): Severe allergic sensitization to an estrogenic cream. *Ohio St. Med. J., 44,* 472.
9. Cronin, E. (1980): Immediate-type hypersensitivity to henna. *Contact Dermatitis, 5,* 198.
10. Daughters, D., Zackheim, H. and Maibach, H.I. (1973): Urticaria and anaphylactoid reactions after topical application of mechlorethamine. *Arch. Dermatol., 107,* 429.
11. Fisher, A.A. (1978): Immediate and delayed allergic contact reactions to polyethyleneglycol. *Contact Dermatitis, 4,* 135.
12. Fisher, A.A. and Dooms-Goossens, A. (1976): Persulfate hair bleach reactions. Cutaneous and respiratory manifestations. *Arch. Dermatol., 112,* 1407.
13. Forsbeck, M. and Skog, E. (1977): Immediate reactions to patch tests with balsam of Peru. *Contact Dermatitis, 3,* 201.
14. François, A., Henin, P., Carli Basset, C. and Ginies, G. (1970): Anaphylactic shock following application of Milian's solution. *Bull. Soc. Franç. Derm. Syph., 77,* 834.
15. Soschin, D. and Leyden, J.J. (1986): Sorbic acid-induced erythema and edema. *J. Am. Acad. Dermatol, 14,* 234–241.
16. Gaul, L.E. (1969): Dermatitis from cetyl and stearyl alcohol. *Arch. Dermatol., 99,* 593.
17. Grunnet, E. (1976): Contact urticaria and anaphylactoid reaction induced by topical application of nitrogen mustard. *Br. J. Dermatol., 94,* 101.
18. Guilhou, J.-J., Barnéon, G., Malbos, S., Peyron, J.-L., Michel, B. and Meynadier, J. (1980): Mucinose folliculaire perforante et hypersensibilité immédiate à la méchloréthamine chez un malade atteint de mycosis fongoïde. *Ann. Derm. Venereol, (Paris), 107,* 59.
19. Guill, A. Goette, K., Knight, C.G., Peck, C.C. and Lupton, G.P. (1979): Erythema multiforme and urticaria. *Arch. Dermatol., 115,* 742.
20. Haustein, U.F. (1976): Anaphylactic shock and contact urticaria after the patch test with professional allergens. *Allergie u. Immunol. (Leipzig), 22,* 349.
21. Henry, J.C., Tschen, E.H. and Becker, L.E. (1979): Contact urticaria to parabens. *Arch. Dermatol., 115,* 1231.
22. Heygi, E. and Dolezalová, A. (1976): Urticarial reaction after patch tests of toothpaste with a sub shock condition: Hypersensitivity to Caraway seed. *Cs. Derm., 51,* 19.
23. Kassen, B. and Mitchell, J.C. (1974): Contact urticaria from vitamin E preparation in two siblings. *Contact Dermatitis Newsl., 16,* 482.
24. Kleinhans, D. and Zwissler, H. (1980): Anaphylaktischer Schock nach Anwendung einer Benzocainhaltigen Salbe. *Z. Hautkr., 55,* 945.
25. Kligman, A.M. (1965): Dimethyl Sulfoxide — Part 2. *J. Am. Med. Assoc., 193,* 151.
26. Kozáková, M. (1976): Sub-shock brought on by epidemic skin test for chloramphenicol. *Cs. Derm., 51,* 82.
27. Lahti, A. (1980): Non-immunologic contact urticaria. *Acta derm.-venereol. (Stockh.), 60,* Suppl. 91, 1.
28. Löwenfeld, W. (1928): Überempfindlichkeit gegen Iodthion mit gleichzeitiger urtikarieller Reaktion. *Derm. Wschr., 78,* 502.
29. Maibach, H.I. and Conant, M. (1977): Contact urticaria to a corticosteroid cream: polysorbate 60. *Contact Dermatitis, 3,* 350.
30. Maibach, H.I. and Johnson, H.L. (1975): Contact urticaria syndrome. *Arch. Dermatol., 111,* 726.
31. Mathews, K.P. and Pan, P.M. (1968): Immediate type hypersensitivity to phenylmercuric compounds. *Am. Dermatol., 79,* 545.
32. Maucher, O.D., (1972): Anaphylakitische Reaktionen beim Epikutantest. *Hautarzt, 23,* 139.

33. Merck Index (1976): Ninth Edition, p.433. Merck and Co. Inc., Rahway, USA.
34. Murrell, T.W. and Taylor, W.M. (1959): The cutaneous reaction to nicotinic acid (niacin)–furfuryl. *Arch. Dermatol., 79,* 545.
35. Nater, J.P., De Jong, M.C.J.M., Baar, A.J.M. and Bleumink, E. (1977): Contact urticarial skin responses to cinnamaldehyde. *Contact Dermatitis, 3,* 151.
36. Odom, R.B. and Maibach, H.I. (1976): Contact urticaria: A different contact dermatitis. *Cutis, 18,* 672.
37. Papa, C.M. and Shelley, W.B. (1974): Menthol hypersensitivity. *J. Am. Med. Assoc., 189,* 546.
38. Pietzcker, F. and Kuner, V. (1975): Anaphylaxie nach epikutanem Ampicillin-Test. *Z. Hautkr., 50,* 437.
39. Ramsay, D.L., Cohen, H.J. and Baer, R.L. (1972): Allergic reaction to benzophenonen. *Arch. Dermatol., 105,* 906.
40. Rietschel, R.L. (1978): Contact urticaria from synthetic cassia oil and sorbic acid limited to the face. *Contact Dermatitis, 4,* 347.
41. Rilliet, A., Hunziker, N. and Brun, R. (1980): Alcohol contact urticaria syndrome (immediate-type hypersensitivity). *Dermatologica (Basel), 161,* 361.
42. Roed-Petersen, J. and Hjorth, N. (1976): Contact dermatitis from antioxidants. *Br. J. Dermatol., 94,* 233.
43. Roupe, G. and Strannegard, C. (1969): Anaphylactic shock elicited by topical administration of bacitracin. *Arch. Derm., 100,* 450.
44. Rudzki, E. and Grzywa, Z. (19760: Immediate reactions to balsam of Peru, cassia oil and ethyl vanillin. *Contact Dermatitis, 2,* 360.
45. Rudzki, E., Rebandel, P. and Rogozinski, T. (1981): Contact urticaria from rat tail, guinea pig, streptomycin and vinyl pyridine. *Contact Dermatitis, 7,* 186.
46. Sikorski, H. (1951): Salvarsan-Allergie der Haut. *Z. Haut-u. Geschlkr., 11,* 341.
47. Tachibana, S., Horio, T. and Hayakawa, M. (1977): Contact urticaria and dermatitis due to fluocinonide cream. *Acta. Derm. (Kyoto), 72,* 141.
48. Temesvári, E., Soos, G., Podányi, B., Kovács, I. and Nemeth, I. (1978): Contact urticaria provoked by balsam of Peru. *Contact Dermatitis, 4,* 65.
49. Tharp, C.K. (1973): Contact urticaria (monoamylamine). *Arch. Dermatol., 108,* 135.
50. Tuft, L. (1975): Contact urticaria from cephalosporins. *Arch. Dermatol., 111,* 1609.
51. Von Liebe, V., Karge, H.J. and Burg, G. (1979): Kontakturtikaria. *Hautarzt, 30,* 544.
52. Lahti, A. and Maibach, H.I. (1990): Immediate contact reactions. In: Menné T. and Maibach, H.I. (Editors), *Exogenous Dermatoses, Environmental Contact Dermatitis.* CRC Press, Boca Raton, 21–35.
53. Burdick, A.E. and Mathias, C.G.T. (1985): The contact urticaria syndrome. *Dermatologic Clinics, 3,* 71–84.
54. Ng, S.K. (1988): Contact urticaria — A review. *Ann. Acad. Med., 17,* 563–568.
55. Maibach, H.I., cited by Andersen, K.E. and Storrs, F.J. (1982): Hautreizungen durch Propylenglykol. *Hautarzt, 33,* 12.
56. De Groot, A.C. and Liem, D.H. (1983): Contact urticaria to rouge. *Contact Dermatitis, 9,* 322.
57. Dooms-Goossens, A., Gevers, D., Mertens, A. and Van der Heyden, D. (1983): Allergic contact urticaria due to chloramine. *Contact Dermatitis, 9,* 319.
58. Von Mayenburg, J. and Rakoski, J. (1983): Contact urticaria to diethyltoluamide. *Contact Dermatitis, 9,* 171.
59. Tkach, J.R. (1982): Allergic contact urticaria to benzoyl peroxide. *Cutis, 29,* 187.
60. Böttger, E.M., Mücke, Chr. and Tronnier, H. (1981): Kontaktdermatitis auf neuere Antimykotika und Kontakturtikaria. *Acta Dermatol., 7,* 70.
61. Gotmann-Lückerath, I. (1982): Kontakturtikaria nach Dermoxin®. Society Proceedings. *Dermatosen, 30,* 124.
62. Maucher, O.M. and Fuchs, A. (1983): Kontakturtikaria im Epikutantest bei Pyrazolonallergie. *Hautarzt, 34,* 383.
63. Clemmensen, O. and Hjorth, N. (1982): Perioral contact urticaria from sorbic acid and benzoic acid in a salad dressing. *Contact Dermatitis, 8,* 1.
64. Warin, R.P. and Smith, R.J. (1982): Chronic urticaria. Investigations with patch and challenge tests. *Contact Dermatitis, 8,* 117.
65. Lindskov, R. (1982): Contact urticaria to formaldehyde. *Contact Dermatitis, 8,* 333.
66. Ryan, M.E., Davis, B.M. and Marks, J.G. (1980): Contact urticaria and allergic contact dermatitis to benzocaine gel. *J. Am. Acad. Dermatol., 2,* 221.
67. Drevets, C.C. and Seebohm, P.M. (1961): Dermatitis from alcohol. *J. Allergy, 32,* 277.
68. Fisher, A.A. (1968): Contact dermatitis. The noneczematous variety. *Cutis, 4,* 567.

69. Fisher, A.A. (1973): *Contact Dermatitis, 2nd Edition,* Lea and Febiger, Philadelphia, p. 284.
70. Rothenborg, H.W., Menné, T. and Sjolin, K.-E. (1977): Temperature dependent primary irritant dermatitis from lemon perfume. *Contact Dermatitis, 3,* 37.
71. Langeland, T. and Nyrud, M. (1982): Contact urticaria to wheat bran bath: a case report. *Acta derm. venereol. (Stockh.), 62,* 82.
72. Katchen, B.R. and Maibach, H.I. (1990): Immediate-type contact reaction: immunologic contact urticaria. In: Menné, T. and Maibach, H.I. (Editors). *Exogenous Dermatoses: Environmental Contact Dermatitis.* CRC Press, Boca Raton, 51–64.
73. Schwarting, H.H. (1983): Berufsbedingte Tetracyclin-Allergie. *Dermatosen Beruf. Umw., 31,* 130.
74. McDaniel, W.R. and Marks, J.G. (1979): Contact urticaria due to sensitivity to spray starch. *Arch. Derm., 115,* 628.
75. Thestrup-Pedersen, K., Christiansen, J.V. and Zachariae, H. (1982): Precautions for personnel applying topical nitrogen mustard to patients with mycosis fungoides. *Dermatologica (Basel), 165,* 108.
76. Marks, J.G. Jr. (1986): Contact urticaria. *Cosmetics and Toiletries, 101,* 59–63.
77. Gollhausen, R. and Kligman, A.M. (1985): Human assay for identifying substances which induce non-allergic contact urticaria: the NICU test. *Contact Dermatitis, 13,* 98–106.
78. Susitaival, P. and Häkkinen, L. (1989): Anaphylactic allergy to chlorhexidine cream. In: Frosch, P.J. et al. (Editors), *Current Topics in Contact Dermatitis.* Springer Verlag, Berlin, pp. 99–103.
79. Okano, M., Nomura, M., Hata, S., Okado, N., Sato, K., Kitano, Y., Tashiro, M., Yoshimoto, Y., Hama, R. and Aoki, T. (1989): Anaphylactic symptoms due to chlorhexidine gluconate. *Arch. Dermatol., 125,* 50–52.
80. De Groot, A.C. and Hoekstra, J.W. (1990): Gecombineerde Type I en type IV allergie voor chloorhexidinegluconat. *Bulletin Contactdermatosen* (ISSN 0921-0625), 4, 154–155.
81. Wong, W.K., Goh, C.L. and Chan, K.W. (1990): Contact urticaria from chlorhexidine. *Contact Dermatitis, 22,* 52.
82. Przybilla, B., Ring, J. and Galosi, A. (1986): Alcohol-induced anaphylaxis: allergy to the ethanol metabolite acetic acid? *Allergologie, 9,* 164–169.
83. Van Hecke, E. and Santosa, S. (1985): Contact urticaria to DNCB. *Contact Dermatitis, 12,* 282.
84. Valsecchi, R., Foiadelli, L., Reseghetti, A. and Cainelli, T. (1986): Generalized urticaria from DNCB. *Contact Dermatitis, 14,* 254–255.
85. Santucci, B., Cristaudo, A. and Picardo, M. (1985): Contact urticaria from papain in a soft lens solution. *Contact Dermatitis, 12,* 233.
86. Corrales Torres, J.L. and de Corres, F. (1985): Anaphylactic hypersensitivity to mercurochrome (merbromin). *Ann. Allergy, 54,* 230–232.
87. Schechter, J.F., Wilkinson, R.D. and Del Carpio, J. (1984): Anaphylaxis following the use of bacitracin ointment. *Arch. Dermatol, 120,* 909–911.
88. Nethercott, J.R., Lawrence, M.J., Roy, A.M. and Gibson, B.L. (1984): Airborne contact urticaria due to sodium benzoate in a pharmaceutical manufacturing plant. *J. Occup. Med., 26,* 734–736.
89. Braun-Falco, O. and Ring, J. (1984): Zur Therapie des atopischen Ekzems. *Hautarzt, 35,* 447–454.
90. Gonçalo, M., Gonçalo, S. and Moreno, A. (1987): Immediate and delayed sensitivity to chlorocresol. *Contact Dermatitis, 17,* 46–47.
91. Frosch, P.J. and Hausen, B.M. (1986): Allergic reactions of the immediate type to the hair dye Henna. *Allergologie, 9,* 351–353.
92. Edwards, E.K. Jr. and Edwards, E.K. (1984): Contact urticaria and allergic contact dermatitis caused by paraphenylenediamine. *Cutis, 34,* 877–878.
93. Goldberg, B.J., Herman, F.F. and Hirata, I. (1987): Systemic anaphylaxis due to an oxidation product of p-phenylenediamine in a hair dye. *Ann. Allergy, 58,* 205–208.
94. Boyle, J. and Kennedy, C.T.C. (1984): Contact urticaria and dermatitis to Alphaderm®. *Contact Dermatitis, 10,* 178.
95. Tuer, W.F., James, W.D. and Summers, R.J. (1986): Contact urticaria to *o*-phenylphenate. *Ann. Allergy, 56,* 19–21.
96. Wilkin, J.K. and Fortner, G. (1985): Ethnic contact urticaria to alcohol. *Contact Dermatitis, 12,* 118–120.
97. Emmons, W.W. and Marks, J.G. Jr. (1985): Immediate and delayed reactions to cosmetic ingredients. *Contact Dermatitis, 13,* 258–265.
98. Rudzki, E. and Grzywa, Z. (1985): The value of a mixture of cassia and citronella oils for detection of hypersensitivity to essential oils. *Dermatosen, 33,* 59–62.

99. Hutt, N., Firdion, O., Abbas, F. and Pauli, G. (1986): A propos d'un cas d'allergie immédiate vraisemblable au cromoglycate disodique. *Rev. Fr. Allergol., 26,* 147–148.
100. Ring, J., Galosi, A. and Przybilla, B. (1986): Contact anaphylaxis from emulgade F. *Contact Dermatitis, 15,* 49–50.
101. Smith, I.L.F. (1969): Acute allergic reaction following the use of toothpaste. *Br. Dental J., 125,* 304–305.
102. Vasecchi, A. (1987): *G. Ital. Derm. Ven., 122,* 55.
103. Goh, C.L. (1986): Anaphylaxis from topical neomycin and bacitracin. *Aust. J. Derm., 27,* 125–126.
104. Horio, T. (1975): Chlorpromazine photoallergy: co-existence of immediate and delayed type. *Arch. Dermatol., 111,* 1469–1471.
105. Lovell, C.R., Cronin, E. and Rhodes, E.S. (1986): Photocontact urticaria from chlorpromazine. *Contact Dermatitis, 14,* 290–291.
106. Masuda, T., Honda, S. and Nakauchi, Y. et al. (1971): Photocontact dermatitis due to bithionol, TBS, diaphene and hexachlorophene. *Jpn. J. Dermatol., 81,* 238–244.
107. Jarmoc, L.M. and Primack, W.A. (1987): Anaphylaxis to cutaneous exposure to milk protein in a diaper rash ointment. *Clin. Pediatr., 26,* 154–155.
108. Grob, J.J., Pommier, G., Robaglia, A., Collet-Vilette, A.M. and Bonerandi, J.J. (1987): Contact urticaria from rifamycin. *Contact Dermatitis, 16,* 284–285.
109. Johansson, G. (1988): Contact urticaria from levomepromazine. *Contact Dermatitis, 19,* 304.
110. Gehse, M., Gehring, W. and Gloor, M. (1988): Berufsbedingte Formaldehyd-Allergie vom Soforttyp. *Dermatosen, 36,* 101–102.
111. Elsner, P., Pevny, I. and Burg, G. (1990): Anaphylaxis induced by topically applied Bacitracin. *Am. J. Contact Dermatitis, 1,* 162–164.
112. Hollmann, B., Rehmann, O. and Bormann, B. (1988): Lebensbedrohliche allergische Reaktionen durch Einsatz von Urocomb-gel®. *Z. Urol. Nephrol., 81,* 715–717.
113. Budde, J., Stary, A. and Beiteke, U. (1989): Kontaktallergie vom Sofort-Typ auf topische Anwendung von Lidocain. *Dermatosen, 37,* 181–182.
114. Tosti, A., Guerra, L. and Bardazzi, F. (1989): Contact urticaria during topical immunotherapy. *Contact Dermatitis, 21,* 196–197.
115. Barth, J.H., Darley, C.R. and Gibson, J.R. (1985): Squaric acid dibutylester in the treatment of alopecia areata. *Dermatologica, 170,* 40–42.
116. Budde, J., Lentner, A., Stary, A. and Beiteke, U. (1989): Anaphylaktischer Schock nach Hautkontakt mit Mezlozillin (Baypen). *Allergologie, 12,* 355–358.
117. Kousa, M., Strand, R., Mäkinen-Kiljunen, S. and Hunnuksela, M. (1990): Contact urticaria from hair conditioner. *Abstract book, Ninth International Symposium on Contact Dermatitis, 17–19 May 1990, Stockholm, Sweden,* p. 26.
118. Safford, R.J., Basketter, D.A., Allenby, C.F. and Goodwin, B.F.J. (1990): Immediate contact reactions to chemicals in the fragrance mix and a study of the quenching action of eugenol. *Br. J. Dermatol., 123,* 595–606.
119. Palungwachira, P. (1991): Contact urticaria syndrome and anaphylactoid reaction from topical clioquinol and bacitracin (Banocin): a case report. *J. Med. Assoc. Thail., 74,* 43–46.
120. Murphy, G.M., White, I.R. and Cronin, E. (1990): Immediate and delayed photocontact dermatitis from isopropyl dibenzoylmethane. *Contact Dermatitis, 22,* 129–131
121. Orlandini, A., Viotti, G. and Magno, L. (1988): Anaphylactoid reaction induced by patch testing with formaldehyde in an asthmatic. *Contact Dermatitis, 19,* 383–384.
122. Revuz, J., Poli, F., Wechsler, J. and Dubertret, L. (1984): Dermite de contact a l'hexamidine. *Ann. Derm. Venereol, 111,* 805–810.
123. Kanzaki, T. and Hori, H. (1991): Late phase allergic reaction of the skin to ethyl alcohol. *Contact Dermatitis, 25,* 252–253.
124. Pigatto, P.D., Riboldi, A., Morelli, M., Altomare, G.F. and Polenghi, M.M. (1985): Allergic contact dermatitis from oxyphenbutazone. *Contact Dermatitis, 12,* 236.
125. Mancuso, G. and Masara, N. (1992): Contact urticaria and severe anaphylaxis from rifamycin SV. *Contact Dermatitis, 27,* 124–125.
126. Loesche, C., Dejobert, Y. and Thomas, P. (1992): Immediate wheal after topical administration of chlorproethazine. *Contact Dermatitis, 26,* 278.
127. Fisher, A.A. (1989): Urticaria, asthma and anaphylaxis due to sodium sulfite in an antifungal cream complicated by treatment with aminophylline in an ethylenediamine-sensitive person. Part 1, *Cutis*, 44, 19–20.

8. Necrosis of the skin and the mucous membranes due to topical drugs

8.1 The following drugs have caused necrosis after contact with the skin or mucous membranes:

Drug	Use	Ref.
arsenious oxide	self medication	5
cetrimonium bromide	antiseptic	1
chlorhexidine	antiseptic	6
clioquinol	antiseptic	13
crystal violet	antiseptic	9
dequalinium	antiseptic	11
fluorouracil	topical cytostatic	7
fuchsin-silver nitrate	marking patch test sites	3
gentian violet	antifungal drug	4
menthol and methyl salicylate	vasodilator antirheumatic preparation	12
phenol	antipruritic agent antiseptic, chemical face peeling	8
povidone iodine	antiseptic	10
silver nitrate	caustic for the treatment of umbilical granulomas	15
triclocarban	antiseptic	2

8.2 REFERENCES

1. August, P.J. (1975): Cutaneous necrosis due to cetrimide application. *Br. Med. J., 1,* 70.
2. Barrière, H. (1973): La dermite cutanéomuceuse caustique du trichlorocabanilide. *Sem. Hôp. Paris, 49,* 685.
3. Björnberg, A. (1977): Toxic reactions to a patch test skin marker containing fuchsin–silver nitrate. *Contact Dermatitis, 3,* 101.
4. Björnberg, A. and Mobacken, H. (1972): Necrotic skin reactions caused by 1% gentian violet and brilliant green. *Acta. Derm-venereol, (Stockh.), 52*, 55.

5. Fakirbhai, M. (1969): Self-medication of herpes zoster with an arsenic paste. *Br. J. Plast. Surg., 22,* 382.
6. Flotra, L., Gjermo, P., Rolla, G. and Waerhang, J. (1971): Side effects of chlorhexidine mouthwashes. *Scand. J. Dent. Res., 79,* 119.
7. Lee, S., Kim, J.C. and Chun, S.I. (1980): Treatment of verruca plana with 5% 5-fluorouracil ointment. *Dermatologica (Basel), 160,* 383.
8. Wenzel, P., Husemann, M. and Goos, M. (1988): Toxische Dermatitis nach hochdosierter Phenol-Applikation. *Akt. Dermatol.,* 334–335.
9. Meurer, H. and Konz, B. (1977): Hautnekrosen nach Anwendung 2%iger Pyoktaninlösung. *Hautarzt, 28,* 94.
10. Shroff, A.P. and Jones, J.K. (1980): Reactions to povidone iodine preparation. *J. Am. Med. Assoc., 243,* 230.
11. Wilkinson, D.S. (1970): Durch Dequalinium hervorgerufene Hautnekrosen. *Hautarzt, 21,* 114.
12. Heng, M.C.Y. (1987): Local necrosis and interstitial nephritis due to topical methyl salicylate and menthol. *Cutis, 39,* 442–444.
13. Peters, K.P., Lechner, T. and Simon, M. Jr. (1986): Schleimhautnekrosen nach lokaler Anwendung von Clioquinol. *Akt. Dermatol., 12,* 87–88.
14. Antrum, R.M. and Kersley, J.B. (1984): An unusual case of skin necrosis due to an adrenaline-containing cream. *Br. J. Clin. Pract., 38,* 191.
15. Chamberlain, J.M., Gorman, R.L. and Young, G.M. (1992): Silver nitrate burns following treatment for umbilical granuloma. *Pediatr. Emergency Case, 8,* 29–30.

9. Acne-folliculitis

9.1 Contact with a great variety of substances can produce a follicular eruption, in which the comedo is the initiating lesion. This type of eruption is called *acne venenata*. The better known varieties are [3,4]:

1. Chloracne, acne venenata caused by chlorinated hydrocarbons. This type of eruption has occurred, among others, in workers manufacturing DDT and weed killers, such as 2,4,5-trichlorophenol. Chlorinated hydrocarbons may also be present in paints, varnish, lacquers and various oils.
2. Acne venenata caused by cutting oils
3. Acne venenata caused by petroleum oil
4. Acne venenata caused by coal tars and pitches
5. Acne venenata caused by topical corticosteroid therapy.

Important for the purpose of this book is another particular form of acne venenata, which has been termed *acne cosmetica* by Kligman and Mills [2]. It is usually a mild eruption, consisting mainly of closed comedones. Blackheads are hard to find; sometimes a number of papulopustules may be seen over the cheeks and the chin. The eruption is seen in adult women and is attributed to the acnegenic properties of cosmetics used by these patients, mainly facial creams. It is stressed that cosmetics are very weak acnegens, and that it is their daily use, year after year, that enables them to induce acne in prone subjects. Two types of reactions may develop in the skin of patients with acne who are using cosmetics. The first is that of true aggravation of acne in which the formation of comedones is promoted, a process that develops slowly over many months. The second is that of a folliculitis in which chemical irritation of the follicular epithelium by the cosmetic product is attended by inflammatory pustules and papules that develop within a relatively short time. The term 'acnegenesis' encompasses the skin reactions of both comedones and follicular inflammation [10].

Pomade acne is a variety of acne venenata, occurring chiefly on the forehead and the temples, seen mostly in adult black males, due to the application of various greases and oils to the scalp as hair-grooming aids [11].

9.2 Assays on the rabbit ear [9] suggested the following compounds for topical use to be comedogenic [2,5,8,12,15,19]. It should be realized that the results of different studies have sometimes varied, which may be due to variations in the test procedures, the interpretation, the materials used and their concentrations.

acetylated lanolin alcohols [18]
ammonium sulfobituminate
butyl stearate [18]
capric/caprylic triglyceride [15]
cetyl alcohol [19]
coal tar
cocoa butter
coconut oil [15]
corn oil
decyl oleate [15,18]
decaglyceryl decaoleate [15]
D & C Red no. 2,6,9,19,21,27,30,36 [18]
ethoxylated lanolin [18]
grape seed oil [15]
hexadecyl alcohol
hexane
hexylene glycol
hybrid safflower oil [15]
hydrogenated lanolin [15]
hydrophilic ointment
isoparaffin C9–11 [15]
isoparaffin C13–16 [15
isopropyl isostearate [18]
isopropyl lanolate [15]
isopropyl linoleate [15]
isopropyl myristate [18]
isopropyl neopentanoate [18]
isopropyl palmitate [15]
isostearic acid [15]
isostearyl alcohol [15]
isostearyl neopentanoate [19]
laneth-10 acetate [15]
lanolic acid [15]
lanolin
lanolin alcohol [19]
laureth-4 [18]
lauryl alcohol
linseed oil
methyl oleate
myreth-3 myristate [15]
myristyl lactate [15,18]
myristyl myristate [18]
myristyl propionate [15]
octanol
octyldodecanol [15]
octyl palmitate [15]
oleic acid
oleyl alcohol [15,18]
olive oil
PPG-2 myristyl propionate [18]
PPG-15 stearyl ether [15]
peach kernel oil [15]
peanut oil
pine tar
polyethylene glycol 300
polyoxyethylene ether of white lanolin
propylene glycol monostearate [18]
red veterinary petrolatum
safflower oil
sesame oil
sodium lauryl sulfate [18]
sorbitan oleate [15]
stearic acid
sulfated castor oil [18]
sulfur (*not* in Ref. [18])
sunscreens, proprietary preparations [6]
sweet almond oil [15]
vitamin E oil [15]

Frank [7] has pointed out that there is no evidence that the rabbit ear model is prophetic of acnegenicity in human subjects, and advised that the dermatologist should reserve judgment as to its prophetic value in the diagnosis and management of the patient with an acne eruption. Indeed, members of an Expert Panel, who provided guidelines for comedogenicity testing [10], deemed such lists of comedogenic substances not necessarily meaningful. Although they may be important for pharmaceutical research and for the formulation of nonacnegenic products, they cannot be translated in what might occur in a final product. The concentrations used in testing are often much greater than those in the final product. Thus it is possible to use concentrations that are lower than the minimal acnegenic level [15]. In addition, vehicles for finished products can increase or decrease the acnegenic potential of individual compounds. It is felt that most cosmetics are adequately tested for their acnegenic potential [10]. Acnegenicity, although a real formulating consideration, can be moderated and even eliminated by use of all but the most severely acnegenic raw materials [15]. Clinical reports of acne cosmetica have included petrolatum [12, 13] although the validity of report 13 was doubted [14]. Scalp comedones have been ascribed to minoxidil [16], but this report was also doubted [17].

Contact acne has also been reported due to a metal spectacle frame in a patient sensitive to nickel sulfate [1].

9.3 REFERENCES

1. Grimalt, F. and Romaguera, C. (1978): Nickel allergy and spectacle frame contact acne. *Contact Dermatitis, 4,* 377.
2. Kligman, A.M. and Mills, O.H. (1972): Acne cosmetica. *Arch. Dermatol., 106,* 843.
3. Plewig, G. and Kligman, A.M. (1975): *Acne, Morphogenesis and Treatment.* Springer Verlag, Berlin, Heidelberg, New York.
4. Weirich, E.G. (1980): Die Kontaktakne: Beispiel einer Zivilisationsdermatose. *Dermatosen Beruf Umw., 26,* 45.
5. Mills, O.H. and Kligman, A.M. (1982): A human model for assessing comedogenic substances. *Arch. Dermatol., 118,* 903.
6. Mills, O.H. and Kligman, A.M. (1982): Comedogenicity of sunscreens. Experimental observations in rabbits. *Arch. Dermatol., 118,* 417.
7. Frank, S.B. (1982): Is the rabbit ear model, in its present state, prophetic of acnegenicity? *J. Am. Acad. Dermatol., 6,* 373.
8. Fulton, J.E. Jr., Bradley, S. and Agundez, A. et al. (1976): Non-comedogenic cosmetics. *Cutis, 17,* 344.
9. Kligman, A.M. and Kwong, T. (1979): An improved rabbit ear model for assessing comedogenic substances. *Br. J. Dermatol., 100,* 1.
10. Strauss, J.S. and Jackson, E.M. (1989): American Academy of Dermatology. Invitational Symposium on Comedogenicity. *J. Am. Acad. Dermatol., 20,* 272–277.
11. Fisher, A.A. (1986): Acne venenata in black skin. *Cutis, 37,* 24–26.
12. Shelley, W.B. and Shelley, E.D. (1986): Chap Stick® acne. *Cutis, 37,* 459–460.
13. Frankel, E.B. (1985): Acne secondary to white petrolatum use. *Arch. Dermatol., 121,* 589–590.
14. English, J.S.C. and Murphy, G. (1985): Acne secondary to white petrolatum use. *Arch. Dermatol., 121,* 1240.
15. Lanzet, M. (1986): Comedogenic effects of cosmetic raw materials. *Cosm. & Toiletries, 101,* 63–72.
16. Baral, J. (1985): Scalp comedones after topical minoxidil. *J. Am. Acad. Dermatol., 13,* 1051.
17. Olsen, E.A. (1985): Reply. *J. Am. Acad. Dermatol., 13,* 1051–1052.
18. Fulton, J.E., Pay, S.R. and Fulton, J.E. III. (1984): Comedogenicity of current therapeutic products, cosmetics and ingredients in the rabbit ear. *J. Am. Acad. Dermatol., 10,* 96–105.
19. Nelson, F.P. and Rumsfield, J. (1988): Cosmetics, Contents and function. *Int. J. Dermatol., 27,* 665–672.

10. Discoloration of the skin and appendages

In § 10.1 topical drugs and cosmetics (ingredients) which have caused (unintended) discoloration of the skin and appendages are listed. Nail pigmentation abnormalities have been reviewed [74].

10.1 Discoloration of the skin and the appendages due to topical drugs and cosmetics

Drug	Use	Side effects	Ref.
ammoniated mercury	formerly used for the treatment of psoriasis	Grey-brown discoloration of the skin and fingernails. Also depigmentation	3 9 17 29
amphotericin B	antibiotic	Yellow discoloration of the nails	48
Arning's tincture	antifungal solution	Brownish discoloration of the nails	51
benzoyl peroxide	acne therapy	Discoloration of the hair and post-inflammatory pigmentation. Hypopigmentation	11 32
BHA (butylated hydroxyanisole)	antioxidant	Depigmentation	25
BHT (butylated hydroxytoluene)	antioxidant	Depigmentation (?)	30
carmustine	cytostatic drug	Pigmentation/hypopigmentation	8 55
chlorhexidine	antiseptic	Discoloration of the teeth and the tongue	7
chrysarobin	psoriasis therapy	Brown-purplish discoloration of the skin, nails and hair	10
cinnamic aldehyde	fragrance compound	Depigmentation	23
clioquinol	antiseptic	Brown discoloration of the nails Yellow discoloration of the nails Green hairy tongue Red discoloration of white hair	48 64 64 64

(continued)

§ **10.1** *(continuation)*

Drug	Use	Side effects	Ref.
cloflucarban	antiseptic	Contact allergy has caused pigmentation of the face *See also* § 4.2 *and* 4.3	24
coal tar dyes	in cosmetics	'Pigmented cosmetic dermatitis' *see also* § 4.2 *and* 4.3. Coal tar dyes having caused pigmented cosmetic dermatitis include: Brilliant lake red R (DC Red 31, CI 15800);	27
		Carbanthrene Blue (DC Blue G);	
		Erythrosine-Al (FDC Red 3, CI 45430);	
		Helindone Pink (DC Red 30, CI 73360)	
		Lithol Red-CA (DC Red 11, CI 15630);	28
		Permanent Orange (DC Orange 17, CI 12075);	
		Red Lake C-Ba (DC Red 9, CI 15585);	
		Toluidine Red (Pigment Red 3, CI 12120);	
corticosteroids	various dermatoses	Hyper- and hypopigmentation	22
dihydroxyacetone	tanning agent	Brown discoloration	21
dinitrochlorobenzene	treatment of alopecia areata and warts	Yellow discoloration of grey hair	12
		Brownish discoloration of the nails	50
		Vitiligo	61
diphencyprone	contact allergen for the treatment of alopecia areata	Vitiligo	58–60
		Dyschromia in confetti	75
dithranol	psoriasis therapy	Brown-purplish discoloration of the skin, nails and hair	47
essential oils (lemon, lime, orange, mandarin, juniper)	fragrance materials	Red discoloration of the skin caused by terpenes	54
estradiol	hormone	Hyperpigmentation provoked by UV-B	72
ethacridine	antiseptic	Brownish discoloration of the nails	51
fluorouracil	topical cytostatic	Hyperpigmentation/hypo-pigmentation	18 42 43
		Melanonychia	56
formaldehyde	various e.g. preservative	Brown discoloration of the nails	48
glutaral	antiperspirant/ antimycotic	Brown discoloration of the skin and nails	14 49

(continued)

§ **10.1** *(continuation)*

Drug	Use	Side effects	Ref.
henna	hair dye	Brown discoloration of the nails and skin	48
hydroquinone	bleaching agent	Exogenous ochronosis Brown discoloration of the finger nails	6 35 36 39 40 46 62
hydroxyquinoline sulfate	antiseptic	Leukoderma	4
iron salts	hemostasis	Brown discoloration (sometimes permanent)	2 41
4-isopropylcatechol	bleaching agent	Reticular hyperpigmentation and depigmentation	5
lead	adstringent in powder	Hyperpigmentation of the nails	67
mechlorethamine hydrochloride	topical cytostatic drug	Pigmentation	33 52
mercuric oxide	bleaching agent	Grey pigmentation of the skin	70
mercury	bleaching agent	Greenish black nail discoloration as a systemic side effect	73
minoxidil	treatment of alopecia androgenetica	Yellow discoloration of white hair, caused by an (unknown) impurity in the minoxidil lotion rather than by minoxidil itself	66
monobenzone (monobenzyl-ether of hydroquinone)	depigmenting agent	Depigmentation and pigmentation (locally and at a distance)	1 34 65
monoethyl ether of hydroquinone	depigmenting agent	Depigmentation locally and at a distance	34 37
musk ambrette	fragrance	pigmented (photo) allergic contact dermatitis	68 71
Perfume ingredients – benzyl alcohol – benzyl salicylate – cananga oil – cinnamic alcohol – geraniol – hydroxycitronellal – jasmin absolute – lavender oil – methoxycitronellal – red zig – sandalwood oil – ylang-ylang oil	in cosmetics	Contact allergy has caused pigmentation of the face (pigmented cosmetic dermatitis). *See also* § 4.2 *and* 4.3	24 27

(continued)

§ **10.1** *(continuation)*

Drug	Use	Side effects	Ref.
petrolatum	vehicle	Hyperpigmentation	20
phenolic compounds	antipruritics, antiseptics	Depigmentation	15
potassium permanganate	wet dressings	Brown discoloration of the skin, brown or yellow discoloration of the nails	48
resorcinol (and monoacetate)	peeling agent	Darkens fair hair	19
		Orange-brown discoloration of (lacquered) nails	48
silver nitrate	in solutions for antisepsis	Grey-brown discoloration of the conjunctiva	16
		Black discoloration of the fingernails	45
		Ulcerating stromal opacification	16
silver sulfadiazine	treatment of burns	Brown-grey discoloration of the skin from silver deposition	69
stilbestrol	hormone	Brown discoloration of the nipples and the linea alba (systemic effects caused by percutaneous absorption. *See* § 16.71)	26
squaric acid dibutylester	treatment of alopecia areata	Vitiligo	63
tetracycline	(topical) antibiotic	Yellow staining	38
thiotepa	in eye drops	Periorbital leukoderma	13
timolol eyedrops	treatment of glaucoma	Nail pigmentation	57
tretinoin	acne therapy	Hypopigmentation	11
		Hyperpigmentation	44
triclocarban	antiseptic	Contact allergy has caused pigmentation of the face. *See also* § 4.2 *and* 4.3	24
vitamin K_1	vitamin	Dark-brown staining in factory workers	31 53

10.2 REFERENCES

1. Bentley-Phillips, B. and Bayler, M.A.H. (1975): Cutaneous reactions to topical application of hydroquinone. *S. Afr. Med. J., 49,* 1391.
2. Brehm, G. (1976): Pigmentierung nach lokaler Anwendung von Eisenchloridlösung. *Akt. Dermatol., 3,* 117.
3. Butterworth, T. and Strean, L.P. (1963): Mercurial pigmentation of nails. *Arch. Dermatol., 88,* 55.
4. Calnan, C.D. (1973): Leucoderma with Quinoderm. *Contact Dermatitis Newsl., 13,* 378.
5. Dong Gil Byen, Young Hoe Kim, Yang Ja Park and Soon Bok Lee (1975): Treatment of hyperpigmented disease with 4-isopropylcatechol (Korean). *Kor. J. Derm., 13,* 5.

6. Williams, H. (1992): Skin lightening creams containing hydroquinone. The case for a temporary ban. *Br. Med. J., 305,* 903–904.
7. Flotra, L. (1973): Different modes of chlorhexidine application and related local side effects. *J. Periodont. Res., 8, Suppl. 12,* 41.
8. Frost, P. and DeVita, V.T. (1966): Pigmentation due to a new antitumour agent. *Arch. Dermatol., 94,* 265.
9. Goeckerman, W.H. (1922): The peculiar discoloration of the skin. *J. Am. Med. Assoc., 70,* 605.
10. Goodman, L.S. and Gilman, A. (1970): *The Pharmacological Basis of Therapeutics,* 4th Ed. The MacMillan Company, London–Toronto.
11. Handojo, I. (1979): The combined use of topical benzoyl peroxide and tretinoin in the treatment of acne vulgaris. *Int. J. Dermatol., 18,* 419.
12. Happle, R., Cebulla, K. and Echternacht-Happle, K. (1978): Dinitrochlorobenzene therapy for alopecia areata. *Arch. Dermatol., 114,* 1629.
13. Harben, D.J., Cooper, P.H. and Rodman, O. (1977): Thiotepa-induced leukoderma. *Arch. Dermatol., 115,* 973.
14. Juhlin, L. and Hansson, H. (1968): Topical glutaraldehyde for plantar hyperhydrosis. *Arch. Dermatol., 97,* 327.
15. Kahn, G. (1970): Depigmentation caused by phenolic germicides. *Arch. Dermatol., 102,* 177.
16. Schirner, G., Schrage, N.F., Salla, S. et al. (1991): Silbernitratverätzung nach Credéscher Prophylaxe. *Klin. Mbl. Augenheilk., 199,* 283–291.
17. Lamar, L.M. and Bliss, B.O. (1966): Localized pigmentation of the skin due to topical mercury. *Arch. Dermatol., 93,* 450.
18. Lee, S., Kim, J.C. and Chun, S.I. (1980): Treatment of verruca plana with 5% 5-fluorouracil ointment. *Dermatologica (Basel), 160,* 383.
19. Loveman, A.B. and Fleigelman, M.T. (1955): Discoloration of the nails. *Arch. Dermatol., 72,* 153.
20. Maibach, H.I. (1978): Chronic dermatitis and hyperpigmentation from petrolatum. *Contact Dermatitis, 4,* 62.
21. Maibach, H.I. and Kligman, A.M. (1960): Dihydroxyacetone: a suntan-simulating agent. *Arch. Dermatol., 82,* 505.
22. Marchand, J.-P., Arnold, J. and Ndiaye, B. (1976): Dépigmentation de la peau du noir africain provoquée par les corticoides. *Bull. Soc. Franç. Derm. Syph., 83,* 17.
23. Mathias, C.G.T., Maibach, H.I. and Conant, M.A. (1980): Perioral leukoderma simulating vitiligo from use of a toothpaste containing cinnamic aldehyde. *Arch. Dermatol., 116,* 1172.
24. Nakayama, H., Harado, R. and Toda, M. (1976): Pigmented cosmetic dermatitis. *Int. J. Dermatol., 15,* 673.
25. Riley, P.A. (1971): Acquired hypomelanosis. *Br. J. Dermatol., 84,* 290.
26. Stoppelman, M.R.H. and Van Valkenburg, R.A. (1955): Pigmentaties en gynecomastie ten gevolge van het gebruik van stilbestrol bevattend haarwater bij kinderen. *Ned. T. Geneesk., 99,* 3925.
27. Nakayama, H., Matsuo, S., Hayakawa, K., Takhashi, K., Shigematsu, T. and Ota, S. (1984): Pigmented cosmetic dermatitis. *Int. J. Dermatol., 23,* 299–305.
28. Sugai, T., Takahashi, Y. and Tagaki, T. (1977): Pigmented cosmetic dermatitis and coal tar dyes. *Contact Dermatitis, 3,* 249.
29. Summa, J.D. (1975): Chronische Quecksilbervergiftung durch Gebrauch kosmetischer Salben. *Münch. med. Wschr., 117,* 1121.
30. Vollum, D.I. (1971): Hypomelanosis from an antioxidant in polyethylene film. *Arch. Dermatol., 104,* 70.
31. Watrous, R.M. (1947): Health hazards of the pharmaceutical industry. *Br. J. Indust. Med., 4,* 111.
32. Yong, C.C. (1979): Benzoyl peroxide gel therapy in acne in Singapore. *Int. J. Dermatol., 18,* 485.
33. Zachariae, H. (1979): Histiocytosis X in two infants treated with topical nitrogen mustard. *Br. J. Dermatol., 100,* 433.
34. Catona, A. and Lanzer, D. (1987): Monobenzone, Superfade, vitiligo and confetti-like depigmentation. *Med. J. Austral., 146,* 320–321.
35. Lawrence, N., Bligard, C.A., Reed, R. and Perret, W.J. (1988): Exogenous ochronosis in the United States. *J. Am. Acad. Dermatol., 18,* 1207–1211.
36. Markey, A.C., Black, A.K. and Rycroft, R.J.G. (1989): Confetti-like depigmentation from hydroquinone. *Contact Dermatitis, 20,* 148–149.
37. Boyle, J. and Kennedy, C.T.C. (1985): Leucoderma induced by monomethyl ether of hydroquinone. *Clin. Exp. Dermatol., 10,* 154–156.

38. Feucht, C.L. (1981): Response to a letter to the Editor. *J. Am. Acad. Dermatol., 5,* 457.
39. Mann, R.J. and Harman, R.R.M. (1983): Nail staining due to hydroquinone skin-lightening creams. *Br. J. Dermatol., 108,* 363.
40. Phillips, J.I., Isaacson, C. and Carman, H. (1986): Ochronosis in black South Africans who use skin lighteners. *Am. J. Dermatopathol., 8,* 14–21.
41. Olmstead, P.M. et al. (1980): Monsel's solution: A histologic nuisance. *J. Am. Acad. Dermatol., 3,* 492.
42. Goette, D.K. and Odom, R.B. (1977): Allergic contact dermatitis to topical fluorouracil. *Arch. Dermatol., 113,* 1058.
43. Goette, D.K. (1981): Topical chemotherapy with 5-fluorouracil. *J. Am. Acad. Dermatol., 4,* 633.
44. Plewig, G. and Kligman, A.M. (1975): *Acne: Morphogenesis and Treatment.* Springer Verlag, Berlin.
45. Krebs, A. (1983): Veränderungen der Nägel durch Arzneimittel. *Dtsch. Apoth. Ztg., 123,* 557.
46. Hull, P.R. and Proctor, P.R. (1990): The melanocyte: An essential link in hydroquinone-induced ochronosis. *J. Am. Acad. Dermatol., 22,* 529–531.
47. Ashton, R.E., Andre, P., Lowe, N.J. and Whitefield, M. (1983): Anthralin: Historical and current perspectives. *J. Am. Acad. Dermatol., 9,* 173.
48. Daniel, C.R. III and Osment, L.S. (1982): Nail pigmentation abnormalities. Their importance and proper examination. *Cutis, 30,* 348.
49. Swinga, D.W. (1970): Treatment of superficial onychomycosis with topically applied glutaraldehyde. *Arch. Dermatol., 102,* 163.
50. Daniel, C.R. III (1982): Nail pigmentation abnormalities: An addendum. *Cutis, 30,* 364.
51. Runne, U. and Orfanos, C.E. (1981): The human nail. *Akt. Probl. Derm., 9,* 102.
52. Hamminga, B., Noordijk, E.M. and van Vloten, W.A. (1982): Treatment of mycosis fungoides. *Arch. Dermatol., 118,* 150.
53. Camarasa, J.G. and Barnadas, M. (1982): Occupational dermatosis by vitamin K3 sodium bisulphite. *Contact Dermatitis, 8,* 268.
54. Shapiro, W.B. (1982): The safety, stability and compatibility of fragrances in skin and hair products. *J. Toxic. Cut. Ocular Toxic., 1,* 211.
55. Zackheim, H.S., Epstein, E.H. Jr. and McNutt, N.S. et al. (1983): Topical carmustine (BCNU) for mycosis fungoides and related disorders. A 10-year experience. *J. Am. Acad. Dermatol., 9,* 363.
56. Baran, R. and Laugier, P. (1985): Melanonychia induced by topical 5-fluorouracil. *Br. J. Dermatol., 112,* 621–625.
57. Feiler-Ofrey, V., Godel, V. and Lazar, M. (1981): Nail pigmentation following timolol maleate therapy. *Opthalmologia, 182,* 153–156.
58. Hatzis, J., Gourgiotou, K., Tosca, A., Varelzidis, A. and Stratigos, J. (1988): Vitiligo as a reaction to topical treatment with diphencyprone. *Dermatologica, 177,* 146–148.
59. Duhra, P. and Foulds, I.S. (1990): Persistent vitiligo induced by diphencyprone. *Br. J. Dermatol., 123,* 415–416.
60. MacDonald-Hull, S.P., Cotterill, J.A.C. and Norris, J.F.B. (1989): Vitiligo following diphencyprone dermatitis. *Br. J. Dermatol., 120,* 323.
61. Hatzis, J., Gourgiotou, K., Tosca, A., Varelzidis, A. and Stratigos, J. (1989): Vitiligo and topical allergens (Reply). *Dermatologica, 179,* 137–138.
62. Tidman, M.J., Horton, J.J. and McDonald, D.M. (1986): Hydroquinone-induced ochronosis - light and electron microscopic features. *Clin. Exp. Dermatol., 11,* 224–228.
63. Valsecchi, R. and Cainelli, T. (1984): Depigmentation from squaric acid dibutylester. *Contact Dermatitis, 10,* 109.
64. Bandmann, H.J. and Speer, U. (1984): Red hair after application of chinoform. *Contact Dermatitis, 10,* 113.
65. Fisher, A.A. (1989): Unusual condom dermatitis. *Cutis, 44,* 365–366.
66. Rebora, A. and Guarrera, M. (1989): Hair discoloration caused by minoxidil lotion. *J. Am. Acad. Dermatol., 21,* 1314.
67. Wenyuan, Z., Mingyu, X., Shengda, H. and Dean, D. (1989): Hyperpigmentation of the nail from lead deposition. *Int. J. Dermatol., 28,* 273–275.
68. Gonçalo, S., Gil, J., Gonçalo, M. and Poiares Baptista, A. (1991): Pigmented photoallergic contact dermatitis from musk ambrette. *Contact Dermatitis, 24,* 229–230.
69. Dupuis, L.L., Shear, N.H. and Zuker, R.M. (1985): Hyperpigmentation due to topical application of silver sulfadiazine cream. *J. Am. Acad. Dermatol., 6,* 1112–1114.

70. Prigent, F., Cohen, J. and Civatte, J. (1986): Pigmentation de paupières probablement secondaire a l'application prolongée d'une pommade opthalmologique contenant du mercure. *Ann. Dermatol Venereol, 113,* 357–358.
71. Hayakawa, R., Matsunaga, K. and Arima, Y. (1987): Airborne pigmented contact dermatitis due to musk ambrette in incense. *Contact Dermatitis, 16,* 96–98.
72. Claudy, A.L. and Perrot, J.L. (1990): Hyperpigmentation induced by UVB at the application site of estradiol. *Dermatologica, 181,* 154–155.
73. Böckers, M., Wagner, R. and Oster, O. (1985): Nageldyschromie als Leitsymptom einer chronischen Quecksilberintoxikation durch ein kosmetisches Bleichmittel. *Z. Hautkr., 60,* 821–829.
74. Daniel, C.R. III. (1985): Nail pigmentation abnormalities. *Dermatologic Clinics, 3,* 431–443.
75. van der Steen, P. and Happle, R. (1992): 'Dyschromia in Confetti' as a side effect of topical immunotherapy with diphenylcyclopropene. *Arch. Dermatol., 128,* 518–520.

11. Stinging sensation due to ingredients of cosmetics and topical pharmaceutical preparations

11.1 Many topical preparations may cause transient burning or itching, especially when applied to diseased skin. Some individuals, mostly women, may experience a stinging sensation due to cosmetics, lasting for up to fifteen minutes and then subsiding. The following ingredients of cosmetics and pharmaceuticals were identified as stinging compounds by Frosch and Kligman [2]:

benzene	1%	phosphoric acid	1%
benzoyl peroxide gel	10%	hydrochloric acid	1.2%
benzoyl peroxide lotion	5%	phenol	1%
coal tar	5%	propylene glycol	
cinoxate	50%	propylene glycol diacetate	
diethyl toluamide (DEET)	undiluted	resorcinol	5%
dimethylacetamide	undiluted	salicylic acid	5%
dimethylformamide	50%	sodium carbonate	15%
dimethyl phthalate	undiluted	sodium hydroxide	1.3%
dimethyl sulfoxide (DMSO)	[1]	trisodium phosphate	5%
2-ethyl-1,3-hexane diol	50%		

Irritation and/or burning may also be caused by benzylidene acetone, hydroxycitronellal, aurantiol and cinnamates [3].

11.2 REFERENCES

1. Calnan, C.D. (1978): Stinging sensation from ethoxyethyl-methoxycinnamate. *Contact Dermatitis, 4,* 294.
2. Frosch, P.J. and Kligman, A.M. (1977): A method for appraising the stinging capacity of topically applied substances. *J. Soc. Cosmet. Chem., 28,* 197.
3. Anonis, D.P. (1973): Perfume and shampoos. *Drug Cosm. Ind., 112,* 32.

12. Miscellaneous side effects

12.1 Miscellaneous side effects of topical drugs

Drug	Use	Side effects	Ref.
acrylic bone cement	fixation of prostheses	Paresthesia of the fingers	11
benzoin	in cosmetics, adhesives and perfumes	Non-eczematous exanthema	36
benzoyl peroxide	treatment of acne	body odour no carcinogenicity	35 59 66
benzyl benzoate	antiscabietic drug	Pemphigoid (?)	41
cantharidin	treatment of warts	Lymphangitis	7
carmustine (BCNU)	topical cytostatic drug	Erythema followed by patchy teleangiectasia; lichenified dermatitis. Mild bone marrow suppression from percutaneous absorption	56
cetrimonium bromide	antiseptic	Matting of the hair	5
chlorhexidine	antiseptic in mouthwashes	Disturbance of taste sensations, swelling of the parotid glands	29
clove oil	topical dental anodyne	Permanent local anesthesia and anhydrosis	46
coal tar	psoriasis therapy	Multiple keratoacanthomas	43 44
cobalt blue	in tattoos	Granulomatous skin reaction with and without cobalt-sensitivity	26
diethyl toluamide (DEET)	insect repellent	Bullous eruption healing with scar formation	50
dimethyl sulfoxide (DMSO)	solvent	Thickening, hardening and desquamation of the skin	18
dinitrochlorobenzene (DNCB)	treatment of alopecia areata and warts	Potentiates sensitization to non-related allergens Mutagenic, carcinogenic (?)	6 45 58

(continued)

§ **12.1** *(continued)*

Drug	Use	Side effects	Ref.
dithranol (anthralin, cignolin)	psoriasis therapy	Bullous pemphigoid (?)	52
		Tumour promotion (?)	53
flourouracil	topical cytostatic drug	Onycholysis	30
		Onychodystrophy	49
		Bullous pemphigoid	54
			2
		'Mental depression'	24
		Telangiectasiae, exacerbation of herpes labialis	4
		Pain, edema and dermatitis of the erythema livedo reticularis-type	
		Hypertrophic scarring	55
		Pigmented purpuric dermatosis	60
		Localized lymphedema	61
hydroquinone	bleaching agent	Ochronosis and colloid milia (sun exposure was required)	10
8-hydroxyquinoline	antimicrobial	Purpuric eruption	34
idoxuridine	antiviral drug	Mutagenic? teratogenic? carcinogenic?	13 38 48
mechlorethamine hydrochloride	topical cytostatic drug	Carcinogenic: increased risk of nonmelanoma skin cancers	19
		Induction of melanoma is unlikely	9
		Focal contact sensitivity on mycosis fungoides plaques	31 51
		Extensive telangiectasia	
mercurial compounds	in tattoos	Granulomatous and lichenoid reaction, both with and without mercury-sensitivity	37 40
monosulfiram	antiseptic	Toxic epidermal necrolysis complicating contact allergy	25
neutral red	photodye therapy for herpes simplex	Carcinogenic?	3
nicotinyl alcohol	rubefacient	acanthosis nigricans	65
petrolatum	vehicle	Lipogranuloma	64
		Myospherulosis	8
		Decrease of inflammatory response in damaged skin	57
p-phenylenediamine	various	Purpuric allergic contact dermatitis	33

(continued)

§ **12.1** *(continued)*

Drug	Use	Side effects	Ref.
podophyllum resin	therapy for condylomata acuminata	Infiltrated hyperplasia reaction Malignant transformation of condylomata acuminata?	23 64
polyethylene glycol	vehicle constituent	Carcinogenic?	14
polysporin ointment	topical antibiotic	Eyelid lipoid granuloma	63
propylene glycol	vehicle constituent	Psoriasis-like reactions	22
retinoic acid	hair growth stimulant	eruptive pyogenic granulomas	47
salicylic acid	keratolytic drug	Lymphangitis, 'Xeroderma pigmentosum'	7 39
salicylic acid 15% lactic acid 15% collodion	wart therapy	Atrophic and partially depigmented scar	12
scopolamine hydrobromide	anticholinergic drug used in ophthalmology	Erythema multiforme	17
selenium sulfide	dandruff medication	Reversible hair loss, oiliness of the scalp	16
sulfonamide	chemotherapeutic in ophthalmic solution	Stevens–Johnson syndrome	28
tar	psoriasis and eczema therapy	Carcinogenic? *See* §18.23	15 42
thiomersal	antiseptic	Acute laryngeal obstruction caused by contact allergy to thiomersal spray	21
tocopherol (vitamin E)	emollient	Sclerosing lipogranuloma of the male genitalia	62
tretinoin	treatment of photodamaged skin	Reversible ectropion teratogenicity [68] very unlikely	67 69 70
triphenylmethane dyes	antiseptics	Carcinogenic? mutagenic?	27
zinc oxide	in topical remedies	Black dermographism in the presence of jewelry	1
zirconium compounds	in antiperspirants	Allergic granulomatous skin reactions	32

12.2 REFERENCES

1. Anderson, K.E. and Maibach, H.I. (1980): Allergic reactions to drugs used topically. *Clin. Toxicol., 16, 415.*
2. Bart, B.J. and Bean, S.F. (1970): Bullous pemphigoid following the topical use of flourouracil. *Arch. Dermatol., 102,* 457.
3. Berger, R.P. and Papa, C.M. (1977): Photodye herpes therapy: Cassandria confirmed? *J. Am. Med. Assoc., 238,* 133.

4. Braunstein, B.L. (1985): Herpes simplex complicating topical 5-fluorouracil therapy. *J. Am. Acad. Dermatol., 12,* 1109.
5. Dawber, R.P.R. and Calnan, C.D. (1976): Bird's nest hair, matting of the scalp hair due to shampooing. *Clin. Exp. Dermatol., 1,* 155.
6. De Groot, A.C., Nater, J.P., Bleumink, E. and De Jong, M.C.J.M. (1981): Does DNCB therapy potentiate epicutaneous sensitization to non-related contact allergens? *Clin. Exp. Dermatol., 6,* 139.
7. Dilaimy, M. (1975): Lymphangitis caused by cantharidin. *Arch. Dermatol., 111,* 1073.
8. Dunlap, C.L. and Barker, B.F. (1980): Myospherulosis of the jaws. *Oral Surg., 50,* 238.
9. Cosnes, A., Revuz, J., Wechsler, J. and Touraine, R. (1984): Mélanome et naevus dysplisiques après 8 ans de caryolysine locale. *Ann. Derm. Venereol., 111,* 127–132.
10. Findlay, G.H., Morrison, J.G.L. and Simson, I.W. (1975): Exogenous ochronosis and pigmented-colloid milium from hydroquinone bleaching creams. *Br. J. Dermatol., 93,* 613.
11. Fisher, A.A. (1979): Paresthesia of the fingers accompanying dermatitis due to methacrylate bone cement. *Contact Dermatitis, 5,* 56.
12. Gaisin, A. (1976): Facial scarring due to topical wart treatment. *Arch. Dermatol., 112,* 1791.
13. Green, J. and Staal, S. (1976): Questionable dermatologic use of iododeoxyuridine. *New Engl. J. Med., 295,* 111.
14. Greene, M.H., Young, T.I. and Eisenbarth, G.S. (1980): Polyethylene glycol in suppositories: Carcinogenic? (letter). *Ann. intern. Med., 93,* 78.
15. Greither, A., Gisbertz, C. and Ippen, H. (1967): Teerbehandlung und Krebs. *Z. Haut- u. Geschlkr., 42,* 463.
16. Grover, R.W. (1956): Diffuse hair loss associated with selenium (Selsun) sulfide shampoo. *J. Am. Med. Assoc., 160,* 1397.
17. Guill, A., Goette, K., Knight, C.G., Peck, C.C. and Lupton, G.P. (1979): Erythema multiforme and urticaria. *Arch. Dermatol., 115,* 742.
18. Kligman, A.M. (1965): Topical pharmacology and toxicology of dimethyl sulfoxide. I and II. *J. Am. Med. Assoc., 193,* 796 and 923.
19. Vonderheid, E.C., Tan, E.T., Kantor, A.F., Shrages, L., Micaily, B. and Van Scott, E.J. (1989): Long term efficacy, curative potential and carcinogenicity of topical mechlorethamine chemotherapy in cutaneous T cell lymphoma. *J. Am. Acad. Dermatol., 20,* 416–428.
20. Lubowe, J.J. (1977): Fluorouracil for skin blemishes and lines. *J. Am. Med. Assoc., 237,* 1312.
21. Maibach, H.I. (1975): Acute laryngeal obstruction presumed secondary to thiomersal (merthiolate) delayed hypersensitivity. *Contact Dermatitis, 1,* 221.
22. Maibach, H.I. (1980): Topical corticoid therapy: a round table discussion. V. The base as a vehicle. *Cutis, 25,* 441.
23. Maxwell, T.B. and Lamb, J.H. (1954): Unusual reaction to application of podophyllum resin. *Arch. Derm. Syph. (Chic.), 70,* 510.
24. Milstein, H.G. (1980): Mental depression secondary to fluorouracil therapy for actinic keratoses. *Arch. Dermatol., 116,* 1100.
25. Monkton Copeman, P.W. (1968): Toxic epidermal necrolysis caused by skin hypersensitivity to monosulfiram. *Br. Med. J., 1,* 623.
26. Rorsman, H., Brehmer-Anderson, E., Dahlquist, I., Ehinger, B., Jacobsson, S., Linell, F. and Rorsman, G. (1969): Tattoo granuloma and uveitis. *Lancet, 2,* 27.
27. Rosenkranz, H.S. and Carr, H.S. (1971): Possible hazard in use of gentian violet. *Br. Med. J., iii,* 5776.
28. Rubin, A. (1977): Opthalmic sulfonamide induced Stevens–Johnson syndrome. *Arch. Dermatol., 113,* 235.
29. Rushton, A. (1977): Safety of Hibitane. II. Human experience. *J. Clin. Periodont., 4,* 73.
30. Shelley, W.B. (1972): Onycholysis due to topical 5-fluorouracil. *Acta Derm.-Venereol. (Stockh.), 52,* 320.
31. Shelley, W.B. (1981): Focal contact sensitivity to nitrogen mustard in lesions of cutaneous T-cell lymphoma (mycosis fungoides). *Acta Derm.-Venereol. (Stockh.), 61,* 161.
32. Shelley, W.B. and Hurley, H.J. (1958): The allergic origin of zirconium deodorant granulomas in man. *Br. J. Dermatol., 70,* 75.
33. Shmunes, E. (1978): Purpuric allergic contact dermatitis to paraphenylenediamine. *Contact Dermatitis, 4,* 225.
34. Sidi, E. and Hincky, M. (1956): *Les manifestations atypiques de l'allergie de contact.* Communication faite á la Societé française d'allergie. Séance du 20 Novembre,. p. 283.
35. Zbinden, G. (1988): Scientific opinion on the carcinogenic risk due to topical administration of benzoylperoxide for the treatment of acne vulgaris. *Pharmacol. Toxicol., 63,* 307–309.
36. Spott, D.A. and Shelley, W.B. (1970): Exanthema due to contact allergen (Benzoin) absorbed through skin. *J. Am. Med. Assoc., 214,* 1881.

37. Taffee, A., Knight, A.G. and Marks, R. (1978): Lichenoid tattoo hypersensitivity. *Br. Med. J., 1,* 616.
38. Thomson, J. and O'Neill, S.M. (1976): Idoxuridine in dimethyl sulfoxide: is it carcinogenic in man? *J. cutan. Path., 3,* 269.
39. Weber, G. and Riegel, A. (1968): 'Xeroderma Pigmentosum' e medicamento. *Z. Haut- u. Geschlkr., 43,* 829.
40. Winkelmann, R.K. and Harris, R.B. (1979): Lichenoid delayed hypersensitivity reactions in tattoos. *J. Cutan. Path., 6,* 59.
41. Wzanicz, A. and Czernielewski, A. (1974): Pemfigoid sprowokowany nowoskabina. *Przegl. derm., 61,* 693.
42. Zackheim, H.S. (1978): Should therapeutic coal-tar preparations be available over the counter? *Arch. Dermatol., 114,* 125.
43. Reid, B.J. and Cheesbrough, M.J. (1978): Multiple keratoacanthoma. *Acta. Derm.-Venereol., (Stockh.), 58,* 169.
44. Vickers, C.F.G. and Ghadially, F.N. (1961): Keratoacanthoma associated with psoriasis. *Br. J. Dermatol., 73,* 120.
45. Wilkerson, M.G., Connor, T.H. and Wilkin, J.K. (1988): Dinitrochlorobenzene is inherently mutagenic in the presence of trace mutagenic contaminants. *Arch. Dermatol., 124,* 396–398.
46. Isaacs, G. (1983): Permanent local anaesthesia and anhidrosis after clove oil spillage (letter). *Lancet, 1,* 882.
47. Baran, R. (1989): Explosive eruption of pyogenic granuloma on the scalp due to topical combination therapy of minoxidil and retinoic acid. *Dermatologica, 179,* 76–78.
48. Koppang, H.S. and Aas, E. (1983): Squamous carcinoma induced by topical idoxuridine therapy? (letter). *Br. J. Dermatol., 108,* 501.
49. Krebs, A. (1983): Veränderungen der Nägel durch Arzneimmittel. *Dtsch. Apoth.-Ztg., 123,* 557.
50. Reuveni, H. and Yagupsky, P. (1982): Diethyltoluamide-containing insect repellent. *Arch. Dermatol., 118, 582.*
51. Hamminga, B., Noordijk, E.M. and van Vloten, W.A. (1982): Treatment of mycosis fungoides. *Arch. Dermatol., 118,* 150.
52. Koerber, W.A., Price, N.M. and Watson, W. (1978): Coexistent psoriasis and bullous pemphigoid. *Arch. Dermatol., 114,* 1643.
53. Ashton, R.E., Andre, P., Lowe, N.J. and Whitefield, M. (1983): Anthalin: Historical and current perspectives. *J. Am. Acad. Dermatol., 9,* 173.
54. Tanebaum, M.H. (1961): Onychodystrophy after topically applied 5-FU for warts. *Arch. Dermatol., 103, 225.*
55. Kaplan, L.A., Walter, J.F. and Macknet, K.D. (1979): Hypertrophic scarring as a complication of fluorouracil therapy. *Arch. Dermatol., 115,* 1452.
56. Zackheim, H.S., Epstein, E.H. Jr. and Crain, W.R. (1990): Topical carmustine (BCNU) for cutaneous T-cell lymphoma: A 15-year experience in 143 patients. *J. Am. Acad. Dermatol., 22,* 802–810.
57. Penneys, N.S., Eaglstein, W. and Ziboh, V. (1980): Petrolatum: interference with the oxidation of arachidonic acid. *Br. J. Dermatol., 103,* 257.
58. Strick, R.A. (1988): The Ames assay and dinitrochlorobenzene. *Arch. Dermatol., 124,* 1570.
59. Molberg, P. (1981): Body odor from topical benzoyl peroxide. *N. Engl. J. Med., 304,* 1366.
60. Voelter, W.W. (1983): Pigmented purpuric dermatosis-like reaction to topical fluorouracil. *Arch. Dermatol., 119,* 875–876.
61. Grattan, C.E.H. and Guerrier, C.J.W. (1985): Reaction to topical fluorouracil of secondary lymphedema. *Arch. Dermatol., 121,* 1484.
62. Foucar, E., Downing, D.T. and Gerber, W.L. (1983): Sclerosing lipogranuloma of the male genitalia from an ointment containing vitamin E: A comparison with classical "paraffinoma". *J. Am. Acad. Dermatol., 9,* 103–110.
63. Moolchandani, J., Kazim, M., Farba, M. and Katowitz, J. (1990): Eyelid lipoid granuloma following topical ointment application. *Opthalmic Plastic Reconstr. Surg., 6,* 133–135.
64. Svinland, H.B. (1984): Malignant transformation of condyloma acuminatum after treatment with podophyllin. *Eur. J. Sexual Transm. Dis., 1,* 165–167.
65. Pascal, J., Roagna, C. and Bonerandi, J.J. (1984): Acanthosis nigricans induit par acide nicotinique local. *Ann. Derm.-Venereol., 111,* 739–740.
66. Hogan, D.J., Wilson, E.R. et al. (1991): A study of acne treatments as risk factors for skin cancer of the head and neck. *Br. J. Dermatol., 125,* 343–348.
67. Brodell, L.P., Asselin, D. and Brodell, R.T. (1992): Reversible ectropion after long-term use of topical tretinoin on photodamaged skin. *J. Am. Acad. Dermatol., 6,* 21–22.
68. Camera, G. and Pregliasco, P. (1992): Ear malformation in baby born to mother using tretinoin cream. *Lancet, 339,* 687.
69. de Wals, P., Bloch, D. and Calabro, A. et al. (1991): Association between holoprosencephaly and exposure to topical retinoids: results of the EUROCAT survey. *Pediat. Perinat. Epidemiol., 5,* 445–457.
70. Thorne, E.G. (1992): Long-term clinical experience with a topical retinoid. *Br. J. Dermatol., 127, (suppl. 41),* 31–36.

13. Drugs used on the mucosae

DRUGS USED ON THE ORAL MUCOSA

General and local effects

13.1 Drugs coming into contact with the oral mucosa may cause (1) general effects, through absorption, and (2) local effects; the latter may consist of:

Irritant reactions
Although the oral mucosa appears to be more resistant to irritants than the skin, chemical injury may occur. This may be produced by contact of undiluted drugs with the mucosa, e.g. aspirin, hydrogen peroxide, silver nitrate. Accidental contact with drugs and subsequent irritation also occurs, especially in children.

Allergic reactions
Many drugs inducing contact allergy when applied to the skin, may also cause contact sensitization when applied to the mucous membranes. Allergic reactions in the oral cavity are relatively rare. This is explained by [1]:

1. Rapid disposal and absorption of the drug
2. Short period of contact with the mucosa
3. Dilution and removal by saliva
4. Lack of recognition of the drug as an allergen

In allergic contact stomatitis, the subjective symptoms are often more prominent than the physical signs. Patients may complain of loss of taste, numbness, a burning sensation and soreness of the affected area. Itching is not a frequent symptom. The appearance of the mucous membrane varies from a barely visible mild erythema to a fiery red colour with or without edema. Lingual papillae may disappear. In the presence of considerable edema the mucosa takes on a smooth, waxy, glazed appearance. Vesiculation of the oral mucosa is rarely seen, because vesicles rupture quickly to form erosions [145].

Other adverse reactions
These are discussed elsewhere in this chapter.

TOOTHPASTES

13.2 Toothpastes may contain abrasives, flavours, colours, preservatives, antiseptics and fluorides. Contact allergic reactions to the constituents of toothpastes seem to be rare. Symptoms may include stomatitis, cheilitis, glossitis, ulceration [126], perioral dermatitis and eczema of the hand holding the toothbrush.

The main sensitizers are the flavouring agents (§ 13.3).

13.3 Contact allergy to ingredients of toothpastes

Ingredient	Patch test conc. & vehicle (§ 5.2)	Ref.
anethole	2–5% pet.	1
azulene	1% pet.	132
carvone	2–5% pet.	1,129,130
chloroacetamide	0.2% pet.	125
cinnamic aldehyde	1% pet.	11,15,21,126
cinnamon oil	2% pet.	13,17
dichlorophene	1% pet.	8
fluorides (?)	toothpaste as is (?)	25
formaldehyde	1% aqua	cited by 128,131
guaiazulene	1% pet	133
hexylresorcinol (?)	0.25% pet.	28
Italian peppermint	2% pet.	1
laurel oil	2% pet.	27
menthol	1-2% pet.	19
oil of anise	0.25% pet.	14
oleum menthae piperitae	2% pet.	13,26
phenyl salicylate (salol)	1% pet.	122
propolis	10% pet.	121
spearmint oil	2% pet.	1
thymol	1% pet.	2

13.4 Other side effects of toothpastes

One case of immediate-type hypersensitivity to caraway seed in a toothpaste has been reported [10]. Sodium lauryl sulfate caused painless oral desquamation in one patient. The desquamation stopped within 24 hours of the use of the incriminated dentifrice, but recurred on use of any brand of toothpaste that contained sodium lauryl sulfate or the related surfactant sodium-*N*-lauroyl-sarcosinate [127]. The flavour in toothpaste has been responsible for bronchospasm in one report [134].

Fluorides

13.5 The possible effects of fluorides in toothpaste are still subject to discussion. The occurrence of acne-like eruptions due to fluorides has been reported [23], but was doubted by other investigators [6]. Ulcerous stomatitis caused by fluorides has been reported by Douglas [5]. Another documented side effect is discoloration of the teeth [3]. The National Registry of possible drug-induced ocular side effects has received two separate case reports of pigmentary macular degeneration in children following dental treatments with fluoride gel [82].

The possibility of contact allergic reactions to fluorides in toothpastes is still under discussion. Seven cases of contact allergy were reported by Shea et al. [25]. Patch test with fluoride-containing toothpaste were positive (2+) in one case, but control tests were not mentioned.

Cinnamic aldehyde

13.6 Contact allergy to cinnamic aldehyde (cinnamal) in toothpaste has been reported to cause perioral leukoderma [16].

ORAL LICHEN PLANUS AND CONTACT ALLERGY

13.7 Several studies suggest that contact allergy to mercury in amalgam fillings may be responsible for some cases of oral lichen planus [147,150,244] and possibly for aphthous ulcers [149]. Other contact allergens held responsible include cinnamic aldehyde and benzoic acid (in food and toothpaste), rosin for repairing broken dentures [243], formaldehyde in toothpaste [150], copper [39], palladium [159] and gold [151] in dental alloys.

BURNING MOUTH SYNDROME

13.8 In the burning mouth syndrome, patients complain of a burning sensation and/or pain in the oral mucosae and/or the tongue, in the absence of evidence of any other specific disease. A mild erythema of the oral mucusae is sometimes observed, but no characteristic histopathologic features are present. The disease occurs most commonly in perimenopausal or postmenopausal women. The pathogenesis is obscure but may include local irritation, contact allergy, systemic diseases (diabetes mellitus, folic acid deficiency), and psychological factors. Frequently, the symptoms arise after dental intervention and the majority of the patients wear dental prostheses [153]. Contact allergens in dentures and dental restoration materials implicated in the burning mouth syndrome include: acrylate monomer [153], benzoyl peroxide [152], butyl methacrylate [154], cobalt chloride [43], *N,N*-dimethyl-4-toluidine [152], formaldehyde [43], glycol dimethacrylate [154], gold chloride [152], nickel sulfate [43], oligoacrylate [152], *p*-phenylenediamine [43], polymethyl methacrylate [33], potassium bichromate [43] and 4-tolyldiethanolamine [152].

Contact allergy to sorbic acid and propylene glycol in foods has also been linked to the burning mouth syndrome [46], as has contact allergy to nicotinic esters in toothpastes [160].

OTHER ORAL MEDICATION

Many other chemicals and drugs may come into contact with the oral mucosa, e.g. chemicals and drugs used in dentistry. Their side effects are listed in § 13.9.

13.9 Side effects of other oral contactants

Contactant	Use	Side effects	Patch test conc. vehicle	Comment	Ref.
benzoyl peroxide	dentures (catalyst)	stomatitis	1% pet.	Patch test conc. used not correct	34
chlorphenol camphor	anti-inflammation	stomatitis	?		35
chrome and cobalt	removable partial denture	generalized dermatitis	0.5% and 1% pet.		32
cinnamic aldehyde (cinnamal)	in mouthwash	swelling of lip and tongue	2% pet. (open test) reading after 15 min.	Contact urticarial reaction	47
clove oil	topical dental anodyne	permanent local anaesthesia and anhidrosis after spillage over the infraorbital skin	–	Possible neurotoxic effects of eugenol in clove oil	42
cobalt chloride	dentures	rhinitis	1% pet.	Rhinitis 3–24 hours after applying dentures	31
epoxy resin	dentures	stomatitis	1% pet.		50
eugenol	impression paste surgical packing cement	dermatitis	1% pet.	Contact allergy in patients and dental personnel	12
fluoride	dental treatment	exacerbation of dermatitis herpetiformis		Causal relation not established	143
9-α-fluoropred-nisolone	corticosteroid	hypokaliaemic alkalosis from permucosal absorption			141
formaldehyde	in paraform-aldehyde containing dental fillings	anaphylactic reactions from type I allergy		Patch and prick tests were negative, specific IgE against formaldehyde was demonstrated	138
glycyrrhiza uralensis	herbal breath refresher	stomatitis	1% alc.		135
gold	dentures	stomatitis	auric trichloride 0.1% aqua	*Cave:* irritant patch test reactions	51
gold	dentures	stomatitis	auric trichloride 0.5% aqua	*Cave:* irritant patch test reactions	36
gold	dentures	stomatitis	potassium dicyanoaurate 0.001% (w/v) ($3.5 \cdot 10^{-5}$ mol/l) ethanol	*Cave:* irritant patch test reactions	38
hexetidine	fungicide	stomatitis	0.1% pet.		48

(continued)

§ **13.9** *(continuation)*

Contactant	Use	Side effects	Patch test conc. vehicle	Comment	Ref.
iodoform	antiseptic in dental dressing	stomatitis dermatitis	potassium iodide 0.5% pet.	Severe iodoform toxicity from iodine absorption leading to coma has been reported [140]	139
mercury amalgam	dental fillings	(lichenoid) allergic stomatitis, allergic dermatitis, systemic contact dermatitis, urticaria. Extracutaneous symptoms: malaise, nausea, headache	mercury 1% pet. ammoniated mercury 1% pet. mercuric chloride 0.1% pet.		7 29 49 52 146
methyldichloro-benzene sulfate	catalyst in impression material (Impregum®)	stomatitis dermatitis	0.1% dibenztoluol	Contact allergy in patients and dental personnel	40 53
methylmethacry-late monomer	dentures	stomatitis	2% pet.		37 46
methyl-*p*-toluene sulfonate	catalyst in material for temporary crowns and bridges (Scutan®)	stomatitis dermatitis	0.1% pet.	Contact allergy in patients and dental personnel	40 45 53
nickel sulfate	dentures	rhinitis	5% pet.	Rhinitis 3–24 hours after applying dentures	31
nickel sulfate	dental prosthesis	stomatitis urticaria systemic contact dermatitis	5% pet.		157 158 249
palladium	dental alloys	swelling of cheek, pain in mouth, generalized itching, dizziness	palladium chloride 1% pet.	Most patients allergic to palladium also react to nickel. When tested with palladium metal, virtually no patient with a positive patch test to palladium chloride also reacts to the metal itself. The relevance of a positive reaction to palladium chloride is very doubtful [155, 156]	44
potassium bichromate	dentures	generalized eczematous dermatitis, intraoral erythema	0.5% pet.		41

(continued)

§ **13.9** *(continuation)*

Contactant	Use	Side effects	Patch test conc. vehicle	Comment	Ref.
proflavine	antiseptic	allergic stomatitis and perioral dermatitis	0.5% pet.		137
propolis	folk medicine	allergic stomatitis	10% pet.		144
tetracaine hydrochloride	local anaesthetic	allergic stomatitis and cheilitis	1% pet.		142

MOUTH FRESHENERS

13.10 A few drops of a mouth freshener to a glass of water makes a mouthwash that is capable of inducing a clean and refreshing feeling to the oral cavity. Mouthwashes can be classified as follows:

1. Cosmetic mouthwashes consisting of water (and usually ethyl alcohol), flavour and colour.
2. Antibacterial mouthwashes: these may contain quaternary ammonium compounds, phenolic derivatives or other antibacterial agents.
3. Astringent mouthwashes: these are formulated for the purpose of flocculating and precipitating proteinaceous materials, so that these can be removed by flushing. The most widely used astringents are zinc and aluminum compounds such as zinc chloride, zinc acetate and aluminum potassium sulphate.
4. Buffered mouthwashes: these depend on their pH for their action. Alkaline mouthwashes may be useful in reducing stringy saliva or in reducing mucinous deposits by dispersion of the protein.
5. Mouthwash concentrates: these must be diluted before use.
6. Deodorizing mouthwashes: these contain antibacterial agents.
7. Therapeutic mouthwashes: these are formulated for specific purposes, e.g. for relieving infection or preventing dental caries.

13.11 A typical formula of a **mouth freshener** is:

Ingredient:	Example:
20% water	water
70% alcohol	ethanol
0.1% sweetener	saccharin
2–10% active ingredients:	
– astringents	myrrha tincture
	ratanhia tincture
– essential oils and fragrances	phenyl salicylate, peppermint oil, thymol, eugenol, clove oil
– antimicrobials	benzalkonium chloride, chlorhexidine digluconate

13.12 Patch tests with toothpastes and mouthwashes may produce false-positive reactions when the preparations are tested undiluted. Dilution and control tests are necessary.

Side effects of mouthwashes

13.13 *Systemic side effects:* Accidental ingestion of mouthwash solution in children has been reported to lead to hypoglycaemia, induced by the ethyl alcohol component [30]. *Local side effects* of ingredients of mouthwashes are listed in § 13.14.

13.14 Local side effects of mouthwashes

Ingredient	Side effect	Ref.
chlorhexidine	discoloration of the teeth	3
	discoloration of the dorsum of the tongue	20
	disturbance of taste sensations, with burning, soreness, dryness	18
	desquamation and ulceration of the oral mucosa	9
	swelling of the parotid glands (reversible)	22
eugenol	allergic contact stomatitis	136
hexetidine	disturbance of taste sensations	24
peppermint oil (2% pet.) – D-limonene (2% pet.) – L-limonene (2% pet.) – α-pinene (15% pet.)	allergic contact dermatitis	4

DRUGS USED ON THE VAGINAL MUCOSA

13.15 Vulvovaginal drugs may cause:

1. Local side effects in and around the vagina, perineum and thighs. In women suffering from pruritus vulvae, many have positive patch test reactions to medicaments: antibacterials (notably neomycin), antiseptics, preservatives and local anaesthetics [161]. Fisher lists fragrances, benzethonium chloride, methyl salicylate, oil of eucalyptus, oxyquinoline, phenyl mercuric acetate and thymol as the sensitizers in vaginal douches [145]. Drugs used on the vaginal mucosa that have caused contact allergy are listed in § 13.16.

2. Systemic side effects. These include:
   a. Systemic eczematous contact-type dermatitis (Chapter 17)
   b. Urticarial eruptions with or without anaphylaxis [162,163]
   c. Erythematous rashes
   d. Other systemic effects.

Other systemic effects: Hydrocortisone and dexamethasone cream were associated with vulvar inflammation and 'toxic shock syndrome' [112]. The local steroid may have facilitated overgrowth of pathogenic staphylococci. The cream also caused irritation which may have enhanced absorption of enterotoxins. Transient eosinophilic pneumonia (Loeffler's syndrome) has been attributed to a vaginal cream containing sulfonamides [116,117]. Vaginally administrated metronidazole may induce disulfiram-type reactions in susceptible patients when alcohol is ingested concurrently [254].

13.16 Contact allergy to vulvovaginal medication

Ingredient	Type of medication	Side effect	Patch test conc./ vehicle (as used in reports referenced)	Comment	Ref.
acetarsol	vaginal tablet	dermatitis of the thigh	not mentioned		114
carbason	vaginal tablet	irritation of vulva and vagina: generalized eruption	1% and 5% pet.		115
chlordantoin	cream	vulvitis	0.1–1% pet.		164
chlorhexidine gluconate	antiseptic cream	urticaria and anaphylaxis	0.002–1% aqua prick test		162 163
cocamidopropyl betaine	cream	vulvitis	1% aqua		166
furazolidone and nifuroxime	vaginal tablet	pruritus and irritation of vulvar and perineal area: generalized eruption	tablet as is	Further testing not performed	113
miconazole	vaginal cream	vulvitis	2% MEK	Cross-reaction to other imidazoles	165
nifuratel	vaginal tablet	vulvitis	1% acet.		247
nifuroxime	vaginal tablet	severe itching around vagina: generalized urticaria with laryngeal edema	not mentioned	Basophil degradation test positive. Combination of type I and IV allergy suggested	111
propyl gallate	cream	vulvitis	1% pet.		167
sulfanilamide	cream	urticarial lesions on vulva, perineum and thighs: generalized eruption		Patch test not performed	113

(continued)

§ **13.16** *(continuation)*

Ingredient	Type of medication	Side effect	Patch test conc./ vehicle (as used in reports referenced)	Comment	Ref.
sulfanilamide	cream	vulvar eczema and spreading dermatitis	sulfanilamide 5% pet.	Systemic eczematous contact-type dermatitis caused by an oral sulfonylurea derivative (Orinase®, an antidiabetic)	118
sulfanilamide and dienoestrol	cream	itching, perivulvar eruption and photodermatitis	cream as is	Positive *photo*patch test	113

DRUGS USED IN OPHTHALMOLOGICAL PRACTICE

13.17 Systemic and local side effects of topical ophthalmic preparations and contact lens solutions may, strictly speaking, not be primarily the concern of the dermatologist. However, in case of local side effects of ophthalmic drugs the advice of a dermatologist is frequently sought. Therefore we have included a text on unwanted effects of ophthalmic preparations; both local and systemic reactions are discussed. A review of systemic effects of topical ophthalmic medication has been documented [100,110]. Reviews of the side effects of beta blockers may be found in Refs. [82, 218 and 228].

Topically applied ophthalmic drugs

13.18 Topically applied ophthalmic drugs:

1. are intended to exert a local therapeutic effect on the eye, to penetrate the cornea and act on internal ocular structures;
2. may cause local side effects;
3. may cause general effects. After being placed in the conjunctival sac a significant amount of the ophthalmic drug may be absorbed and give rise to systemic effects [98].

Absorption takes place by several routes:

1. The drug diffuses into the circulation via conjunctival, episcleral and intraocular vessels. These vessels drain by facial and ophthalmic veins and the sinus cavernosus into the vena cava superior and the right atrium.
2. The drug is absorbed through the mucous membranes. The ophthalmic sac is connected with the nasal mucosa by the nasolacrimal duct and the puncta of the eye. Absorption across the nasal mucous membranes takes place rapidly, in the case of phenylephrine HCl almost as rapidly as by intravenous injection [73,105].
3. After the drug has traversed the nasolacrimal duct and the nasopharynx, access to the gastrointestinal tract occurs; if the drug survives the acidity of the stomach, the gastrointestinal tract forms an important pathway of absorption.

The amount of absorption is influenced by several factors:
1. The dosage and the concentration of the drug.
2. The condition of the conjunctival sac; the lax eyelids of older people makes more retention possible [81].
3. The condition of the eye. If it is dry (which happens under general anaesthesia), hyperaemic or in a pathologic condition, absorption will be increased [95].
4. Paediatric and geriatric patients are more prone to develop symptoms of systemic effects [86].
5. The position of the patient. In the upright position an approximately tenfold loss of drug occurs [101].
6. Simultaneous use of other ophthalmic medications.
7. Degradation of the drug in the course of time.
8. Alteration of the potency, e.g. by the addition of preservatives [91].

Among the most useful pharmacologic agents in ophthalmic practice are the topically applied autonomic drugs that produce mydriasis, miosis and cycloplegia. These drugs (§ 13.19) are commonly used for examination of the eye, control of glaucoma and relief of minor symptoms.

13.19 Topical ophthalmic autonomic drugs

I. Adrenergic
- A. Sympathomimetic
  - 1. Epinephrine (adrenaline)
  - 2. Phenylephrine
- B. Anticholinergic
  - 1. Atropine
  - 2. Scopolamine
  - 3. Homatropine
  - 4. Cyclopentolate
  - 5. Tropicamide

II. Parasympathomimetic, cholinergic
- A. Direct acting
  - 1. Pilocarpine
  - 2. Cabachol
- B. Indirect acting
  - 1. Reversible
    - a. Physostigmine
  - 2. Irreversible
    - a. Echothiopate
    - b. Demecarium bromide

III. Beta-adrenergic antagonists
- 1. Timolol
- 2. Betaxolol
- 3. Levobunolol

IV. Carbonic anhydrase inhibitors
- 1. Acetazolamide
- 2. Methazolamide
- 3. Dichlorphenamide [242]

SYSTEMIC EFFECTS

Sympathomimetic drugs

13.20 Epinephrine (adrenaline)

Epinephrine is used topically in a 1–2% solution. Systemic side effects from ocular instillation are most frequently cardiovascular. Hypertension, tachycardia, arrhythmias, headache, tremor, pallor, perspiration and faintness have been reported [77,95]. Most serious systemic side effects occur in older patients suffering from hypertension, hyperthyroidism, coronary artery disease, advanced cerebral arteriosclerosis or diabetes mellitus. Patients with primary open-angle glaucoma may be more responsive to ocular and systemic side effects of epinephrine. If they also have a preexisting cardiac disease, they should be monitored for premature ventricular contractions [105]. Other reported side effects include [242] bronchodilatation and an increased respiratory rate.

13.21 Phenylephrine hydrochloride

Phenylephrine hydrochloride differs from epinephrine only in the lack of a hydroxyl group on the benzene ring. Systemic absorption from the nasal mucosa is almost as rapid as by intravenous injection [105]. Systemic side effects of phenylephrine are dose-dependent. Severe hypertension, sometimes accompanied by palpitations, tachycardia, bradycardia, severe occipital headaches and tachypnea have been reported [95,105]. The systemic side effects are more marked if phenylephrine hydrochloride is instilled in an eye affected by conjunctival hyperaemia, extensive bleeding or some disruption of corneal epithelium. Patients with cardiac disease, hypertension, advanced cardiovascular or cerebral arteriosclerosis and/or cerebral aneurysm are particularly susceptible to develop an acute increase in systolic and diastolic blood pressure. Phenylephrine has been reported as the cause of hypertension leading to severe and sometimes fatal myocardial infarctions, primarily in older patients with preexisting cardiac disease. It has also been incriminated as the cause of subarachnoid haemorrhage [81,82], ventricular arrhythmias, cardiac arrest [103], coronary artery spasm [219], rupture of aneurysms [220], ventricular arrhythmia [221], acute pulmonary edema [222] and pulmonary embolism [223]. More details and literature data are given in Refs. [100] and [218].

Anticholinergic drugs

13.22 Atropine

In children receiving eyedrops containing 1% atropine, the following systemic side effects have been noted: dryness of skin and mouth, fever, tachycardia, irritability and flushing of the face [103]. Other reported side effects in children are: abdominal distension, arrhythmias, loss of neuromuscular coordination, ataxia, dysarthria, mental aberration, delirium and visual hallucinations [89], precipitation of asthma and convulsions [103]. In adults, fever and tachycardia have been reported. The confusional psychosis with ataxia, dysarthria and visual hallucinations which can be observed after parenteral administration of belladonna derivatives has also been reported after (repeated) ocular topical administration of atropine [75].

13.23 Scopolamine

Elderly patients may exhibit a severe confusional state after instillation of scopolamine-containing eyedrops. The central nervous system syndrome includes confusion, disorientation, hallucinations and disturbances in the level of consciousness [84]. Overdosage may lead to similar reactions in young adults [217].

13.24 Homatropine

Homatropine is similar to atropine in its actions and systemic side effects. It is, however, a weaker drug with about 1/50 the toxicity of atropine [93]. Tachycardia [215] and confusion [216] from ophthalmic homatropine have been observed.

13.25 Cyclopentolate hydrochloride [218]

There is a great similarity in the effects and side effects of atropine and cyclopentolate. Side effects of cyclopentolate include central nervous system symptoms: slurred speech, ataxia, hallucinations, hyperactivity, seizures and syncope [92]. These side effects are seen particularly in the very young and very old. Nonspecific psychotic behaviour (hallucinations, confusion and disturbances of affect and gait) have also been reported in the elderly [92]. In children the symptoms include clouding of the sensorium, hallucinatory phenomenons and disorganization [92]. Symptoms develop about 30–40 minutes after instillation of the drug. Grand mal seizures [224] and necrotising enterocolitis [225] associated with decreased gastric acid secretion and volume [226] have been observed.

13.26 Tropicamide

Systemic side effects of this parasympatholytic drug include hallucinations and psychotic behaviour (in children and in adults), nausea, vomiting, pallor, headache, tachycardia, muscle rigidity, and even vasomotor and cardiorespiratory collapse [103].

Parasympathomimetic drugs

13.27 Pilocarpine

Pilocarpine, used in a 4% eyedrop solution, is rapidly absorbed in the systemic circulation. Reports on systemic reactions are rare. Systemic side effects are characterized by exaggeration of the parasympathomimetic effects. In asthmatic patients a reduction of the vital capacity due to bronchial musculature stimulation occurs; a typical asthmatic attack may even be precipitated. Other effects are increased tone and motility of the intestines resulting in nausea, vomiting and/or diarrhoea; enhanced tone and motility of the ureter, urinary bladder, gall bladder and biliary tract. Diaphoresis, salivation and lacrimation also occur as well as muscle tremors. The cardiovascular symptoms are hypotension, bradycardia [80] and atrioventricular block [242]. Other reported side effects include profuse sweating, tremor and mental status change [242].

13.28 Carbachol

The systemic side effects of carbachol are similar to, but more severe than, those of pilocarpine [77].

13.29 Physostigmine

Physostigmine is readily absorbed from the nasal mucosa and the gastrointestinal tract. The action of physostigmine is similar to that of acetylcholine: side effects include bronchoconstriction, increased tracheal, bronchial and salivary secretion, autonomic stimulation and symptoms of the central nervous system [89].

13.30 Echothiopate

Echothiopate is an anticholinesterase drug which is rapidly absorbed by all routes: the conjunctiva, the gastrointestinal tract, mucous membranes and the skin. Toxicity is generally cumulative and the toxic systemic symptoms generally do not appear for weeks or months after the start of the therapy. The relation between the systemic toxic symptoms and the ocular use of echothiopate is frequently unrecognized. The toxic symptoms include [100]:

1. Gastrointestinal disturbances: diarrhoea, nausea, abdominal cramps, weakness. This may simulate an acute abdominal condition.
2. Cardiovascular symptoms. They reflect both the ganglionic and postganglionic effects of accumulated acetylcholine. The wide variety of haemodynamic effects include bradycardia, hypotension and predomination of decreased cardiac output. Cardiac arrest has occurred.
3. Respiratory symptoms are rhinorrhea, cough, dyspnea, laryngospasm, bronchoconstriction, bronchorrhea, pulmonary edema, central respiratory depression and failure.
4. Central nervous system symptoms include confusion, slurred speech, ataxia, loss of reflexes, Cheyne–Stokes respiration, central respiratory depression and coma.
5. Neuromuscular effects are fatigability, generalized to severe weakness, fasciculation, convulsion and paralysis. Further details and data are given by Selvin [100].

13.31 Demecarium bromide

Demecarium bromide is a cholinesterase inhibitor for local ophthalmological use. Absorption and adverse systemic effects are identical to echothiopate.

Beta-adrenergic antagonists [228]

13.32 At the time of their introduction into general ophthalmologic practice some 15 years ago, topical beta blockers offered a unique alternative to topical agents such as pilocarpine or epinephrine in the treatment of glaucoma. Both topical and systemic side effects from ophthalmic beta blockers have been reported [228], similar to the side effects of systemic beta blockers. The presence of serious systemic reactions from ocular application of beta blockers, including several deaths, has led to more prudent use, particularly in patients with contraindications to systemic beta blockade [228]. Ophthalmic beta blockers include timolol (the prototype) [82], metipranolol, pindolol, betaxolol, levobunolol, and befunolol. Their reported side effects are shown in Table 13.33

Table 13.33 Systemic effects of topical beta blockers used in the eye [82,218,228,239,242]

Effect	Comment	Ref.
Cardiovascular System		
bradycardia	sometimes leading to heartblock	229
conduction arrhythmias		
hypotension		
Raynaud's phenomenon		
fluid retention		
congestive heart failure	especially in patients already compromised	229, 231
Pulmonary System		
bronchoconstriction/spasm		229
asthma		
dyspnea		
respiratory arrest		240
Neurologic System		241
amnesia		
depression		232
confusion		
headache		
migraine prophylaxis		
impotence, decreased libido		237, 238
insomnia		
myasthenia gravis		
lethargy		
transient ischemic attacks		235
Gastrointestinal System		
diarrhoea		
nausea		
dry mouth		

(continued)

§ **13.33** *(continuation)*

Effect	Comment	Ref.
Skin and Appendages		
alopecia (areata)		236
nail pigmentation		213
urticaria		229
Other		
muscle cramps		
hypoglycaemia		233
haematologic reactions		
death from status asthmaticus or cardiac failure		234
amaurosix fugax		235

In general, the spectra of side effects from various beta blockers are quite similar, though quantitative differences exist. By far the most reactions have been observed from the use of timolol, but this may well be because it is the most extensively used ophthalmic beta blocker.

13.34 Carbonic anhydrase inhibitors [242]

Acetazolamide, methazolamide and dichlorphenamide are used as adjunctive treatment of refractory primary open-angle glaucoma. Acetazolamide commonly causes a range of adverse systemic side effects which require discontinuance of the drugs in 50% of the patients treated. It is often a symptom complex of malaise, fatigue, weight loss, anorexia, depression and decreased libido. Patients with symptoms have systemic acidosis. Other more serious adverse reactions to carbonic anhydrase inhibitors include respiratory acidosis, acceleration of osteomalacia in patients taking phenytoin chronically, and aplastic anaemia and agranulocytosis [242].

MISCELLANEOUS DRUGS

13.35 Topical ocular anaesthetic drugs

Topical ocular anaesthetic drugs rarely cause systemic adverse reactions. In markedly apprehensive or emotionally agitated persons symptoms such as fainting, convulsions or personality changes may occur, probably an idiosyncratic or exaggerated emotional response [82].

13.36 Corticosteroids

Topically applied ocular corticosteroids may, after absorption, infrequently give rise to systemic effects. More details are given by Nutsall [66] and Burch [67]. Corticosteroid-induced ocular hypertension occurs especially in glaucoma patients [214].

13.37 Chloramphenicol

Topical ocular chloramphenicol rarely produces systemic symptoms of haematopoietic toxicity [68,218,253].

13.38 Sulfacetamide sodium

Cases of Stevens–Johnson syndrome from an ophthalmic preparation containing sulfacetamide sodium 10% have been reported [90,253].

LOCAL SIDE EFFECTS

13.39 Contact allergy

Drugs that have caused contact allergy in topical ophthalmic preparations and contact lens solution are listed in § 13.40. A suggested ophthalmic tray for patch testing is shown in Table 13.39 [194]. The literature has been reviewed [194]. *Other local side effects* of drugs used in topical ophthalmic preparations are listed in § 13.41.

Table 13.39. Suggested ophthalmic tray [194]

Compound	Patch test (%) concentration	Vehicle
Preservatives		
Benzalkonium chloride	0.1	aq.
Benzethonium chloride	1	aq.
Chlorhexidine gluconate	1	aq.
Cetalkonium chloride	0.1	aq.
Sodium EDTA	1	aq.
Sorbic acid	2.5	pet.
Thimerosal (merthiolate)	0.1	pet.
Beta adrenergic blocking agents		
Befunolol	1	aq.
Levobunolol HCl	1	aq.

(continued)

§ **13.39** *(continuation)*

Compound	Patch test (%) concentration	Vehicle
Metipranolol	2	aq.
Metoprolol	3	aq.
Timolol	0.5	aq.
Mydriatics		
Atropine sulfate	1	aq.
Epinephrine HCl	1	aq.
Phenylephrine HCl	10	aq.
Scopolamine hydrobromide	0.25	aq.
Antibiotics		
Bacitracin	5	pet.
Chloramphenicol	5	pet.
Gentamicin sulfate	20	pet.
Kanamycin	10	pet.
Neomycin sulfate	20	pet.
Polymyxin B Sulfate	20	pet.
Antiviral drugs		
Idoxuridine	1	pet.
Trifluoridine	5	pet.
Antihistaminics		
Chlorpheniramine maleate	5	pet.
Sodium cromoglycate	2	aq.
Anaesthetics		
Benzocaine	5	pet.
Procaine	5	aq.
Oxyburprocaine	0.5	aq.
Proxymetacaine	0.5	aq.
Enzymatic cleaners (for soft contact lenses)		
Papaine	1	pet.
Tegobetaine	1	aq.
Miotics		
Pilocarpine	1	aq.
Tolazoline	10	aq.
Echothiopate iodine	1	aq.
ε-aminocaproic acid	1	aq.

13.40 Contact allergy to topical ophthalmic preparations and contact lens solutions

Drug	Patch test conc./vehicle	Cross-reactions	Comment	Ref.
ε-aminocaproic acid	1% aqua		fibronolysin	177
amlexanox	1% pet.		antiallergic	172
antazoline phosphate	1% pet.	aminophylline	antihistamine. Injection of aminophylline caused generalized dermatitis	72
atropine sulfate	1% pet./aqua	homatropine	mydriatic agent	79 187
bacitracin	20% pet.		antibiotic	123
befunolol	1% aqua		β-blocker	189 190 248
benoxinate (oxybuprocaine)	0.5% pet.		local anaesthetic	196
benzalkonium chloride	0.05% aqua	cetrimonium bromide	preservative. *Cave:* irritant patch test reactions	54 85 97
benzethonium chloride	0.1% aqua		preservative in contact lens solution	64
benzocaine	5% pet.		local anaesthetic	196
betamethasone valerate	5% pet.		corticosteroid	74
cetalkonium chloride	0.01% aqua		preservative	195
chloramphenicol	5% pet.		antibiotic	123 169
chlorhexidine digluconate	0.5% aqua and pet.		in preserving liquids for soft contact lenses	109
chlorpheniramine maleate	5% pet.		antihistamine	178
cinnamic aldehyde (cinnamal)	1% pet.		fragrance	197
cobalt chloride	1% pet.	concomitant reaction to nickel sulphate	impurity in contact lens solution	171
cocamidopropyl betaine	1% aqua		amphoteric surfactant	168
cromoglycate disodium	2% aqua		antiallergic	175
echothiopate iodide	0.25–1% aqua		cholinergic	96
EDTA (edetic acid)	1% pet.		preservative	123

(continued)

§ **13.40** *(continuation)*

Drug	Patch test conc./vehicle	Cross-reactions	Comment	Ref.
ephedrine	1% pet.			102
epinephrine bitartrate	1% aqua			99
epinephrine chloride	1% aqua	epinephrine borate, diisopropyl fluorophosphate (?)		74 88
erythromycin glucoheptonate	5% pet.			197
fluorescein	10% aqua		photoallergic reaction. Dye for angiography	185
fragrance, unspecified	?			176 88
framycetin	20% pet.	possibly *from* other aminoglycosides	antibiotic	197
gentamicin sulfate	20% pet.		antibiotic	197
idoxuridine	1% pet.		antiviral drug	108 169 180
kanamycin	20% pet.	possibly *from* other aminoglycosides	antibiotic	197
metipranolol	2% aqua	L-penbutolol	β-blocker; the 0.6% commercial preparation caused many side effect including granulomatous anterior uveitis and was removed from the market in many countries	192
metoprolol	3% aqua	propranolol, practolol, timolol	β-blocker	94
neomycin	20% pet.		antibiotic	97 170
nickel sulfate	5% pet.	concomitant reaction to cobalt chloride	impurity in contact lens solution	171
nitrofurazone	1% pet.		antibiotic	179
parabens	3% pet.		preservative	97
d-penicillamine	1% aqua	*not* to penicillin	prevention of corneal fibrosis	173

(continued)

§ 13.40 *(continuation)*

Drug	Patch test conc./vehicle	Cross-reactions	Comment	Ref.
phenylephrine	5% aqua		α-adrenergic receptor stimulant. Also allergen in eardrops [256]	124
phenylmercuric nitrate	0.05% pet.		in contact lens solution	64
pilocarpine	4% pet.	also *photo*contact allergy	cholinomimetic used in the treatment of glaucoma	186
polymyxin B	3% pet.		antibiotic	123
procaine HCl	1% pet.		local anaesthetic	195
proparacaine hydrochloride	2% aqua		anaesthetic	76
prednisolone-21-trimethyl-acetate	1% pet.		*not* to prednisolone-21-monoacetate	182
rubidium iodide	1% pet.		prevention of cataracts	174
scopolamine hydrobromide	0.25% pet.		mydriatic	196
sisomicin sulfate	not specified	gentamicin	*systemic* contact dermatitis	183
sorbic acid	2.5% pet.		preservative	195
sulfonamides	5% pet.		antibiotics	123
thiomersal	0.1% pet.		also in preserving liquids for soft contact lenses. Occupational allergy, *see* [198]	64 104 107
timolol maleate	1% aqua		β-blocker	188
tixocortol pivalate	0.1% pet.	see § 5.31	corticosteroid	193
tobramycin	20% pet.		*systemic* contact dermatitis	184
tolazoline hydrochloride	10% aqua		α-sympathicolytic drug. Test concentration used slightly irritant	169
trifluorthymidine	5% pet.		antiviral drug. The allergy in case [78] probably represents a cross-reaction to primary IDU sensitization	78 181
tropicamide	1% pet.		anticholinergic	188
wool wax alcohols	30% pet.		vehicle ingredients	123

13.41 Other local side effects of topical ophthalmic preparations

Drug	Side effect	Comment	Ref.
amphotericin B	subconjunctival nodules and yellow discoloration		251
benoxinate	keratitis		70
benzalkonium chloride	corneal damage cicatrization of the conjunctiva due to allergy and irritation		87 97
chloramphenicol	toxic conjunctivitis		227
chlorhexidine	corneal damage from accidental eye contact		245
cinnamic aldehyde (cinnamal)	cicatrization of the conjunctiva due to allergy and irritation		97
corticosteroids	glaucoma, keratitis from infection due to immunosuppression [255]		71
cromoglycate disodium	acute chemotic reaction: redness, swelling and itching of the conjunctiva	allergy tests inadequately performed	63
epinephrine	melanosis of the conjunctiva and staining of the cornea		69
idoxuridine	punctal or canalicular stenosis	also with trifluorthymidine	250
isofluorophate	depigmentation around one eye		60
neomycin	cicatrization of the conjunctiva due to allergy and irritation		
papain	conjunctivitis angioedema contact lens intolerance contact urticarial reaction	papain is an enzyme cleanser in contact lens solutions	64 199 201
parabens	cicatrization of the conjunctiva due to allergy and irritation		97
phenylmercuric nitrate	band keratopathy		250
propamidine isethionate	intraepithelial microcysts		252
proparacaine	allergic keratitis	prolonged use of topical ocular anaesthetic agents can cause severe keratitis and permanent reduction of vision	200
sorbic acid	contact lens intolerance	contact urticarial reactions	64
thiomersal	cicatrization of the conjunctiva due to allergy and irritation		97
thiotepa	periorbital leukoderma		58
timolol	superficial punctate keratitis corneal epithelial erosions dry eyes cataracts	 causal relationship not established [229]	229 230 229

13.42 The mucous membranes of the nose and bladder

Topical drugs may also be used on the mucosae of the nose and the urine bladder. Their reported side effects are listed in Table 13.42.

Table 13.42 Side effects of drugs applied to the mucous membranes of the nose and the urine bladder

Drug	Function	Patch test conc./vehicle	Side effect	Comments	Ref.
ambroxol HCl	mucolytic drug	0.5% aqua	contact allergy		211
apomorfine	treatment of Parkinson's disease	0.05% aqua	contact allergy		246
budesonide	corticosteroid	1% pet.	contact allergy		205
corticosteroids				*See* § 5.31	
dexamethasone	corticosteroid		nasal septal perforation		203
disodium cromoglycate	mast cell stabilizer	powder pure	contact urticaria	symptoms included nasal congestion, rhinorrhea and bronchospasm	212
flunisolide	corticosteroid		nasal septal perforation	causal relationship not proven	202
gentian violet	antimicrobial		haemorrhagic cystitis	accidental injection of gentian violet through the urethra. Mucosal ulceration has also been reported [208]	207
lidocaine	local anaesthetic		contact urticaria syndrome	lubricant gel used for bladder catheterization	209
mitomycin C	antitumour antibiotic	0.1% pet.	systemic allergic contact dermatitis	frequency estimated to be 8–9% in patients treated with intravesical instillations of mitomycin C	204
propipocaine	local anaesthetic	1% pet.	contact urticaria with anaphylaxis	lubricant gel used for bladder catheterization	210
tixocortol pivalate	corticosteroid	1% pet.	contact allergy	cross-reaction to hydrocortisone	206

13.43 REFERENCES

1. Andersen, K.E. (1978): Contact allergy to toothpaste flavors. *Contact Dermatitis, 4,* 195.
2. Beinhauer, L.G. (1940): Cheilitis and dermatitis from toothpaste. *Arch. Dermatol., 41,* 892.
3. Dolles, O.K., Eriksen, H.M. and Gjermo, P. (1979): Tooth staining during 2 years' use of chlorhexidine and fluoride-containing dentifrices. *Scand. J. Dent. Res., 87,* 268.
4. Dooms-Goossens, A., Degreef, H., Holvoet, C. and Maertens, M. (1977): Turpentine-induced hypersensitivity to peppermint oil. *Contact Dermatitis, 3,* 304.
5. Douglas, T.E. (1975): Fluoride dentrifice and stomatitis. *Northw. Med. (Seattle), 56,* 107.
6. Epstein, E. (1976): Fluoride toothpastes as a cause of acne-like eruptions. *Arch. Dermatol., 112,* 1033.
7. Veien, N.K. (1990): Stomatitis and systemic dermatitis from mercury in amalgam dental restorations. *Dermatologic Clinics, 8,* 157-160.
8. Fisher, A.A. and Tobin, I. (1953): Sensitivity to compound G-4('Dichlorophene') in dentrifices. *J. Am. Med. Assoc., 151,* 998.
9. Flotra, L., Gjermo, O., Rolla, G. and Waerhaug, J. (1971): Side effects of chlorhexidine mouth washes. *Scand. J. Dent. Res., 79,* 119.
10. Heygi, E. and Dolezalova, A. (1976): Urticarial reaction after patch tests of toothpaste with a subshock condition: Hypersensitivity to caraway seed. *Cs. Derm., 51,* 19.
11. Kirton, V. and Wilkinson, D.S. (1975): Sensitivity to cinnamic aldehyde in a toothpaste. 2. Further studies. *Contact Dermatitis, 1,* 77.
12. Koch, G., Magnusson, B. and Nyquist, G. (1971): Contact allergy to medicaments and materials used in dentistry. *Odont. Revy, 22,* 275.
13. Laubach, J.L., Malkinson, F.D. and Ringrose, E.J. (1953): Cheilitis caused by cinnamon (Cassia) oil in toothpaste. *J. Am. Med. Assoc., 152,* 404–405.
14. Loveman, A.B. (1938): Stomatitis venenata, report of a case of sensitivity of the mucous membranes and the skin to oil of anise. *Arch. Derm. Syph., 37,* 70.
15. Magnusson, B. and Wilkinson, D.S. (1975): Cinnamic aldehyde in toothpaste. 1. Clinical aspects and patch tests. *Contact Dermatitis, 1,* 70.
16. Mathias, C.G.T., Maibach, H.I. and Conant, M.A. (1980): Perioral leukoderma simulating vitiligo from use of a toothpaste containing cinnamic aldehyde. *Arch. Dermatol., 116,* 1172.
17. Millard, L. (1973): Acute contact sensitivity to a new toothpaste. *J. Dentistry, 1,* 168.
18. O'Neil, T.C.A. (1976): The use of chlorhexidine mouthwash in the control of gingival inflammation. *Br. Dent. J., 141,* 276.
19. Hjorth, N. (1961): Eczematous allergy to balsalms. *Acta. Derm. Venereol., 41, (suppl. 46),* 136
20. Prayitno, S. and Addy, M. (1979): An in vitro study of factors affecting the development of staining associated with the use of chlorhexidine. *J. Periodont. Res., 14,* 397.
21. Romaguera, C. and Grimalt, G. (1978): Sensitization to cinnamic aldehyde in toothpaste. *Contact Dermatitis, 4,* 377.
22. Rushton, A. (1977): Safety of hibitane. II. Human experience. *J. Clin. Periodont., 4,* 73.
23. Saunders, M.A. (1975): Fluoride toothpastes; a cause of acne-like eruptions. *Arch. Derm., 111,* 793.
24. Schaupp, H. and Wohnaut, H. (1978): Geschmackstörungen durch Munddesinfizienten. *HNO (Berl.), 26,* 335.
25. Shea, J.J., Gillespie, S.M. and Waldbott, G.L. (1967): Allergy to fluoride. *Ann. Allergy, 25,* 241.
26. Smith, I.L.F. (1969): Acute allergic reaction following the use of toothpaste. *Br. Dent. J., 125,* 304.
27. Spier, H.W. and Sixt. I. (1953): Laurel as a hitherto little recognized allergen in contact eczema. *Derm. Wschr., 128,* 805.
28. Templeton, H.J. and Lunsford, C.J. (1932): Cheilitis and stomatitis from ST 37 toothpaste. *Arch. Derm. Syph., 25,* 439–443.
29. White, I.R. and Smith, B.G.N. (1984): Dental amalgam dermatitis. *Br. Dent. J., 156,* 259–261.
30. Varma, B.V. (1978): Mouthwash-induced hypoglycemia. *Am. J. Dis. Child., 132,* 930.
31. Bork, K. (1978): Fließschnupfen durch Metallteile von Zahnprothesen. *Z. Hautkr., 53,* 814.
32. Brendlinger, D.L. and Tarsitano, J.J. (1970): Generalized dermatitis due to sensitivity to a chrome cobalt removable partial denture. *J. Am. Dent. Assoc., 81,* 392.
33. Lamey, P.J. and Lamb, A.B. (1988): Prospective study of etiologic factors in burning mouth syndrome. *Br. Med. J., 296,* 1243–1246.
34. Danilewicz-Stysiak, Z. (1971): Allergy as a cause of denture sore mouth. *J. Prosth. Dent., 25,* 16.

35. Datschev, B. (1971): Allgemeine und Kontakt-Allergie in der Mundhöhle verursacht durch stomatologische Medikamente und Materialen. *Allergie u. Immunol., 17,* 239.
36. Elgart, M.L. and Higdon, R.S. (1971): Allergic contact dermatitis to gold. *Arch. Dermatol., 103,* 649.
37. Corazza, M., Virgili, A. and Martina, S. (1992): Allergic contact stomatitis from methyl methacrylate in a dental prosthesis, with a persistent patch test reaction. *Contact Dermatitis, 26,* 210–211.
38. Fregert, S., Kollander, M. and Poulsen, J. (1979): Allergic contact stomatitis from gold dentures. *Contact Dermatitis, 5,* 63.
39. Frykholm, K.O., Frithiof, L. and Fernström, A.I.B. et al. (1969): Allergy to copper derived from dental alloys as a possible cause of oral lesions of lichen planus. *Acta Derm.-Venereol. (Stockh.), 49,* 268.
40. Fisher, A.A. (1985): Allergic stomatitis from dental impression compounds. *Cutis, 36,* 295–296.
41. Hubler, W.R. Jr. and Hubler, W.R. Sr. (1983): Dermatitis from a chromium dental plate. *Contact Dermatitis, 9,* 377.
42. Isaacs, G. (1983): Permanent local anaesthesia and anhidrosis after clove oil spillage. *Lancet, 1,* 882.
43. Kaaber, S., Thulin, H. and Nielsen, E. (1979): Skin sensitivity to denture base materials in the burning mouth syndrome. *Contact Dermatitis, 5,* 90.
44. van Joost, Th. and Roesyanto-Mahadi, I.D. (1990): Combined sensitization to palladium and nickel. *Contact Dermatitis, 22,* 227–228.
45. Kulenkamp, D., Hausen, B.M. and Schulz, K.H. (1977): Berufliche Kontakallergie durch neuartige, zahnärzlich verwendete Abdruckmaterialien. *Hautarzt, 28,* 353.
46. Lamey, P.J., Lamb, A.B. and Forsyth, A. (1987): Atypical burning mouth syndrome. *Contact Dermatitis, 17,* 242–243.
47. Mathias, C.G.T., Chappler, R.R. and Maibach, H.I. (1980): Contact urticaria from cinnamic aldehyde. *Arch. Dermatol., 116,* 74.
48. Merk, H., Ebert, L. and Goerz, G. (1982): Allergic contact dermatitis due to the fungicide hexetidine. *Contact Dermatitis, 8,* 216.
49. James, J., Ferguson, M.M. and Forsyth, A. (1985): Mercury allergy as a cause of burning mouth. *Br. Dent. J., 21,* 392.
50. Nathanson, D. and Lockhart, P. (1979): Delayed extraoral hypersensitivity to dental composite materials. *Oral Surg., 47,* 329.
51. Schöpf, E., Wex, O. and Schulz, K.K. (1970): Allergische Kontaktstomatitis mit spezifischer Lymphocytenstimulation durch Gold. *Hautarzt, 21,* 422.
52. von Mayenburg, J. (1990): Amalgam-Allergie mit Stomatitis und perioralem Ekzem. *Allergologie, 13,* 389–391.
53. Kulenkamp, D., Hausen, B.M. and Schulz, K.H. (1976): Berufliche Kontaktallergie durch neuartige Abdruckmaterialen in der zahnärztlichen Praxis (Scutan und Impregum) *Zahnärztl. Prax., 66,* 968.
54. Fisher, A.A. (1987): Allergic contact dermatitis and conjunctivitis from benzalkonium chloride. *Cutis, 39,* 381–383.
55. Barber, K.A. (1983): Allergic contact eczema to phenylephrine. *Contact Dermatitis, 9,* 274.
56. Fratto, C. (1978): Provocation of bronchospasm by eye-drops. *Ann. Intern. Med., 88,* 362.
57. Fraunfelder, F.T. and Scafidi, A.F. (1978): Possible adverse effects from topical ocular 10% phenylephrine. *Am. J. Ophthal., 85,* 447.
58. Harben, D.J., Cooper, P.H. and Rodman, O. (1977): Thiotepa-induced leukoderma. *Arch. Derm., 115,* 973.
59. Henkes, H.E. and Waubke, T.N. (1978): Keratitis from abuse of corneal anaesthetics. *Br. J. Ophthal, 62,* 62.
60. Koldys, K.W. and Frye, L. (1973): A perplexing pigmentary problem. *Cutis, 12,* 420.
61. Lipmann, M. and Rogoff, R.C. (1974): Clinical evaluation of pyridostigmine bromide in the reversal of pancuronium. *Anesth. Analg. Curr. Res., 53,* 20.
62. Morton, W.R., Drance, S.M. and Fairclough, M. (1969): Effect of echothiopate iodide on the lens. *Am. J. Ophthal., 68,* 1003.
63. Ostler, H.B. (1982): Acute chemotic reaction to cromolyn. *Arch. Ophthal., 100,* 412.
64. Podmore, P. and Storrs, F.J. (1989): Contact lens intolerance; allergic conjunctivitis? *Contact Dermatitis, 20,* 98–103.
65. Velez, G.J. (1968): Jaundice and Floropryl. Report of a case. *J. Pediat. Ophthal., 5,* 179.
66. Nursall, J.F. (1965): Systemic effects of topical use of ophthalmic corticosteroid preparations. *Am. J. Ophthal., 59,* 29.
67. Burch, P.G. and Migeon, C.J. (1968): Systemic absorption of topical steroids. *Arch. Ophthal., 79,* 174.

68. Fraunfelder, F.T., Bagby, G.O. and Kelly, D.J. (1982): Fatal aplastic anaemia following topical administration of ophthalmic chloramphenicol. *Am. J. Ophthalmol., 93,* 356–359.
69. Schuster, H. (1974): Uber eine seltene Nebenwirkung von Adrenalin–Augentropfen. *Klin. Mbl. Augenheilk., 165,* 517.
70. Henkes, H.E. and Waubke, T.N. (1978): Keratitis from abuse of corneal anaesthetics. *Br. J. Ophthal., 62,* 62.
71. Eisenlohr, J.E. (1983): Glaucoma following the prolonged use of topical steroid medication to the eyelids. *J. Am. Acad. Dermatol., 8,* 878.
72. Berman, B.A. and Ross, R.N. (1983): Ethylenediamine systemic eczematous contact-type dermatitis. *Cutis, 31,* 594.
73. Adriani, J. and Campbell, D. (1956): Fatalities following topical application of local anesthetics to mucous membranes. *J. Am. Med. Assoc., 162,* 1527.
74. Alani, S.D. and Alani, M.D. (1976): Allergic contact dermatitis and conjunctivitis from epinephrine. *Contact Dermatitis, 2,* 147.
75. Baker, J.P. and Farley, J.D. (1958): Toxic psychosis following atropine eyedrops. *Br. Med. J., 2,* 390.
76. Bandmann, H.J., Breit, R. and Mutzeck, E. (1974): Allergic contact dermatitis from Proxymetacaine. *Contact Dermatitis Newsl., 15,* 451.
77. Benjamin, K.W. (1979): Toxicity of ocular medications. *Int. Ophthal. Clin., 19,* 199.
78. Millán-Parilla, F. and de la Cuadra, J. (1990): Allergic contact dermatitis from trifluoridine in eyedrops. *Contact Dermatitis, 22,* 289.
79. van der Willigen, A.H., de Graaf, Y.P. and van Joost, Th. (1987): Periocular dermatitis from atropine. *Contact Dermatitis, 17,* 56–57.
80. Epstein, E. and Kaufman, I. (1965): Systemic pilocarpine toxicity from overdosage. *Am. J. Ophthal., 59,* 109.
81. Fraunfelder, F.T. (1976): Extraocular fluid dynamics; how best to apply topical ocular medication. *Trans. Am. Ophthal. Soc., 74,* 457.
82. Fraunfelder, F.T. and Meyer, S.M. (1987): Systemic side effects from ophthalmic timolol and their prevention. *J. Ocular Pharmacol., 3,* 177–184.
83. Fregert, S. and Möller, H. (1962): Hypersensitivity to the cholinesterase inhibitor di-iso-propoxy-phosphorylfluoride. *J. Invest. Derm., 38,* 371.
84. Freund, M. and Merin, S. (1970: Toxic effects of scopolamine eye-drops. *Am. J. Ophthal., 70,* 637.
85. Klein, G.F., Sepp, N. and Fritsch, P. (1991): Allergic reactions to benzalkonium chloride? Do the use test. *Contact Dermatitis, 25,* 269–270.
86. Friedman, T.S. and Patton, T.F. (1976): Differences in ocular penetration of pilocarpine in rabbits of different ages. *J. Pharm. Sci., 65,* 1095.
87. Gasset, A.R. (1977): Benzalkonium chloride toxicity to the human cornea. *Am. J. Ophthal., 84,* 169.
88. Gibbs, R.C. (1970): Allergic contact dermatitis to epinephrine. *Arch. Dermatol., 101,* 92.
89. Goodman, L.S. and Gilman, A. (Eds) (1980): *The Pharmacological Basis of Therapeutics,* 6th ed., MacMallian Publishing Co., New York.
90. Gottschalk, H.R. and Stone, O.J. (1976): Stevens–Johnson syndrome from ophthalmic sulfonamide. *Arch. Dermatol., 112,* 513.
91. Haddad, N.J., Moyer, N. and Riley, F. (1970): Mydriatic effect of phenylephrine hydrochloride. *Am. J. Ophthal., 70,* 729.
92. Havener, W.H. (1979): *Ocular Pharmacology,* 4th ed., pp. 40–50. C.V. Mosby Co., St. Louis.
93. Hoefnagel, D. (1961): Toxic effects of atropine and homatropine eye-drops in children. *New Engl. J. Med., 264,* 168.
94. Van Joost, Th., Middlekamp Hup. J. and Ros, F.E. (1980): Dermatitis as a side-effect of long-term topical treatment with certain beta-blocking agents. *Br. J. Dermatol., 101,* 171.
95. Lansche, R.K. (1966): Systemic reactions to topical epinephrine and phenylephrine. *Am. J. Ophthal., 61,* 95.
96. Mathias, C.G.T., Maibach, H.I., Irvine, A. and Adler, W. (1979): Allergic contact dermatitis to echothiopate iodide and phenylephrine. *Arch. Ophthal., 97,* 286.
97. Ostler, H.B., Okumoto, M., Daniels, T. and Conant, M.A. (1983): Drug-induced cicatrisation of the conjunctiva. *Contact Dermatitis, 9,* 155.
98. Patton, T.F. and Francoeur, M. (1978): Ocular bioavailability and systemic loss of topically applied ophthalmic drugs. *Am. J. Ophthal., 85,* 225.
99. Romaguera, C. and Grimalt, F. (1980): Contact dermatitis from epinephrine. *Contact Dermatitis, 6,* 364.

100. Selvin, B.L. (1983): Systemic effects of topical ophthalmic medications. *Sth. Med. J., 76,* 349.
101. Sieg, J.W. and Robinson, J.R. (1974): Corneal absorption of fluorometholone in rabbits. *Arch. Ophthal., 92,* 240.
102. Spencer, G.A. (1945): Hypersensitivity to ephedrine. *Arch. Dermatol. Syph., (Chic.), 51,* 48.
103. Stokes, H.R. (1979): Drug reactions reported in a survey of South Carolina. *Am. Ophthal., 86,* 161.
104. Tosti, A. and Tosti, G. (1988): Thimerosal: a hidden allergen in ophthalmology. *Contact Dermatitis, 18,* 268–273.
105. Vaughan, R.W. (1973): Ventricular arrhythmias after topical vasoconstrictors. *Anesth. Analg., 52,* 161.
106. Alani, S.D. and Alani, M.D. (1976): Allergic contact dermatitis and conjunctivitis to corticosteroids. *Contact Dermatitis, 2,* 301.
107. Bang Pedersen, N. (1978): Allergic contact conjunctivitis from merthiolate in soft contact lenses. *Contact Dermatitis, 4,* 165.
108. Van Ketel, W.G. (1979): Allergy to idoxuridine eyedrops. *Contact Dermatitis, 5,* 106.
109. Rapaport, M. (1991): Contact dermatitis secondary to chlorhexidine in contact lens cleansing solutions. *J. Am. Acad. Dermatol., 2,* 65–66.
110. Palmer, E.A. (1982): Drug toxicity in pedriatric ophthalmology. *J. Toxic.-Cut. Ocul. Toxic., 1,* 181.
111. Aaronson, Ch. M. (1969): Generalized urticaria from sensitivity to nifuroxime. (Letter). *J. Am. Med. Ass., 210,* 557.
112. Dutton, A.H., Hayes, P.C., Shepherd, A.N. and Geirsson, R. (1983): Vulvovaginal steroid cream and toxic shock syndrome. *Lancet, 1,* 938.
113. Goette, D.K. and Odom, R.B. (1980): Vaginal medications as a cause for varied widespread dermatitides. *Cutis, 26,* 406.
114. Robin, J. (1978): Contact dermatitis to acetarsol. *Contact Dermatitis, 4,* 309.
115. Verburgh-van der Zwan, N. and van Ketel, W.G. (1981): Contactallergie voor een arseen bevattend intravaginaal toegepast geneesmiddel. *Ned. T. Geneesk., 125,* 1718.
116. Donlan, Ch. J. Jr. and Scutero, J.V. (1975): Transient eosinophilic pneumonia secondary to use of vaginal cream. *Chest, 67,* 232.
117. Klinghoffer, J.F. (1954): Loeffler's syndrome following use of a vaginal cream. *Ann. Intern. Med., 40,* 343.
118. Fisher, A.A. (1982): Systemic contact dermatitis from Orinase® and Diabinese® in diabetics with para-amino hypersensitivity. *Cutis, 29,* 551.
119. Mathias, C.G.T., Chappler, R.R. and Maibach, H.I. (1980): Contact urticaria from cinnamic aldehyde. *Arch. Derm., 116,* 74.
120. Merk, H., Ebert, L. and Goerz, G. (1982): Allergic contact dermatitis due to the fungicide hexetidine. *Contact Dermatitis, 8,* 555.
121. Young, E. (1987): Sensitivity to propolis. *Contact Dermatitis, 16,* 49–50.
122. Marchand, B., Barbier, P. and Ducombs, G., et al. (1982): Allergic contact dermatitis to various salols (phenyl salicylates). *Arch. Dermatol. Res., 272,* 61.
123. Kruijswijk, M.R.J. and Polak, B.C.P. (1980): Contactallergie na toepassing van oogdruppels en oogzalven. *Ned. T. Geneesk., 124,* 1449.
124. Añibarro, B., Barranco, P. and Ojeda, J.A. (1991): Allergic contact blepharoconjunctivitis caused by phenylephrine eyedrops. *Contact Dermatitis, 25,* 323–324.
125. Machácková, J. and Smid, P. (1991): Allergic contact cheilitis from toothpastes. *Contact Dermatitis, 24,* 311.
126. Lamey, P.J., Rees, T.D. and Forsyth, A. (1990): Sensitivity reaction to the cinnamon aldehyde component of toothpaste. *Br. Dental. J., 168,* 115–118.
127. Rubright, W.C., Walker, J.A., Karlsson, U.F. and Diehl, D.L. (1978): Oral slough caused by dentifrice detergents and aggravated by drugs with antisialic activity. *J. Am. Dent. Assoc., 97,* 215–220.
128. Loewenthal, K. (1952): Eczematous contact dermatitis of the palm due to toothpaste. *N. York State J. Med., 52,* 1437–1438.
129. Hausen, B.M. (1984): Zahnpasta-Allergie. *Deutsche Med. Wschr., 109,* 300–302.
130. Hausen, B.M. (1986): Zahnpasta-Allergie durch L-Carvon. *Akt. Dermatol., 12,* 23–24.
131. Ormerod, A.D. and Main, R.A. (1985): Sensitization to "sensitive teeth" toothpaste. *Contact Dermatitis, 13,* 192–193.
132. Balato, N., Lembo, G., Nappa, P. and Ayala, F. (1985): Allergic cheilitis to azulene. *Contact Dermatitis, 13,* 39–40.
133. Angelini, G. and Vena, G.A. (1984): Allergic contact cheilitis to guaiazulene. *Contact Dermatitis, 10,* 311.
134. Spurlock, B.W. and Dailey, T.M. (1990): Shortness of (fresh) breath — toothpaste-induced bronchospasm. *N. Engl. J. Med., 323,* 1845–1846.

135. Kim, S.C., Hong, K.T. and Kim, D.H. (1988): Contact stomatitis from a breath refresher (Eundan®). *Contact Dermatitis, 19,* 309.
136. Vilaplana, J., Grimalt, F., Romaguera, C. and Conellana, F. (1991): Contact dermatitis from eugenol in mouthwash. *Contact Dermatitis, 24,* 224.
137. Lim, J., Goh, L. and Lee, C.T. (1991): Perioral and mucosal oedema due to contact allergy to proflavine. *Contact Dermatitis, 25,* 195.
138. Ebner, H. and Kraft, D. (1991): Formaldeyde-induced anaphylaxis after dental treatment? *Contact Dermatitis, 24,* 307–308.
139. Maurice, P.D.L., Hopper, C., Punnia-Moorthy, A. and Rycroft, R.J.G. (1988): Allergic contact stomatitis and cheilitis from idoform used in a dental dressing. *Contact Dermatitis, 18,* 114–116.
140. O'Connor, A.F.F., Freeland, A.P., Heal, D.J. and Rossouw, D.S. (1977): Iodoform toxicity following the use of BIPP; a potential hazard. *J. Laryngol. Otol., 91,* 903–907.
141. Scarpa, C. and Gentilli, G. (1983): Alcalosi ipocaliemica da 9-alfa-fluoroprednisolone applicato local mente in corso di penfigo volgare. *Giorn. It. Derm. Vener., 118,* 179–181.
142. Kleinhans, D. and Fuchs, Th. (1983): Akute allergische Kontaktstomatitis durch Tetracain. *Akt. Dermatol, 9,* 241–242.
143. Bovenmyer, D.A. (1985): Aggravation of dermatitis herpetiformis by dental fluoride treatments. *J. Am. Acad. Dermatol, 12,* 719–720.
144. Ayala, F., Lembo, G., Nappa, P. and Balato, N. (1985): Contact dermatitis from propolis. *Contact Dermatitis, 12,* 181–182.
145. Fisher, A.A. (1987): Reactions of the mucous membrane to contactants. *Clinics in Dermatol., 5,* 123–136.
146. von Mayenburg, J., Rakoski, J. and Szliska, C. (1991): Patch testing with amalgam at various concentrations. *Contact Dermatitis, 24,* 266–269.
147. Nordlind, K. and Liden, S. (1992): Patch test reactions to metal salts in patients with oral mucosal lesions associated with amalgam restorations. *Contact Dermatitis, 27,* 3.
148. Mobacken, H., Hersle, K., Sloberg, K. and Thilander, H. (1984): Oral lichen planus: hypersensitivity to dental restoration material. *Contact Dermatitis, 10,* 11–15.
149. Garioch, J., Todd, P., Lamey, P.J., Forsyth, A. and Rademaker, M. (1990): The significance of a positive patch test to mercury in oral disease. *Br. J. Dermatol., 123,* (suppl. 37): 25–26.
150. Todd, P., Garioch, J., Lamey, P.J., Lewis, M., Forsyth, A. and Rademaker, M. (1990): Patch testing in lichenoid reactions of the mouth and oral lichen planus. *Br. J. Dermatol., 123,* (suppl. 37): 26.
151. Izumi, A.K. (1982): Allergic contact gingivostomatitis due to gold. *Arch. Derm. Res., 272,* 387–389.
152. Dutrée-Meulenberg, R.O.G.M., Kozel, M.M.A. and van Joost, Th. (1992): Burning mouth syndrome: A possible etiologic role for local contact hypersensitivity. *J. Am. Acad. Dermatol., 26,* 935–940.
153. Lindmaier, A. and Lindemayr, H. (1989): Probleme mit Zahnprothesen und Zahnfüllungsmaterialen: Epicutantestergebnisse. Konsequenzen und Nachbeobachtung. *Z. Hautkr., 64,* 24–30.
154. Ali, A., Bates, J.F., Reynolds, A.J. et al. (1986): The burning mouth sensation related to the wearing of acrylic dentures: an investigation. *Br. Dent. J., 161,* 444–447.
155. Todd, D.J. and Burrows, D. (1992): Patch testing with pure palladium metal in patients with sensitivity to palladium chloride. *Contact Dermatitis, 26,* 327–331.
156. de Fine Olivarius, F. and Menné, T. (1992): Contact dermatitis from metallic palladium in patients reacting to palladium chloride. *Contact Dermatitis, 27,* 71–73.
157. Romaguera, C., Vilaplana, J. and Grimalt, F. (1989): Contact stomatitis from a dental prosthesis. *Contact Dermatitis, 21,* 204.
158. Espana, A., Alonso, M.L., Soria, C., Guimarens, D. and Ledo, A. (1989): Chronic urticaria after implantation of a nickel-containing dental prosthesis in a nickel-allergic patient. *Contact Dermatitis, 21,* 204–205.
159. Downey, D. (1989): Contact mucositis due to palladium. *Contact Dermatitis, 21,* 54.
160. Haustein, U.F. (1988): Burning mouth syndrome due to nicotinic acid esters and sorbic acid. *Contact Dermatitis, 19,* 225–226.
161. Doherty, V.R., Forsyth, A. and McKie, R.M. (1990): Pruritus vulvae: a manifestation of contact hypersensitivity? *Br. J. Dermatol., 123,* (suppl. 37): 26–27.
162. Susitaival, P. and Häkkinen, L. (1989): Anaphylactic allergy to chlorhexidine cream. In: Frosch, P.J. et al. (Editors), *Current Topics in Contact Dermatitis*, Springer, Berlin. 99–103.
163. Okano, M., Nomura, M. and Hata, S. (1989): Anaphylactic symptoms due to chlorhexidine gluconate. *Arch. Dermatol., 125*, 50–52.

164. Helander, I., Hollmén, A. and Hopsu-Havu, V.K. (1979): Allergic contact dermatitis to chlordantoin. *Contact Dermatitis, 5,* 54–55.
165. Baes, H. (1991): Contact sensitivity to miconazole with ortho-chloro cross-sensitivity to other imidazoles. *Contact Dermatitis, 24,* 89–93.
166. Bonneau, J.C. (1990): Allergie à la Tégobétaine: à propos d'un cas. *Allergie et Immunologie, 22,* 195.
167. Valsecchi, R. and Cainelli, T. (1988): Contact allergy to propyl gallate. *Contact Dermatitis, 19,* 380–381.
168. Sertoli, A., Lombardi, P., Palleschi, G.M., Gola, M. and Giorgini, S. (1987): Tegobetaine in contact lens solutions. *Contact Dermatitis, 16,* 111–112.
169. Frosch, P.J., Olbert, D. and Weickel, R. (1985): Contact allergy to tolazoline. *Contact Dermatitis, 13,* 272.
170. Mariani, R., Tardio, M., Bassi, R. and Alessandrini, F. (1991): Allergic contact conjunctivitis without eyelid involvement. *Contact Dermatitis, 24,* 227.
171. Vilaplana, J., Romaguera, C. and Grimalt, F. (1991): Contact dermatitis from nickel and cobalt in a contact lens cleaning solution. *Contact Dermatitis, 24,* 232–233.
172. Kabasawa, Y. and Kanzaki, T. (1991): Allergic contact dermatitis from amlexanox (Elics®) ophthalmic solution. *Contact Dermatitis, 24,* 148.
173. Coenraads, P.J., Woest, T.E., Blanksma, L.J. and Houtman, W.A. (1990): Contact allergy to d-penicillamine. *Contact Dermatitis, 23,* 371–372.
174. Cameli, N., Bardazzi, F., Morelli, R. and Tosti, A. (1990): Contact dermatitis from rubidium iodide eyedrops. *Contact Dermatitis, 23,* 377–378.
175. Kudo, H., Tanaka, T., Miyachi, Y. and Imamura, S. (1988): Contact dermatitis from sodium cromoglycate eyedrops. *Contact Dermatitis, 19,* 312–313.
176. Meynadier, J.M., Meynadier, J., Peyron, J.L. and Peyron, L. (1986): Formes cliniques des manifestations cuntanées d'allergie aux parfums. *Ann. Dermatol. Venereol., 113,* 31–39.
177. Shono, M. (1989): Allergic contact dermatitis from epsilon-aminocaproic acid. *Contact Dermatitis, 21,* 106–107.
178. Tosti, A., Bardazzi, F. and Piancastelli, E. (1990): Contact dermatitis due to chlorpheniramine maleate in eyedrops. *Contact Dermatitis, 22,* 55.
179. Ancora, A. (1985): Allergic contact dermatitis to nitrofurazone. *Contact Dermatitis, 13,* 35.
180. Senff, H., Engelmann, L., Kunze, J. and Hausen, B.M. (1990): Allergic contact dermatitis from idoxuridine. *Contact Dermatitis, 23,* 43–45.
181. Naito, T., Shiota, H. and Mimura, Y. (1987): Side effects in the treatment of herpetic keratitis. *Curr. Eye Res., 6,* 237–239.
182. Schmoll, M. and Hausen, B.M. (1988): Allergische Kontaktdermatitis auf Prednisolon-21-trimethylacetate. *Z. Hautkr., 63,* 311–313.
183. Katayama, I. and Nishioka, K. (1987): Systemic contact dermatitis medicamentosa induced by topical eye lotion (sisomicin) in a patient with corneal allograft. *Arch. Dermatol., 123,* 436–437.
184. Tanaka, I., Sasaki, T., Oozeki, H. et al. (1978): Clinical studies in tobramycin eye lotion. *Jpn. Rev. Clin. Ophthalmol., 22,* 822–828.
185. Hochsattel, R., Gall, H., Weber, L. and Kaufmann, R. (1990): Photoallergic reaction to fluorescein. *Contact Dermatitis, 22,* 42–44.
186. Helton, J. and Storrs, F.J. (1991): Pilocarpine allergic contact and photocontact dermatitis. *Contact Dermatitis, 25,* 133–134.
187. Yoshikawa, K. and Kawahara, S. (1985): Contact allergy to atropine and other mydriatic agents. *Contact Dermatitis, 12,* 56–57.
188. Romaguera, C., Grimalt, F. and Vilaplana, J. (1986): Contact dermatitis by Timolol. *Contact Dermatitis, 14,* 248.
189. Kanzaki, T., Kato, N., Kabasawa, Y., Mizuno, N., Yuguchi, M. and Majima, A. (1988): Contact dermatitis due to the β-blocker timolol in eyedrops. *Contact Dermatitis, 19,* 388.
190. Schultheiss, E. (1989): Überempfindlichkeit gegenüber Levobunolol. *Dermatosen, 37,* 185–186.
191. de Groot, A.C. and Conemans, J. (1988): Contact allergy to metipranolol. *Contact Dermatitis, 18,* 107–108.
192. D'Arcy, P.F. (1990): Drug reactions and interactions. *Int. Pharmacy J., 4,* 244–245.
193. Foussereau, J. and Jelen, G. (1986): Tixocortol pivalate — an allergen closely related to hydrocortisone. *Contact Dermatitis, 15,* 37–38.
194. Herbst, R.A. and Maibach, H.I. (1991): Contact dermatitis caused by allergy to ophthalmic drugs and contact lens solutions. *Contact Dermatitis, 25,* 305–312.
195. Maucher, O.M. (1974): Periorbitalekzem als iatrogene Erkrankung. *Klin. Monatsbl. Augenheilkd., 164,* 350–356.

196. Haetinen, A., Teraesvirta, M. and Fraeki, J.E. (1985): Contact allergy to components in topical ophthalmologic preparations. *Acta. Derm.-Venereol., 63,* 424–426.
197. Frosch, P.J., Weickel, R., Schmitt, T. and Krastel, H. (1988): Nebrenwirkungen von ophthalmologischen Externa. *Z. Hautkr., 63,* 126–136.
198. De Groot, A.C., van Wynen, W.G. and van Wynen-Vos, M. (1990): Occupational contact dermatitis of the eyelids, without ocular involvement from thimerosal in contact lens fluid. *Contact Dermatitis, 23,* 195.
199. Bernstein, D.I., Gallagher, J.S., Grad, M. and Bernstein, I.L. (1984): Local ocular anaphylaxis to papain enzyme contained in a contact lens cleansing solution. *J. All. Clin. Immunol., 74,* 258–260.
200. Brent, M.H., Slomovic, A.R. and Easterbrook, M. (1987): Keratitis associated with the use of proparacaine hydrochloride. *Can. Med. Assoc. J., 136,* 380–381.
201. Santucci, B., Cristuado, A. and Picardo, M. (1985): Contact urticaria from papain in a soft lens solution. *Contact Dermatitis, 12,* 233.
202. Soderberg-Warner, M.L. (1984): Nasal septal perforation associated with topical corticosteroid therapy. *J. Pediat., 105,* 840–841.
203. Miller, F.F. (19750: Occurence of nasal septal perforation with use of intranasal dexamethasone aerosol. *Ann. Allergy, 34,* 107–109.
204. De Groot, A.C. and Conemans, J.M.H. (1991): Systemic allergic contact dermatitis from intravesical instillation of the antitumor antibiotic mitomycin C. *Contact Dermatitis, 24,* 201–209.
205. Faria, A., Marote, J. and de Freitas, C. (1992): Contact allergy to budesonide in nasal spray. *Contact Dermatitis, 27,* 57.
206. Bircher, A.J. (1990): Short induction phase of contact allergy to tixocortol pivalate in a nasal spray. *Contact Dermatitis, 22,* 237–238.
207. Walsh, C. and Walsh, A. (1986): Haemorrhagic cystitis due to gentian violet. *Br. Med. J., 293,* 732.
208. John, R.W. (1968): Necrosis of oral mucosa after local application of crystal violet. *Br. Med. J., i,* 157–158.
209. Budde, J., Stary, A. and Beiteke, U. (1989): Kontaktallergie vom Sofort-Typ auf topische Anwendung von Lidocain. *Dermatosen, 37,* 181–182.
210. Hallmann, B., Rehmann, O. and Bormann, B. (1988): Lebensbedrohliche allergische Reaktionen durch Einsatz von Urocomb-Gel®. *Z. Urol. Nephrol., 81,* 715–717.
211. Mancuso, G. and Berdondini, R.M. (1989): Contact allergy to ambroxol. *Contact Dermatitis, 20,* 154.
212. Hutt, N., Firdion, O., Abbas, F. and Pauli, G. (1986): A propos d'un cas d'allergie immédiate vraisemblable au cromoglycate disodique. *Rev. Fr. Allergol., 26,* 147–148.
213. Feiler-Ofrey, V., Godel, V. and Lazar, M. (1981): Nail pigmentation following timolol maleate therapy. *Ophthalmologia, 182,* 153–156.
214. Akingbehin, T. (1986): Corticosteroid-induced ocular hypertension. *J. Toxicol.-Cut. Ocular Toxicol., 5,* 45–53.
215. Anonymous. (1989): Tachycardia precipitated by topical homatropine. *Br. Med. J., 299,* 795–796.
216. Fale, W.J. and Boyd, D.L. (1988): Homatropine-associated confusion in an elderly patient. *J. Am. Geriatr. Soc., 36,* 649.
217. Birkhimer, L.J., Jacobson, P.A., Olson, J. and Guyette, D.M. (1984): Ocular scopolamine-induced psychosis. *J. Family Practice, 18,* 464–469.
218. Fraunfelder, F.T. and Meyer, S.M. (1987): Systemic reactions to ophthalmic drug preparations. *Med. Toxicol,* 287–293.
219. Adler, A.G., McElwain, G.E. and Martin, J.H. (1981): Coronary artery spasm induced by phenylephrine eyedrops. *Arch. Intern. Med., 141,* 1384–1385.
220. Cass, E., Kadar, D. and Stein, H.A. (1979): Hazards of phenylephrine topical medication in persons taking propranolol. *Can. Med. Assoc. J., 20,* 1261–1262.
221. Vaughan, R.W. (1973): Ventricular arrhythmias after topical vasoconstrictors. *Anesthesia and Analgesia, 52,* 161–165.
222. Matthews, T.G., Wilczek, A.M. and Shenan, A.T. (1977): Eyedrop induced hypertension. *Lancet, 2,* 827.
223. Wesley, R.E., Blount, W.C. and Arterberry, J.F. (1981): Pulmonary embolism in a diabetic patient after ocular 10% phenylephrine. *Ann. Ophthalmol., 13,* 311–313.
224. Kennerdell, J.S. and Wucher, F.P. (1972): Cyclopentolate associated with two cases of grand mal seizure. *Arch. Ophthalmol., 87,* 634–635.
225. Hermansen, M.C. and Sullivan, L.S. (1985): Feeding intolerance following ophthalmologic examination. *Am. J. Dis. Child., 139,* 367–368.
226. Isenberg, S.J., Abrams, C. and Hyman, P.E. (1985): Effects of cyclopentolate eyedrops on gastric secretory function in pre-term children. *Ophthalmol., 92,* 698–700.

227. Buckley, S.A. (1990): Survey of patients taking topical medication at their first presentation to eye casualty. *Br. Med. J., 300,* 1497–1498.
228. Novack, G.D. and Leopold, I.H. (1987): The toxicity of topical ophthalmic beta-blockers. *J. Toxicol., 6,* 283–297.
229. Van Buskirk, E.M. (1980): Adverse reactions from timolol administration. *Ophthalmol., 87,* 447–450.
230. Fraunfelder, F.T. and Meyer, S.M. (1986): Corneal complications of ocular medications. *Cornea, 5,* 55–59.
231. Ball, S. (1987): Congestive heart failure from betaxolol. *Arch. Ophthalmol., 105,* 320–323.
232. Orlando, R.G. (1986): Clinical depression associated with betaxolol. *Am. J. Ophthalmol., 102,* 275–278.
233. Velde, T.M. and Kaiser, F.E. (1983): Ophthalmic timolol treatment causing altered hypoglycemic response in a diabetic patient. *Arch. Intern. Med., 143,* 1627–1629.
234. Nelson, W.L., Fraunfelder, F.T., Sills, J.M., Arrowsmith, J.B. and Kuritsky, J.N. (1986): Adverse respiratory and cardiovascular events attributed to timolol ophthalmic solution, 1978–1985. *Am. J. Ophthalmol., 102,* 606–611.
235. Coppeto, J.R. (1985): Transient ischemic attacks and amaurosis fugax from timolol. *Ann. Ophthalmol., 17,* 64–65.
236. Fraunfelder, F.T. and Meyer, S.M. (1990): Alopecia possibly secondary to topical ophthalmic β-blockers. *JAMA., 263,* 1493–1494.
237. Fraunfelder, F.T. and Meyer, S.M. (1985): Sexual dysfunction secondary to topical ophthalmic timolol. *JAMA., 253,* 3092–3093.
238. Katz, J.M. (1986): Sexual dysfunction and ocular timolol. *JAMA., 255,* 37–38.
239. Munroe, W.P., Rindone, J.P. and Kershner, R.M. (1985): Systemic side effects associated with the ophthalmic administration of timolol. *Drug Intell. Clin. Pharmacy, 19,* 85–89.
240. Botet, C., Grau, J., Benito, P., Coll, J. and Vivancos, J. (1986): Timolol ophthalmic solution and respiratory arrest. *Ann. Intern. Med., 165,* 306–307.
241. Shore, J.H., Fraunfelder, F.T. and Meyer, S.M. (1987): Psychiatric side effects from topical ocular timolol, a beta-adrenergic blocker. *J. Clin. Psychopharmacol, 7,* 264–267.
242. Everitt, D.E. and Avorn, J. (1990): Systemic effects of medication used to treat glaucoma. *Ann. Intern. Med., 112,* 120–125.
243. Garcia-Bravo, B., Pons, A. and Rodriguez-Pichardo, A. (1992): Oral lichen planus from colophony. *Contact Dermatitis, 26,* 279.
244. Laine, J., Kalimo, K., Forssel, H. and Happonen, R.P. (1992): Resolution of oral lichenoid lesions after replacement of amalgam restorations in patients allergic to mercury compounds. *Br. J. Dermatol., 126,* 10–15.
245. Tabor, E., Bostwick, D.C. and Evans, C.C. (1989): Corneal damage due to eye contact with chlorhexidine gluconate. *JAMA, 261,* 557–558.
246. van Laar, T., Kruyswyk, M.R.J. and Jansen, E.N.H. (1992): Nasolabiale allergische reactie op intranasale toediening van apomorfine by de ziekte van Parkinson. *Ned. Tijdschr. Geneesk., 136,* 702–704.
247. Corazza, M., Virgili, A. and Mantovani, L. (1992): Vulvar contact dermatitis from nifuratel. *Contact Dermatitis, 27,* 273–274.
248. Mancuso, G. (1992): Allergic contact dermatitis due to befunolol in eyedrops. *Contact Dermatitis, 27,* 198.
249. Trombelli, L., Virgili, A., Corazza, M. and Lucci, R. (1992): Systemic contact dermatitis from an orthodontic appliance. *Contact Dermatitis, 27,* 259–260.
250. Wilson, F.M. (1979): Adverse external ocular effects of topical ophthalmic medications. *Surv. Ophthalmol., 24,* 57–58.
251. Bell, R.W. and Ritchey, J.P. (1973): Subconjunctival nodules after amphotericin B injection. *Ophthalmol., 90,* 402–404.
252. Johns, K.J., Head, S. and O'Day, D.M. (1988): Corneal toxicity of propamidine. *Arch. Ophthalmol., 106,* 68–69.
253. Stern, G.A. and Killingsworth, D.W. (1989): Complications of topical antimicrobial agents. *Int. Ophthalmol. Clinics, 29,* 137–142.
254. Plosker, G.L. (1987): Possible interaction between ethanol and vaginally administrated metronidazole. *Clin. Pharmacy, 6,* 189–193.
255. Egbert, J.E., Feder, J.M., Rapoza, P.A., Chandler, J.W. and France, T.D. (1990): Keratitis associated with Pseudomonas mesophilien in a patient taking topical corticosteroids. *Am. J. Ophthalmol., 110,* 445–446.
256. Bardazzi, F., Tardio, M., Mariani, R., Rapacchiale, S. and Valenti, R. (1991): Phenylephrine in eardrops causing contact dermatitis. *Contact Dermatitis, 24,* 56.

14. Local side effects of corticosteroids

14.1 Topical steroids have the following effects on the skin [33], in that they:

1. inhibit proliferation and regeneration of epidermis (inhibition of DNA synthesis);
2. inhibit collagen synthesis;
3. inhibit elastin synthesis;
4. cause atrophy of adipose tissue;
5. cause vasoconstriction;
6. seal and stabilize the cell walls;
7. cause follicular hyperkeratosis;
8. cause focal degeneration of follicular epithelium;
9. stimulate hair growth;
10. inhibit antigen–antibody reactions;
11. inhibit leukocyte migration and proliferation;
12. inhibit antibody production and proliferation of immunocompetent cells;
13. depress or stimulate melanogenesis.

Table 14.2 provides a guide to the clinical potency of commonly used topical steroids [28].

14.2 Relative potency of topical steroid products [28]

	Drug*	Available forms	Concentration (%)
I.	Betamethasone dipropionate in optimized vehicle	Cream, ointment, lotion	0.05
	Clobetasol propionate	Cream, ointment	0.05
	Diflorasone diacetate	Ointment	0.05
II.	Amcinonide	Cream, ointment	0.1
	Betamethasone dipropionate	Cream, ointment, lotion	0.05
	Desoximetasone	Cream, ointment	0.25
	Diflorasone diacetate	Cream, ointment	0.05
	Fluocinolone acetonide	Cream	0.2

(continued)

§ **14.2** *(continuation)*

	Drug*	Available forms	Concentration (%)
	Fluocinonide	Cream, ointment, solution, gel	0.05
	Halcinonide	Cream, ointment, solution	0.1
	Triamcinolone acetonide	Cream, ointment	0.5
III.	Betamethasone benzoate	Cream, ointment, gel, lotion	0.025
	Betamethasone valerate	Cream, ointment, lotion	0.1
	Desoximetasone	Cream, gel	0.05
	Flurandrenolide	Cream, ointment, lotion	0.05
	Halcinonide	Cream	0.025
	Triamcinolone acetonide	Cream, ointment, lotion	0.1
IV.	Betamethasone valerate	Cream	0.01
	Clocortolone pivalate	Cream	0.1
	Fluocinolone acetonide	Cream, ointment	0.025
	Flurandrenolide	Cream, ointment	0.025
	Hydrocortisone valerate	Cream, ointment	0.2
	Triamcinolone acetonide	Cream, ointment, lotion	0.025
V.	Alclometasone dipropionate	Cream, ointment	0.05
	Desonide	Cream, ointment	0.05
	Fluocinolone acetonide	Cream, solution	0.01
VI.	Dexamethasone	Aerosol, cream, gel	0.01–0.1
	Hydrocortisone	Aerosol, cream, gel, lotion, ointment	0.25–2.5
	Methylprednisolone acetate	Ointment	0.25–1.0

*Group I is the most potent, and potency decreases with each group, so that drugs in group VI are the least potent. There is no significant difference among agents in any given group.
Adapted from Cornell R.C. and Stoughton R.B. (1984): The use of topical steroids in psoriasis. *Dermatol. Clin.*, *2*, 397–409.

TOPICAL CORTICOSTEROID PREPARATIONS

14.3 The activity of topical corticosteroid preparations has been investigated by various methods. One of the most important bioassay methods is the vasoconstrictor test. The assay is based on an alleged relationship between the ability of a corticosteroid to induce vasoconstriction and its clinical effectiveness. Differences in concentration of a particular corticosteroid are not always reflected as significant differences in vasoconstrictor potency [45]. Other bioassay methods are: in vitro fibroblast inhibition, antimitotic effect on human epidermis, the effect on damaged skin, the reaction to inflammation induced by various sources (UV light, croton oil, kerosene, allergic contact dermatitis) and the reduction of the size of histamine-induced wheals. A review of bioassays used in the development of topical steroid preparations has been provided by Behrendt and Korting [15]. Although the results of these methods may serve as a useful guide to topical anti-inflammatory and anti-mitotic activity, clinical assessment remains necessary.

Penetration and effectiveness

14.4 Factors influencing the penetration and clinical effectiveness (and also the possible occurrence of side effects) include [27]:

1. *Anatomical site.* Corticosteroids penetrate the skin through hair follicles and by transepidermal routes: absorption is increased in regions with large or numerous hair follicles. The scalp absorbs 3.5 times, the forehead 6 times and the scrotum 36 times the quantity of hydrocortisone as compared with the ventral aspect of the forearm. Absorption is decreased in regions of the skin having thickened stratum corneum [13].
2. *Vehicle formulation.* Improper formulation may diminish or completely abolish the clinical activity of the corticosteroid. The addition of penetrants may facilitate absorption, e.g. salicylic acid or urea.
3. *Concentration of the corticosteroid.* A 10-fold increase in concentration induces a 4-fold increase in hydrocortisone absorption from the skin of the forearm [21].
4. *Occlusive (polyethylene) dressing.* This may enhance penetration approximately 10 to 100-fold, lessens the differences in potency between the corticosteroids and reduces the influence of the vehicle on the penetration [18]. In skin folds, occlusion from the anatomical situation also increases penetration.
5. *Age.* The thin skin of children and aged people enhances percutaneous absorption.
6. *Chemical structure of the steroid.*

14.5 The question whether the side effects of corticosteroids are related to the incorporation of halogens in the molecule is still in debate. Dermatitis perioralis (a frequently reported side effect of halogenated corticosteroids) has also been reported after the use of non-halogenated steroids [6]. Furthermore, it must be stressed that less potent steroids may produce many of the same side effects as do more potent ones. Even prolonged application of 1% hydrocortisone, generally considered innocuous, may cause local side effects in vulnerable skin areas, though generally less than found following use of the more potent corticosteroids [14]. The skin of the face seems to be particularly susceptible to the effects of corticosteroids. In general, the more potent the corticosteroids, the more liable they are to induce side effects. Possibly, nonfluorinated double-ester type corticosteroids such as prednicarbate, may have an improved benefit/risk ratio [50], although prednicarbate also causes steroid-induced rosacea [7]. Ammonium lactate [51] and all-*trans*-retinoic acid [9] may be useful in mitigating the atrophy induced by corticosteroids.

Side effects

14.6 The following side effects of locally applied corticosteroids have been reported [5, 16,28,33,47].

1. *Effects on the pilosebaceous unit*

- Perioral dermatitis [38]: This condition is characterized by a symmetrical eruption of erythematous papules, papulo-pustules and vesicles on the chin and the nasolabial folds, with a clear perilabial zone. When stopping the application of the topical corticosteroid a rebound phenomenon may frequently be noted. Some authors believe that the *halogenated* corticosteroids play an important part in the pathogenesis of perioral dermatitis. The dermatosis has, however, also been reported in patients treated with hydrocortisone and hydrocortisone butyrate [6,14]. In children, perioral dermatitis may also be associated with the topical use of corticosteroids [52]. Perioral dermatitis is not always associated with the topical application of corticosteroids. Three cases have been observed after ingestion of the spices marjoram, bay leaf and cinnamon. The eruption cleared on a diet without these spices [12]. Some authors [44] prefer to restrict the term 'perioral dermatitis' to those patients presenting with the well-known perioral rash who have *not* used topical corticosteroids. If dermal steroids have been used, Cohen [44] prefers the term 'rosacea-like dermatitis'.
- Rosacea-like dermatitis: This term has been used as a synonym for perioral dermatitis, but Cohen [44] distinguishes it from (not steroid-induced) perioral dermatitis by the presence of teleangiectasia and a reddish hue. Steroid-induced papulopustular lesions, morphologically similar to perioral dermatitis but located on other parts of the face, may also be termed rosacea-like dermatitis [7]. A 'lupoid' form has been described in children [22].
- Steroid acne: This side effect of topical corticosteroids is not necessarily limited to the area of application. Steroid acne may also be induced by systemic administration of corticosteroids. The eruption is characterized by crops of comedones; its onset is usually rather sudden [29].
- Exacerbation of pre-existing rosacea; also, prerosacea may become manifest under corticosteroid treatment.
- Hypertrichosis of the face.
- Perianal comedones [42].

2. *Atrophy of underlying tissues*

There is clinical and experimental evidence that the initial atrophy caused by topical steroids is reversible [41], but long-term application may lead to more permanent changes. Even discontinuous application may lead to atrophic changes [25]. Skin atrophy is mostly due to a decrease in collagen synthesis [24]. Clinical manifestations of steroid-induced atrophy include:

- 'Cigarette paper wrinkling' of the skin
- Teleangiectasias
- Petechiae, ecchymoses
- Striae rubrae distensae, mainly occurring in the inguinal and axillary region (occlusion effect)
- Susceptibility of the skin to minor trauma
- Fragile skin in surgery

– Delayed wound healing
– Exacerbation of existing ulceration
– Fingertip atrophy ('disappearing digit') [30]
– Loss of fingerprints (epidermal ridges) [35]

3. *Effects on skin colour* [1]
– Hypopigmentation
– Hyperpigmentation

4. Effects on the immunological system
– Masking of the pre-existing disease
– Aggravation of pre-existing disease
– Inhibition of immunological mechanisms

Clinical examples of the effects on the immunological system are:
– Aggravation of pre-existing folliculitis
– Development of extensive, but unrecognized dermatophytic infections, so-called tinea incognito [17]
– Perpetuation of masked infections with candida albicans
– Conversion of scabies into the 'Norwegian' type [26]
– Extensive mollusca contagiosa eruption
– 'Galloping' impetigo
– Worsening of demodex folliculorum infection (?) [31]
– Development of generalized pustular psoriasis [32]
– Spreading of malignant skin lesions
– Suppression of pruritus

5. *Ocular and nasal effects*
– Ocular hypertension
– Open angle glaucoma [13,46]
– Uveitis
– Posterior subcapsular cataracts, either from application around the eye or from systemic absorption [39]
– Nasal septal perforation (steroid aerosol)
– Amaurosis (only tabulated, Ref. [5])

6. *Allergic effects* (see also Chapter 5):
– Allergic contact dermatitis (*cave:* allergic reactions to vehicle constituents, preservatives, etc.) Formerly considered to be rare, corticosteroids now are a frequent cause of (worsening of) allergic contact dermatitis [47]
– Generalized urticaria [49]

7. *Miscellaneous side effects*
– Tachyphylaxis [8]: This is acute tolerance to the vasoconstriction effect of topically applied corticosteroids.
– Milia [34]: degeneration of collagen probably plays a role in the pathogenesis.
– Granuloma gluteale infantum [2]: this condition is characterized by multiple red or reddish-brown nodules in the napkin area in young infants. Local steroid treatment as well as candidiasis are held responsible.
– Pseudo-cicatrices stellaires spontanées: This condition is characterized by scarring

purpura and skin atrophy on the back of the forearms of elderly people after long-term steroid application [4].
- Elastoidosis cutanée nolulaire à cystes et à comédons Favré–Racouchot: This dermatosis is localized mainly in the periorbital and neck region and is presumably caused by solar or senile degeneration of the skin: in addition, it has been reported after topical application of corticosteroids [33].
- Erythrosis interfollicularis colli. This entity is localized on the sides of the neck and upper breast and is usually caused by actinic degeneration. Topical application of corticosteroids may worsen these changes [33].
- Cutis linearis punctata colli or 'stippled skin': Prominent sebaceous glands on atrophic skin are the cause of this condition. It has also been reported as a side effect of systemic steroid therapy [11].
- Photosensitivity: Long-term topical corticosteroid treatment leads to an atrophy of the epidermis which in turn increases its sensitivity to light [33].
- Erythema craquelé: This effect occurred after *cessation* of long-term continuous steroid application to normal skin [43].
- Angina bullosa haemorrhagica [48].
- Transepidermal elimination of altered collagen [40].

TOPICAL CORTICOSTEROID–ANTIBIOTIC PREPARATIONS

14.7 The use of topical corticosteroid-antibiotic preparations in the treatment of dermatoses is still in debate. Critics state that the use of such combinations is not without hazards. The risks are [19]:
- Shifts in the existing ecological situation, with the possible establishment of pathogenic organisms
- Proliferation of resistant organisms
- Development of resistance of such organisms to antibiotics related to the one used
- Sensitization to the antibiotic in the topical preparation
- Masking of the sensitization to the antibiotic or other ingredients of the preparation
- Development of cross-sensitization to related antibiotics

In fact, most of these events may also develop after use of a topical antibiotic preparation alone.

14.8 Topical corticosteroid–antibiotic preparations may be used in the treatment of:
- Primary pyodermic skin diseases (e.g. impetigo, folliculitis).
- Chronic skin diseases in which a shift in the ecological situation has resulted in the invasion of pathogens.

In primary pyodermic skin diseases the addition of a corticosteroid to an antibiotic preparation adds nothing to the efficacy of the therapy. In cases of chronic skin diseases secondarily infected by pathogens, the use of combined preparations has been advocated [23]. Other authors are not convinced that the benefit of this addition outweighs the possible risks.

14.9 The discussion is complicated by the fact that the diagnosis of secondary infection of a skin disease is not always easily made. This leads to the question whether the isolation of a pathogen may be considered sufficient evidence for the presence of 'infection'. The lesions of eczema, particularly in atopic subjects, are very readily colonized by staphylococci, and even the normal skin of patients with eczema carries a larger bacterial population than that of controls. It has been assumed that the moist conditions in the lesions favour bacterial multiplication and that treatment should be 'directed at the skin lesions rather than at eradication of micro-organisms'. Eczema does indeed favour colonization and multiplication, but the critical question is whether such colonization increases the severity or duration of the lesions so that they can logically be regarded as 'infected' [10]. The traditional clinical criteria for judging infection are considered unreliable for this purpose. The diagnosis is only possible with certainty by performing a quantitative bacteriological analysis [20]. It is, however, seldom possible to obtain quantitative bacteriological reports, but semi-quantitative reports are often provided.

14.10 The following directions for the management of secondarily infected dermatoses have been given [10,20,36]:

1. Clinical evidence of secondary infection of eczema such as impetiginous crusting or pustulation, or a report that *Staphylococcus aureus* is present in abundance, may justify the use of a steroid–antibiotic combination. The application should be of short duration, e.g. 7–10 days.
2. The choice of the antibiotic depends on the nature and the sensitivity of the micro-organism.
3. Intermittent resumption of the combination therapy may be justified, e.g. in atopic subjects.
4. Prolonged continuous application must always be avoided.
5. It must be kept in mind that the risk of contact sensitization is especially present in the treatment of eczema or ulcus of the lower legs.
6. The corticosteroid in the preparation may mask the development of contact sensitization.

14.11 REFERENCES

1. Allen, B.R. and Hunter, J.A.A. (1975): Abnormal facial pigmentation associated with the prolonged use of topical corticosteroids. *Scot. Med. J., 20,* 277.
2. Bruckner-Tuderman, L. (1986): Granuloma gluteale Infantum. *Hautarzt, 37,* 347–349.
3. Bevis Cubey, R. (1976): Glaucoma following the application of corticosteroid to the skin of the eye lids. *Br. J. Dermatol., 95,* 207.
4. Braun-Falco, O. and Balda, B.R. (1970): Sogenannte pseudo-cicatrices stellaires spontanées. *Hautarzt, 21,* 509.
5. Takeda, K., Arase, S. and Takahashi, S. (1988): Side effects of topical corticosteroids and their prevention. *Drugs, 36,* (suppl. 5): 15–23.
6. Cotterill, J.A. (1979): Perioral dermatitis. *Br. J. Dermatol., 101,* 259.
7. Lubach, D. and Platschek, H. (1990): Steroidbedingte Gesichtshautschädigungen nach Anwendung von Prednicarbat. *Hautarzt, 41,* 43–45.
8. Du Vivier, A. and Stoughton, R.B. (1975): Tachyphylaxis to the action of topically applied corticosteroids. *Arch. Dermatol., 111,* 58.
9. Lesnik, R.H., Mezick, J.A., Capetola, R. and Kligman, L.H. (1989): Topical all-*trans*-retinoic acid prevents corticosteroid-induced skin atrophy without abrogating the anti-inflammatory effect. *J. Am. Acad. Dermatol., 21,* 186–190.
10. Editorial (1977): Steroid–antibiotic combinations. *Br. Med. J., 1,* 1303.
11. Even-Paz, Z. and Sagher, F. (1963): Cutis punctata linearis colli: stippled skin. *Dermatologica (Basel), 126,* 1.

12. Farkas, J. (1981): Perioral dermatitis from marjoram, bay leaf and cinnamon. *Contact Dermatitis, 7,* 121.
13. Feldmann, R.J. Maibach, H.I. (1967): Regional variation in percutaneous penetration of 14C cortisol in man. *J. Invest. Derm., 48,* 181.
14. Guin, J.D. (1981): Complications of topical hydrocortisone. *J. Am. Acad. Dermatol., 4,* 417.
15. Behrendt, H. and Korting, H.C. (1990): Klinische Prüfung von erwünschten und unerwünschten Wirkungen topisch applizierbarer Glukokortikosteroide am Menschen. *Hautarzt, 41,* 2–8.
16. Hill, C.J.H. and Rostenberg, A. (1978): Adverse effects from topical steroids. *Cutis, 21,* 624.
17. Ive, F.A. and Marks, R. (1968): Tinea incognito. *Br. med. J., 3,* 149.
18. Kaidbey, K.H. and Kligman, A.M. (1976): Assay of topical corticosteroids. *Arch. Dermatol., 112,* 808.
19. Leyden, J.J. and Marples, R.R. (1973): Ecologic principles and antibiotic therapy in chronic dermatoses. *Arch. Dermatol., 107,* 208.
20. Leyden, J.J. and Kligman, A.M. (1977): The case for steroid–antibiotic combinations. *Br. J. Dermatol., 96,* 179.
21. Maibach, H.I. and Stoughton, R.B. (1973): Topical corticosteroids In: *Steroid Therapy* pp. 174–190. Editor: D.L. Azarnoff, W.B. Saunders, Philadelphia.
22. Marghescu, S. (1988): Lupoide Form der Rosazea-artigen Dermatitis. *Hautarzt, 39,* 382–383.
23. Marples, R.R., Peborn, A. and Kligman, A.M. (1973): Topical steroid–antibiotic combinations. *Arch. Dermatol., 108,* 237.
24. Oikarinen, A. and Autio, P. (1991): New aspects of the mechanism of corticosteroid-induced dermal atrophy. *Clin. Exp. Dermatol., 16,* 416–419.
25. Lubach, D., Bensmann, A. and Bornemann, U. (1989): Steroid-induced dermal atrophy investigations on discontinuous application. *Dermatologica, 179,* 67–72.
26. Millard, L.G. (1977): Norwegian scabies developing during treatment with fluorinated steroid therapy. *Acta Derm.-Venereol., (Stockh.), 57,* 86.
27. Miller, J.A. and Munro, D.D. (1980): Topical steroids, clinical pharmacology and therapeutic use. *Drugs, 19,* 119.
28. Prawer S.E. and Katz, H.I. (1990): Guideline for using superpotent topical steroids. *AFP., 41,* 1531–1538.
29. Hurwitz, R.M. (1989): Steroid acne. *J. Am. Acad. Dermatol., 21,* 1179–1181.
30. Requena, L., Zamora, E. and Martin, L. (1990): Acroatrophy secondary to long-standing applications of topical steroids. *Arch. Dermatol., 126,* 1013–1014.
31. Sakuntabhai, A. and Timpatanpong, P. (1991): Topical steroid induced chronic demodicosis. *J. Med. Assoc. Thailand, 74,* 116–119.
32. Telfer, N.R. and Dawber, R. (1987): Generalized pustular psoriasis associated with withdrawal of topical clobetasol-17-propionate. *J. Am. Acad. Dermatol., 17,* 144–145.
33. Schöpf, E. (1975): Side effects from topical corticosteroid therapy. *Ann. Clin. Res., 7,* 353.
34. Iacobelli, D., Hashimoto, K., Kato, I., Ito, M. and Suzuki, Y. (1989): Clobetasol-induced milia. *J. Am. Acad. Dermatol., 21,* 215–217.
35. Gean, C.J., Hiatt, G.F.S. and Maibach, H.I. (1983): Complete eradication of fingerprints associated with topical corticosteroids. *Semin. Dermatol., 2,* 257–261.
36. Wachs, G.N. and Maibach, H.I. (1976): Co-operative double-blind trial of an antibiotic/corticoid combination in impetiginized atopic dermatitis. *Br. J. Dermatol., 95,* 323.
37. Weber, S. (1976): Perioral dermatitis, an important side-effect of corticosteroids. *Dermatologica (Basel), 152, suppl. 1,* 161.
38. Wilkinson, D.S., Kirton, V. and Wilkinson, J.D. (1979): Perioral dermatitis: a 12-year review. *Br. J. Dermatol., 101,* 245.
39. Costaglioga, C., Cati-Giovanelli, B., Piccirillo, A. and Delfino, M. (1989): Cataracts associated with long-term topical steroids. *Br. J. Dermatol., 120,* 472–473.
40. Katz, R. and Hood, A.F. (1985): Transepidermal elimination following the use of a topical adrenal steroid. *Arch. Dermatol., 121,* 412–413.
41. Lubach, D., Grüter, H., Behl, M. and Nagel, C. (1989): Investigations on the development and regression of corticosteroid-induced thinning of the skin in various parts of the human body during and after topical application of amcinonide. *Dermatologica, 178,* 93–97.
42. Oliet, E.J. and Estes, S.A. (1982): Perianal comedones associated with chronic topical fluorinated steroid use. (Letter to the Editor). *J. Am. Acad. Dermatol., 7,* 405.
43. Björnberg, A. (1982): Erythema craquelé provoked by corticosteroids on normal skin. *Acta Derm.-Venereol. (Stockh.), 62,* 147.
44. Cohen, H.J. (1981): Perioral dermatitis (Letter to the editor). *J. Am. Acad. Dermatol., 4,* 739.

45. Gibson, J.R., Kirsch, J., Dartey, C.R. and Burke, C.A. (1983): An attempt to evaluate the relative clinical potencies of various diluted and undiluted proprietary corticosteroid preparations. *Br. J. Dermatol.*, 109, (Suppl. 25), 114.
46. Eisenlohr, J.E. (1983): Glaucoma following the prolonged use of topical steroid medication to the eyelids. *J. Am. Acad. Dermatol., 8,* 878.
47. Lauerma, A.I. (1992): Contact hypersensitivity to glucocorticosteroids. *Am. J. Contact Dermatitis, 3,* 112–132.
48. Higgins, E.M. and Du Vivier, A.W.P. (1991): Angina bullosa haemorrhagica — a possible relation to steroid inhalers. *Clin. Exp. Dermatol.*, 16, 244–246.
49. Breneman, D.L., Davis, M., Berger, V. and Chaney, R. (1992): A double-blind trial comparing the efficacy and safety of augmented betamethasone dipropionate lotion with fluocinonide solution in the treatment of severe scalp psoriasis. *J. Derm. Treatm., 3,* 19–21.
50. Korting, H.C., Kerscher, M.J. and Schäfer-Korting, M. (1992): Topical glucocorticoids with improved benefit/risk ratio: do they exist? *J. Am. Acad. Dermatol., 27,* 87–92.
51. Lavker, R.M., Kaidbey, K. and Leyden, J.J. (1992): Effects of topical ammonium lactate on cutaneous atrophy from a potent topical corticosteroid. *J. Am. Acad. Dermatol., 26,* 535–544.
52. Manders, S.M. and Lucky, A.W. (1992): Perioral dermatitis in childhood. *J. Am. Acad. Dermatol., 27,* 688–692.

15. Percutaneous absorption of topically applied drugs

15.1 Several drugs for topical use on the skin and mucous membranes are capable of producing systemic side effects. Whether such events happen or not and, if so, to what extent, usually depends on the degree of absorption of the chemical through the skin or mucous membranes. In this chapter the factors influencing the absorption of topically applied drugs will be discussed [2–4].

Although the surface of the skin is only slightly permeable, many substances are capable of penetrating the skin to some degree. Absorption is greatly increased if the epidermis is diseased or damaged. The stratum corneum layer of the epidermis acts as the skin's main barrier; a few substances, however, may encounter a second barrier in the dermal–epidermal basement membrane. Although absorption mainly depends on the transepidermal route, follicular orifices and sweat gland ducts may provide alternate or additional pathways for absorption.

FACTORS INFLUENCING ABSORPTION

15.2 Several factors influence the degree of absorption of a particular substance:

1. **Physicochemical properties of the substance**
   Of importance are:
   - Molecular size — usually, absorption decreases with increasing molecular size.
   - Water- and lipid-solubility of the drug.
   - Solubility of the penetrant within the vehicle; greater solubility in the stratum corneum than in the vehicle promotes penetration.

2. **Use of occlusive dressings**
   An occlusive covering over the skin enhances the penetration of topical drugs by a factor of 10 or more, caused by:
   - increased water retention in the stratum corneum layer;
   - increased blood flow;
   - increased temperature;
   - increased surface area after prolonged occlusion.

3. **The vehicle in which the substance is incorporated**
   Of importance are:
   - The degree of affinity of the vehicle for the drug — increased affinity reduces percutaneous absorption.

- The physical properties of vehicles, especially the degree of occlusion they produce — greases, oils and collodion are very occlusive vehicles (see under 'use of occlusive dressings').
- Structural or chemical damage in the barrier layer, caused by the vehicle used.

In this respect, percutaneous absorption is increased by using vehicles such as dimethyl sulfoxide, dimethyl acetamide and dimethyl formamide. Certain solvents such as acetone, ethanol, methanol and ether may also cause damage.

4. **Drug concentration**
   In general, high concentrations enhance penetration

5. **Site of application**
   Regional differences in permeability of skin largely depend on the thickness of the intact stratum corneum. According to the findings of a study by Feldman and Maibach [1], the highest total absorption of hydrocortisone is that from the scrotum, followed (in decreasing order) by absorption from the forehead, scalp, back, forearms, palms and plantar surfaces.

6. **Age**
   The impression now exists that the skin of children, whether normal or inflamed, is more permeable than that of adults.

7. **Temperature**
   Increasing temperature of the skin usually enhances penetration (see under 'use of occlusive dressings'.)

8. **Integrity of the barrier**
   Increase of percutaneous absorption may result from the loss of barrier integrity caused by:
   - removal of the stratum corneum layer (e.g. 'stripping');
   - damage due to alkalis, acids, etc.;
   - irritation or endogenous inflammation of the skin, e.g. in psoriaris, atopic dermatitis, seborrhoeic dermatitis and exfoliative dermatitis.

15.3 REFERENCES

1. Feldman, R.J. and Maibach, H.I. (1967): Regional variation in percutaneous penetration of 14C-cortisol in man. J. Invest. Derm., 48, 181.
2. Malkinson, F.D. and Gehlman, L. (1977): Factors affecting percutaneous absorption. In: Cutaneous Toxicity, pp. 63–81. Editors: V.A. Drill and P. Lazar. Academic Press Inc., New York.
3. Rasmussen, J.E. (1979): Percutaneous absorption in children. In: Year Book of Dermatology. Editor: R.L. Dobson. Year Book Medical Publishers, Chicago.
4. Freeman, S. and Maibach, H.I. (1992): Systemic toxicity in man secondary to percutaneous absorption. In: The Environmental Threat to the Skin, pp. 249–263. Editors: R. Marks and G. Plewig. Martin Dunitz, London.

16. Systemic side effects caused by topically applied drugs and cosmetics

Some systemic side effects are the result of the *toxic action* of the chemicals applied, whereas others require an acquired *hypersensitivity state* of the organism, as seen e.g. in contact urticaria and anaphylaxis caused by bacitracin and the insect repellent diethyltoluamide.

ANAPHYLACTIC REACTIONS TO TOPICALLY APPLIED DRUGS AND COSMETICS

16.1 Several topical drugs and cosmetic ingredients have caused anaphylactic shock reactions, usually as part of the 'contact urticaria syndrome' (see § 7.1). Such reactions have been reported from contact with:

- aminophenazone
- ammonium persulfate
- ampicillin
- bacitracin
- benzocaine
- caraway seed oil
- chloramphenicol
- chlorhexidine digluconate
- mechlorethamide hydrochloride
- Millan's solution (gentian violet and methyl green)
- neomycin
- propipocaine
- rifamycine

For further information on this subject, the reader is referred to Chapter 7 on contact urticaria.

TOXIC ACTION OF TOPICALLY APPLIED DRUGS AND COSMETICS

Systemic side effects have been reported on the topical application of a number of chemicals, which will be discussed below.

Arsenic

16.2 Arsenical keratoses and malignancies are well-recognized long-term adverse reactions to oral administration of arsenic, previously employed widely in the treatment of psoriasis. However, Roemeling et al. [127] have reported on the development of consecutive multifocal malignancies of the large bowel, bladder, rectum and skin of a psoriatic patient who had been treated *externally* with Fowler's solution more than 20 years before. According to the authors, this may indicate that arsenic can be absorbed percutaneously in amounts sufficient to lead to later occurrence of internal cancers.

Benzocaine

16.3 Methaemoglobinaemia has been reported following the topical application of benzocaine on both the skin [254] and the mucous membranes [126,217,219,255, 256]. However, this is an uncommon occurrence [253]. The preponderance of reported cases occurred in infants and it has been suggested that this might be due to a deficiency of DPNH-dependent methaemoglobin reductase, resulting in a diminished capacity to physiologically protect against methaemoglobin-inducing foreign compounds. Cases of methaemoglobinaemia in older children [217] and adults [218] have also been reported.

Boric acid

16.4 Boric acid (H_3BO_3) is a colourless, odourless compound available as crystals, granules, and as a white powder. It is usually prepared by the action of sulphuric acid on borax (sodium borate, $Na_2B_4O_7 \cdot 10H_2O$).

Boric acid was first employed as an antiseptic by Lister in 1875 and for many years it enjoyed great popularity in medical practice; although it had an unwarranted reputation as a germicide, it is, however, only mildly bacteriostatic, even in saturated aqueous solution.

In the past, boric acid was erroneously considered a relative non-toxic substance; nevertheless, it has often proved poisonous, both on ingestion and following topical use. Little boric acid penetrates the intact skin, but it is readily absorbed through inflamed or otherwise damaged skin or through mucous membranes.

Valdes-Dapena and Arey [158] collected 172 cases of boric acid intoxication from the literature, including 83 fatal cases (see below). In this series there were 37 deaths after external use of boric acid, including 23 children with napkin rashes.

Summary of 172 cases of boric acid intoxication

	Fatal (n = 83)	Non-fatal (n = 89)	Total (n = 172)
Patients:			
adults	28	50	78
children	55	39	94
Exposure:			
diaper area	23	7	30
accidental ingestion (in formula or as medicine or infusion)	35	36	71
other routes (deliberate)	25	46	71

The most common clinical side effects of boric acid, independent of the route of administration, are seen on the skin, in the gastrointestinal tract and the central nervous system [64,89,136,198,296].

The *skin rash* consists of an intense erythematous eruption, often covering the entire body, and followed in one or two days by extensive desquamation. The palms and soles are often particularly red. Some authors observed an initial erythema around the mouth, buttocks and perineum. Mucous membranes are often involved, especially in young infants, in whom the mouth, pharynx and conjunctivae are inflamed. The skin lesions may resemble Ritter's disease [178], Leiner's disease or scarlet-fever, and be confused with these affections. Cyanosis may be present in the most severe cases. Other skin signs of borate intoxication include psoriasiform lesions and bullae [198].

Gastrointestinal symptoms have been described after topical use of boric acid; the incidence via this route of intoxication is unknown. After ingestion, a typical clinical picture starts with persistent vomiting which terminally becomes bloody, and diarrhoea (mucous and bloody, with a bluish-green colour). Nausea, vomiting and epigastric pain have been reported.

Central nervous system manifestations, particularly in the younger patients, consist of signs of meningeal irritation, convulsions, delirium and coma; in the infant, a high-pitched cry, exaggerated startled reflex, opisthotonus and apprehensive facial expression have been noted.

Acute *tubular necrosis* with oliguria or anuria may also occur, followed by hyperthermia, a fall in blood pressure, tachycardia and shock.

Occupational *toxic alopecia* due to absorption of borax from a hand washing powder containing nearly 80% crystalline borax was reported by Tan [146]. Ingestion of boric acid has also caused alopecia [249].

Undoubtedly the use of borates should be abandoned because of their very limited therapeutic value and high toxicity. Few cases of borate intoxications seem to have been published recently, which may reflect the rapid disappearance of these chemicals from medical use, or greater awareness of the possible adverse effects to those still employing the drug.

Calcipotriol

16.5 Calcipotriol is a new vitamin D_3 analogue with a potent effect on cell differentiation and proliferation. When applied topically, it has been shown to be of benefit in psoriasis [456]. Irritation/irritant dermatitis is a frequent side effect and the ointment should not be used on the face. Systemic effects on calcium metabolism have been observed only in patients who far exceeded the maximum weekly dose of 100 gram [456,457]. Symptoms of hypercalcaemia include malaise, headaches, drowsiness, constipation, polydipsia, polyuria, muscle weakness, fatigue, irritability, nausea and vomiting. Chronic hypercalcaemia (not reported from topical calcipotriol) may result in urinary stones, soft tissue calcification in blood vessels, myocardium and cornea, nephrocalcinosis and renal failure [458].

Camphor

16.6 Camphor is a pleasant-smelling cyclic ketone of the hydroaromatic terpene group. When rubbed on the skin, camphor is a rubefacient but, if not vigorously applied, produces a feeling of coolness. It is an ingredient of a large number of over-the-counter remedies (with a camphor content of 1–20%), taken especially for symptomatic relief of 'chest congestion' and muscle aches, but its effectiveness is rather dubious.

Camphor is readily absorbed from all sites of administration, including topical application to the skin. The compound is classified as a Class IV chemical, i.e. a very toxic substance. Hundreds of cases of intoxications have been reported, usually after accidental ingestion in children [26,209]. The symptomatology of camphor poisoning is given below [26].

Symptomatology of camphor poisoning

1. nausea and vomiting
2. feeling of warmth, headache
3. confusion, vertigo, excitement, restlessness, delirium and hallucinations
4. increased muscular excitability, tremors and jerky movements
5. tremors, progression to epileptiform convulsions, followed by depression
6. coma, CNS depression and finally either:
7. death from respiratory failure or from status epilepticus, or;
8. slow convalescence

Skoglund et al. [137] documented systemic adverse reactions after *cutaneous* contact with camphor: a 15-month-old child had crawled through spirits-of-camphor, containing 10% camphor. Over the ensuing 48 hours the child became progressively ataxic and had some brief generalized major motor seizures. The seizures persisted for two days despite appropriate therapy. Over a 15-day period he slowly improved; recovery in motor and mental function was complete. The child has no further seizures until one year later, when a camphorated vaporizer preparation containing 4.81% camphor was administered by the mother. Concurrent with this inhalation, a brief major motor seizure occurred. Two other children of 4 and 6 weeks old have been described showing signs of camphor intoxication from topical camphor-containing preparations due to percutaneous absorption. Signs and symptoms included; paleness, cyanosis, shallow breathing, apnea and muscular dystony [209]. Gossweiler warns that repeated applications of camphor-containing ointments to young babies has led to poisonings with coma, convulsions and breathing difficulties. These preparations should therefore not be used in newborns and small infants [209].

Capsicain

16.7 Capsicain is the active ingredient in hot peppers. In topical formulations capsicain has been used for the symptomatic treatment of post-herpetic neuralgia and painful diabetic neuropathy with some success [455]. Burning and irritant dermatitis are frequent local side effects. Over 10% of patients treated complain of coughing and sneezing, which probably reflects "caking" of dried capsicain residue on the skin with subsequent aerolization and inhalation [455].

Carmustine (BCNU)

16.8 Topical carmustine (BCNU) has been used for the treatment of cutaneous T-cell lymphoma, lymphomatoid papulosis and parapsoriasis en plaques [288]. Percutaneous absorption of BCNU has been demonstrated in man [289]. Zackheim et al. [288] treated 143 patients with cutaneous T-cell lymphoma with topical BCNU. Mild to moderate reversible bone marrow depression occurred in 7 patients. In this study there were no apparent long-term effects on the haematopoietic system or internal organs.

Castellani's solution

16.9 Castellani's solution (or paint) is an old medicine, mainly used for the local treatment of fungal skin infections. It contains boric acid 5.0, fuchsin 5.0, resorcinol 100.00, water 705.0, phenol 40.0 (90%), acetone 50.0 and spirit 100.0.

Lundell and Nordman [95] reported a case in which two applications of Castellani's solution severely poisoned a 6-week old boy. The infant became cyanotic with 41% of methaemoglobin. According to the authors, this case history demonstrates that the application of Castellani's solution to napkin eruptions and other areas where it can be rapidly absorbed may cause serious complications.

Another case report states that hours after the application of Castellani's paint to the entire body surface, except the face, of a six-week old infant for severe seborrhoeic eczema, the child became drowsy, had shallow breathing and was passing blue urine. Phenol was detected in the urine of 4 out of 16 children treated with Castellani's paint [128].

The reader is also referred to the paragraphs on resorcinol (§ 16.57), boric acid (§ 16.4), and phenol (§ 16.51), in this chapter.

Chloramphenicol

16.10 Oral administration of chloramphenicol may lead to aplastic anaemia. This condition is quite rare, occurring about once in every 18,000 to 50,000 subjects thus treated [164]. Although it has been stated that parenteral administration of chloramphenicol does not induce aplastic anaemia [174], at least 4 such cases have been described [50].

A case of marrow aplasia with a fatal outcome after *topical* application of chloramphenicol in eye ointment has been described by Abrams et al. [2]. It is remarkable that very small amounts of chloramphenicol could induce such very serious adverse reactions. There have been 3 earlier reports of bone marrow aplasia after the use of chloramphenicol-containing eyedrops.

Clindamycin

16.11 Topical antibiotics are widely used for the treatment of acne vulgaris. Topical clindamycin, erythromycin, tetracycline and lincomycin hydrochloride are considered more or less efficacious and without significant systemic side effects [144]. However, it is estimated that an average of 4–5% clindamycin hydrochloride is absorbed systemically, but greater amounts may be absorbed in some individuals [204]. The degree of absorption largely depends on the vehicle, ranging from 0.13%

(acetone) to 13.92% (DMSO) in one study [221]. Several cases of topical clindamycin hydrochloride-associated diarrhoea have been reported [144,163,220]. Percutaneous absorption of clindamycin *phosphate* has been reported to be less than 1% [297,298]. However, when applied intravaginally, more than 10% of the applied dose may enter the circulation [299]. No significant changes in intestinal microflora, as reflected by changes of *Clostridium difficile* or *B. fragilis* have been observed after topical clindamycin phosphate treatment of acne [300].

Pseudomembranous colitis is a well-recognized side effect of systemic administration of clindamycin [147] as well as of other antibiotics such as ampicillin, erythromycin, tetracyclines and cephalosporins.

A case of pseudomembranous colitis after *topical* administration of clindamycin hydrochloride has been reported by Milstone et al. [103]. Abdominal cramping and diarrhoea developed in a 24-year-old woman with facial acne vulgaris five days after she had started local therapy with 1% clindamycin hydrochloride. A stool specimen contained a significant titer of a toxin produced by *C. difficile*. Findings from sigmoidoscopy and a colonic biopsy specimen were consistent with pseudomembranous colitis. The patient became asymptomatic after 10 days of supportive care and oral vancomycin hydrochloride therapy. The authors conclude that all patients receiving topical clindamycin should be warned to discontinue therapy and consult their physician if intestinal symptoms occur. A similar case of pseudomembranous colitis caused by clindamycin *phosphate* has been reported [297].

Coal tar

16.12 A case of methaemoglobinaemia in an infant following the application of an ointment containing 2.5% crude coal tar and 5% benzocaine in a water-soluble base to about half the body surface was reported by Goluboff and MacFadyen [65]. On the fifth day of treatment the infant suddenly became critically ill, cyanotic and anoxic; death appeared imminent. Methylene blue i.v., 1.5–2 ml of 1% solution brought about a dramatic cure. The clinical diagnosis of methaemoglobinaemia was confirmed by examination of a blood specimen taken shortly after the methylene blue had been given. Though the child had been treated with several other medicaments as well, the authors believe that the coal tar–benzocaine ointment was the most likely factor to have caused the methaemoglobinaemia. (*See also* § 16.3 on benzocaine)

Cocaine

16.13 Cocaine, the active alkaloid in coca leaf, is widely used as a local anaesthetic for otolaryngologic procedures and for local anaesthesia in children. A healthy 14-month old boy was given 30 mg topical cocaine through a bronchoscope during surgery to remove a foreign body [445]. On submission to the recovery room the patient was fully awake with dilated pupils, hyperactive, with euphoric excitement, marked hyperventilation and continuous movements of the extremities. The maximum safe dose of topical cocaine is said to be 3 mg/kg, but the patient had received less [445]. Electrocardiographic and enzymatic documented acute myocardial infarction developed in a healthy 28-year-old woman undergoing closed reduction of a nasal fracture with topical cocaine anaesthesia [446]. The topical anaesthetic TAC (tetracaine, adrenaline, cocaine) applied to the oral mucosa in a 6-month-old baby caused respiratory distress and seizures. A urinary drug screen was positive for the cocaine metabolite benzoylecgonine [447]. Direct application of TAC to the mucous membranes has even led to the death of two children [447,448].

Corticosteroids

16.14 It has been amply documented that topically applied glucocorticosteroids are absorbed through the skin and gain access to the systemic circulation [272]. Factors favouring the penetration of corticosteroids have been discussed in Chapter 14. Systemic absorption of topically applied corticosteroids in quantities sufficient to cause adrenocortical suppression is not uncommon [301,302,312]. However, iatrogenic Cushing's syndrome resulting from the use of topical steroids is rare. Table 16.14 summarizes the relevant data of some of the reported cases. For other case reports see references [166,274–277,310,315]. Systemic side effects from occupational contact with inhalation of steroids has been reported [313].

Table 16.14. Iatrogenic hypercorticism due to topical corticosteroids. Relevant data of 12 cases (Adapted from Pascher, [267])

Age	Diagnosis	Steroid	Occlusion	Therapy	Side effects	Ref.
5 years	chronic eczema	HC ointment 1%	0	16 months	pseudotumour cerebri, retarded growth	260
2 months	eczema (generalized)	HC ointment 1%	0	3 months	arrested growth	261
3 weeks	epidermolysis bullosa	HC lotion 0.25%	0	10 days	cushingoid features	262
2 months	eczema (widespread)	betamethasone valerate cream 0.01%	0	2 weeks	failure to thrive	
18 months	napkin dermatitis	fluocortolone and fluocortolone caproate 0.25%	semi-occlusion (diapers)	14 months	growth inhibition	264
11 weeks	seborrhoeic dermatitis (disseminated)	betamethasone valerate 0.05%	0	7 weeks	Cushing's syndrome	265
42 years	psoriasis (exfoliative)	betamethasone valerate cream 0.1% diluted 1:8 with bland cream	0	2 years	Cushing's syndrome	
54 years	mycosis fungoides	betamethasone valerate (vehicle?) 0.1%	0	2.5 years	osteoporosis muscle atrophy	268

(continued)

§ **16.14** *(continuation)*

Age	Diagnosis	Steroid	Occlusion	Therapy	Side effects	Ref.
11 years	epidermolytic hyperkeratosis	triamcinolone acetonide cream 0.05%	0	1 month	cushingoid facies	
8 years	erythroderma ichthysiforme congenita	betamethasone valerate ointment 0.1%	0	7.5 years	Cushing's syndrome osteoporosis growth retardation	
57 years	seborrhoeic eczema of the face	betamethasone valerate cream 0.1%	0	11 years	Cushing's syndrome glaucoma	273
36 years	psoriasis	desoximethasone cream 0.25%	0	1 year	Cushing's syndrome	271

Systemic side effects caused by topical corticosteroids occur more frequently in children than in adults [47], which can be accounted for by the relatively large surface area and possibly the increased absorption through the thin skin in children. Patients with liver disease are more prone to develop systemic side effects due to retardation of the degradation of systemically absorbed drugs [275,304,315]. The side effects may remain subclinical [59]. Metabolic indexes of glucocorticoid action may provide useful parameters for assessing systemic absorption of topical glucocorticosteroids [271,302]. The two main causes of systemic side effects are hypercorticism leading to an iatrogenic Cushing's syndrome and suppression of the hypothalamic–pituitary–adrenal axis [98]. Very potent and readily absorbed corticosteroids may induce these two conditions at the same time.

The iatrogenic Cushing's syndrome includes benign intracranial hypertension, glaucoma, subcapsular cataract, diabetes [311], pancreatitis, aseptic necrosis of the bones, panniculitis, obesity, facial rounding, psychiatric symptoms, edema, delayed wound healing and to a lesser degree hypertension, acne, disorders of sexual functions, hirsutism, virilism, striae and plethora. Cases of avascular necrosis of the bones [303–305] due to topical corticosteroid treatment have been reported. Application of steroids with mineralocorticoid activity such as 9-α-fluoroprednisolone may lead to hypertension [307] and pseudohyperaldosteronism: hypertension, hypokalaemia, depressed plasma renin activity and absence of aldosterone hypersecretion [269,308–309]. In some cases, rhabdomyolysis developed secondary to hypokalaemia [306].

16.15 Skin symptoms of long-term systemic absorption of corticosteroids are:
- symmetrical steroid striae
- steroid acne
- widespread skin atrophy
- purpura
- ecchymoses

In one exceptional case, intrauterine growth retardation was ascribed to topical use of triamcinolone acetonide [263].

16.16 It is not easy to provide data on 'safe' doses of topical corticosteroids. Hydrocortisone is generally accepted to be safe except for small infants with severe and extensive skin disease [320], although a mild effect on the pituitary–adrenal axis is not uncommon [270]. Indeed, in several countries including the USA, Canada, the UK and the Scandinavian countries, hydrocortisone (acetate) preparations 0.5–1% are available as non-prescription (over-the-counter) drugs [321]. As for clobetasol-17-propionate, currently considered to be the most potent corticosteroid available, it has been recommended to limit the dosage to 50 g of the 0.05% ointment weekly. Larger doses entail a risk of suppression of the hypothalamic–pituitary–adrenal axis [159]. However, suppression of plasma cortisol levels were detected in 20% of psoriasis patients treated with 50 g/week clobetasol propionate ointment [316]. Moreover, amounts as low as 15 g/week have been reported to induce adrenal suppression [312,317]. Depressed cortisol levels usually return to normal within 1–3 weeks of stopping treatment and may also return to normal in some patients while treatment is continued, presumably due to suppression of the skin disease and consequent restoration of skin barrier function and reduced percutaneous steroid absorption [319]. The suppressive effect of topical steroids on cortisol levels is of little clinical significance with normal usage [318]. *See also* Chapter 19 on side effects of systemic drugs (§ 19.1).

Diethyl toluamide

16.17 Diethyl toluamide (DEET) has been used as an insect repellent since 1957. It is especially active against mosquitoes, but also repels biting flies, gnats, chiggers, ticks and other insects. After application, diethyl toluamide remains effective against insects for several hours. Local side effects including contact urticaria (§ 7.5) and irritant reactions with burning, erythema and bullae, sometimes followed by ulceration and scarring have been observed after application of 50–75% DEET [235]. DEET is absorbed through the skin: approximately 50% of each topically applied dose of diethyl toluamide is absorbed in six hours [322] and 10–15% is excreted unchanged in the urine within one hour [322,323]. DEET is used by 50 100 million persons each year in the USA [324] and preparations containing less than 50% DEET are almost free of side effects when applied to the skin of adults [325]. In contrast, encephalopathy has followed the repeated and extensive application of (lower concentrations of) DEET in children: slurred speech, staggering gait, agitation, tremors, convulsions and death resulted [236,237,326–328]. Ingestion of DEET rapidly causes respiratory depression, severe hypotension and convulsions: the case fatality may be as great as 40% [329,330]. Acute manic psychosis following dermal application of DEET in an adult has been reported [331].

When used sensibly insect repellents are advantageous and safe, but the potential toxicity of DEET is high and the use of repellents containing more than 50% DEET should be avoided in infants and young children. Frequent total body application of DEET for days or weeks should be avoided [325].

Dimethyl sulfoxide

16.18 The toxicology of topical dimethyl sulfoxide (DMSO) has been investigated by Kligman [86]. In this study, 9 ml of 90% dimethyl sulfoxide were applied twice daily to the entire trunk of twenty healthy volunteers for three weeks. The following laboratory tests were done; complete bloodcount, urinalysis, blood sedimentation rate, SGOT, BUN and fasting blood sugar determinations. At the end of the study, all laboratory values had remained normal. Except for the appearance of cutaneous signs such as erythema, scaling, contact urticaria, stinging and burning sensations, the drug was tolerated well by all but two individuals, who developed systemic symptoms. In one, a toxic reaction developed on the 12th day which was characterised by a diffuse erythematous and scaly rash accompanied by severe abdominal cramps; the other had a similar rash and complained of nausea, chills and chest pains. However, these signs abated in spite of continued administration of the drug.

To investigate possible side effects of *chronic* exposure to dimethyl sulfoxide another twenty volunteers were painted with 9 ml of 90% dimethyl sulfoxide applied to the entire trunk, once daily for a period of 26 weeks. Neither clinical nor laboratory investigations showed adverse effects of the drug. However, most subjects did experience the well-known DMSO-induced disagreeable oyster-like breath odour, to which they eventually became insensitive.

In a trial of treating digital ulcers in patients with systemic sclerosis with 70% DMSO (thrice-daily soaking in the study solution for 15 minutes), over 25% of the patients were withdrawn from the study because of severe skin reactions including cracking, blistering, sloughing and burning [332]. Two cases of peripheral neuropathy ascribed to the combination of topical DMSO and oral sulindac have been reported [333, 334]. One fatality, possibly due to a hypersensitivity reaction to DMSO, has been observed [290].

Dinitrochlorobenzene (DNCB)

16.19 Dinitrochlorobenzene (DNCB), a potent contact allergen, has been used with some success for the treatment of recalcitrant alopecia areata; today, however, its use has been discouraged because suspicion has been aroused that DNCB may be mutagenic. Another drawback for its use is its ability to potentiate epicutaneous sensitization to non-related allergens [222]. DNCB is absorbed in substantial amounts through the skin, and about 50% of the applied dose is ultimately recoverable in the urine [223].

A possible systemic reaction to DNCB has been reported [201]: a 25-year-old man was treated with 0.1% DNCB in an absorbent ointment base for alopecia areata after prior sensitization. After two months of daily applications the patient experienced generalized urticaria, pruritus and dyspepsia; discontinuance of the drug led to cessation of all symptoms, which recurred after reintroduction of DNCB therapy.

Diphenhydramine hydrochloride

16.20 Caladryl® is a topical antipruritic preparation containing 1% diphenhydramine (an H_1 antihistamine), 2% alcohol and 2% menthol. Two children aged 4 and 9 developed systemic toxicity from diphenhydramine by treatment of varicella with Caladryl® [442,443]. They were both agitated, frightened, confused and had visual and auditory hallucinations. The pupils were dilated. In one child, the serum toxic screen revealed a serum diphenhydramine level of 1.4 µg/ml (most patients with documented diphenhydramine intoxication have serum levels >0.6 µg/ml). The symptoms and signs were similar to those of overdose of oral diphenhydramine [442]. Another case of poisoning, again in a child treated for varicella with Caladryl® was described more recently [444].

Diphenylpyraline hydrochloride

16.21 Diphenylpyraline hydrochloride, an antihistamine, has been used topically in Germany for the treatment of eczematous and other itching dermatoses. Symptomatic psychosis apparently due to percutaneous absorption has been observed in 12 patients, 9 of which were children. The amounts of the active drug applied ranged from 225–1350 mg. The first symptoms of intoxication were psychomotoric restlessness in all cases, usually within 24 hours. Other symptoms included disorientation and optic and acoustic hallucinations. Most patients displayed anxiety, which was sometimes converted into aggressiveness. After discontinuation of the topical medication all symptoms disappeared within 4 days [215].

Dithranol (cignolin, anthralin)

16.22 Although the topical use of dithranol, which has been used since 1916 for the treatment of psoriasis, may lead to local side effects such as irritant dermatitis, discoloration of the skin and the appendages and to contact allergic reactions [36], its use is generally considered to be devoid of systemic side effects.

Gay et al. [57] studied a group of 40 psoriatic patients, treated with dithranol paste or ointment 0.1–0.4%. Creatinine clearance, chemistry profile, complete blood cell count and urinalysis were performed on all patients before treatment and after 1 and 3 months of continuous dithranol therapy. No evidence of systemic toxicity was found. No changes in renal function were observed in two dithranol-treated patients with renal disease, which, according to the authors, suggests that even renal disease if not necessarily a contradiction to the use of topically administered dithranol in low concentrations [57].

Farber and Harris [45] reported no toxicity in 25 hospitalized patients treated with topical dithranol paste for an average of 11 days. Their toxicity studies included serum electrolytes, total protein and globulin, total bilirubin, alkalic phosphatase, ASAT, blood urea nitrogen, fasting blood glucose and urinalysis.

Although according to the *Merck Index* [99] application of *chrysarobin*, which is chemically closely related to dithranol, to large areas of skin may lead to percutaneous absorption and 'renal irritation', no cases of renal or hepatic damage due to dithranol have yet been reported. Only one possible case of systemic side effect of dithranol has been reported; a patient had a fixed drug eruption, which was attributed to percutaneous absorption of dithranol [20].

Ethyl alcohol

16.23 Twenty-eight children with alcohol intoxication from percutaneous absorption were described by Giménez et al. [60] from Buenos Aires, Argentina. Apparently, in that area it is (or was) a popular procedure to apply alcohol-soaked cloths to the abdomen of babies as a home-remedy for the treatment of disturbances of the gastrointestinal tract such as cramps, pain, vomiting and diarrhoea, or because of crying, excitability and irritability. The children were of both sexes and ranged in age from 33 months to 1 year (mean: 12 months, 27 days). Alcohol-soaked cloths had been applied on the babies' abdomen under rubber panties and the number of applications varied from one to three; it was estimated that each application contained approximately 40 cc ethanol. Medical consultation took place from 1 to 23 hours after application. Alcoholic breath and abdominal erythema were valuable clues to the diagnosis. Signs and symptoms and their relative frequency are listed below.

Symptoms of percutaneous alcohol intoxication

Symptom	No. of patients (n = 28)	%
CNS depression (+ to ++++)	28	100
abdominal erythema	25	89
alcoholic breath	24	86
miosis	24	86
hypoglycaemia	15	54
convulsions	5	18
respiratory depression	5	18
mydriasis	4	14
acidosis	3	11
death	2	7

These symptoms may be interpreted as a consequence of the alcohol absorption and secondary hypoglycaemia. Quantitative determination for alcohol in the blood was made upon admission in 11 cases, with results ranging from 0.6 to 1.49 g%. Of the 2 children who died one was autopsied: the findings were consistent with ethyl alcohol intoxication. As the local population became more aware of the consequences of this practice of topical application of large amounts of alcohol, there was a resultant decrease in the number of cases. More recently a case of acute ethanol intoxication in a preterm infant of 1800 g due to local application of alcohol-imbued compresses on the legs as a treatment for puncture haematomas was reported [291].

Topically applied ethanol in tar gel [294] and beer-containing shampoo [295] has caused antabuse effects in patients on disulfiram for alcoholism, through percutaneous absorption.

5-Fluorouracil

16.24 Topical 5-fluorouracil is used for the treatment of warts, actinic keratoses and sometimes psoriasis. A patient who treated psoriatic nails for 110 days with this cytostatic drug (total dose of 325 mg) was found to have elevated creatine phosphokinase, ASAT and lactic dehydrogenase, with the elevation of the latter principally due to the isoenzyme. The patient did not experience myalgia or muscular weakness, and no muscular tenderness was found on palpation. Application of 5FU was immediately discontinued and all enzymatic abnormalities returned to normal within 14 days. The authors suggest that percutaneous absorption of 5-fluorouracil has been responsible for this case of rhabdomyolysis [434].

Fumaric acid monoethyl ester

16.25 The effect of topically administered fumaric acid monoethyl ester (ethyl fumarate) on psoriasis was studied by Dubiel and Happle [40] in six patients. Two patients who had been treated with locally applied ointments, consisting of 3% or 5% ethyl fumarate in petrolatum, developed symptoms of renal intoxication.

Gentamicin

16.26 Ototoxicity is a well-known hazard of systemic gentamicin administration. However, topical application to large thermal injuries of the skin has similarly caused ototoxic effects, ranging from mild to severe loss of hearing, with an associated decrease of vestibular function [35]. In the two patients described, serum levels of gentamicin measured were 1.0–3.0 μg/ml and 3.3–4.3 μg/ml, respectively.

Drake [39] described a woman who developed tinnitus each time she treated her paronychia with gentamicin sulfate cream 0.1%. Use of gentamicin in ear drops may also be associated with ototoxic adverse reactions [104]. See also § 16.49 on neomycin.

The *local* adverse reactions to topical use of gentamicin and other aminoglycosides are discussed elsewhere in this book.

Henna dye and *p*-phenylenediamine

16.27 The use of a henna dye is traditional in Islamic communities. The dye is used on nails, skin and hair by married ladies and it is also traditionally used by the major participants in marriage ceremonies, when the bridegroom and best man also apply henna to their hands.

Henna consists of the dried leaves of *Lawsonia alba* (family Lythraceae), a shrub that is cultivated in North Africa, India and Sri Lanka. The colouring matter, lawsone, is hydroxynaphthoquinone and this is associated with fats, resin and henna-tanin in the leaf. Dying hair or skin with powdered henna is a somewhat lengthy procedure and to speed up this process, Sudanese ladies mix a 'black powder' with henna; this accelerates the fixing process of the dye to merely a matter of minutes. This 'black powder' is paraphenylenediamine. The combination of henna and 'black powder' is particularly toxic and over 20 cases of such toxicity, some fatal, have been noted in Khartoum alone in a 2-year period. Initial symptoms are those of angioneurotic edema with massive edema of the face, lips, glottis, pharynx, neck and bronchi. These occur within hours of the application of the dye-mix to the skin. The symptoms may then progress on the second day to anuria and acute renal failure with death occurring on the third day. Dialysis has helped some patients, but others have died from renal tubular necrosis [230]. Whether this toxicity is due to *p*-phenylenediamine *per se* (probably grossly impure) or whether its toxicity is potentiated in its combination with henna powder is unknown. Systemic administration of the 'black powder' leads to similar symptoms and several deaths due to ingestion with suicidal intent have been reported [231]. In another report [335] two cases of cutaneous vasculitis and renal disease were (very unconvincingly) ascribed to *p*-phenylenediamine in hair dyes.

Hexachlorophene

16.28 Hexachlorophene (2,2′-methylenebis (3,4,6-trichlorophenol) has been used extensively in hospital nurseries since 1961, mainly for reducing the incidence of staphylococcal infections among newborns. In addition, it has been an ingredient of many medical preparations, cosmetics and other consumer goods.

Hexachlorophene readily penetrates excoriated or otherwise damaged skin [94], but absorption of this antiseptic through intact skin has also been demonstrated [3,32,155]. If hexachlorophene is applied in high concentrations or at frequent intervals to the intact skin, excoriation will result.

16.29 In 1972, in France, 6.3% of hexachlorophene was accidentally added to batches of baby talcum powder [115,180]; 204 babies fell ill and 26 died owing to respiratory arrest. Symptoms of intoxication included a severe rash in the diaper area [337], gastro-enteritis, pronounced hyperexcitability and lethargy. In addition, several babies showed hyperaesthesia, hypertonicity, opisthotonus, pyramidal tract signs, clonic movement of the extremities and papilloedema. High blood levels of hexachlorophene were demonstrated. Distribution of symptoms and signs in 224 hexachlorophene poisoning episodes among 204 children was as follows [180]:

Systemic and skin features:	
– Erythema of buttocks	209 (93%)
– Other cutaneous signs	38 (17%)
– Fever	99 (44%)
– Vomiting	77 (34%)
– Refusal of food	75 (33%)
– Diarrhoea	65 (29%)
Neurological features:	
– Drowsiness	83 (37%)
– Irritability	75 (33%)
– Coma	55 (25%)
– Seizures	39 (17%)
– Babinski signs	24 (11%)
– Decerebration	22 (10%)
– Weakness or paralysis	17 (8%)
– Opisthotonus	9 (4%)

This report was followed by animal experiments with hexachlorophene, confirming a relationship between the drug and morphological and functional disturbances of the nervous system. Consequently, the FDA in 1972 banned all non prescription use of hexachlorophene, restricting it to prescription use only, as a surgical scrub and handwash product for health care personnel. Hexachlorophene was excluded from cosmetics except as a preservative in levels not exceeding 0.1%.

Neurotoxicity

Several studies (e.g. by Powell et al. [118], Shuman et al. [133]) have confirmed the assumption that hexachlorophene does indeed have a high neurotoxic potential. It must be added that symptoms of neurotoxicity have been observed only after dermal application to large burned [336] or otherwise damaged skin areas or after the use of high doses on intact skin. Hexachlorophene neurotoxicity leads to cerebral edema, exclusively affecting the white matter of the brain and spinal cord, producing a spongiform encephalopathy which transforms the matter into a network of cystic spaces lined by fragments of myelin. There is a degeneration of myelin; nerve cells are unaffected. This process has been shown to be reversible. The clinical symptoms include nausea, vomiting, spasms, coma and finally apnea and death.

Teratogenicity and carcinogenicity

There has been concern about possible teratogenicity of hexachlorophene after the report of Halling [70,71]: Swedish medical personnel apparently had a high number of malformed babies in association with hexachlorophene hand washing during the first trimester of pregnancy. Other authors have also raised suspicion [245,246]. A detailed study [43], however, could not confirm this assumption, whereas animal experiments on teratogenicity provide conflicting evidence. As for carcinogenicity, this possible adverse effect of hexachlorophene cannot be assessed on the basis of data currently available [7].

Contraindications

Because of the high absorption through damaged skin and the proven neurotoxicity, hexachlorophene is contraindicated for the treatment of burns or application on otherwise damaged skin; premature infants are also at risk. Although it has been stated that hexachlorophene should no longer be used for routine bathing of babies [155], this point remains controversial [180,181]. Gluck [247] indicates that there is no evidence that any full-term baby with normal skin, even with the total body washed in the usual manner, has ever shown any untoward effects. However, the prophylactic efficacy of a technique using 0.5% hexachlorophene powder instead of the usual 3% emulsion has been demonstrated [248], which may indicate that preparations containing a lower hexachlorophene concentration are preferable [182].

For reviews of benefit and risks of hexachlorophene, see also Plueckhahn et al. [116] and Hopkins [79].

4-Homosulfanilamide

16.30 4-Homosulfanilamide (sulfamylon acetate) is a topical sulfonamide which was formerly used for the treatment of large burns. Unfortunately, the drug frequently produces a rash, and is associated with severe pain on application. Sulfamylon as well as para-sulfamoylbenzoic acid, an important metabolite, are carboanhydrase inhibitors. Inhibition of renal carbonic acid anhydrase decreases reabsorption of bicarbonate. Thus, hyperchloraemic metabolic acidosis has been observed in patients with extensive burns undergoing topical treatment with 4-homosulfanilamide [111,212], caused by percutaneous absorption of the drug. Reversible pulmonary complications have been associated with the drug when applied to patients with large burns [176]. It has been suggested that the respiratory failure might be the result of a hypersensitivity reaction, the lung being the shock organ, or the result of high doses of carbonic anhydrase inhibitors formed from the mafenide acetate and its metabolic products.

Ohlgisser et al. [108] reported methaemoglobinaemia as a possible side effect of 4-homosulfanilamide in two children who were treated with topical 4-homosulfanilamide for extensive burns.

Nowadays, 4-homosulfanilamide has largely been replaced by sulfadiazine silver (see § 16.64).

Iodine

16.31 Alexander [4] reported on a case of fatal dermatitis following the use of a 2.5% solution of resublimated iodine in pure industrial alcohol before a surgical operation. The reaction was thought to be due to idiosyncrasy to iodine.

Skin disinfection with iodine has caused goitre and hypothyroidism in 5 of 30 newborns under intensive care [22]. See also § 16.53 on povidone–iodine.

Isopropyl Alcohol

16.32 The topical use of isopropyl alcohol for fever control in children was once an accepted paediatric practice. Since the late 1950s, this practice has been discouraged following reports of neurotoxic effects that include stupor, narcosis, coma and even death [449]. Unfortunately, sponging with rubbing alcohol remains a fairly common method for fever control in children in some communities and a recent case of coma reminds us of the dangers of the procedure [449]. Isopropyl alcohol is hardly absorbed percutaneously, inhalation being the most likely route of entry. However, in patients with multiple skin lesions, percutaneous absorption may occur [450].

Lead

16.33 *Surma* is a topical preparation used in Asian communities in the United Kingdom; it is applied to the eye, apparently for medicinal purposes, and has the appearance of mascara. However, application is not to the outside of the eyelid, but to the conjunctival surface. In addition, it is the custom to apply a small dot of the material on the forehead of a Muslim child to ward off the 'evil eye'.

A case of lead poisoning in a 4-year-old Asian child has been reported [8], which appeared to be attributable to the use of a Surma; this preparation was found to contain 86% lead as lead sulfide. In this case, Surma had been applied to larger areas of the skin, and for prolonged periods of time. Various Surmas were investigated by the authors and 36% of these had lead concentrations in excess of 50%. Chronic lead poisoning has been caused by unguentum diachylon on leg ulcer [451] and even by the use of a lead soap [441].

Lidocaine

16.34 Lidocaine has been used as a local anaesthetic agent since 1948. Lidocaine is also prescribed as a local anaesthetic preparation for application to the mucous membranes and the skin. Cutaneous absorption of lidocaine is negligible through normal skin after short-term application. However, when applied to erosive lesions over large body areas, significant absorption may occur [338]. When the drug is applied to mucous membranes, blood levels simulate those resulting from intravenous injection [224]. The major toxic effects of lidocaine involve the central nervous system. Toxic manifestations first appear at a serum lidocaine concentration of 5 mg/l and worsen progressively at higher levels [225,338]. Early symptoms (at serum lidocaine concentrations of 5–10 mg/l) are dizziness, drowsiness, tinnitus and perioral paraesthesia. More severe symptoms are disorientation, delirium, convulsions, coma (at concentrations of 10–20 mg/l) and cardiorespiratory arrest (>20 mg/l). Lidocaine intoxication has been reported with various routes of administration; severe and even lethal intoxications have been described after local application to mucous membranes or after ingestion [191,226,339,340,343].

Topical administration of lidocaine to the nasal mucosa occasionally causes severe methaemoglobinaemia in patients who have the heterozygous form of NADH-methaemoglobin reductase deficiency [341,342]. See also under Prilocaine (§ 16.54).

Lindane

16.35 Lindane is the γ-isomer of 1,2,3,4,5,6-hexachlorocyclohexane and is widely used in the treatment of scabies and pediculosis, usually in a lotion containing 1% γ-benzene hexachloride, which is applied to the entire body surface and left on for 24 hours (in cases of scabies). The percutaneous absorption of the drug has been studied by Feldmann and Maibach [48]: after applying lindane in acetone to intact human skin (forearm), at least 9.3% of the substance was found to be absorbed and excreted in the urine during the following five days. There was a marked individual variation relative to transcutaneous lindane absorption in the subjects studied, who were male volunteers.

Ginsburg et al. [61] studied the percutaneous absorption of lindane in children suffering from scabies: mean levels of γ-benzene hexachloride found at 2 and 48 hours after application were 0.015 and 0.006 μg/ml, respectively. These levels tended to be higher in younger and smaller infants and children. In another study [190] plasma lindane levels of 10.3±2.2 ng/ml were determined 3 days after a therapeutic application of 1% lindane cream. Topical treatment with lindane of lactating women may result in a 30-fold increase of lindane concentrations in mother's milk [348].

16.36 Lindane is a potentially toxic agent, and the hazards of excessive industrial exposure and accidental ingestion have been well-documented. Signs and symptoms of intoxication include [140]:

1. *Nervous system disorders:* convulsions, headache, vertigo, mental confusion, dysarthria and death
2. *Gastrointestinal disorders:* nausea, vomiting, diarrhoea, stomatitis, intestinal colic, depressed liver function

3. *Miscellaneous:* respiratory failure with cyanosis, blood dyscrasias and hemopoietic depression, altered menses, cardiac arrhythmias, myalgia, blindness.

Transient pancytopenia has also been ascribed to excessive topical application of lindane for scabies [347]

16.37 Intoxication from *excessive topical therapeutic applications* of lindane has been documented. Six such patients were reported [91]: adverse reactions included seizures (4), nervousness, irritability, anxiety and insomnia (1), and dizziness and amblyopia (1). Seizures after excessive topical application of lindane have been reported by Telch and Jarvis [197].

A 2-month-old male infant was found dead in his crib after excessive application of a 1% lindane lotion [175]. Lindane was identified in the brain at a concentration of 110 ppb. The brain level was three times higher than the levels found in the central nervous system. The authors admitted that the relationship of the pesticide exposure to the fatal outcome in this case was conjectural.

The issue of possible toxic adverse reactions *to a single therapeutic application* of lindane, notably central nervous system toxicity, has not been settled yet.

Several poorly documented cases of convulsions following topical treatment with the drug have been reported to the Division of Drug Experience of the United States Food and Drug Administration [46].

Lee and Groth [91] mentioned the case of a 4-year-old boy who started to vomit approximately 8.5 hours after total body application of lindane cream and slowly drifted into unconsciousness. He subsequently had a convulsion and stopped breathing; complete recovery ensued. A 7-year-old boy with tuberous sclerosis had two petit mal seizures within 12 hours after a single total body application of 1% lindane lotion [196]. Pramanik and Hansen [120] reported on a premature, malnourished infant with scabies who developed increased muscle tone, poor orientation to a visual animate stimulus and frequent side-to-side head movements two days after one application of 1% lindane lotion. The patient, who also had a ventriculoseptal defect and was treated for pneumonia and congestive heart failure (which drugs were used?), was diagnosed as having 'clinical seizure'; this latter effect was ascribed to treatment with lindane. Nausea, vomiting, epileptiform convulsions and muscular spasms have been observed after proper administration of lindane to a 3-year-old boy with nonbullous congenital ichthyosiform erythroderma [344]. A compromised epidermal barrier function is likely to have facilitated percutaneous absorption in this case. Only one report associated seizures *in adults* with lindane therapy [349]. Nineteen elderly residents of a chronic-care ward of a small general hospital were treated with a single application (30–60 ml) of 1% lindane lotion. Three of them had a single seizure of 5–10 minutes duration at 5.5 and 4 days after the lindane application. None of the nineteen patients had a past history of seizures [349]. With peak levels of lindane after 4–8 hours and a half-life time of 21 hours [350], the causal relationship between lindane and the observed seizures is not very likely.

Urinary bladder retention has been observed in a 47-year-old woman who had been treated with lindane. Anatomical and functional outlet obstruction as well as bladder denervation was excluded radiologically and urodynamically. Urinary retention was supposed to be a side effect of lindane [351].

16.38 Most authors seem to agree that the benefits to be derived from the continued use of lindane as a scabicide and pediculicide outweighs the risks involved [140,194, 195,239,345,346]. Alternatives for lindane include crotamiton, benzyl benzoate, permethrin and sulfur. Their safety has not been established [195]. Although a potential for adverse reactions from application of lindane preparations therapeutically does exist if the preparations are not used properly, the risk of toxicity appears minimal *when used properly and according to directions* [199]. Children with severe underlying cutaneous disease may be at greater risk for developing toxicity [195, 344], which is also true for premature, emaciated and malnourished children as well as those with a history of seizure disorders [195]. Continued use of lindane because of its beneficial effects, however, does not mean that steps should not be taken to minimize potential risks.

Solomon et al. [140], for example, in their review on lindane toxicity give the following observations and recommendations "which may have some merit":

1. Lindane should *not* be applied after a hot bath.
2. The regimen of application for 24 hours may be unnecessarily long; 8–12 hours may be sufficient exposure [195].
3. A concentration weaker than 1% may suffice, particularly for badly excoriated patients.
4. Lindane 1% should be used with extreme caution, if at all, in pregnant women, very small infants and people with massively excoriated skin. Rasmussen [195] does not agree, pointing out that there are no reported instances of fetal malformation or spontaneous abortions following the use of lindane.
5. Lindane treatment should not be repeated within eight days, and then only if active organisms can be demonstrated.

Malathion

16.39 Malathion is used in the treatment of lice, a single application of 0.5% in a solution being customary. Used in this way, it is generally safe, although the same compound has caused fatal poisoning when used as a pesticide in the environment. Ramu et al. [124] reported on 4 children with an intoxication following hair washing with a solution containing malathion (50% in xylene) for the purpose of louse control. One case is described in detail. The patient was in coma and did not respond to painful stimuli. Other symptoms included severe dyspnea, audible extensive moist rales over both lung fields, voluminous frothy saliva and mucous filling the nose, mouth and pharynx, pinpoint pupils not responding to light, excess lacrimation and fasciculation in the upper eyelids, flaccid limbs and absence of tendon reflexes. Hyperglycaemia and glucosuria were found in all cases. Their presence may, according to the author, lead to the erroneous diagnosis of diabetic hypersmolar coma if other symptoms of organophosphate poisoning are overlooked.

In view of the increasing use of malathion for the control of lice it must be kept in mind that malathion is a weak, but definite sensitizer [102].

Mercury and mercurial compounds

16.40 For several centuries the most popular remedy for syphilis consisted of mercury in the form of an ointment rubbed into the skin. The original preparation was called 'unguentum saracenicum' from its Arabian origin, and contained one-ninth part mercury. If it was used for too long or too frequently, the absorption of mercury through the skin led to extensive symptoms of intoxication. These included ulcerations of the jaws, loosening of the teeth, swelling of the tongue, lips and palate, ptyalism, 'salivation', fetid breath and symptoms of renal intoxication. It has been suggested that, through the centuries, mercury has killed more patients than any other medicament.

16.41 Mercury can be found in three basic states:

1. *Elemental mercury*, as liquid or vapour. This is used in dental fillings.
2. *Inorganic mercury* (mercurous and mercuric salts)
   - ammoniated mercury (mercury ammonium chloride)
   - mercuric chloride (mercury bichloride, mercury perchloride)
   - mercurous chloride (calomel)

   Ammoniated mercury may be employed in ointments, used as an antiseptic or ectoparasiticide, in contraceptive jellies, in haemorrhoidal remedies and in 'bleach creams' [25,169]. When incorporated in ointments this compound dissolves slowly, forming very toxic mercuric ions. Mercurous chloride (calomel) may still be part of laxatives in some countries. It has also been used as diuretic, an antiseptic and in the treatment of syphilis.
3. *Organic mercury* (in human medicine: aryl mercurials)
   - phenylmercuric acetate
   - phenylmercuric nitrate
   - merbromin
   - thimerosal (thiomersal, merthiolate)
   - nitromersol.

These compounds are used for different purposes:

- as preservatives, e.g. in eyedrops, ointments, vaccines, sera and other injection liquids
- as disinfectants
- in the treatment of infection of the skin, mouth, vagina etc.
- in contraceptive jellies
- in haemorrhoidal remedies

The toxicity of organic mercury compounds has been reviewed [380].

16.42 With a few exceptions, the use of mercury in medicine is considered to be outdated. However, attention should be paid to the possibility of mercurial poisoning even nowadays, as mercury may still be present in many drugs and in many countries even in over-the-counter remedies, often without mention on the label.

Although there are considerable differences between various mercurials regarding the rate of absorption through the skin, all mercurial preparations are a potential hazard and may cause intoxication. Metallic mercury is readily absorbed through intact skin: absorption of ammoniated mercury in psoriatic patients was demonstrated by Bork et al. [19].

16.43 Symptoms of chronic mercurial poisoning include [25,90,100]:

–*Nervous system disturbances:* emotional deviations, irritability, hypochondria, psychosis, impaired memory, insomnia, tremors, dysarthria, involuntary movements, vertigo, hypacusis, neuritis optica, mononeuropathy, polyneuropathy, paresthesias of the extremities, headache, mad hatters disease.

– *Gastrointestinal disturbances:* anorexia, nausea, vomiting, epigastric pain, diarrhoea, constipation, discoloration of the gums and the mucosa of the mouth, stomatitis, ulcerations of the mouth, foetor ex ore.

– *Cardiovascular symptoms:* hypertension, hypotension, arteritis of the legs.

– *Blood disorders:* hypochromic anaemia, erythrocytosis, lymphocytosis, neutropenia, aplastic anaemia.

– *Skin disorders:* tylotic eczema, dryness of the skin, skin ulcerations, erythroderma.

– *Renal damage:* nephrotic syndrome.

– *Disorders of the eye:* corneal opacities and ulcerations, conjunctivitis.

– *Endocrine abnormalities:* dysmenorrhoea, hyperthyroidism.

– *Miscellaneous:* acrodynia ('pink disease'; see below), loose teeth.

Acrodynia ('pink disease')

Topical mercurial-containing remedies such as teething powders, lotions, ointments and napkin rinses have caused acrodynia [34,41,166] in children between the ages of 3 months and 8 years. This distinctive syndrome usually begins with restlessness and irritability. Other early symptoms include fever, tachycardia and hypotonia. After 2 to 3 weeks one may observe swelling and reddening of the hands and the feet, which are cold to the touch owing to peripheral vasoconstriction. Other dermatological symptoms include skin rashes, usually macular or maculopapular, and the hands and feet may show desquamation. The child may complain of burning and itching; the skin is often excoriated. In addition, excessive sweating, diarrhoea and renal disturbances may be noticed. In severe cases, stomatitis with loosening of the teeth and dystrophic changes of the nails and the hair have occurred. The mortality rate is high: 10% of all affected children die of infections.

After prohibition of mercurial teething powders in 1965 acrodynia has become very rare in Great Britain. Nevertheless, a new case is occasionally reported, as other sources of mercury such as house paint may induce the same syndrome [78].

Case reports

Young [172] examined 70 psoriatic patients treated with ointment containing ammoniated mercury before, during and after treatment. Symptoms or signs of mercurial poisoning could be detected in 33 of them; these consisted of:

albuminuria	11	conjunctivitis	1
headache	8	epistaxis	1
gingivitis	5	keratitis	1
erythroderma	4	tremor	1
nausea	2	neuritis	1
dizziness	2	haematological changes	1
precordial pain	2	metallic taste in mouth	1
contact dermatitis	2	purpura	1

Mercury in dental fillings probably does not contribute much to toxicity (although it may be a health hazard to dentists [376,377]), but convincing cases have been reported of mercury amalgam-induced generalized allergic reactions [56, 151].

A case has been reported of a 24-year-old man who, whilst using an ammoniated mercury-containing ointment for his psoriasis, developed a nephrotic syndrome. The predominant lesion was focal membranous glomerulonephritis. As this was thought to be due to mercury, the application was stopped; thereafter, slow, but progressive recovery ensued [134, *see also* 154]. Nephrotic syndrome due to topical mercury was also reported by Lyons et al. [259]. Even the use of a mercury-containing skin lightening cream has caused renal damage [379].

Stanley-Brown and Frank [141] described a child with an omphalocele treated with merbromin. The patient produced pink urine, and diffuse sclerema and anuria developed. Respiratory arrest occurred on the 5th day and the infant died. Another child died from intoxication caused by thimerosal ear irrigations [383].

Apparently even nowadays cases of mercury intoxication from use of topical mercurial antiseptics still occur [139,375]. A premature child had 4 applications of 10% merbromin to an omphalocele; three days later bradycardia developed and the child died [205]. Serum mercury levels were reported as greater than 260 µg/dl (normal <10 µg/dl). For other recent case reports see Refs. [381,384,462].

16.44 In view of the risks of both systemic side effects and contact allergic reactions to mercurials, there hardly seems to be any justification for continuing the use of these drugs in dermatological therapy [378].

Minoxidil

16.45 Minoxidil (2,4-diamino-6 piperidinopyrimidine-3 oxide) is a potent antihypertensive drug. It is a peripheral vasodilator, especially enhancing the cutaneous blood flow. It does not reduce the blood pressure of normotensive individuals. Side effects of systemic minoxidil include fluid retention, reflex cardiac stimulation, ECG-changes, angina pectoris, tachycardia, nausea, fatigue, dyspnoea and gynaecomastia. Another prominent side effect is hypertrichosis, which occurs over the forehead, periorbital area, ears, face, extremities and lower back in at least 80% of the patients [357,358]. Stimulated by case reports on regrowth of hair in baldness during systemic minoxidil treatment [359], *topical* application of minoxidil was introduced for alopecia areata (and some years later) for male pattern baldness [362]) in 1981 [360]. Whereas minoxidil does induce some hair growth in androgenic alopecia, results in alopecia areata have generally been disappointing [370].

In the USA, Rogaine® (Upjohn), containing 2% minoxidi,l has been approved by the FDA for the treatment of alopecia androgenitica.

Topical treatment with minoxidil has a potential for systemic side effects: 1–4% of the applied dose may be absorbed percutaneously [361]. Systemic doses in the range of 2.4 to 5.4 mg/day can be anticipated if application is made to the entire scalp [361].

Hypotension

Although some authors have reported hypotension in normotensive individuals from topical minoxidil [363,369] most investigators have found no effect on blood pressure in normotensive individuals [364–368]. However, hypertensive patients may develop reduced blood pressure from topical minoxidil [370]. Rebound increase in the blood pressure of 2 patients with alopecia areata following discontinuation of minoxidil has been observed, but may have been coincidental [357].

Other cardiovascular effects

Most patients treated with minoxidil have been normotensive and they did not have any cardiovascular disease or severe systemic illness. No major cardiovascular effects have been observed in the therapeutic trials reported [368]. Ankle oedema [370] and palpitations and chest pain [371] have rarely been described. 'Minor' ECG changes have been observed [374]. In one study, possible cardiac effects of topical minoxidil were recorded using quantitative echocardiography [367]. In a double-blind, randomized study for two parallel groups (n = 20 for minoxidil, n = 15 for placebo) blood pressure did not change during 6 months of follow-up. Minoxidil increased heart rate by 3–5 beats per minute. Compared with placebo, topical minoxidil caused significant increases in left ventricular (LV) end-diastolic volume, in cardiac output (by 0.75 L/min) and in LV mass (by 5 g/m^2). It was concluded that, in healthy subjects, short-term use of topical minoxidil is likely not to be detrimental. However, safety needs to be established regarding ischaemic symptoms in patients with coronary artery disease as well as for the possible development of LV hypertrophy in healthy subjects during years of therapy [367].

Death

Several cases of (sudden) death of patients using topical minoxidil have been reported [372,373]. No causal relationship could be demonstrated, and considering the low levels of minoxidil from topical application, such a causal relationship seems to be highly unlikely.

Smoking intolerance

Smoking intolerance has been observed in two patients [463]. The relationship between treatment with minoxidil and smoking intolerance was emphasized by stopping treatment and the disappearance of the smoking intolerance, and then by rechallenge in both patients [463].

Monobenzone

16.46 Monobenzone (monobenzyl ether of hydroquinone) is used topically by patients with extensive vitiligo to depigment their remaining normally pigmented skin. A patient who had been applying the drug for one year had an anterior linear deposition of pigment in both corneas. Of 15 additional patients with vitiligo, 11 of whom were using monobenzone, acquired conjunctival melanosis in two patients and pingueculae in 3 may have been related to monobenzone use. Light and electron microscopy of one corneal epithelial scraping and 12 conjunctival biopsy specimens revealed pleomorphic, single-membrane-limited intracytoplasmic inclusions within the corneal epithelium and within the epithelium fibrocytes, histiocytes and vascular endothelium of the conjunctiva. The ultrastructural aspects of the inclusions suggested that they are residual bodies containing lipid and lipofuscin [214].

Monosulfiram

16.47 Monosulfiram (sulfiram, tetraethyl thiurammonosulfide) is used for the topical treatment of scabies. After repeated treatment, the ingestion of alcohol may rarely lead to an antabuse effect with generalized flushing, malaise and rhinorrhoea [432,453]. Conversely, an antabuse effect of topically applied alcohol in beer-containing shampoo was observed in an individual with implanted disulfiram (Antabuse®) [433].

2-Naphthol

16.48 Since its introduction about a century ago, 2-naphthol (β-naphthol) has been used for the treatment of various dermatoses, including psoriasis, scabies, rosacea and acne. Nowadays its use is restricted to acne; however, a considerable proportion of 2-naphthol from peeling paste is absorbed percutaneously, and Harkness and Beveridge [74] reported the isolation from the urine of about 10% of the 2-naphthol applied in such a peeling paste to the skin of a young man. This observation was confirmed by Hemels [76], who showed that on average 5% of a cutaneous dose of 2-naphthol is excreted, mostly in the first 24 hours after application. Also, a brownish-red discoloration of the urine may be noted after systemic or topical administration of this drug. The external application of 2-naphthol ointments has been responsible for systemic side effects, including vomiting and death [99,110].

Hemels [76] concludes that 2-naphthol-containing pastes should be applied only for short periods of time and to a limited area not exceeding 150 cm^2.

Neomycin

16.49 Not only is ototoxicity a well-known hazard of parenteral neomycin administration, but deafness has also been reported after almost any form of local treatment, including treatment of skin infections and burns, use of neomycin as an intestinal antiseptic or for the control of intestinal infections, application as an aerosol for inhalation, instillation into cavities, irrigation of large wounds and use of neomycin-containing eardrops.

Aerosols

In the late seventies, the Committee on Safety of Medicines in Britain warned about the use of aerosol preparations containing neomycin, after receiving reports of deafness following the use of these preparations in the treatment of extensive skin damage such as burns [6,55].

Wound treatment

Acute renal failure and total deafness as a result of intermittent 7-day lavage of a surgical cavity with neomycin in one patient were described by Masur et al. [97]. Peritoneal dialysis promoted complete recovery of the renal function, but the patient remained deaf. Quante [122] described a case of deafness after treatment of a 2 × 2 cm Pyocyaneus-infected wound with daily neomycin solutions. A total of 30 g was given over a period of 3 months, during which time the patient became deaf. A case of progressive auditory impairment leading to almost total deafness after topical irrigation of decubitus ulcers with neomycin had already been reported in 1969 by Kelly et al. [84]. Ototoxicity from treatment of ulcera cruris in 2 patients was reported from Germany [353]. For deafness and biochemical imbalance following burns treatment, see Bamford and Jones [10].

Ear drops

Antibiotic eardrops are widely used in the treatment of aural discharge, and have sometimes been used in cases with perforated tympanic membranes.

In response to a leading article in the *British Medical Journal* on neomycin ototoxicity following the topical use of this antibiotic, Murphy [106], in a letter, stated that he had seen many cases of mixed deafness in children with chronic suppurative otitis media, presumably due to eardrops containing chloramphenicol or neomycin. Use of eardrops containing neomycin and polymyxin for some days in patients with a perforated tympanic membrane caused ototoxicity in 2 patients in Belgium [63]. Kellerhals [83] reported on an inquiry among the members of an otolaryngological society; this revealed 15 cases of inner ear damage caused by this practice, the frequency of this complication being assessed as one case per 1000–3000 treatments. Eight patients had a total loss of hearing in the affected ear. Neomycin and framycetin were incriminated in 13 cases. The paper in question concludes that in cases with perforated tympanic membranes one should not use these drops (or those containing chloramphenicol, colistin or polymyxin) for periods longer than 10 days. The antibiotics concerned may diffuse into the perilymph of the inner ear and attain dangerous levels on continuous use. A German study reported 7 cases of ototoxicity in children from the use of neomycin (n = 4) and from neomycin and gentamicin (n = 3) ointment for burns [352,353].

Use of neomycin on intact skin

In a young girl with chronic dermatomyositis approximately 30% of the body surface was treated with an ointment containing 1% neomycin and 11% dimethyl sulfoxide during a period of 3 months. Vertigo, nystagmus and complete loss of hearing occurred [77]. DMSO has probably enhanced percutaneous absorption of neomycin in this case. Although in theory the ototoxic effects may have been due to dimethyl sulfoxide, it was regarded as being very likely that neomycin was the causative agent (see § 16.18 on dimethyl sulfoxide).

16.50 Application of topical neomycin (and probably other aminoglycosides) should be discouraged for the following reasons:

1. risk of inducing bacterial resistance with an associated risk of cross-resistance with other aminoglycosides, including life-saving drugs such as kanamycin and tobramycin;
2. risk of inducing hypersensitivity with an associated risk of cross-allergy with other aminoglycosides;
3. risk of systemic eczematous contact-type dermatitis (see § 17.2);
4. potential risk of causing or increasing drug-induced ototoxicity or nephrotoxicity.

Phenol (carbolic acid)

16.51 Phenol is a strong but also a toxic bactericide. It is not used as an antiseptic at the present time, but in dilutions of 0.5–2% it is sometimes prescribed as an antipruritic in the form of various topical medicines. Experimental studies in human volunteers have shown a rise of blood phenol to about 0.4 mg/100 ml after the application of 2% phenol in either calamine lotion or liquid paraffin [130]. Skin absorption of phenol from aqueous solutions was investigated by Baranowska [177]; the concentration of phenol, time of exposure and temperature all influenced the degree of absorption. It was shown that as much as 25% of phenol was absorbed from 2 ml of a solution of 2.5 g phenol/l water applied to the skin of the forearm and left on for 60 minutes. Phenol skin absorption in men from acetone solutions containing ^{14}C-labelled phenol has previously been documented [240].

Case reports

Phenol-induced ochronosis has been reported in the older literature [241]; the disorder occurred in patients who for many years (10–40) had treated leg ulcers with applications of wet dressings containing phenol in various concentrations. Many patients with phenol ochronosis were noted to have dark urine, much like patients with alkaptonuria. The pigmentation persists for life.

Johnstone [81] reported a fatal reaction in a 22-year-old man who accidentally spilled a bottle of carbolic acid, saturating the right leg, right side of the abdomen and the chest. Fellow employees immediately removed his shirt and threw water over the upper part of his body. The man then walked across the street to a physician's office without difficulty but collapsed and died within 15 minutes of his arrival. Autopsy revealed, in addition to local first and second degree burns, hyperaemia and edema of the lower lobes of both lungs, of both kidneys, the pancreas and the spleen. There was no change in the heart or liver.

Cronin and Brauer [30] described a case of fatal poisoning in a 10-year-old boy who was treated for kerosene burns with a preparation called 'Foille', composed of 2.36% phenol, together with traces of a number of other chemicals, in corn oil.

A fatal phenol reaction following the application to wounds was reported by Deichmann [37]. There were symptoms of abdominal pain, dizziness, haemoglobinuria, cyanosis and coma. According to Woolley [168] the *prolonged* use of phenol may produce ochronosis with darkening of the cornea and of the skin of the face and the hands.

Ruedemann and Deichmann [130] reported a case in which repeated applications of 1 or 2% phenol in calamine lotion produced dizziness and collapse in an elderly woman. Serious systemic effects caused by topically applied phenol in 2 newborn infants were reported by Von Hinkel and Kintzel [160]: a 1-day-old child died after the application of 2% phenol to the umbilicus. A marked cyanosis was noted after 6 hours. The other child, 6 days old, developed methaemoglobinaemia, circulatory failure and cerebral symptoms. Recovery ensued after exchange transfusions.

Phenol face peels

Several cases of acute death and intra- and postoperative complications have been reported after phenol face peels [38]. Laryngeal edema with respiratory stridor, hoarseness, and tachypnea within 24 hours after a chemical face peel has been reported in 3 patients [242], but it was uncertain whether these effects were due to phenol or one of the other constituents of the face peel. The toxic dose for adults has been estimated to be 8 to 15 g. In fatal cases, death usually results within 24 hours or less from respiratory failure, but the prognosis is guarded even after this period of time.

Major cardiac arrhythmias were noted by Truppman and Ellerby [153] in 10 out of 43 patients during phenol face peels; 9 of them had no previous ECG abnormalities, but needed intravenous lidocaine and/or propranolol for cardiac rhythm conversion. However, this item is rather controversial, and some authors feel that when the procedure is done in more than one hour, and when the dose applied is carefully monitored, phenol face peels are not risky [243,244]. Nevertheless, of 54 patients treated by Gross in 1984, 39% developed some form of cardiac arrhythmia. The next 100 patients had half the face treated on consecutive days, with a 22% incidence of arrhythmias. All forms of arrhythmias were encountered. Cardiac toxicity would first manifest itself by tachycardia and premature contractions. In severe cases, these would progress to ventricular tachycardia or atrial fibrillation [435]. For a suggested protocol to prevent such reactions, see [436].

Local complications of chemical face peeling include [213]: hypopigmentation, hyperpigmentation, phenol bleaching, blotchy pigmentation, demarcation, milia, persistent erythema, skin pore prominence, teleangiectasia and scarring.

For additional information on side effects of chemical face peeling see §20.3.

p-Phenylenediamine

See under Henna (§ 16.35)

Podophyllum resin

16.52 Podophyllum resin is extracted from the dried rhizome of *Podophyllum peltatum* (mandrake or may apple). It contains numerous lignins and flavonols, including podophyllotoxin and α- and β-peltatins. Podophyllum resin is a powerful skin irritant which is widely used in the local treatment of condylomata acuminata. As a potent antimitotic agent it has been extensively used as a cytotoxic drug. Systemic toxicity from local podophyllin treatment has occurred when the drug has been applied to extensive areas of the skin in excessive amounts, has been allowed to remain in contact with the skin for an extended period of time, and from intralesional injection [464]. Features of systemic toxicity include nausea and vomiting, respiratory stimulation, peripheral neuropathy, fever, acute confusional states, tachycardia, oliguria, anuria, adynamic ileus, coma, and death.

To prevent systemic side effects, the following recommendations have been suggested [67]:
1. applications should be limited to small areas of intact skin;
2. extended periods of contact time should be avoided;
3. alcoholic beverages should be avoided for several hours after treatment;
4. podophyll in resin should not be used on buccal mucosa or tongue.

Signs and symptoms of systemic podophillin toxicity include [29,67,208]:

respiratory	respiratory stimulation
cardiovascular	tachycardia, cyanosis [132]
nervous system	fever, seizures, acute confusional state, peripheral neuropathy, coma, death [29]
haematological	leukocytosis, leukopenia, anaemia, thrombocytopenia [142,206]
liver	elevation of liver enzymes
gastrointestinal	nausea, vomiting, abdominal pain, adynamic ileus
urinary system	oliguria, anuria, haematuria
skin and appendages	urticaria
second generation effects	teratogenicity: skin tags on the ear and cheek, simian crease, preauricular skin tags, limb malformations, polyneuritis, intra-uterine death [23,82]

Povidone-iodine

16.53 Povidone-iodine is a water-soluble iodine complex, which is said to retain the non-selective broad-range microbicidal activity of iodine without the undesirable effects of iodine tincture. Betadine products are said to kill both gram-positive and negative bacteria, including antibiotic-resistant organisms, as well as fungi, viruses, protozoa and yeasts. Apparently povidone-iodine has a more prolonged germicidal action than ordinary iodine solutions, and maintains its effectiveness in the presence of blood, serum and pus.

Several studies have shown that povidone-iodine, or at least iodine, may be absorbed from damaged skin, such as burns [17,114,192,250], from the vaginal mucosa [162], from the oral mucosa [49], but also from normal skin in children [18,121].

Effects on thyroid function

Absorption of povidone-iodine may lead to elevation of iodine blood levels [162], elevation of protein-bound iodine [27], and thyroid function abnormalities [18,49]. Usually there are no clinical manifestations [389], but both hyperthyroidism [386,388] and hypothyroidism [387] have been observed. Skin disinfection with *iodine* has caused goitre and hypothyroidism in 5 of 30 newborns under intensive care [22], and there is concern that absorption of povidone-iodine may give rise to similar adverse reactions. In this regard, children would seem to constitute a high-risk group.

Application of povidone-iodine to pregnant women

A very rapid absorption of povidone-iodine from the vaginal mucosa, after only two minutes vaginal disinfection, resulting in an increase in serum concentration of total iodine and inorganic iodine up to 5 to 15-fold, has been documented by Vorherr et al. [162]. Etling et al. [44] noted that after vaginal povidone-iodine application during pregnancy, levels of total iodine in amniotic fluid were increased 10 to 150 times over the control values. As an overload of iodine can suppress thyroid hormonogenesis [22], Vorherr et al. [162] advised not to treat vaginitis in pregnant women with povidone-iodine because of the possible development of iodine-induced goitre and hypothyroidism in the fetus and the newborn. Moreover, Utiger [157] has reported that repeated vaginal application of povidone-iodine has resulted in goitre and hypothyroidism, with sequelae of airway obstruction, mental and physical retardation, and neurological disturbances. Less dramatic transient hypothyroidism after prenatal and perinatal exposure to povidone-iodine has been noted in a 'significant' number of newborns [202]. The authors suggested not using iodine in pregnancy or neonatology, when follow-up of the newborn is not guaranteed.

Application of povidone-iodine to neonates

The thyroid function of very-low-birthweight (VLBW; below 1500 g) infants admitted to neonatal intensive-care units was studied at two hospitals; one routinely used topical iodinated antiseptic agents and the other used chlorhexidine-containing antiseptics. Serial monitoring of urinary iodine excretion and serum thyrotropin and thyroxine levels was undertaken from birth for the first 4 weeks of life. Urinary iodine excretion rose dramatically in the 54 iodine-exposed infants and was up to fifty times greater than in the 29 non-exposed infants. Within 14 days, 25% (9 of 36) of the infants exposed to iodine had serum thyrotropin levels above 20 mIU/l, compared with none of the control group. The mean serum thyroxine level in these 9 infants (44·1 nmol/l) was significantly lower than that in exposed infants with normal thyrotropin levels (83·1 nmol/l) and in the non-exposed control group (83·0 nmol/l); thyroxine levels fell before serum thyrotropin rose. These disturbances in thyroid function correlated positively with urinary iodine excretion and hence iodine absorption. Thyroid function had returned to normal by the time of discharge from hospital. It was concluded that iodine absorption, from topical iodine-containing antiseptics, may cause hypothyroidism during a critical period of neurological development in the newborn infant. The routine use of iodine antisepsis in VLBW infants should, according to Smerckly et al. [21], be avoided because of this effect.

In one patient with a perineal fistula has prolonged therapy with topical application of povidone-iodine solution and iodoform-impregnated packing strips led to hypothyroidism [119]. Topical povidone-iodine applied to an abdominal wound has also caused transient thyroid suppression [251].

Neutropenia

A case of neutropenia, presumably due to topical treatment with povidone-iodine was reported by Alvarez [5]: his patient had deep second-degree burns, involving about 50% of the body surface, which were treated with betadine helafoam twice a day.

Renal effects

A 50-year-old woman with chronic renal insufficiency was admitted to hospital for treatment of an extensive decubitus ulcer, gram-negative septicemia and increasing azotemia. The ulcer was packed every 4 hours with PVP-I-soaked gauze. From the 17th day she developed unexplained oliguria, decreasing renal function, hypochloremic metabolic acidosis and cardiovascular instability, which were apparently due to iodide retention (11,200 μg/dl). The authors suggest monitoring serum iodide concentrations if topical povidone-iodine therapy is to be used in patients with renal insufficiency or on large areas of denuded skin [292].

Metabolic acidosis

Metabolic acidosis was attributed to povidone-iodine in the report of Pietsch and Meakins [114]. Two patients, one with a 75% burn, the second with a 35% burn, were treated topically with povidone-iodine. In both patients severe metabolic acidosis developed, which could not be attributed to sepsis, hypervolemia, renal failure, lactic acidemia, etc. The acidosis associated with the 75% burn required large amounts of sodium bicarbonate to maintain pH at 7.35 and a serum bicarbonate concentration of 15 mmol/l (mEq/l); serum iodine was 48,000 μg/dl (normal 4–8.5 μg/dl). Acidosis in the second patient was not as severe, and serum iodine concentration reached 17,600 μg/dl. Haemodialysis was very effective in reducing serum iodine concentration. According to the authors, the acidosis could have been caused by absorption of the iodine or the acidic povidone-iodine. They suggest that, until the etiology of the acidosis and renal damage is more clear, iodophores should not be used topically for burns greater than 20% of the body surface, or in the presence of renal failure. A similar case, in which metabolic acidosis, hypernatremia and renal insufficiency were ascribed to topical treatment of decubitus ulcers (only 2–3% of the body surface), was described more recently [385].

Iododerma

A case of generalized iododerma caused by absorption of povidone-iodine has been described by Bishop and Garcia [17].

Prilocaine

16.54 Emla® is the trade name for a local anaesthetic cream containing prilocaine 25 g/l and lidocaine 25 g/l in an oily base. It is widely used for reducing the pain of venepuncture and other minor skin procedures in children, and its efficacy is well established [356]. The recommended dose of Emla is 1.5–3.0 g/10 cm^2, with a maximum of 5 g. Prilocaine is associated with methaemoglobinaemia, two of its metabolites, 4-hydroxy-2-methylaniline and 2-methylaniline (*o*-toluidine) having been implicated in this condition [356]. Application of 5 g Emla cream under occlusion for 2 hours in children aged 1–6 years resulted in a small but significant increase in methaemoglobin concentration, well within safe limits [356]. As some children may be at special risk owing to pre-existing anaemia, coadministration of sulfonamide antibiotics or reduced renal excretion of metabolites of prilocaine, the minimum effective dose should be used in all children requiring daily application of the cream [356]. The most alarming report of methaemoglobinaemia after the use of prilocaine-lignocaine cream concerned a 3-month-old infant who became cyanosed after 5 g of the cream was applied. His methaemoglobin concentration was 28%, although this may have been partly due to concomitant sulfonamide drug treatment [75].

Promethazine

16.55 A 16-month-old male (weight 11.5 kg) was treated with 2% promethazine cream for generalized eczema. After approximately 15–20 g of the cream had been applied the child fell asleep; a few hours later he awoke with abnormal behaviour, loss of balance, inability to focus, irritability, drowsiness and failure to recognize his mother. One day later all symptoms had spontaneously disappeared. A diagnosis of promethazine toxicity through percutaneous absorption was made [188]. Two more cases of young infants in which dermal absorption resulted in a toxic neurologic syndrome were reported from Canada [437]. The symptoms included central nervous system depression, acute excitomotor manifestations, ataxia and visual hallucinations. In addition, peripheral anticholinergic effects occurred. Widespread application of promethazine 2% cream may even endanger adults [438]. Known symptoms of promethazine toxicity include disorientation, hallucinations, hyperactivity, convulsions, and coma.

Quinine analogs

16.56 Thrombocytopenia due to quinine analogs, although well known from oral administration, has only rarely been described after topical application.

Khaleeli [85] observed thrombocytopenia in a female patient with extensive bilateral varicose ulcers and myxedema who was treated with Quinaband-dressings. (Quinaband contains zinc oxide paste 9.25%, gum acacia 18.5%, clioquinol 1%, calamine 5.75%, boric acid 2%, glycerol 27%, propyl hydroxybenzoate 0.0625% and aqua). The patient was hospitalized for surgical treatment of her ulcers. Medication was limited to thyroxine, multivitamin and ferrous sulfate tablets, and Quinaband dressings were applied to the leg ulcers. During hospitalization she lapsed into a myxedematous coma. She was treated with triiodothyronine and intravenous hydrocortisone. Because sputum had grown *Staphylococcus aureus*, the patient in addition received intramuscular ampicillin and flucloxacillin. The platelet count dropped from 250×10^9 to 100×10^9 and purpura was noted on the chest. She was transfused with 2 units of packed cells but the platelet count continued to fall (to 30×10^9): haematuria and nose bleeding occurred. Patch tests with Quinaband were negative. Shortly after discontinuation of the Quinaband application the patient received 2 units of fresh blood and the platelet count rapidly returned to normal values. Though conclusive evidence is definitely lacking the author ascribes the thrombocytopenia to the use of Quinaband dressings and, more specifically, to the clioquinol contained therein.

There can be no doubt, however, that absorption of halogenated hydroxyquinolines does occur: in a child with generalized psoriasis who had received topical treatment with clioquinol-containing ointment 18.1 mg/100 ml of the conjugated (glucuronic acid) ester of the drug was traced in the urine [72]. Fischer and Hartvig [52] reported on percutaneous absorption of clioquinol: four patients with widespread dermatitis were treated with an ointment containing 3% clioquinol and a corticosteroid. A body area of 40% was treated with 15–20 g of the ointment twice daily. The serum concentration increased to 0.8–1.2 μg/ml within four hours of application, remained constant during treatment and then fell to zero within four days. Urinary excretion measured in one case comprised 15–20 mg conjugated metabolites daily. This topical treatment thus gave about the same urinary excretion as would a daily oral dose of 0.25 g (one tablet) of clioquinol. The authors estimate that 3–4% of the applied clioquinol was absorbed percutaneously. Stohs et al. [354] calculated that a far higher percentage of topically applied clioquinol is absorbed percutaneously, notably 40%. They suggested that the methodology of Fischer and Hartvig [52] and others who suggested percutaneous absorption to be 3–4% was inadequate, as only urinary excretion data were used, but far more of the drug is excreted in the faeces [355].

As chronic oral use of this drug may lead to serious neurological adverse events, notably subacute myelo-optic neuropathy, concern has been raised about the safety of extensive topical application of clioquinol [73].

An abnormal protein-bound iodine after topic application of clioquinol has been recorded by Upjohn et al. [156].

Systemic side effects of topical clioquinol in a previously sensitized individual were described by Simpson [135]: a woman known to react to ingested quinine applied 3%, clioquinol cream to her submammary region. Twelve hours after the first application she developed a generalized erythema and, within hours, had bronchospasm which required oral and intravenous steroids.

The Committee on Drugs of the American Academy of Pediatrics has advised against the topical use of clioquinol and iodiquinol in children [460].

Resorcinol

16.57 Resorcinol (*m*-dihydroxybenzene) is used for its keratolytic and 'peeling' properties in the treatment of acne vulgaris; also, it is a constituent for the antifungal Castellani's solution. Formerly, leg ulcers were treated with external application of resorcinol-containing preparations.

Case reports

Resorcinol can penetrate human skin [227,228] and an extensive review of the industrial toxicity of resorcinol has been reported [229]. It has been estimated that less than 3% resorcinol in a hydroalcoholic vehicle applied to the skin is absorbed percutaneously [227]. Although the drug is chemically unrelated to any of the known groups of antithyroid drugs, resorcinol has an antithyroid activity similar to that of methyl thiouracil. Consequently, several cases of myxedema caused by percutaneous absorption of resorcinol, especially from ulcerated surfaces, have been described [15,150]. Two cases of resorcinol-induced hypothyroidism were described by Berthezene et al. [15]. All symptoms disappeared after discontinuation of the treatment with resorcinol. The authors assume that resorcinol produced a defect in the organic binding of iodine and in the release of thyroid hormones. This latter effect may be due to a defect in the coupling of iodotyrosines. In the report of Thomas and Gisburn [150] resorcinol-induced myxedema was associated with ochronosis.

Methaemoglobinaemia in children, caused by the absorption of resorcinol applied to wounds has been reported by Flandin et al. [53] and by Murray [107]. Cunningham [31] reported a case in which the application of an ointment containing 12.5% resorcinol to the napkin area of an infant produced cyanosis, a maculopapular eruption, haemolytic anaemia, and haemoglobinuria. In the literature, this author found seven cases of acute poisoning in babies, as a consequence of topical resorcinol application, in some instances to limited areas; five fatalities were recorded.

Wuthrich et al. [170] reported on two young adults who were treated for pustular acne with a peeling paste containing 40% resorcinol. After three to four weeks of treatment with one application daily, adverse reactions were noted consisting of pallor, dizziness, cold sweat, tremors, collapse and violet-black urine.

A case of severe poisoning of a six-week-old infant due to two applications of Castellani's paint (containing basic fuchsin, boric acid, phenol, resorcinol, acetone and alcohol) was described by Lundell and Nordman [95].

Although the use of resorcinol in young children and for leg ulcers should be avoided, topical resorcinol, when used for acne vulgaris, appears to be safe [227].

Salicylic acid

16.58 In 1874, salicylic acid became widely available as the result of its production by a synthetic process. Since that time it has been widely used in dermatology for topical application because of its keratolytic properties.

As early as 1880 Beyer [16,171] reported the presence of salicylates in the urine following application to the skin. Cases of salicylate poisoning after topical use of salicylic acid have been reported several times. Taylor and Halprin [257] used 6% salicylic acid in a gel base under plastic suit occlusion in adults with extensive psoriasis. During their 5-day study, serum salicylates never exceeded 5 mg/100 ml and no patient developed toxicity. However, toxicity was noted by von Weis and Lever; they found serum salicylate levels ranging from 46 to 64 mg/100 ml. Salicylic acid therapy for extensive lesions may be especially dangerous for children. An unpublished review [258] revealed 13 deaths associated with the widespread use of salicylic acid preparations, and all but 3 occurred in children. This compound should not be used on large areas (more than 25%) of the skin of a child [258].

16.59 The *signs and symptoms of intoxication* vary according to the level of salicylic acid in the plasma, although considerable differences exist in individual susceptibility [68]. Symptoms may be present with levels of salicylic acid in the plasma as low as 10 mg/100 ml. Ordinarily, symptoms that occur at levels below 35 mg/100 ml are quite mild. The clinical manifestations of intoxication with salicylic acid include gastrointestinal, respiratory, renal, metabolic, neural and psychic disturbances [161]. The first symptoms are, according to Gorter [66], paleness, fatigue and drowsiness, and a modification of the respiration, which becomes more frequent and at the same time deeper, and can be heard from a distance. Other early signs of intoxication with salicylic acid are nausea, vomiting, changes in the ability to hear, and mental confusion [161]. Several deaths have been recorded, mainly in children.

The treatment of mild to moderate intoxication with salicylic acid consists of discontinuing the salicylic acid ointment, giving large amounts of fluids to promote excretion, and administering sodium bicarbonate, either orally or intravenously, in order to ensure an alkaline pH of the urine [109]. The pH of the urine is a significant factor in the occurrence of intoxication with salicylic acid. In severe renal damage salicylic acid is poorly excreted [69].

Case reports

In 1952 Young collected 8 fatal cases of salicylate poisoning with symptoms of vomiting, tinnitus, stupor, Cheyne–Stokes respiration and nuchal rigidity. Von Weiss and Lever [161] reported on 3 adults with extensive psoriasis who were treated with an ointment containing 3% or 6% salicylic acid 6 times daily. Between the second and fourth day, symptoms of salicylism developed in all 3 patients. The outstanding symptoms were *nausea*, *dyspnea*, *decreased ability to hear*, *confusion* and *hallucinations*.

Other signs included:

- *Gastrointestinal*: vomiting, thirst, anorexia, diarrhoea
- *Neurological*: headache, dizziness, tinnitus, slurred speech
- *Psychic*: agitation, disorientation, lethargy, delusions, belligerence, retrograde amnesia, depression, feeling of unreality
- *Other*: fever, profuse sweating.

The levels of salicylic acid in the serum ranged from 46 to 64 mg/100 ml. Within one day after discontinuation of the ointment, the symptoms had largely disappeared. The serum salicylic acid decreased to zero within a few days. The same authors also recorded 13 deaths resulting from intoxication with salicylic acid following the application of salicylic ointment to the skin, reported in literature up to 1964, and several non-fatal intoxications. The 13 deaths included 3 patients with psoriasis, 5 cases of scabies, 3 of dermatitis, one of lupus vulgaris and one of congenital ichthyosiform erythroderma. Ten of the fatal cases occurred in children, 3 of them being under 3 years of age.

The most dramatic account in the literature is that of 2 plantation workers in Bougainville, in the Solomon Islands, who were painted twice a day with an alcoholic solution of 20% salicylic acid for tinea imbricata involving about 50% of the body. The victims were comatose within 6 hours and died within 28 hours [92].

Wechselberg [167] reported a 3-month-old baby with scaly erythroderma treated in a hospital with 1% salicylic acid in soft paraffin. After 10 days the child began to vomit and lose weight. Later hyperpnoea developed and an increasing somnolence. When the treatment was stopped the child recovered rapidly.

More recently, a case of salicylic acid intoxication leading to coma in an adult patient with psoriasis, who had been treated with 20% salicylic acid in petrolatum, was described [152]. Lipman et al. [93] summarized the electrolyte changes that occur in salicylate intoxication as follows: "A hyperpnoea due to the central stimulatory effect of the salicyl radical produces a respiratory loss of carbon dioxide, altering the ratio of carbonic acid to sodium bicarbonate in the direction of increased alkalinity. This then is a state of respiratory alkalosis and represents the first stage of salicylate intoxication. The next stage is a state of compensated acidosis caused by ketosis resulting from altered carbohydrate metabolism and the presence of retained acid anions in the blood and tissue fluids. The final stage is that of decompensated acidosis, with depletion of the alkali reserve, decrease in the blood pH and failure of the respiratory centre in its attempt to achieve compensation."

Salicylic acid in higher concentrations, combined with ammoniated mercuric chloride ('ammoniated mercury'), can severely irritate the skin because free mercuric chloride is formed.

Selenium sulfide

16.60 Ransone et al. [125] reported a case of *systemic* selenium toxicity in a woman who had been shampooing her hair 2 or 3 times weekly for 8 months with selenium sulfide suspension. One hour after a shampoo the patient noticed a mild non-rhythmical tremor of the arms and hands over a period of 3 or 4 minutes. This was followed by severe perspiration and an increasingly severe generalized tremor. Two hours after the shampoo she noticed a metallic taste in the mouth and others noted that her breath smelled of garlic, though none had been eaten. The tremor lasted for eight hours and was followed by a dull continuous pain in the lower abdomen. For the next three days she felt quite weak, lethargic and anorectic, and occasionally vomited. The patient denied headaches, speech, visual or gait disturbances and skin eruptions except for an excoriated crusted and scaling eruption, 5×12 cm, on the scalp.

Sex hormones

Estrogens

16.61 Topical application of estrogen-containing externa may lead to resorption of these hormones and systemic estrogenic effects.

Beas et al. [13] reported on seven children with *Pseudoprecocious puberty* due to an ointment containing estrogens. The common fact found in every patient was the use of the same ointment for treatment or prevention of ammoniacal dermatitis for a period of 2 to 18 months with 2 to 10 daily applications. Endocrinological and radiological studies had excluded other possible causes of sexual precocity. The most important clinical signs were: intense pigmentation of the mammillary areola, linea alba of the abdomen and the genitals, mammary enlargement and the presence of pubic hair. Three female patients also had vaginal discharge and bleeding. Estrogenic contamination of the ointment was suspected and confirmed by a biological test of the vaginal opening of castrated female guinea pigs. After discontinuation of the incriminated topical drug all symptomatology progressively disappeared in every patient. Pseudoprecocious puberty has also been observed in young girls after contact with hair lotions and other substances containing estrogens [14,88,123]. Such contact has lead to gynaecomastia in young boys

[143,199]. Gynaecomastia in a 70-year-old man from exposure to 0.01% dienestrol cream used by his wife for atrophic vaginitis and as a lubricant before intercourse has been reported [189].

Estrogen cream for the treatment of baldness has also caused gynaecomastia, which was persistent in the reported case [238]. In adult males both oral and topical administration of estrogens may result first in pigmentation of the areola and then in gynaecomastia [12,62] and also in loss of libido, impotence and galactorrhoea. More recent similar cases are described and cited in Refs. [430,431, 454]. *See also* § 16.71.

Testosterone

16.62 Topical testosterone is the standard treatment for vulvar lichen sclerosus et atrophicus. Increased libido, clitoral hypertrophy and pubic hirsutism have been reported as common side effects. Uncommon side effects include thinning of the scalp hair in elderly patients, one case of slight facial acne, and, rarely, voice change. Several cases of mild hirsutism have been reported, and one case of severe hirsutism with other signs of virilization (large, masculine-appearing upper trunk with muscular extremities) [461]. *See also* § 16.76.

Silver nitrate

16.63 Ternberg and Luce [148] observed fatal *methaemoglobinaemia* in a three-year-old girl suffering from extensive burns, involving 82% of the body surface, who was treated with silver nitrate solutions. Two weeks after admission a transient episode of cyanosis was noted, for which no definite diagnosis was established. Ten days later, she became progressively cyanotic, respiratory rate and pulse increased and then the patient became hypothermic and died. In a post-mortem blood specimen methaemoglobin was found to constitute 70% of the haemoglobin. Known causes of methaemoglobinaemia were excluded. Presumably nitrate had been reduced by *Aerobacter cloacae,* cultured from her wounds, into nitrite, which was absorbed and subsequently caused methaemoglobinaemia (nitrite is prominent among the agents capable of producing methaemoglobin).

Other cases of silver nitrate-induced methaemoglobinaemia were reported by Cushing and Smith [33], Aberman [1], Strauch et al. [145] and Geffner et al. [202]. It is stated that the appearance of cyanosis in burn patients treated with silver nitrate should suggest the possibility of methaemoglobinaemia, especially when the cyanosis persists despite oxygen treatment.

Another complication of the use of silver nitrate in the treatment of large burns is *electrolyte disturbance*, especially in children. Due to the hypotonicity of the silver nitrate dressings hyponatremia, hypokalemia and hyperchloremia may develop [28,42]. Also, loss of other water-soluble minerals and vitamins may occur. Post-mortem examinations of patients treated with silver nitrate have revealed that silver has been deposited in internal organs, showing that absorption of silver from topical preparation does occur [9]. It should be mentioned that the excessive use of silver-containing drugs has led to local and systemic argyria [87] and to renal damage involving the glomeruli with proteinuria [173]. Generalized argyria from uncontrolled silver nitrate application to bleeding gingiva during a period of 2.5 years was reported by Marshall and Schneider [96].

Sulfadiazine silver

16.64 Sulfadiazine silver cream is widely used for the topical treatment of burns. Intended primarily for the control of *Pseudomonas* infections, this bactericidal agent acts on the cell membranes and the cell walls of a variety of gram-positive and gram-negative bacteria as well as on yeasts. Its relative freedom from appreciable side effects such as electrolyte and acid-base disturbances, staining and pain on application, has contributed to its popularity. In a series of 314 burn patients treated with sulfadiazine silver the incidence of drug reactions was only 1.3% [113].

Absorption of sulfonamide from burns treated with sulfadiazine silver has been studied [238]. In 3 patients with 17–46% burned surface area, approximately 20–25% of the daily topical dose could be accounted for as conjugated sulfonamide. Unconjugated drug represented from 35–95% of the total output. Total plasma sulfonamide concentration did not exceed 10 μg/ml.

Silver deposition (Argyria)

Silver sulfadiazine was applied to the wounds of 509 burn patients. Eleven patients with burns covering more than 20% of the body surface showed silver deposits in the mucosa of the lips, gingiva and cheeks. Silver sulfadiazine had been applied topically for between 4 and 12 days as a paste-like suspension in distilled water with concentration of 20–50%. Silver deposits were seen between 9 and 32 days (mean 25 days) after application. The colour of the burn wound was also slightly darker than in patients not treated with silver compounds. The darker colour spontaneously disappeared during the year following discharge [372]. This report was criticized by Fox [393] who suggested that the silver deposits may have been caused by oral administration, as some patients had also received sulfadiazine silver to burns on the face.

Nephrotic syndrome and leukopenia

Nephrotic syndrome following topical therapy with this drug has been reported by Owens et al. [112], but this observation has not been confirmed since [390,391]. Several authors have, however, reported leukopenia during treatment with sulfadiazine silver [24,54]. This side effect appears to run a typical course: sulfadiazine-induced leukopenia reaches a nadir within 2–4 days of starting therapy, with a characteristic drop in the neutrophil count and a relative increase in the number of band forms. The erythrocyte count is not affected. Two to three days after the onset of leukopenia, the leukocyte count returns to normal levels. Recovery is not affected by the continuation of therapy, from which no complications are reported [80].

Owing to the circumstances under which topical sulfadiazine therapy is instituted (ill patient, septic conditions, additional medication), it is very difficult to prove a causal relationship between the drug and the event. However, there are several arguments in favour of such a relationship [54]: (1) no observations of leukopenia associated with other burn therapies, such as mafenide acetate and silver nitrate soaks, have been reported; (2) sulfadiazine is absorbed to a considerable extent following the topical administration of sulfadiazine silver (serum levels up to 20 μg/ml); (3) sulfadiazine is a known cause of leukopenia, agranulocytosis, and other blood dyscrasias; (4) the leukopenic response follows a predictable course; (5) a positive rechallenge has been demonstrated while attempting to reinstitute therapy. Current evidence, therefore, suggests a causal relationship of sulfadiazine silver with leukopenia. The mechanism of this reaction is unknown [80].

Miscellaneous

Reports on the occurrence of respiratory tract infections and pneumonia [394] and toxicity against human protozoa [395] presumably caused by silver sulfadiazine, have been published.

Five patients with burns involving 7–62% of the body surface and treated with sulfadiazine silver developed anuric acute renal failure. Concomitantly, severe neurological abnormalities appeared that progressed relentlessly into irreversible coma and death. These events were ascribed (but not very convincingly) to diethyleneglycol(stearate) present in the sulfadiazine silver preparation [452].

In one case report, acute haemotolytic anaemia developed in a patient with glucose-6-phosphatase dehydrogenase deficiency, and treated with sulfadiazine silver on 35% body surface area burns [465].

Sulfur [439]

16.65 Though its efficacy is sometimes questioned, sulfur is still widely used in the treatment of acne vulgaris and seborrhoeic conditions: no toxicity is to be feared from this practice. However, sulfur has been used in the treatment of scabies [440], and some authors recommend the use of this 'alternative scabicide' in young children, pregnant patients and in patients with massively excoriated skin, because of the alleged neurotoxic effects of treatment with the most commonly used scabicide, lindane (see § 16.35). It must, therefore, be mentioned that the safety of application of sulfur-containing topical remedies over large parts of the body has not been established.

Experimental studies

The percutaneous absorption of sulfur was studied by Geivitz and Wust [58]: after the application of sulfur in a cream base to the skin of healthy subjects, the substance was traced two hours later in the urine. It was estimated that approximately 1% of the sulfur had been absorbed. The application of 25% sulfur in petrolatum to abraded guinea pig skin led to total anorexia and paralysis with demonstrable blood levels of hydrogen sulfide in the experiments of Basch [11]. This same author also reported on clinical evidence of poisoning in patients with scabies treated with sulfur ointments, and even noted fatal toxicity in babies after application of sulfur to large areas of the skin.

Tretinoin

16.66 Of 245 patients treated for various dyskeratotic states (ichthyosis, callosities, palmoplantar keratoderma, acne, and verrucae plantares), 19 (7.8%) had mildly elevated liver function test results of serum transaminase levels, both of which were reversible with cessation of treatment [232]. These changes were seen in patients who had an 'erythematous effect' from treatment. The significance of the data from this study is unclear. In a multicentre study, 44 patients treated for various keratinizing dermatoses showed no elevation in liver function tests [233]. Physiologic levels of vitamin A have been measured in the dermis after the topical application of tretinoin [234]. Theoretically, increased dermal blood flow (erythema) might lead to the absorption of sufficient amounts of tretinoin to cause temporary alteration in liver function. However, only the one study mentioned above has reported changes in liver function tests, so the risk of liver toxicity from tretinoin that is not in an ointment base, used in a patient who does not have a severe erythematous process, would appear to be negligible [234].

Triclocarban

16.67 Triclocarban (trichlorocarbanilide, TCC) is a bacteriostatic agent used to reduce microbial skin flora, and has been present in antimicrobial toilet soap bars since 1956. Its chemistry and antimicrobial properties have been described by Roman et al. [129]. The percutaneous penetration of TCC has been studied by Scharpf et al. [131]: after a single shower employing a whole body lather with approximately 6 g of soap containing 2% TCC, about 0.23% of the applied dose of TCC was recovered in the faeces after six days, and 0.16% of the dose in the urine after two days. At all sampling times blood levels of radioactivity were below the detection limit of 10 ppb.

Methaemoglobinaemia

In 1962 the Subcommittee on Accidental Poisoning called attention to occurrences of methaemoglobinaemia in premature and full-term newborn infants whose diapers were autoclaved after a final laundry rinse with triclocarban. Subsequent reports in the paediatric literature confirmed and added to these 'epidemics' of neonatal methaemoglobinaemia (e.g. Fisch et al. [51]), and suggested that aniline — a well-known cause of methaemoglobinaemia — resulting from the breakdown of TCC during autoclaving, was absorbed from diapers and other nursery clothing through the skin of the infants. A more recent report of methaemoglobinaemia presumably induced by topical TCC was documented by Ponte et al. [117]: Five neonates with methaemoglobinaemia were seen by the authors. In each case, the family history of methaemoglobinaemia was negative; other possible causes, such as drugs, were excluded. A cure was obtained rapidly after injection of methylene blue, completed in some cases by exchange transfusions; no relapses were noted during the following months. In four cases, TCC-containing solutions had been used during delivery either for antisepsis of the perineum of the pregnant woman, or by the obstetrician for hand washing. In the fifth case, 2% TCC containing ointment had been applied to the neonate's umbilicus. The authors assume that triclocarban has caused methaemoglobinaemia in these cases, although they admit that a causative relationship between the drug and the adverse event could not be convincingly demonstrated. Currently, the issue of triclocarban and methaemoglobinaemia is still unsettled.

Triphenylmethane dyes

16.68 Gentian violet and methyl green are triphenylmethane dyes, formerly used for topical antisepsis. A systemic reaction to these drugs in a previously sensitized individual was described by Michel et al. [101]: a woman became cyanosed and then collapsed after the application of a 1% solution of gentian violet and methyl green to a stasis ulcer. An epicutaneous test with the solution was positive.

TRANSDERMAL DRUG DELIVERY SYSTEMS

16.69 Percutaneous absorption of skin contactants, usually an undesirable effect, may also be exploited for therapeutic purposes. Classic examples are nitroglycerin and scopolamine. The drug, which is intended to exert a systemic effect, may be applied to the skin in an ointment base, a solution, or in an especially developed 'transdermal drug delivery system'. The transdermal drug delivery system consists in principle of a reservoir with a microporous membrane, which is applied with an adhesive layer to a hairless part of the skin. The drug is presented to the skin in a continuous rate, which is controlled by the semipermeable microporous membrane of the reservoir and not by the permeability of the skin. This prevents unintended high plasma concentrations of the drugs in patients with unusually permeable skin [138,428,429].

Clonidine

16.70 Clonidine in a transdermal therapeutic system (clonidine-TTS) has been used for the treatment of mild to moderate hypertension. Systemic side effects reported include drowsiness (less than with the oral preparation), dry mouth [293,405], and rebound hypertension after discontinuation of transdermal clonidine therapy [40]. Sexual disturbance, cold extremities, obstipation and fatigue have rarely been ascribed to clonidine [408]. Plasma dilution may be caused by increased water intake due to dry mouth [409]. Paediatric intoxication from accidental ingestion and skin contact with clonidine transdermal patches with drowsiness and awakening only to painful stimuli has been reported [403].

Contact dermatitis (allergic and irritant) may occur in many of the patients treated [405,407], sometimes necessitating discontinuance of therapy. Patients sensitized to topical clonidine usually tolerate subsequent oral administration of clonidine well [406].

The occurrence of 7 cases of urticaria and 1 case of angioedema has been (wrongly) cited by Holdiness [407]. Irritation from transdermal clonidine may trigger recurrent herpes simplex in sites previously affected and can cause marked hyperpigmentation [410].

Estrogens

16.71 Transdermal estradiol can elicit many of the desirable actions of estrogens in postmenopausal women while avoiding the pharmacologic effects of oral estrogens on hepatic proteins [411].

No systemic side effects have been reported from estradiol transdermal therapeutic systems, but topical treatment of 114 postmenopausal women with a hydroalcoholic gel containing 17-β-estradiol led to breast tenderness in 7 (6.1%) and vaginal bleeding in 3 (2.6%) [412]. Skin reactions were observed in 24%, but only 4% required discontinuation of therapy [413]. Contact allergic reactions may be caused by estradiol [415,459], but more often by hydroxypropyl cellulose [414], other components of the reservoir, or the adhesive [407,415]. Post-inflammatory hyperpigmentation is frequent in pigmented patients [416]. *See also* § 16.61.

Glycopyrrolate

16.72 The quaternary ammonium compound glycopyrrolate has been used topically for the treatment of facial gustatory sweating and flushing (Frey syndrome). This syndrome occurs in 60% of patients after parotidectomy with facial nerve dissection. Side effects due to the anticholinergic action of glycopyrrollate include blurred vision and dry mouth. The incidence of these side effects is low when compared to topical scopolamine [286].

Nicotine

16.73 Nicotine TTS is used to help heavy smokers give up their addition by systematic and continuous nicotine application. Intoxication from topical application may occur after cutaneous contact with nicotine, characterized by nausea, vomiting, abdominal cramps, lethargy, constricted pupils and absent deep tendon reflexes [419]. Such effects have not been observed from nicotine TTS. Contact allergy to nicotine may develop in 3% of patients treated [418].

Nitroglycerin

16.74 Nitroglycerin acts directly on the smooth muscles of both arterial and venous vessels causing relaxation. Sublingual (buccal) administration of nitroglycerin has been the treatment of choice for angina pectoris. Because of its extremely short half-life of 3–5 minutes, nitroglycerin in this way is not suitable for continuous prophylaxis. A disadvantage of oral administration is the rapid metabolization to inactive metabolites. A possibility to overcome this 'liver first-pass effect' of oral administration is application to the skin. From industrial use it is known that nitroglycerin easily penetrates the intact epidermis [285]. An ointment formulation of nitroglycerin to be applied under occlusive dressing has been available for many years [279]. However, dosage delivery of the drug is not very accurate, bearing the risk of unnecessarily high plasma concentrations of nitroglycerin. These disadvantages of the ointment have led to the development of several nitroglycerin transdermal delivery systems [287]. Side effects of the nitroglycerin transdermal delivery systems include: headache, pressure feeling in the head, nausea, vomiting, dizziness, tiredness, and black-outs [282]. One case of a cutaneous burn-like reaction with resultant atrophic changes has been reported [423]. Nitroglycerin patches may explode when patients are defibrillated [427]. Gastrointestinal side effects are said to occur very frequently in healthy individuals exposed to the system [287]. The causal relationship between transdermal nitroglycerin, penile erection and spousal headache in one report [424] was seriously doubted [425]. Ageusia (loss of taste) may have been caused by transdermal nitroglycerin in one patient [426]. Contact allergy to the adhesive [280,282] has been reported, as has irritation [105] and post-inflammatory hyperpigmentation [422]. Contact allergy to the active drug is infrequent [407,422].

Scopolamine (Hyoscine)

16.75 The use of scopolamine for prevention of motion-sickness is well-established. In tablet or injectable form scopolamine frequently causes (in addition to the intended antiemetic effect) adverse effects due to its anticholinergic action: dry mouth, hypotension, drowsiness, cycloplegia, bradycardia (low doses), and tachycardia (high doses). These frequently occurring adverse reactions stimulated the development of a transdermal delivery system, which is also used to prevent postoperative emesis [284]. Other uses have included prevention of chemotherapy-induced emesis, treatment of vertigo and reduction of gastric acid secretion [399]. Transdermal scopolamine is reported to have a lower incidence of adverse effects that the oral form. Nevertheless, side effects involving the central nervous system (CNS), vision, bladder, and skin have been described, as have withdrawal symptoms that occur after the patch is removed [278] (Table 16.75).

Table 16.75. Side effect of transdermal scopolamine [278]

CNS effects	*Urinary retention*
confusion	
disorientation	*Dry mouth*
dizziness	
drowsiness ([396]	*Constipation*
excitability	
hallucinations	*Cutaneous effects*
memory disturbances [396]	erythema
restlessness	rash
Ocular effects	*Withdrawal symptoms*
cycloplegia [398]	dizziness
anisocoria [397]	headaches
mydriasis	nausea
acute narrow-angle glaucoma	vomiting

The most common side effects are dry mouth (65%), drowsiness, mydriasis and impaired ocular accommodation [399,400]. Toxic psychosis has been reported several times [278,399,402]. Several factors predispose to CNS side effects, including advanced age, pre-existing psychiatric disease, and concurrent treatment with medications that possess anticholinergic activity [278]. Children may also be more susceptible to unwanted effects [401].

Irritant skin reactions occur in 25% of the patients treated [407], and few isolated case reports of contact allergy have been published [407]. Quite surprisingly, in one Israeli study 16 of 164 (10%) male naval crew members treated for seasickness became sensitized to the patch and the active drug [417].

Testosterone

16.76 Transdermal testosterone is used for the treatment of male hypogonadism [420]. Of 12 men treated with topical testosterone 100 mg daily (not a TTS) for experimental male contraception, 5 female partners developed moderate hair growth on the upper lip and on the inner side of the thighs [421]. *See also* § 16.62.

16.77 REFERENCES

1. Aberman. A. (1969): Oxygentension in methemoglobinemia (letter). *New Engl. J. Med., 281*, 1020.
2. Abrams, S.M., Degnan, T.J. and Vinciguerra, V. (1980): Marrow aplasia following topical application of chloramphenicol eye ointment. *Arch. Intern. Med., 140,* 576.
3. Alder, V.D., Burman, D., Coroner-Beryl, D. and Gillespie, W.A. (1972): Absorption of hexachlorophene from infant's skin. *Lancet, 2*, 384.
4. Alexander, R.C. (1930): Fatal dermatitis following the use of iodine spirit solution. *Br. Med. J., 2*, 100.
5. Alvarez, E. (1979): Neutropenia in a burned patient being treated topically with povidone-iodine foam. *Plast. Reconstr. Surg., 63*, 839.
6. Anonymous (1977): Warning on aerosols containing neomycin. *Lancet, 1,* 1115.
7. Anonymous (1980): Hexachlorophene. *JARC Monographs on the Evaluation of the Carcinogenic Risk of Chemicals to Humans, 20,* 241.
8. Aslam. M., Davis, S.S. and Healy, M.A. (1979): Heavy metals in some Asian medicines and cosmetics. *Publ. Hlth (Lond.), 93,* 274.
9. Bader, K.F. (1966): Organ deposition of silver following silver nitrate therapy of burns. *Plast. Reconstr. Surg., 37,* 550.
10. Bamford, M.F.M. and Jones, L.F. (1978): Deafness and biochemical imbalance after burns treatment with topical antibiotics in young children. *Arch. Dis. Childh., 53,* 326.
11. Basch, F. (1926): Über Schwefelwasserstoffvergiftung bei äusserlicher Applikation von elementarem Schwefel in Salbenform. *Arch. Exp. Path. Pharm., 111,* 126.
12. Bazex, A., Salvader, R., Dupre, A. and Christol, B. (1967): Gynecomastie et hyperpigmentation aréolaire après oestrogénotherapie locale antiséborrhéque. *Bull. Soc. Fr. Derm. Syph., 74,* 466.
13. Beas, F., Vargas, L., Spada, R.P. and Merchak, N. (1969): Pseudoprecocious puberty in infants caused by a dermal ointment containing estrogens. *J. Pediat., 75,* 127.
14. Bertaggia, A. (1968): A case of precocious puberty in a girl following the use of an oestrogen preparation on the skin. *Pediatria (Napoli), 76,* 579.
15. Berthezène, F., Fournier, M., Bernier, E. and Mornex, R. (1973): L'Hypothyroidie induite par la résorcine. *Lyon Med., 230,* 319.
16. Beyer (1880): Cited by Young (1952) (Ref. 171).
17. Bishop, M.E. and Garcia, R.L. (1978): Iododerma from wound irrigation with povidone-iodine. *J. Am. Med. Assoc., 240,* 249.
18. Block, S.H. (1980): Thyroid function abnormalities from the use of topical betadine solution on intact skin of children. *Cutis, 26,* 88.
19. Bork, K., Morsches, B. and Holzmann, H. (1973): Zum Problem der Quecksilber-Resorption aus weisser Präzipitatsalbe. *Arch. Derm. Forsch., 248,* 137.
20. Brenn, H. and Röckl, H. (1954): Fixes Exanthem durch perkutane Resorption von Cignolin. *Hautarzt, 5,* 250.
21. Smerckly, P., Boyages, S.C., Wu, D. et al. (1989): Topical iodine-containing antiseptics and neonatal hypothyroidism in very-low-birthweight infants. *Lancet, ii*, 661–664.
22. Chabrolle, J.P. and Rossier, A. (1978): Goitre and hypothyroidism in the newborn after cutaneous absorption of iodine. *Arch. Dis. Childh., 53,* 495.
23. Chamberlain, M.J., Reynolds, A.L. and Yoeman, W.B. (1972): Toxic effects of podophyllum application in pregnancy. *Br. Med. J., 3*. 391.
24. Wilson, P., George, R. and Raïne, P. (1986). Topical silver sulphadiazine and profound neuropenia in a burned child. *Burns, 12*, 295–296.
25. Ciaccio, E.I. (1971): Mercury: therapeutic and toxic aspects. *Semin. Drug Treatm., 1,* 177.

26. Committee on Drugs (1978): Camphor — Who needs it? *Pediatrics, 62,* 404.
27. Connell Jr., J.F. and Rousselot, L.M. (1964): Povidone-iodine, extensive surgical evaluation of a new antiseptic. *Am. J. Surg., 108,* 849.
28. Connely, D.M. (1970): Silver nitrate — ideal burn wound therapy? *N.Y. St. J. Med., 70,* 1642.
29. Conard, P.F., Hanna, N., Rosenblum, M. and Gross, J.B. (1990): Delayed recognition of podophyllum toxicity in a patient receiving epidural morphine. *Anesth. Analg., 71,* 191–193.
30. Cronin, T.D. and Brauer, R.O. (1949): Death due to phenol contained in Foille®. *J. Am. Med. Assoc., 139,* 777.
31. Cunningham, A.A. (1956): Resorcin poisoning. *Arch. Dis. Childh., 31,* 173.
32. Curley. A., Hawk, R.E., Kimbrough, R.D., Nathenson, G. and Finberg, L. (1971): Dermal absorption of hexachlorophene in infants. *Lancet, 2,* 296.
33. Cushing, A.H. and Smith, S. (1969): Methemoglobinemia with silver nitrate therapy of a burn: Report of a case. *J. Pediat., 74,* 613.
34. Dathan, J.G. and Harvey, C.C. (1965): Pink disease ten years after. *Brit. Med. J., 1,* 1181.
35. Dayal, V.S., Smith, E.L. and McCain, W.G. (1974): Cochlear and vestibular gentamicin toxicity: a clinical study of systemic and topical usage. *Arch. Otolaryng., 100,* 338.
36. De Groot, A.C. and Nater, J.P. (1981): Contact allergy to dithranol. *Contact Dermatitis,* 7, 5.
37. Deichmann, W.B. (1949): Local and systemic effects following skin contact with phenol — a review of the literature. *J. Industr. Hyg., 31,* 146.
38. Del Pizzo, A. and Tanski, E. (1980): Chemical face peeling — Malignant therapy for benign disease? (editorial). *Plast. Reconstr. Surg., 66,* 121.
39. Drake, T.E. (1974): Reaction to gentamycin sulfate cream. *Arch. Dermatol., 110,* 638.
40. Dubiel, W. and Happle, R. (1972): Behandlungsversuch mit Fumarsaure mono-äthylester bei Psoriasis vulgaris. Z. *Haut- u. Ceschlkr., 47,* 545.
41. Editorial (1963): New source of mercury poisoning. *New Engl. J. Med., 269,* 926.
42. Editorial (1965): Burns and silver nitrate. *J. Am. Med. Assoc., 193,* 230.
43. Ericsson, A. and Kallen, B. (1978): *Report on a study of deliveries in women employed in medical occupations.* Report to the National Board of Health and Welfare, Sweden, 28 September 1978.
44. Etling. N., Gehin-Fouque, F., Vielh, J. P. et al. (1979): The iodine content of amniotic fluid and placental transfer of iodinated drugs. *Obstet. Gynecol., 53,* 376.
45. Farber, E.M. and Harris, D.R. (1970): Hospital treatment of psoriasis. *Arch. Dermatol., 101,* 381.
46. FDA Drug Bulletin (1976): Gamma benzene hexachloride (Kwell) and other products alert, *6,* 28.
47. Feiwell, M., James, V.H.T. and Barnett, E.S. (1969): Effect of potent topical steroids on plasmacortisol levels of infants and children with eczema. *Lancet, 1,* 485.
48. Feldmann, R.J. and Maibach, H.I. (1974): Percutaneous penetration of some pesticides and herbicides in man. *Toxicol. Appl. Pharmacol., 28,* 126.
49. Ferguson, M.M., Geddes, D.A.M. and Wray, D. (1978): The effect of a povidone-iodine mouthwash upon thyroid function and plaque accumulation. *Br. Dent. J., 144,* 14.
50. Fink, Th.J. and Gumps, D.W. (1978): Chloramphenicol: an inpatient study of use and abuse. *J. Infect. Dis., 138,* 690.
51. Fisch, R.O., Berglund, E.B., Bridge, A.G., Finley, P.R., Quie, P.G. and Raile, R. (1963): Methemoglobinemia in a hospital nursery. *J. Am. Med. Assoc., 185,* 760.
52. Fischer, T. and Hartvig, P. (1977): Skin absorption of 8-hydroxyquinolines. *Lancet, 1,* 603.
53. Flandin, C., Rabeau, H. and Ukrainczyk, M. (1953): Intolérance à la résorcine. Test cutane. *Soc. Derm. Syph., 12,* 1804.
54. Fraser, G.L. and Beaulieu, J.T. (1979): Leukopenia secondary to sulfadiazine silver. *J. Am. Med. Assoc., 241,* 1928.
55. Friedmann, I. (1977): Aerosols containing neomycin. *Lancet, 1,* 1662.
56. Gasser, F. (1974): Allergien durch zahnärztliche Fremdstoffe. In: *Arzneimittelallergie,* pp. 197–202. Editors: M. Werner and W. Gronemeyer. Gustav Fischer Verlag, Stuttgart.
57. Gay, M.W., Moore, W.J., Morgan, J.M. and Montes, L.F. (1972): Anthralin toxicity. *Arch. Dermatol., 105,* 213.
58. Geivitz, W. and Wust, H. (1955): Über die Resorption von anorganischen Stoffen durch die menschliche Haut. *Z. Ges. Exp. Med., 125,* 587.
59. Gill, K.A. and Baxter, D.L. (1964): Plasma cortisol suppression by steroid creams. *Arch. Dermatol., 89,* 734.

60. Gimenez, E.R., Vallejo, N.E., Roy, E., Lis, M., Izurieta, E.M., Rossi, S. and Capuccio, M. (1968): Percutaneous alcohol intoxication. *Clin. Toxicol., 1,* 39.
61. Ginsburg, C.M., Lowry, W. and Reisch, J.S. (1977): Absorption of lindane (gamma benzene hexachloride) in infants and children. *J. Pediat., 91,* 998.
62. Goebel, M. (1969): Mamillenhypertrophie mit Pigmentierung nach lokaler Oestrogentherapie im Kindesalter. *Hautarzt, 20,* 521.
63. Goffinet, M. (1977): A propos de la toxicité cliniquement presumable de certaines gouttes otiques. *Acta Oto-rhino-laryng. Belg., 31,* 585.
64. Goldbloom, R.B. and Goldbloom, A. (1953): Boric acid poisoning. Report of four cases and a review of 104 cases from the world literature. *J. Pediat., 43,* 631.
65. Goluboff, N. and MacFadyen, D.J. (1955): Methemoglobinemia in an infant. *J. Pediat., 47,* 222.
66. Gorter, E. (1949): On salicylate poisoning in children. *Acta Paediat. (Uppsala), 37,* 170.
67. Miller, R.A. (1985): Podophyllin. *Int. J. Dermatol., 24*, 491–498.
68. Graham, J.D.P. and Parker, W.A. (1948): Toxic manifestations of sodium salicylate therapy. *Quart. J. Med. (new series), 17*, 153.
69. Gross, H. and Greenberg, L.A. (1948): *Salicylates: Critical Bibliographic Review.* Hillhouse Press, New Haven, Connecticut.
70. Halling, H. (1977): Misstänkt samband mellan hexaklorophenexposition och missbildningsbörd. *Läkartidningen, 74,* 542.
71. Halling, H. (1979): Suspected link between exposure to hexachlorophene and malformed infants. *Ann. N.Y. Acad. Sci., 320,* 426.
72. Hansson, O. (1963): Acrodermatitis enterophatica. *Acta Derm.-Venereol. (Stockh.). 43,* 465.
73. Hansson, O. (1977): Vioform condemned. *Pediatrics, 60*, 769.
74. Harkness, R.A. and Beveridge, G.W. (1966): Isolation of p-naphthol from urine after its application to skin. *Nature (Lond.), 211*, 413.
75. Jakobson, B. and Nilsson, A. (1985): Methaemoglobinaemia associated with a prilocaine-lidocaine cream and trimethoprin-sulphamethoxazole. A case report. *Acta Anaesthesiol. Scand., 29*, 453–455.
76. Hemels, H.G.W.M. (1972): Percutaneous absorption and distribution of 2-naphthol in man. *Br. J. Dermatol., 87*, 614.
77. Herd, J.K., Cramer, A., Hoak, F.C. and Norcross, B.N. (1967): Ototoxicity of topical neomycin augmented by dimethyl sulfoxide. *Pediatrics, 40*, 905.
78. Hirschman, S.Z., Feingold, M. and Boylen, G. (1963): Mercury in house paints as a cause of acrodynia. Effect of therapy with N-acetyl-D,L-penicillamine. *New Engl. J. Med., 269*, 889.
79. Hopkins, J. (1979): Hexachlorophene: more bad news than good. *Food Cosm. Toxicol., 17,* 410.
80. Fuller, F.W. and Engler, P.E. (1988): Leukopenia in non-septic burn patients receiving topical 1% silver sulfadiazine cream therapy. A survey. *J.B.C.R., 9*, 606–609.
81. Johnstone, R.T. (1948): *Occupational Medicine and Industrial Hygiene*, p. 216, C.V. Mosby Co., St. Louis, MO.
82. Karol, K.D., Conner, Ch.S., Watanabe, A.S. and Murphey, K.J. (1980): Podophyllum: suspected teratogenicity from topical application. *Clin. Toxicol., 16*, 283.
83. Kellerhals, B. (1978): Hörschäden durch ototoxische Ohrtropfen. Ergebnisse einer Umfrage. *HNO (Berl.), 26*, 49.
84. Kelly, D.R., Nilo, E.N. and Berggren, R.B. (1969): Deafness after topical neomycin wound irrigation. *New Engl. J. Med., 280*, 1338.
85. Khaleeli, A.A. (1976): Quinaband-induced thrombocytopenic purpura in a patient with myxoedema. *Br. Med. J., 2*, 562.
86. Kligman, A.M. (1965): Dimethyl sulfoxide. Part 2. *J. Am. Med. Assoc., 193*, 151.
87. Krückemeyer, K. (1972): Argyrosis universalis nach Langzeittherapie mit silberhaltigen Präparaten. *Ärztl. Praxis, 24, 18.*
88. Landolt, R. and Mürset, G. (1968): Vorzeitige Pubertätsmerkmale als Folge unbeabsichtigter Östrogenverabreichung. Schweiz. Med. Wschr., 98, 638.
89. Leading Article (1966): Boric acid and babies. *Lancet, 2,* 188.
90. Leclercq, A., Melennec, J. and Proteau, J. (1973): Intoxication mercurielle. *Concours Med., 95*, 6055.
91. Lee, B. and Groth, P. (1977): Scabies: Transcutaneous poisoning during treatment. *Pediatrics, 59*, 643.
92. Lindsey, C.P. (1968): Two cases of fatal salicylate poisoning after topical application of an antifungal solution. *Med. J. Aust., 1*, 353.

93. Lipman et al. (1952): Cited by Young (1952) (Ref. 171).
94. Lockart, J.D. (1972): How toxic is hexachlorophene? *Pediatrics, 50,* 229.
95. Lundell, E. and Nordman, R. (1973): A case of infantile poisoning by topical application of Castellani's solution. *Ann. Clin. Res., 5*, 404.
96. Marshall, J.P. and Schneider, R.P. (1977): Systemic argyria secondary to topical silver nitrate. *Arch. Dermatol., 113,* 1072.
97. Masur, H., Whelton, P. K. and Whelton, A. (1976): Neomycin toxicity revisited. *Arch. Surg., 3,* 822.
98. May, Ph., Stern, E.J., Ryter, R.J., Hirsch, F.S., Michel, B. and Levy, R.P. (1976): Cushing syndrome from percutaneous absorption of triamcinolone cream. *Arch. Intern. Med., 136,* 612.
99. Merck Index (1976): Ninth Edition, p. 291. Merck and Co., Inc., Rahway, N.J., U.S.A.
100. Meyboom, R.H.B. (1975): Metals. In: *Meyler's Side Effects of Drugs. Vol. VIII*, pp. 517–522. Editor: M.N.G. Dukes. Excerpta Medica, Amsterdam.
101. Michel, P.J., Buyer, R. and Delorme, G. (1958): Accidents géneraux (cyanose, collapsus cardiovasculaire) par sensibilisation à une solution aqueuse de violet de gentiane et vert de méthyle en applications locales. *Bull. Soc. Fr. Dermatol. Syph., 65,* 183.
102. Milby, T.H. and Epstein, W.L. (1964): Allergic contact sensitivity to malathion. *Arch. Environm. Hlth., 9,* 434.
103. Milstone, E.B., McDonald, A.J. and Scholhamer, C.F. (1981): Pseudomembranous colitis after topical application of clindamycin. *Arch. Dermatol., 117,* 154.
104. Mittelman, H. (1972): Ototoxicity of 'ototopical' antibiotics: past, present, and future. *Trans. Am. Acad. Ophthal. Otolaryng., 76,* 1432.
105. Vaillant, L., Biette, S., Machet, L., Constans, T. and Monpère, C. (1990): Skin acceptance of transcutaneous nitroglycerin patches: a prospective study of 33 patients. *Contact Dermatitis, 23*, 142–145.
106. Murphy, K.W.R. (1970): Deafness after topical neomycin (letter). *Br. Med. J., 2*, 144.
107. Murray, M.C. (1926): Analysis of sixty cases of drug poisoning. *Arch. Pediat., 43*, 193.
108. Ohlgisser, M., Adler, M., Ben-Dov, B., Taitelman, U., Birkhan, H. J. and Bursztein, S. (1978): Methaemoglobinaemia induced by mafenide-acetate in children. A report of two cases. *Br. J. Anaesth.*, 50, 299.
109. Oliver, T.K. and Dyer, M.E. (1960): Prompt treatment of salicylism with sodium bicarbonate. *Am. J. Dis. Child., 99,* 553.
110. Osol, A. and Farrar Jr., G.E. (1947): *The Dispensatory of the United States of America,* 24th Edition. Lippincott, Philadelphia.
111. Otten, H. and Plempel, M. (1975): Antibiotika und Chemotherapeutika in Einzeldarstellungen. Chemotherapeutika mit breitem Wirkungsbereich. Sulfonamide, pp. 110–145. In: *Antibiotika-Fibel.* Editors: H. Otten, M. Plempel and W. Siegenthaler. G. Thieme Verlag, Stuttgart.
112. Owens, C.J., Yarbrough, D.R. and Brackett, N.R. (1974): Nephrotic syndrome following topically applied sulfadiazine therapy. *Arch. intern. Med., 134,* 332.
113. Pegg, S.P., Ramsay, K., Meldrum, L. and Laundy, M. (1979): Clinical comparison of maphenide and silver sulphadiazine. *Scand. J. Plast. Reconstr. Surg., 13,* 95.
114. Pietsch, J. and Meakins, J.L. (1976): Complications of povidone-iodine absorption in topically treated burn patients. *Lancet, 2,* 280.
115. Pines, W.I. (1972): Hexachlorophane: Why FDA concluded that hexachlorophane was too potent and too dangerous to be used as it once was? *FDA Consumer, 6,* 24.
116. Plueckhahn, V.D., Ballard, B.A., Banks, J.M., Collins, R.B. and Flett, P.T. (1978): Hexachlorophene preparations in infant antiseptic skin care: benefit. risks and the future. *Med. J. Aust., 2,* 555.
117. Ponté, C., Richard, J., Bonte, C., Lequien, P. and Lacombe, A. (1974): Méthémoglobinémies chez le nouveau-né. Discussion du rôle étiologique du trichlorcarbanilide. *Ann. Pédiat., 21,* 359.
118. Powell, H., Swarner, O., Gluck, L. and Lamper, P. (1973): Hexachlorophene myelinopathy in premature infants. *J. Pediat., 82,* 976.
119. Prager. E.M. and Gardner, R.E. (1979): Iatrogenic hypothyroidism from topical iodine-containing medication. *West. J. Med., 130,* 553.
120. Pramanik, A.K. and Hansen, R.C. (1979): Transcutaneous gamma benzene hexachloride absorption and toxicity in infants and children. *Arch. Derm., 115,* 1224.
121. Pyati, S., Ramamurthy, R., Krause, M. et al. (1977): Absorption of iodine in the neonate following topical use of povidone-iodine. *J. Pediat., 91,* 825.
122. Quante, M. (1976): Taubheit mit lokaler Neomycinapplikation. *HNO (Berl.), 24,* 127.
123. Ramos, A.S. and Bower, B.F. (1969): Pseudoisosexual precocity due to cosmetics ingestion. *J. Am. Med.*

Assoc., 207, 369.
124. Ramu. A., Slonim, E.A. and Egal, F. (1973): Hyperglycemia in acute malathion poisoning. *Israel J. Med. Sci., 9,* 631 (cited acc. to WHO, VBC/Tox/74.12. p. 24).
125. Ransone, J.W., Scott, N.M. and Knoblock, E.C. (1961): Selenium sulfide intoxication. *New Engl. J. Med., 264,* 384.
126. Buquet, S., Driencourt, J.B., La Condamine, S., Cannamela, A., Szymanovicz, A. and Carton, M.J. (1987): Méthémoblobinémie toxique par lotion gingivale à base de benzocaine et résorcine. *Ann. Pédiat. (Paris), 34,* 339.
127. Roemeling, R.V., Hartwich, G. and König, H. (1979): Multilokuläre Krebsentstehung nach Arsentherapie. *Forum Clin., 30,* 1928.
128. Rogers, S.C.F., Burrows, D. and Neill, D. (1978): Percutaneous absorption of phenol and methyl alcohol in magenta paint B.P.C. *Br. J. Dermatol., 98,* 559.
129. Roman, D.P., Barnett, E.H. and Balske, R.J. (1957): Cutaneous antiseptic activity of 3,4,4′-trichlorocarbanilide. *Proc. Sci. Sect. Toilet Goods Assoc., 28,* 1213.
130. Ruedemann, R. and Deichmann, W.B. (1953): Blood phenol level after topical application of phenol-containing preparations. *J. Am. Med. Assoc., 152,* 506.
131. Scharpf, L.G., Hill, I.D. and Maibach, H.I. (1975): Percutaneous penetration and disposition of triclocarban in man. *Arch. Environm. Hlth., 30,* 7.
132. Sundharam, J.A. (1990): Podophyllin and its use in the treatment of condylomata aluminata. *Indian J. Dermatol. Venereol. Leprol., 56,* 10–14.
133. Shuman, R.M., Leech, W.R. and Alvord, E.C. (1974): Neurotoxicity of hexachlorophene in the human. 1. A clinicopathologic study of 248 children. *Pediatrics, 54,* 689.
134. Silverberg, D.S., McCall, J.T.and Hunt, J.C. (1967): Nephrotic syndrome with use of ammoniated mercury. *Arch. Intern. Med., 120,* 581.
135. Simpson, J.R. (1974): Reversed cross-sensitization between quinine and iodochlohydroxyquinoline. *Contact Dermatitis Newsl., 15,* 431.
136. Skipworth, G.B., Goldstein, N. and McBride, W.P. (1967): Boric acid intoxication from 'medicated talcum powder'. *Arch. Dermatol. Syph., 95,* 83.
137. Skoglund, R.R., Ware Jr., L.L. and Schanberger, J.E. (1977): Prolonged seizures due to contact and inhalation exposure to camphor. *Clin. Pediatr., 16,* 901.
138. Boddé, H., Verhoeven, J. and van Driel, L.M.J. (1989): The skin compliance of transdermal drug delivery systems. *CRC Critical Reviews in Therapeutic Drug Carrier Systems, 6,* 87–115.
139. Slee, P.H.T.J., Den Ottolander. G.J. and De Wolff, F.A. (1979): A case of merbromin (mercurochrome) intoxication possibly resulting in aplastic anemia. *Acta Med. Scand., 205,* 463.
140. Solomon, L.M., Fahrner, L. and West, D.P. (1977): Gamma benzene hexachloride toxicity. A review. *Arch. Dermatol., 113,* 353.
141. Stanlcy Brown, E.G. and Frank, J.E. (1971). Mercury poisoning from application to omphalocele (Letter to the Editor). *J. Am. Med. Assoc., 216,* 2144.
142. Stoehr, G.P., Petersen, A.L. and Taylor, W.J. (1978): Systemic complications of local podophyllin therapy. *Ann. Intern. Med., 89,* 362.
143. Stoppelman, M.R.H. and Van Valkenburg, R.A. (1955): Pigmentaties en gynecomastie ten gevolge van het gebruik van stilboestrol bevattend haarwater bij kinderen. *Ned. T. Geneesk., 99,* 3925.
144. Stoughton, R.B. (1979): Topical antibiotics for acne vulgaris: Current usage. *Arch. Dermatol., 115,* 486.
145. Strauch, B., Buch, W., Grey, W. and Laub, D. (1969): Successful treatment of methemoglobinemia secondary to silver nitrate therapy. *New Engl. J. Med., 281,* 257.
146. Tan, G.T. (1970): Occupational toxic alopecia due to Borax. *Acta Derm.-Venereol. (Stockh.), 50,* 55.
147. Tedesco, F.J. (1977): Clindamycin and colitis: A review. *J. Infect. Dis., 135* (suppl.), 95.
148. Ternberg, J.L. and Luce, E. (1968): Methemoglobinemia: A complication of the silver nitrate treatment of burns. *Surgery, 63,* 328.
149. *The Merck Index* (1976): Ninth Edition. Merck and Co. Inc., Rahway, N.J., U.S.A.
150. Thomas, A.E. and Gisburn, M.A. (1961): Exogenous ochronosis and myxoedema from resorcinol. *Br. J. Dermatol., 73,* 378.
151. Thompson, J. and Russell, J.A. (1970): Dermatitis due to mercury following amalgam dental restorations. *Br. J. Dermatol., 82,* 292.
152. Treguer, G., Le Bihan, G., Coloignier, M., Le Roux, P. and Bernard, J.P. (1980): Intoxication salicylée par application locale de vaseline salicylée a 20% chez un psoriasique. *Nouv. Presse Méd., 9.* 192.

153. Truppman, E.S. and Ellerby, J.D. (1979): Major electrocardiographic changes during chemical face peeling. *Plast. Reconstr. Surg., 63,* 44.
154. Turk, J.L. and Baker, H. (1968): Nephrotic syndrome due to ammoniated mercury. *Br. J. Dermatol., 80,* 623.
155. Tyrala, E.E., Hillman, L.S., Hillman, R.E. and Dodson, W.E. (1977): Clinical pharmacology of hexachlorophene in newborn infants. *J. Pediat., 91,* 481.
156. Upjohn, A.C., Galbraith, H.J.B. and Solomons, B. (1971): Raised serum protein bound iodine after topical clioquinol. *Postgrad. Med., 47,* 515.
157. Utiger, R. D. (1979): Hypothyroidism. In: *Endocrinology,* pp. 471–488. Editor: L.J. de Groot. Grune and Stratton Inc., New York.
158. Valdes-Dapena, M.A. and Arey, J.B. (1962): Boric acid poisoning: three fatal cases with pancreatic inclusions and a review of the literature. *J. Pediat., 61,* 531.
159. Van der Harst, L.C.A., Smeenk, G., Burger, P.M., Van der Rhee, H.J. and Polano, M.K. (1978): Waardebepaling en risicoschatting van de uitwendige behandeling met clobetasol-17-propionaat (Dermovate). *Ned. T. Geneesk., 122,* 219.
160. Von Hinkel, G.K. and Kintzel, H.W. (1968): Phenolvergiftungen bei Neugeborenen durch kutane Resorption. *Dtsch. Gesundh.- Wes., 23,* 240.
161. Von Weiss, J.F. and Lever, W.F. (1964): Percutaneous salicylic acid intoxication in psoriasis. *Arch. Dermatol., 90,* 614.
162. Vorherr, H., Vorherr, U., Mehta, P., Ulrich, J.A. and Messer, R.H. (1980): Vaginal absorption of povidone-iodine. *J. Am. Med. Assoc., 244,* 2628.
163. Voron, D.A. (1978): Systemic absorption of topical clindamycin. *Arch. Dermatol., 114,* 798.
164. Wallerstein, R.O., Condit, P.K., Brown, J.W. and Morrison, F.R. (1969): Statewide study of chloramphenicol-therapy and fatal aplastic anemia. *J. Am. Med. Assoc., 208,* 2045.
165. Bargman, H. (1988): Is podophyllin a safe drug to use and can it be used during pregnancy? *Arch. Dermatol., 124,* 1718–1720.
166. Ward, O.C. and Hingerty, D. (1967): Pink disease from cutaneous absorption of mercury. *J. Irish Med. Assoc., 60,* 94.
167. Wechselberg, K. (1969): Salizylsäure-Vergiftung durch perkutane Resorption 1%-iger Salizylvaseline. *Anästh. Prax., 4,* 103.
168. Woolley, P.B. (1952): Exogenous ochronosis. *Br. Med. J., 4,* 760.
169. Wustner, H., Orfanos, C.E., Steinbach, H., Kaferstein, H. and Herpers, H. (1975): Nagelverfarbung und Haarausfall. *Dtsch. Med. Wschr., 100,* 1694.
170. Wuthrich, B., Zabrodsky, S. and Storck, H. (1972): Percutaneous poisoning by resorcinol, salicylic acid and ammoniated mercury. *Pharm. Acta Helv., 45,* 453.
171. Young, C.J. (1952): Salicylate intoxication from cutaneous absorption of salicylic acid. Citing Beyer (1880) and Lipman et al. (1952). *Sth. Med. J. (Bgham., Ala.), 45,* 1075.
172. Young, E. (1960): Ammoniated mercury poisoning. *Br. J. Dermatol., 72,* 449.
173. Zech, P., Colon, S., Labeeuw, R., Blanc-Brunat, N., Richard, P. and Porol, M. (1973): Syndrome néphrotique avec dépôt d'argent dans les membranes glomérulaires au cours d'une argyrie. *Nouv. Presse Med., 2,* 161.
174. Weinstein, L. (1975): Antimicrobial agents: Tetracyclines and chloramphenicol. In: *The Pharmacological Basis of Therapeutics, 5th Edition,* Chapter 59, p. 1196. Editors: L. Goodman and A. Gilman. Macmillan Publishing Co., Inc. New York, Toronto, London.
175. Davies, J.E., Dedhia, H.V., Morgade, C. et al. (1983): Lindane poisonings. *Arch. Dermatol., 119,* 142.
176. Albert, Th.A., Lewis, N.S. and Warpeha, R.L. (1982): Late pulmonary complications with use of mafenide acetate. *J. Burn Care Rehabil., 3,* 375.
177. Baranowska-Dutkiewicz, B. (1981): Skin absorption of phenol from aqueous solutions in men. *Int. Arch. Occup. Environm. Health, 49,* 99.
178. Rubenstein, A.D. and Musher, D.M. (1970): Epidemic boric acid poisoning simulating staphylococcal toxic epidermal necrolysis of the newborn infant: Ritter's disease. *J. Pediat., 77,* 884.
179. Martin-Bouyer, G., Lebreton, R., Toga, M. and Stolley, P.D. (1982): Outbreak of accidental hexachlorophene poisoning in France. *Lancet, 1,* 91.
180. Editorial (1982): Hexachlorophene today. *Lancet, 1,* 87.
181. Goldstein, G.S. (1982): Hexachlorophene poisoning (Letter). *Lancet, 1,* 500.
182. García-Buñuel, L. (1982): Toxicity of hexachlorophene (Letter). *Lancet, 1,* 1190.

183. Fisher, A.A. (1980): Irritant and toxic reactions to phenol in topical medications. *Cutis, 26*, 363.
184. Rubin, M.B. and Pirozzi, D.J. (1973): Contact dermatitis from carbolated vaseline. *Cutis, 12*, 52.
185. Birmingham, B.K., Greene, D.S. and Rhodes, C.T. (1979): Systemic absorption of topical salicylic acid. *Int. J. Dermatol., 18*, 228.
186. Baer, R.I., Serri, F. and Weissenbach-Vidal, C. (1955): Studies on allergic sensitization to certain topical therapeutic agents. *Arch. Dermatol., 71*, 19.
187. Andrews, G.C. and Domonkos, A.N. (1971): *Diseases of the Skin*, p. 87. W.B. Saunders, Philadelphia.
188. Bloch, R. and Beysovec, L. (1982): Promethazine toxicity through percutaneous absorption. *Contin. Practice, 9*, 28.
189. DiRaimondo, C.V., Roach, A.C. and Meador, C.K. *(1980):* Gynecomastia from exposure to vaginal estrogen cream (Letter). *New Engl. J. Med., 302*, 1089.
190. Hosler, J., Tschanz, C., Higuite, C. et al. (1980): Topical application of lindane cream (Kwell) and antipyrine metabolism. *J. Invest. Dermatol., 74*, 51.
191. Giard, M.J., Uden, D.L. and Whitlock, D.J. (1983): Seizures induced by oral viscous lidocaine. *Clin. Pharmacy, 2,* 110.
192. Hunt, J.L., Sato, R., Heck, F.L. and Baxter, C.R. (1980): A critical evaluation of povidone-iodine absorption in thermally injured patients. *J. Trauma*, 20, 127.
193. Delaveau, P. and Freidrich-Noué, P. (1977): Absorption cutanée et élimination urinaire d'une combination sulfadiazine-argent utilisée dans le traitement des brûlures. *Therapie, 32*, 563.
194. Shacter, B. (1981): Treatment of scabies and pediculosis with lindane preparations: An evaluation. *J. Am. Acad. Dermatol., 5*, 517.
195. Rasmussen, J.E. (1987): Lindane. A prudent approach. *Arch. Dermatol.*, 123, 1008–1110.
196. Matsuoka, L.Y. (1981): Convulsions following application of gamma benzene hexachloride. *J. Am. Acad. Dermatol., 5*, 98.
197. Telch, J. and Jarvis, D.A. (1982): Acute intoxication with lindane (gamma benzene hexachloride). *Can. Med Assoc. J., 126*, 662.
198. Schillinger, B.M., Bernstein, M., Goldberg, L.A. and Shalita, A.R. (1982): Boric acid poisoning. *J. Am. Acad. Dermatol., 7*, 667.
199. Edidin, D.V. and Levitsky, L.L. (1982): Prepubertal gynecomastia associated with estrogen-containing hair cream. *Am. J. Dis. Child., 136*, 587.
200. Gabrilove, J.L. and Luria, M. (1978): Persistent gynecomastia resulting from scalp inunction of estradiol: A model for persistent gynecomastia. *Arch. Dermatol., 114*, 1672.
201. McDaniel, D.H., Blatchley, D.M. and Welton, W.A. (1982): Adverse systemic reaction to dinitrochlorobenzene (Letter). *Arch. Dermatol., 118*, 371.
202. Geffner, M.E., Powars, D.R. and Choctaw, W.T. (1981): Acquired methemoglobinemia. *West. J. Med., 1347*, 7.
203. Binstock, J.H. (1982): Safety of chemical face peels (Letter). *J. Am. Acad. Dermatol., 7*, 137.
204. Barza, M., Goldstein, J.A., Kane, A. et al. (1982): Systemic absorption of clindamycin hydrochloride after topical application. *J. Am. Acad. Dermatol., 7*, 208.
205. Clark, J.A., Kasselberg, A.G., Glick, A.D. and O'Neill, J.A. Jr. (1982): Mercury poisoning from merbromin (Mercurochrome®) therapy of omphalocele. *Clin. Pediat. (Philad.). 21*, 445.
206. Leslie, K.O. and Shitamoto, B. (1982): The bone marrow in systemic podophyllin toxicity. *Am. J. Clin. Pathol., 77*, 478.
207. Von Krogh, G. (1982): Selbstbehandlung von Condylomata acuminata mit 0.5%-iger Podophyllotoxinlösung. *Hautarzt, 33*, 571.
208. Cassidy, D.E., Drewry, J. and Fanning, J.P. (1982): Podophyllum toxicity: a report of a fatal case and a review of the literature. *J. Toxicol. Clin. Toxicol., 19*, 35.
209. Gossweiler, B. (1982): Kampfervergiftungen heute. *Schweiz. Rundschau. Med. (PRAXIS), 71*, 1475.
210. Von Krogh, G. (1982): Podophyllotoxin in serum: absorption subsequent to three-day repeated applications of a 0.5% ethanolic preparation on Condylomata acuminata. *Sex. Transm. Diseases, 9*, 26.
211. Meynadier, J. and Peyron, J.-L. (1982): Résorption transcutanée des médicaments. *Rev. Pract. (Paris), 32*, 41.
212. Liebman, P.R., Kennelly, M.M. and Hirsch, E.F. (1982): Hypercarbia and acidosis associated with carbonic anhydrase inhibition: a hazard of topical mafenide acetate use in renal failure. *Burns, 8*, 395.
213. Litton, C. and Trinidad, G. (1981): Complications of chemical face peeling as evaluated by a questionnaire. *Plast. Reconstr. Surg., 67*, 738.

214. Hedges, T.R. III, Kenyon, K.R., Hanninen, L.A. and Mosher, D.B. (1983): Corneal and conjuctival effects of monobenzone in patients with vitiligo. *Arch. Ophthal.*, 101, 64.
215. Cammann, R., Hennecke, H. and Beier, R. (1971): Symptomatische Psychosen nach Kolton-Gelee-Applikation. *Psychiat. Neurol. Med. Psychol., 23*, 426.
216. Goluboff, N. and MacFayden, D.J. (1955): Methemoglobinemia in an infant. *J. Pediat., 47*, 222.
217. Bloch, A. (1965): More on infantile methemoglobinemia due to benzocaine suppository. *J. Pediat., 67,* 509.
218. Bernstein, B.M. (1952): Cyanosis following the use of anesthesin (Ethyl Aminobenzoate). *Rev. Gastroent.*, 19, 411.
219. Steinberg, J.B. and Zepernick, R.G. (1962): Methemoglobinemia during anesthesia. *J. Pediat., 61*, 885.
220. Becker, L.E., Bergstresser, P.R., Whiting, D.A. et al. (1981): Topical clindamycin therapy for acne vulgaris: A cooperative clinical study. *Arch. Dermatol., 117*, 482.
221. Franz, T.J. (1983): On the bioavailability of topical formulations of clindamycin hydrochloride. *J. Am. Acad. Dermatol., 9*, 66.
222. De Groot, A.C., Nater, J.P., Bleumink, E. and de Jong, M.C.J.M. (1981): Does DNCB therapy potentiate epicutaneous sensitization to non-related contact allergens? *Clin. Exp. Dermatol., 6*, 139.
223. Feldman, R.J. and Maibach, H.I. (1970): Absorption of some organic compounds through the skin in man. *J. Invest. Dermatol., 54*, 399.
224. Adriani, J. and Zepernick, R. (1964): Clinical effectiveness of drugs used for topical anesthesia. *J. Am. Med. Assoc.,118*, 711.
225. Seldon, R. and Sasahara, A.A. (1967): Central nervous system toxicity induced by lidocaine. *J. Am. Med. Assoc., 202*, 908.
226. Mofenson, H. C., Caraccio, T. R., Miller, H. and Greensher, J. (1983): Lidocaine toxicity from topical mucosal application. *Clin. Pediat., 22*, 190.
227. Yeung, D., Kantor, S., Nacht, S. and Gans, E.H. (1983): Percutaneous absorption, blood levels and urinary excretion of resorcinol applied topically in humans. *Int. J. Dermatol., 22*, 321.
228. Roberts, M.S., Anderson, R.S. and Swarbrick, J. (1977): Permeability of human epidermis to phenolic compounds. *J. Pharm. Pharmacol., 29*, 677.
229. Flickinger, C.W. (1976): The benzenediols: A review of the industrial toxicity and current industrial exposure limit. *Am. Industr. Hyg. Assoc. J., 37*, 596.
230. D'Arcy, P.F. (1982): Fatalities with the use of a henna dye. *Pharmacy Int., 3*, 217.
231. El-Ansary, E.H., Ahmed, M.E.K. and Clague, H.W. (1983): Systemic toxicity of para-phenylenediamine. *Lancet, 1,* 1341.
232. Günther, S. and Freitag, F. (1975): Therapeutic value and side-effects of retinoic (vitamin A) acid on human patients and animal experimental investigations on rats. *Derm. Mschr., 161*, 137.
233. Muller, S.A., Belcher, R.W., Esterly, N.B. et al. (1977): Keratinizing dermatoses: Combined data from four centers on short-term topical treatment with tretinoin. *Arch. Dermatol., 113*, 1052.
234. Thomas, J.R. III and Doyle, J.A. (1981): The therapeutic uses of topical vitamin A acid. *J. Am. Acad. Dermatol., 4,* 505.
235. Reuveni, H. and Yagupsky. P. (1982): Diethyltoluamide-containing insect repellent. Adverse effects in worldwide use. *Arch. Dermatol., 118*, 582.
236. Grybowksy, J., Weinstein, D. and Ordway, N. (1961): Toxic encephalopathy apparently related to the use of an insect repellent. *New Engl. J. Med., 264*, 289.
237. Zadicoff, C. (1979): Toxic encephalopathy associated with use of insect repellent. *J. Pediat., 95*, 140.
238. Gabrilove, J.L. and Luria, M. (1978): Persistent gynecomastia resulting from scalp inunction of estradiol: A model for persistent gynecomastia. *Arch. Dermatol., 114*, 1672.
239. Kramer, M.S., Hutchinson, T.A., Rudnick, S.A. et al. (1980): Operational criteria for adverse drug reactions in evaluating suspected toxicity of a popular scabicide. *Clin. Pharmacol. Ther., 27*, 149.
240. Feldman, R.J. and Maibach, H.I. (1970): Absorption of some organic compounds through the skin in man. *J. Invest. Dermatol., 54*, 399.
241. Cullison, D., Abele, D.C. and O'Quinn, J.L. (1983): Localized exogenous ochronosis. Report of a case and review of the literature. *J. Am. Acad. Dermatol., 8*, 882.
242. Klein, D.R. and Little, J.H. (1983): Laryngeal edema as a complication of chemical peel. *Plast. Reconstr. Surg., 71,* 149.
243. Tromovitch, T.A. (1982): Safety of chemical face peels (Letter). *J. Am. Acad. Dermatol., 7*, 137.
244. Baker, T.J. (1979): The voice of polite dissent. *Plast. Reconstr. Surg. 63*, 262.
245. Check, W. (1978): New study shows hexachlorophene is teratogenic in humans. *J. Am. Med. Assoc., 240*, 513.

246. Janerich, D.T. (1979): Environmental causes of birth defects. The hexachlorophene issue. *J. Am. Med. Assoc., 241*, 830.
247. Gluck, L. (1980): Hexachlorophene: a useful and lifesaving drug. In: *Controversies in Therapeutics,* p. 436. Editor: L. Lasagna. Saunders, Philadelphia.
248. Plueckhahn, V.D. (1980): Hexachlorophene preparations and the newborn infant. *Aust. Paediat. J., 16*, 40.
249. Stein, K.M., Odom, R.B., Justice, G.R. and Martin, G.C. (1973): Toxic alopecia from ingestion of boric acid. *Arch. Dermatol., 108*, 95.
250. Hunt, J.L. et al. (1980): The systemic effects of a burn ointment. *Emergency Med., 12*, 159.
251. Lyen, K.R., Finegold, D., Orsini, R. et al. (1982): Transient thyroid suppression associated with topically applied povidone-iodine. *Am. J. Dis. Child., 136*, 369.
252. Gee, S. (1979): Topical burn agents. *Am. Pharmacy, 19,* 30.
253. AMA Drug Evaluations (1977). 3d Edition, p. 269. Publishing Sciences Group, Inc., Littleton, MA.
254. Haggerty, R.J. (1962): Blue baby due to methemoglobinemia. *New Engl. J. Med., 267*, 1303.
255. Adriani, J. and Zepernick, R.: Summary of methemoglobinemia: Study of child receiving benzocaine. Letter to the Commissioner in OTC, Volume 060150.
256. Olson, M.L. and McEvoy, G.K. (1981): Methemoglobinemia induced by local anesthetics. *Am. J. Hosp. Pharm., 38*, 89.
257. Taylor, J.R. and Halprin, K. (1975): Percutaneous absorption of salicylic acid. *Arch. Dermatol., 106*, 740.
258. United States Department of Health, Education and Welfare, Food and Drug Administration, OTC Antimicrobial II Advisory Panel. Quoted by Rasmussen, J.E. (1979): Percutaneous absorption in children. In: *Year Book of Dermatology, 1979*, p. 28. Editor: R.L. Dobson. Year Book Medical Publishers, Inc., Chicago.
259. Lyons, T.J., Christer, C.N. and Larsen, F.S. (1975): Ammoniated mercury ointment and the nephrotic syndrome. *Minn. Med., 58*, 383.
260. Benson, P.F. and Pharoah, P.O.D. (1960): Benign intracranial hypertension due to adrenal steroid therapy. *Guy's Hosp. Rep., 109,* 202.
261. Fanconi, G. (1962): Hemmung des Wachstums bei einem Säugling durch die zu intensive Anwendung einer 1%-igen Hydrocortisonsalb auf der Haut bei generalisierten Ekzem. *Helv. Paediat. Acta, 17,* 267.
262. Feinblatt, B.I., Aceto, T. Jr., Bechhorn, G. and Bruck, E. (1966): Percutaneous absorption of hydrocortisone in children. *Am. J. Dis. Child., 112*, 218.
263. Katz, V.L., Thorp, J.M. and Bowes, W.A. (1990): Severe symmetric intrauterine growth retardation associated with the topical use of triamcinolone. *Am. J. Obstet. Gynecol., 162*, 396–397.
264. Johns, A.M. and Bower, R.D. (1970): Wasting of napkin area after repeated use of fluorinated steroid ointment. *Br. Med. J., 111,* 347.
265. Keipert, J.A. and Kelly, R. (1971): Temporary Cushing's syndrome from percutaneous absorption of betamethasone 17 valerate. *Med. J. Aust., 11,* 542.
266. Young, C.A., Williams, I.R. and McFarlane, I.A. (1991): Unrecognised Cushing's syndrome and adrenal suppression due to topical clobetasol propionate. *Br. J. Clin. Practice, 45*, 61–62.
267. Pascher, F. (1978): Systemic reactions to topically applied drugs. *Int. J. Dermatol., 17*, 768.
268. Rimbaud, P., Serre, H., Meynadier, J. and Baumelou, H. (1973): Accidents cortisonique graves après corticotherapie locale prolongée pour M.F. avec xanthomatisation des lesions. *Bull. Soc. Fr. Dermatol. Syph., 80*, 176.
269. Marin, F., González Quintela, A., Moya, M., Suarez, E. and de Zárraga, M. (1989): Pseudohyperaldosteronism due to application of an antihemorrhoid cream. *Nephron, 52*, 281–282.
270. Turpeinen, M. (1989). Adrenocortical response to adrenocorticotropic hormone in relation to duration of topical therapy and percutaneous absorption of hydrocortisone in children with dermatitis. *Eur. J. Pediat., 148*, 729–731.
271. Cook, L.J., Freinkel, R.K., Zugerman, Ch. et al. (1982): Iatrogenic hyperadrenocorticism during topical steroid therapy: assessment of systemic effects by metabolic criteria. *J. Am. Acad. Dermatol.,* 6, 1054.
272. Feldmann, R.J. and Maibach, H.I. (1965): Penetration of ^{14}C hydrocortisone through normal skin. *Arch. Dermatol., 91,* 661.
273. Leu, F. (1983): Complications from prolonged topical steroid therapy (Letter to the Editor). *J. Am. Acad. Dermatol., 8*, 425.
274. May, P. and Stein, E.J. (1976): Cushing's syndrome from percutaneous absorption of triamcinolone cream. *Arch. intern. Med., 136*, 612.

275. Burton, T.T., Cunliffe, W.J., Holti, G. and Wright, W. (1974): Complications of topical corticosteroid therapy in patients with liver disease. *Br. J. Dermatol., 9 (Suppl. 10),* 22.
276. Staughton, R.C.D. and August, P. (1975): Cushing's syndrome and pituitary adrenal suppression due to clobetasol propionate. *Br. Med. J., 2,* 419.
277. Himathongkam, T., Dasanabhairochana, P., Ninlawan, P. and Sriphrapradang, A. (1978): Florid Cushing's syndrome and hirsutism induced by desoximetasone. *J. Am. Med. Assoc., 239,* 430.
278. Ziskind, A.A. (1988): Transdermal scopolamine-induced psychosis. *Postgrad. Med., 84,* 73–76.
279. Davies, J.A. and Wiesel, B.H. (1955): The treatment of angina pectoris with a nitroglycine ointment. *Am. J. Med. Sci., 230,* 259.
280. Garnier, B., Imhof, P., Spinell, F. and Jost, H. (1982): Die Behandlung der Angina Pectoris mit einem neuen transdermalen therapeutischen System von Nitroglycerin unter Praxisbedingungen. *Schweiz. Rundschau Med. (Praxis), 71,* 511.
281. Lepore, F.E. (1982): More on cycloplegia from transdermal scopolamine. *New Engl. J. Med., 307,* 824.
282. Müller, P., Imhof, P. F., Burkart, F., Chu, L.-C and Gerardin, A. (1982): Human pharmacological studies of a new transdermal system containing nitroglycerin. *Eur. J. Clin. Pharmacol., 22,* 473.
283. Osterholm, R.K. and Camoriano, J. (1982): Transdermal scopolamine psychosis. *J. Am. Med. Assoc., 247,* 3081.
284. Tigerstedt, I., Salmela, L. and Aromaa, U. (1988): Double-blind comparison of transdermal scopolamine, droperidol and placebo against postoperative nausea and vomiting. *Acta Anaethesiol. Scand., 32,* 454–457.
285. Schwartz, A.M. (1946): The cause, relief and prevention of headaches arising from contact with dynamite. *New Engl. J. Med.,* 235, 541.
286. Hays, L.L., Novack, A.J. and Worsham, J.C. (1982): The Frey syndrome: A simple, effective treatment. *Otolaryngol. Head Neck Surg., 90,* 419.
287. Olivari, M.-T. and Cohn, J. N. (1983): Cutaneous administration of nitroglycerin: a review. *Pharmacotherapy, 3,* 149.
288. Zackheim, H. S., Epstein, E.H. and Crain, W.R. (1990): Topical carmustine (BCNU) for cutaneous T cell lymphoma: A 15-year experience in 143 patients. *J. Am. Acad. Dermatol., 22,* 802–810.
289. Zackheim, H.S., Feldman, R.J., Lindsay, C. and Maibach, H.I. (1977): Percutaneous absorption of 1,3-bis(2-chloroethyl)-1-nitrosurea (BCNU, carmustine) in mycosis fungoides. *Br. J. Dermatol., 97,* 65.
290. Bennett, C.C. (1980): Dimethyl sulfoxide. *J. Am. Med. Assoc., 244,* 2768.
291. Castot, A., Garnier, R., Lanfranchi, C. et al. (1980): Effets systématiques indésirables des médicaments appliqués sur la peau chez l'enfant. *Thérapie, 35,* 423.
292. Aronoff, G.R., Friedman, S.J., Doedens, P.J. et al. (1980): Increased serum iodide concentration from iodine absorption through wounds treated topically with povidone-iodine. *Am. J. Med. Sci., 279,* 173.
293. Chen, S. and Vidt, D.G. (1989): Patient acceptance of transdermal clonidine. *Clev. Clin. J. Med., 56,* 21–26.
294. Ellis, C.N., Mitchell, A.J. and Beardsley, G.R. Jr. (1979): Tar gel interaction with disulfiram. *Arch. Dermatol., 115,* 1367.
295. Stoll, D. and King, L.E. Jr. (1980): Disulfiram — alcohol skin reaction to beer-containing shampoo (Letter). *J. Am. Med. Assoc., 244,* 2045.
296. Siegel, E. and Wason, S. (1986): Boric acid toxicity. *Ped. Clinics North America, 33,* 363–367.
297. Parry, M.F. and Rha, C.-K. (1986): Pseudomembranous colitis caused by topical clindamycin phosphate. *Arch Dermatol., 122,* 583–584.
298. Borglund, E., Hagermark, O. and Nord, C.E. (1984): Impact of topical clindamycin and systemic tetracycline on the skin and colon microflora in patients with acne vulgaris. *Scand. J. Infect. Dis., 43 (suppl.),* 76–81.
299. Borin, M.T. (1990): Systemic absorption of clindamycin following intravaginal application of clindamycin phosphate 1% cream. *J. Clin. Pharmacol., 30,* 33–38.
300. Siegle, R., Fekety, R., Sarbone, P., Finch, R.N., Deery, H.G. and Voorhees, J.J. (1986): *J. Am. Acad. Dermatol., 15,* 180–185.
301. Shohat, M., Mimouni, M., Shuper, A. and Varsano, I. (1986): Adrenocortical suppression by topical application of glucocorticosteroids in infants with seborrheic dermatitis. *Clin. Pediatr., 25,* 209–212.
302. Garden, J.M. and Freinkel, R.K. (1986): Systemic absorption of topical steroids. Metabolic effects as an index of mild hypercortisolism. *Arch. Dermatol., 122,* 1007–1010.
303. Hogan, D.J., Sibley, J.T. and Lane, P.R. (1986): Avascular necrosis of the hips following long-term use of clobetasol propionate. *J. Am. Acad. Dermatol., 14,* 515–517.
304. Cunliffe, W.J., Burton, J.I., Hold, G. and Wright, V. (1975): Hazards of steroid therapy in hepatic failure.

Br. J. Dermatol., *93*, 183–185.
305. Tang, S.C., Chan, K.C. and Chow, S.P. (1986): Osteonecrosis of femoral head after topical steroid therapy. *J. Roy. Coll. Surg. (Edinburgh)*, *31*, 321–323.
306. Mijares, R.P. (1986): Hypokalemic rhabdomyolysis secondary to pseudohyperaldosteronism due to the use of a lotion containing 9-α-fluoroprednisolone. *Nephron*, *43*, 232–233.
307. Bartorelli, A. and Rimondini, A. (1984). Severe hypertension in childhood due to prolonged skin application of a mineralocorticoid ointment. *Hypertension*, *6*, 586–588.
308. Mantero, F., Armanini, D., Opocher, G. et al. (1981): Mineralocorticoid hypertension due to a nasal spray containing 9-α-fluoroprednisolone. *Am. J. Med.*, *71*, 352–357.
309. Lauzurica, R., Bonal, J., Bonet, J. et al. (1988). Rhabdomyolysis, oedema and arterial hypertension: different syndromes related to topical use of 9-alpha-fluoroprednisolone. *J. Human Hypertension*, *2*, 183–186.
310. Dhein, S. (1986): Cushing-Syndrom nach externer Glukokortikoid-Applikation bei Psoriasis. *Z. Hautkr.*, *61*, 161–166.
311. Gomez, E.C. and Frost, P. (1976): Induction of glycosuria and hyperglycemia by topical corticosteroid therapy. *Arch. Dermatol.*, *112*, 1559–1562.
312. Ohman, E.M., Rogers, S., Meenan, F.O. and McKenna, T.J. (1987): Adrenal suppresion following low-dose topical clobetasol propionate. *Roy. Soc. Med.*, *80*, 422–424.
313. Pezzarossa, A., Angiolini, A., Cimicchi, M.C., D'Amato, L., Valenti, G. and Gnudi, A. (1987): Adrenal suppression after long-term exposure to occupational corticosteroids followed by rapid recovery. *Lancet*, *i*, 515.
314. Novak, E., Francom, S.F. and Schlagel, C.A. (1983): Adrenal suppression with high-potency corticosteroid ointment formulation in normal subjects. *Clin. Therapeut.*, *6*, 59–71.
315. Lawlor, F. and Ramabala, K. (1984): Iatrogenic Cushing's syndrome — a cautionary tale. *Clin. Exp. Dermatol.*, *9*, 286–289.
316. Katz, H.I., Hien, N.T., Prawer, S.E., Mastbaum, L.I., Mooney, J.J. and Samsom, C.R. (1987): Superpotent topical steroid treatment of psoriasis vulgaris — clinical efficacy and adrenal function. *J. Am. Acad. Dermatol.*, *16*, 804–811.
317. Olsen, E.A. and Cornell, R.C. (1986): Topical clobetasol-17-propionate: Review of its clinical efficacy and safety. *J. Am. Acad. Dermatol.*, *15*, 246–255.
318. Dahl, M.G.C. (1985): Hazards of topical steroid therapy. *Adverse Drug Reaction Bull., no. 115 (Dec.)*, 428–430.
319. Turpeinen, M., Mashkilleyson, N., Björkstén, F. and Salo, O.P. (1988): Percutaneous absorption of hydrocortisone during exacerbation and remission of atopic dermatitis in adults. *Acta Derm.-Venereol. (Stockh.)*, *68*, 331–335.
320. Turpeinen, M., Salo, O.P. and Leisti, S. (1986): Effect of percutaneous absorption of hydrocortisone on adrenocortical responsiveness in infants with severe skin disease. *Br. J. Dermatol.*, *115*, 475–484.
321. Pflugshaupt, C. (1987): Freigabe hydrokortison-haltiger Topika für den OTC-Markt? *Hautarzt*, *38*, 629–630.
322. Laurie, A.A., Gleiberman, S.E. and Tsizin, Y.S. (1979): Pharmacokinetics of insect repellent N,N-diethyltoluamide. *Med. Parazitol.*, *47*, 72–76.
323. Wu, A., Pearson, M.L., Shekoski, D.L., Soto, R.J. and Stewart, R.D. (1979): High resolution gas chromatography/mass spectrometric characterization of urinary metabolites of N,N-diethyl-m-toluamide (DEET) in man. *J. High Resol. Chromatogr., Chromatogr. Commun.*, *2*, 558–562.
324. Anon. (1989): Seizures temporally associated with use of DEET insect repellent — New York and Connecticut. *Arch. Dermatol.*, *125*, 1619–1620.
325. Editorial (1988): Are insect repellents safe? *Lancet*, *ii*, 610–611.
326. Heick, H.M.C., Shipman, R.T., Norman, M.G. et al. (1980): Reye-like syndrome associated with use of insect repellent in a presumed heterozygote for ornithine carbamoyl transferase deficiency. *J. Pediatr.*, *97*, 471–473.
327. Roland, E.H., Jan, J.E. and Rigg, J.M. (1985): Toxic encephalopathy in a child after brief exposure to insect repellents. *Can. Med. Assoc. J.*, *132*, 155–156.
328. Edwards, D.L. and Johnson, C.E. (1987): Insect-repellent-induced toxic encephalopathy in a child. *Clin. Pharm.*, *6*, 496–498.
329. Tenenbein, M. (1987): Severe toxic reactions and death following the ingestion of diethyltoluamide-containing insect repellents. *JAMA*, *258*, 1509–1511.

330. Konovalov, G.A. and Romanov, A.N. (1980): Early hemodialysis in the treatment of severe poisonings with repellents DETA, benphthalate and dimethylphthalate. *Anesteziol. Reanimatol., 2*, 54–55.
331. Snyder, J.W., Poc, R.O., Stubbins, J.F. and Garrettson, L.K. (1986): Acute manic psychosis following the dermal application of N,N-diethyl-m-toluamide (DEET) in an adult. *Clin. Toxicol., 24*, 429–439.
332. Williams, H.J., Furst, D.E., Dahl, S.L. et al. (1985): Double-blind, multicenter controlled trial comparing topical dimethyl sulfoxide and normal saline for treatment of hand ulcers in patients with systemic sclerosis. *Arthr. Rheumat., 28*, 308–314.
333. Reinstein, L., Mahon, R. Jr. and Russo, G.L. (1982): Peripheral neuropathy after concomitant dimethyl sulfoxide use and sulindac therapy. *Arch. Phys. Med. Rehabil., 63*, 581–584.
334. Swanson, B.N.,, Ferguson, R.K., Raskin, N.H. and Wolf, B.A. (1983): Peripheral neuropathy after concomitant administration of dimethyl sulfoxide and sulindac. *Arthr. Rheumat., 26*, 791–793.
335. Brown, J.H., McGeown, M.G., Conway, B. and Hill, C.M. (1987): Chronic renal failure associated with topical application of paraphenylenediamine. *Br. Med. J., 294*, 155.
336. Marquardt, E.D. (1986): hexachlorophene toxicity in a pediatric burn patient. *Drug Intell. Clin. Pharm., 20*, 624.
337. Larrègue, M., Laidet, B., Ramdene, P. and Djeridi, A. (1984): Dermite caustique du siege et encéphalite secondaires à l'application de talc contaminé par l'hexachlorophène. *Ann. Dermatol. Venereol., 111*, 789–797.
338. Lie, R.L., Vermeer, B.J. and Edelbrock, P.M. (1990): Severe lidocaine intoxication by cutaneous absorption. *J. Am. Acad. Dermatol., 23*, 1026–1028.
339. Amitai, Y., Whitesell, L. and Lovejoy, F.H. (1986): Death following accidental lidocaine overdose in a child. *N. Engl. J. Med., 314*, 182–183.
340. Rothstein, P., Dornbosch, J., Shaywitz, B.A. (1982): Prolonged seizures associated with the use of viscous lidocaine. *J. Pediatr., 101*, 461–463.
341. Kotler, R.L., Hansen-Flaschen, J. and Casey, M.P. (1989): Severe methaemoglobinaemia after flexible fiberoptic bronchoscopy. *Thorax, 44*, 234–235.
342. Olson, M.L. and McAvoi, G.K. (1981): Methemoglobinemia induced by local anesthetics. *Am. J. Hosp. Pharm., 38*, 89–93.
343. Kirkpatrick, M.B. (1989): Lidocaine topical anesthesia for flexible bronchoscopy. *Chest, 96*, 965–966.
344. Friedman, S.J. (1987): Lindane neurotoxic reaction in nonbullous congenital ichthyosiform erythroderma. *Arch. Dermatol., 123*, 1056–1058.
345. Wilkinson, C. (1988): Is the treatment of scabies hazardous? *J. Roy. Coll. Gen. Pract., 38*, 468–469.
346. Burns, D.A. (1991): The treatment of human ectoparasite infection. *Br. J. Dermatol., 125*, 89–93.
347. Berry, D.H., Brewster, M.A., Watson, R. and Neuberg, R.W. (1987): Untoward effects associated with lindane abuse. *Am. J. Dis. Childh., 141*, 125–126.
348. Senger, E., Menzel, I. and Holzmann, H. (1989). Therapiebedingte Lindan-Konzentration in der Muttermilch. *Dermatosen, 37*, 167–170.
349. Tenebein, M. (1991): Seizures after lindane therapy. *J. Am. Ger. Soc., 39*, 394–395.
350. Lange, M., Nitzsche, K. and Zesch, A. (1981): Percutaneous absorption of lindane in healthy volunteers and scabies patients. *Arch. Derm. Res., 271*, 387–399.
351. Martinez, E., Aragona, F. and Caparrós, J. (1984): Retención urinaria como complicación de un tratamiento anti-escabiasis. *Actas Fund. Puigvert Urolog. Nefrolog. Androlog., 3*, 51–55.
352. Heidemüller, B. and Berger, K. (1985): Hörschäden nach Lokalbehandlung mit Aminoglycosidantibiotika. *Z. Klin. Med., 40*, 1899–1902.
353. Martin, J., Heidemüller, B., Berger, K. and Dietel, K. (1985): Gefahren der Lokalbehandlung von thermischen Schäden der Haut am Beispiel ototoxischer Erscheinungen durch Neomycin. *Kinderärtztl. Praxis, 53*, 597–601.
354. Stohs, S.J., Ezzedeen, F.W., Anderson, A.K., Baldwin, J.W. and Makoid, M.C. (1984): Percutaneous absorption of iodochlorohydroxyquin in humans. *J. Invest. Dermatol., 82*, 195–198.
355. Stohs, S.J., Ezzedeen, F.W., Anderson, A.K., Baldwin, J.W. and Makoid, M.C. (1984): Absorption of iodochlorohydroxyquin in humans. *J. Invest. Dermatol., 84*, 79.
356. Frayling, I.M., Addison, G.M., Chattergee, K. and Meakin, G. (1990): Methaemoglobinaemia in children treated with prilocaine-lignocaine cream. *Br. Med. J., 301*, 153–154.
357. Frentz, G. (1985): Topical minoxidil for extended areate alopecia. *Acta Derm. Venereol., 65*, 172–175.
358. Burton, J.L. and Marshall, A. (1979): Hypertrichosis due to minoxidil. *Br. J. Dermatol., 101*, 393–395.
359. Zappacosta, A.R. (1980): Reversal of baldness in a patient receiving minoxidil for hypertension. *N. Engl.*

J. Med., *303*, 1480–1481.

360. Weiss, V.C., West, D.P. and Mueller, C.E. (1981): Topical minoxidil in alopecia areata. *J. Am. Acad. Dermatol.*, *5*, 224–226.
361. Franz, T.J. (1985): Percutaneous absorption of minoxidil in man. *Arch. Dermatol.*, *121*, 203–206.
362. De Villez, R.L. (1985): Topical minoxidil therapy in hereditary androgenetic alopecia. *Arch. Dermatol.*, *121*, 197–202.
363. Ranchoff, R.E. and Bergfeld, W.F. (1985): Topical minoxidil reduces blood pressure. *J. Am. Acad. Dermatol.*, *12*, 586–587.
364. Van der Veen, E.E. and Ellis, C.N. (1985): Topical minoxidil reduces blood pressure. Reply. *J. Am. Acad. Dermatol.*, *12*, 587.
365. Van der Veen, E.E., Ellis, C.N., Kang, S. et al. (1984): Topical minoxidil for hair regrowth. *J. Am. Acad. Dermatol.*, *11*, 416–421.
366. Feinstein, R.P. (1985): The effect of topical minoxidil on blood pressure. *J. Am. Acad. Dermatol.*, *13*, 673–674.
367. Leenen, F.H.H., Smith, D.L. and Unger, W.P. (1988): Topical minoxidil: cardiac effects in bald men. *Br. J. Clin. Pharmacol.*, *26*, 481–485.
368. Katz, H.I. (1989): Topical minoxidil: Review of efficacy and safety. *Cutis*, *43*, 94–98.
369. Alanis, A., Barbara, F., Meurehy, C., Montes de Oca, F. and Ramirez, L. (1991): Double-blind comparison of 2% topical minoxidil and placebo in early male pattern baldness. *Curr. Ther. Res.*, *49*, 723–730.
370. White, S.I., Friedmann, P.S. (1985): Topical minoxidil lacks efficacy in alopecia areata. *Arch. Dermatol.*, *121*, 591–595.
371. Yates, V.M., King, C.M. and Harrop, B. (1984): Topical minoxidil in the treatment of alopecia areata. *Br. Med. J.*, *288*, 1087–1089.
372. Baral, J. (1985): Minoxidil and sudden death. *J. Am. Acad. Dermatol.*, *13*, 297–298.
373. Spindler, J.R. (1987): Deaths occurring during clinical studies of topical minoxidil. *J. Am. Acad. Dermatol.*, *16*, 725–729.
374. Olsen, E.A., Weiner, M.S., Delong, E.R. and Pinnell, S.R. (1985): Topical minoxidil in early male pattern baldness. *J. Am. Acad. Dermatol.*, *13*, 185–192.
375. Mucklow, E.S. (1988): Mercury as a health hazard. *Arch. Dis. Child.*, *63*, 1416–1417.
376. Störtebecker, P. (1989): Mercury poisoning from dental amalgam through a direct nose–brain transport. *Lancet*, *i*, 1207.
377. Nylander, M. (1986): Mercury in pituitary glands of dentists. *Lancet*, *1*, 442.
378. Aberer, W. (1991): Topical mercury should be banned — dangerous, outmoded, but still popular. *J. Am. Acad. Dermatol.*, *24*, 150–151.
379. Oliveira, D.B.G., Foster, G., Savill, J., Syme, P.D. and Taylor, A. (1987): Membranous nephropathy caused by mercury-containing skin lightening cream. *Postgrad. Med. J.*,. *63*, 303–304.
380. Winship, K.A. (1986): Organic mercury compounds and their toxicity. *Adv. Drug React. Acute Pois. Rev.*, *3*, 141–180.
381. Van Tittelboom, T., Mostin, M., Govaerts-Lepicard, M. and Knockaert, D. (1985): A propos de deux cas d'intoxication à la pommade mercurielle (PBIV). *J. Toxicol. Clin. Exper.*, *5*, 185–193.
382. De Bont, B., Lauwerys, R., Gavaerts, H. and Moulin, D. (1986): Yellow mercuric oxide ointment and mercury intoxication. *Eur. J. Pediatr.*, *145*, 217–218.
383. Rohyans, J., Watson, P.D., Wood, G.A., MacDonald, W.A. (1992): Mercury toxicity following merthiolate ear irrigations. *J. Pediatr.*, *104*, 311–313.
384. Bourgeois, M., Dooms-Goossens, A., Knockaert, D., Sprengers, D., van Boven, M. and van Tittelboom, T. (1986): Mercury intoxication after topical application of a metallic mercury ointment. *Dermatologica*, *172*, 48–51.
385. De la Cruz, F., Harper Brown, D., Leikin, J.B., Franklin, C. and Hryhrczuk, D.O. (1987): Iodine absorption after topical administration. *West. J. Med.*, *146* , 43–45.
386. Böckers, M., Klee, W., Bräuninger, W. and Bork, K. (1986): Das Hyperthyreoserisiko durch Lokaltherapie mit PVP-Jod. *Akta Dermatol.*, *12*, 155–157.
387. Prager, E.M. and Gardner, R.F. (1979): Iatrogenic hypothyroidism from topical iodine-containing medication. *West. J. Med.*, *130*, 553–555.
388. Rajatanavin, R., Safran, M., Stoller, W.A. et al. (1984): Five patients with iodine-induced hyperthyroidism. *Am. J. Med.*, *77*, 378–384.
389. Glöbel, B., Glöbel, H. and Andres, C. (1984): Resorption von Jod aus PVP-Jod-Präparaten nach Anwen-

dung am Menschen. *Dtsch. Med. Wschr., 37*, 1401–1404.
390. Kulick, M.I., Wong, R., Okarma, T.B., Falces, E. and Berkowitz, R.L. (1985): Prospective study of side effects associated with the use of silver sulfadiazine in severely burned patients. *Ann. Plast. Surg., 14*, 407–419.
391. Nangia, A.K., Hung, C.T. and Lim, J.K.C. (1987): Silver sulfadiazine in the management of burns — an update. *Drugs of Today, 23*, 21–30.
392. Wang, X-W., Zang, N.Z. and Zhang, O.Z. (1985): Tissue deposition of silver following topical use of silver sulphadiazine in extensive burns. *Burns, 11*, 197–201.
393. Fox, C.L. (1985): Letter to the Editor. *Burns, 11*, 306.
394. Pegg, S.P., Ramsay, K., Meldrum, L. and Laundy, M. (1979): Clinical comparison of maphenide and silver sulfadiazine. *Scand. J. Plast. Reconstr. Surg., 13*, 95–102.
395. Linn, P.S. Chang, T.W. (1980): Effect of silver sulfadizine on human protozoa. *Curr. Chemother. Infect. Dis. Proc. Intl. Cong. Chemother., 1*, 549–552.
396. Parrott, A.C. (1987): Transdermal scopolamine: effects of single and repeated patches upon psychological task performance. *Neuropsychobiology, 17*, 53–59.
397. Price, B.H. (1985): Anisocoria from scopolamine patches. *JAMA, 253*, 1561.
398. Lugaresi, A., Uncini, A., Chiarelli, F. and Cortelli, P. (1989): Transdermal scopolamine cycloplegia in juvenile diabetes. *Ital. J. Neurol. Sci., 10*, 203–205.
399. Mego, D.M., Omori, D.J.M. and Hanley, J.F. (1988): Transdermal scopolamine as a cause of transient psychosis in two elderly patients. *South. Med. J., 81*, 394–395.
400. Clissold, S.P. and Heel, R.C. (1985): Transdermal hyoscine (scoplamine). *Drugs., 29*, 189–207.
401. Sennhauser, F.H. and Schwarz, H.P. (1986): Toxic psychosis from transdermal scopolamine in a child. *Lancet, ii*, 1033.
402. Rozzini, R., Inzoli, M. and Trabucchi, M. (1988): Delirium from transdermal scopolamine in an elderly woman. *JAMA, 260*, 478.
403. Hamblin, J.E. and Martin, C.A. (1987): Transdermal patch poisoning. *Pediatrics, 79*, 161.
404. Metz, S., Klein, C. and Morton, N. (1987): Rebound hypertension after discontinuation of transdermal clonidine therapy. *Am. J. Med., 82*, 17–19.
405. Editorial (1987): Transdermal antihypertensive drugs. *Lancet, i*, 79–80.
406. Maibach, H.I. (1987): Oral substitution in patients sensitized by transdermal clonidine treatment. *Contact Dermatitis, 16*, 1–8.
407. Holdiness, M.R. (1989): A review of contact dermatitis associated with transdermal therapeutic systems. *Contact Dermatitis, 20*, 3–9.
408. Groth, H., Vetter, H., Knüsel, J. et al. (1983): Clonidin-TTS bei essentieller Hypertonie: Wirkung und Verträglichkeit. *Schweiz. Med. Wschr., 113*, 1841–1845.
409. Zawada, E.T. Jr., Jensen, R.A., Williams, L., Zeigler, D.W. and Kauker, M.L. (1989): Plasma dilution during transdermal clonidine antihypertensive monotherapy. *Int. J. Artif. Organs, 121*, 200–203.
410. Wiser, T.H., Kazakis, A.M. and La Civita, C.L. (1987): Transdermal clonidine: An association with recurrent herpes simplex and hyperpigmentation. *J. Am. Acad. Dermatol., 17*, 143–144.
411. Chetkowski, R.J., Meldrum, D.R., Steingold, K.A. et al. (1986): Biologic effects of transdermal estradiol. *New Engl. J. Med., 314*, 1615–1620.
412. Keller, P.J. (1989): Die perkutane Östrogen therapie in der Postmenopause. *Schweiz. Med. Wschr., 119*, 999–1004.
413. Utain, W.H. (1987): Transdermal estradiol overall safety profile. *Am. J. Obstet. Gynecol., 156*, 1335–1338.
414. Schwartz, B.K. and Clendenning, W.E. (1988): Allergic contact dermatitis from hydroxypropyl cellulose in a transdermal estradiol patch. *Contact Dermatitis, 18*, 106–107.
415. McBurney, E.I., Noel, S.B. and Collins, J.H. (1989): Contact dermatitis to transdermal estradiol system. *J. Am. Acad. Dermatol., 20*, 508–510.
416. Sentrakul, P., Chompootaweep, S., Sintupak, S. et al. (1991): Adverse skin reactions to transdermal oestradiol in tropical climate. *Maturitas, 13*, 151–154.
417. Gordon, C.R., Shupak, A., Doweck, I. and Spitzer, O. (1989): Allergic contact dermatitis caused by transdermal hyoscine. *Br. Med. J., 298*, 1220–1221.
418. Transdermal Nicotine Study Group. Transdermal nicotine for smoking cessation. *JAMA, 266*, 3133–3138.
419. Benowitz, N.L., Lake, T., Keller, K. and Lee, B.L. (1987): Prolonged absorption with development of tolerance to toxic effects after cutaneous exposure to nicotine. *Clin. Pharmacol. Ther., 42*, 119–120.
420. Editorial (1989): Transdermal testosterone. *Lancet, i*, 652.

421. Delanoe, D., Fougeyrollas, B., Meyer, L. and Thonneau, P. (1984): Androgenisation of female partners of men on medroxyprogesterone acetate/percutaneous testosterone contraception. *Lancet, i*, 276.
422. Harari, Z., Sommer, J. and Knobel, B. (1987): Multifocal contact dermatitis to Nitroderm TTS-5 with extensive postinflammatory hypermelanosis. *Dermatologica, 174*, 249–252.
423. Letendre, P.W., Barr, C. and Williams, K. (1984): Adverse dermatologic reaction to transdermal nitroglycerin. *Drug Intell. Clin. Pharm., 18*, 69–70.
424. Talley, J.D. and Crawley, I.S. (1985): Transdermal nitrate, penile erection, and spousal headache. *Ann. Intern. Med., 103*, 804.
425. Becker, G.J. and Hicks, M.E.(1986): Side effects of transdermal nitrate. *Ann. Intern. Med., 104*, 590.
426. Ewing, R.C., Janda, S.M. and Henann, N.E. (1989): Ageusia associated with transdermal nitroglycerin. *Clin Pharmacy, 8*, 146–147.
427. Kuhnen, R., Nitsch, J. and Luederitz, B. (1985): Explosion von Nitroplastern bei De-fibrillation. *Dtsch. Med. Wschr., 110*, 37.
428. Ledger, P.W. and Nichols, K.C. (1989): Transdermal drug delivery devices. *Clin Dermatol., 7*, 25–31.
429. Niedner, R. (1988): Transdermale therapeutische Systeme (TTS). *Hutarzt, 39*, 761–766.
430. Gottswinter, J.M., Korth-Schütz, S., Tümmers, B. and Ziegler, R. (1984): Gynäkomastie durch östrogenhaltiges Haarwasser. *Med. Klin., 79*, 181–183.
431. Anon. (1985): Estrogens in cosmetics. *Medical Letter on Drugs and Therapeutics, 23 August*, 54–55.
432. Plouvier, B., Lemoine, X., de Coninck, P., Bachet, J.L. and François, M. (1982): Effet antabuse lors de l'application d'un topique à base de monosulfirame. *Nouv. Press Med., 11*, 3209.
433. Stoll, D. and King, L.E. Jr. (1980): Disulfiram–alcohol skin reaction to beer-containing shampoo. *JAMA, 244*, 2045.
434. Schmied, E. and Levy, P.M. (1986): Transient rhabdomyolysis connected with topical use of 5-fluorouracil in a patient with psoriasis of the nails. *Dermatologica, 173*, 257–258.
435. Gross, B.G. (1984): Cardiac arrhythmias during phenol face peeling. *Plast. Reconstr. Surg., 73*, 590–594.
436. Botta, S.A., Straith, R.E. and Goodwin, H.H. (1988): Cardiac arrhythmias in phenol face peeling: a suggested protocol for prevention. *Aesth. Plast. Surg., 12*, 115–117.
437. Shawn, D.H. and McGuigan, M.A. (1984): Poisoning from dermal absorption of promethazine. *Can. Med. Assoc. J., 130*, 1460–1461.
438. Gonzalez Quintela, A. and Anuncibay, P.G. (1989): Topical promethazine intoxication. *DICP, The Annals of Pharmacotherapy, 23*, 89.
439. Lin, A.N., Reimer, R.J. and Carter, D.M. (1988): Sulfur revisited. *J. Am. Acad. Dermatol., 18*, 533–538.
440. Avila-Romay, A., Alvarez-Franco, M. and Ruiz-Maldonado, R. (1991): Therapeutic efficacy, secondary effects and patient acceptability of 10% sulfur in either pork fat or cold cream for the treatment of scabies. *Pediatr. Dermatol., 8*, 64–66.
441. Alleman, M.-H., Cosendey, B., Lob, M. and Saegesser, F. (1986): Saturnisme par résorption cutanée médicamenteuse. *Schweiz. Med. Wschr., 116*, 888–891.
442. Filloux, F. (1986): Toxic encephalopathy caused by topically applied diphenhydramine. *J. Pediatr., 108*, 1018–1020.
443. Patrarellea, P. (1987): Toxicité par la diphénhydramine contenue dans l'applications de Caladryl®. *Ann. Dermatol. Venereol., 114*, 494.
444. Reilly, J.F. and Weisse, M.E. (1990): Topically induced diphenhydramine toxicity. *J. Emerg. Med., 8*, 59–61.
445. Schou, H., Krogh, B. and Knudsen, F. (1987): Unexpected cocaine intoxication in a fourteen month old child following topical administration. *Clinical Toxiciol., 25*, 419–422.
446. Chiu, Y.C., Brecht, K., Das Gupta, D.S. and Mhoorn, E (1986): Myocardial infarction with topical cocaine anesthesia for nasal surgery. *Arch. Otolaryngol. Head Neck Surg., 112*, 988–990.
447. Tipton, G.A., De Witt, G.W. and Eisenstein, S.J. (1989): Topical TAC (tetracaine, adrenaline, cocaine) solution for local anesthesia in children: prescribing inconsistency and acute toxicity. *South. Med. J., 82*, 1344–1346.
448. Dailey, R.H. (1988): Fatality secondary to misuse of TAC solution. *Ann. Emerg. Med., 17*, 159–160.
449. Arditi, M. and Killner, M.S. (1987): Coma following use of rubbing alcohol for fever control. *Am. J. Dis. Child., 141*, 237–238.
450. McGrath, R.B. and Einterz, R. (1989): Absorption of topical isopropyl alcohol in an adult. *Critical Care Med., 1*, 1233.
451. Alleman, M.-H. (1986): Bleivergiftung durch Unguentum diachylon. *Schweiz. Med. Wschr., 116*, 888–890.

452. Cantarell, M.C., Fort, J., Camps, J. et al. (1987): Acute intoxication due to topical application of diethylene glycol. *Ann. Intern. Med., 106*, 478–479.
453. Blanc, D. and Deprez, Ph. (1990): Unusual adverse reaction to an acaricide. *Lancet, i*, 1291–1292.
454. Langer, J. (1989): Gynäkomastie durch Pharmaka. *Dermatosen, 37*, 121–147.
455. The Capsicain Study Group (1991): Treatment of painful diabetic neuropathy with topical capsicain. *Arch. Intern. Med., 151*, 2225–2229.
456. Cunliffe, W.J., Berth-Jones, J., Claudy, A. et al. (1992): Comparative study of calcipotriol (MC 903) ointment and betamethasone 17-valerate ointment in patients with psoriasis vulgaris. *J. Am. Acad. Dermatol., 26*, 736–743.
457. Dwyer, C. and Chapman, R.S. (1991): Calcipotriol and hypercalcaemia. *Lancet, 338*, 764–765.
458. Berth-Jones, J. and Hutchinson, P.E. (1992): Vitamin D analogues and psoriasis. *Br. J. Dermatol., 127*, 71–78.
459. Carmichael, A.J. and Foulds, I.S. (1992): Allergic contact dermatitis from oestadiol in oestrogen patches. *Contact Dermatitis, 26*, 194–195.
460. Committee on Drugs (1990): Clioquinol (iodochlorhydroxyquin, Vioform) and iodoquinol (diiodohydroxyquin): Blindness and neuropathy. *Pediatrics, 86*, 797–798.
461. Parker, L.U. and Bergfeld, W.F. (1991): Virilization secondary to topical testosterone. *Cleveland Clinic J. Med., 58*, 43–46.
462. Kern, F., Roberts, N. Ostlere, L., Langtry, J. and Staughton, R.C.D. (1991): Ammoniated mercury ointment as a cause of peripheral neuropathy. *Dermatologica, 183*, 280–282.
463. Trattner, A. and Ingber, A. (1992): Topical treatment with minoxidil 2% and smoking intolerance. *Ann. Pharmacother., 26*, 198–199.
464. Tomczak,R.L. and Hake, D.H. (1992): Near fatal systemic toxicity from local injection of podophyllin for pedal verrucae treatment. *J. Food Surg., 31*, 36–42.
465. Eldad, A., Neuman, A., Weinberg, A. et al. (1991): Silver sulphadiazine-induced haemolytic anaemia in a glucose-6-phosphatase dehydrogenase-deficient burn patient. *Burns, 17*, 430–432.

17. Systemic eczematous contact-type dermatitis medicamentosa

17.1 In patients with a delayed-type hypersensitivity to a certain drug, oral or parenteral administration of this drug or chemically related compounds may lead to the following side effects [69]:

1. Focal flares at sites of previous dermatitis (and sites of patch testing)
2. Dyshidrotic eruptions.
3. Generalized eruptions, including generalized urticaria and erythroderma. The distribution of such generalized eruptions may be diagnostic. The major feature may be a diffuse erythema of the buttocks ('baboon syndrome') and an erythema of the upper inner surface of the thighs, possibly accompanied by erythema of the axillae [67].
4. Vasculities [90,91]
5. Systemic effects such as nausea, vomiting, generalized itching, fever, headache, diarrhoea, hot flush and syncope.

Such reactions were termed "hämatogenes Kontaktekzem" by Binder [5], and "endogenic contact eczema" by Pirilä [42]. The title of this chapter is derived from the terminology used by Fisher [15].

Systemic contact dermatitis is usually caused by oral or intravenous administration of drugs, sometimes by inhalation [85], intravesical instillation [84] or application to the eye [82,83]. These effects may be provoked in some, but not all, sensitized subjects; they may be produced not only by the sensitizing drug, but also by chemically related substances.

The most frequent reactions are focal flares at sites of previous dermatitis or occasionally dyshidrotic eruptions, but generalized eruptions may occur, sometimes accompanied by systemic effects. Sometimes reactions are noted within hours after the administration of the allergen, which suggests that both an immediate and a delayed type of hypersensitivity may be involved.

A list of drugs that have caused systemic eczematous contact-type dermatitis is given in § 17.2.

17.2 Systematic eczematous contact-type dermatitis medicamentosa [69,94–96]

Delayed-type hypersensitivity to:	Use	Substance that caused the eruption	Comment	Ref.
alprenolol	β-adrenergic blocking agent	alprenolol		92
p-aminobenzoic acid	sunscreen	*p*-aminobenzoic acid		10
amlexanox	anti-allergic drug	amlexanox		109
antazoline	antihistamine	pyribenzamine	Both drugs are ethylenediamine derivatives	45
antazoline	antihistamine in eye drops	aminophylline	Antazoline is an ethylenediamine derivative; aminophylline contains ethylenediamine	58
arsphenamine	organic arsenical	neoarsphenamine	Inhalation of neoarsphenamine caused asthma, fever, urticaria and gastrointestinal symptoms	53
balsam Peru	various	orange marmalade, vanilla sugar, fruits and ices, balsam Peru		27 28 42 87
beclomethasone dipropionate	corticosteroid	prednisolone		103
benzocaine	local anaesthetic	chlorpropamide	Both drugs are PARA-compounds	59
betamethasone	corticosteroid	betamethasone		105
betamethasone valerate	corticosteroid	prednison		102
BHA (butylated hydroxyanisole)	antioxidant	butylated hydroxyanisole		18 44
BHT (butylated hydroxytoluene)	antioxidant	butylated hydroxyanisole and butylated hydroxytoluene		44
chloral hydrate	scalp medication, hypnotic	chloral hydrate		2 8
chlorpromazine	sedative	chlorpromazine	Accidental contact in a nurse	40
cinnamon oil	flavour	cinnamon oil	Flare-up of previous eczema of the hands	35
clonidine	antihypertensive drug	clonidine	Most patients sensitized to topical clonidine do *not* react to the oral drug	93

(continued)

§ **17.2** *(continuation)*

Delayed-type hypersensitivity to:	Use	Substance that caused the eruption	Comment	Ref.
corticosteroids (many)	corticosteroids	triamcinolone acetonide		103
corticosteroid (unclassified)	corticosteroid	methylprednisolone budesonide		75 101
desoxymethasone	corticosteroid	triamcinolone acetonide		104
dibucaine	local anaesthetic	*p*-aminophenylsulfamide		46
dimethyl sulfoxide (DMSO)	solvent, anticystitis drug	dimethyl sulfoxide	Systemic contact dermatitis from intravesical installation	86
diphenhydramine hydrochloride	antihistamine	diphenhydramine hydrochloride		57
disulfiram (tetra-ethylthiuram disulfide)	in cosmetics, foods and rubber industry	disulfiram (Antabuse®)	Both patients had been sensitized for previous disulfiram implants for alcoholism. Antabuse® may also cause a flare-up of dermatitis in patients allergic to nickel [72] or cobalt [73]	33 70
ephedrine	nasal decongestant	pseudoephedrine HCl, norephedrine citrate		80
ethyl alcohol	antiseptic, in beverages	alcohol		12
ethylenediamine	solvent, emulsifier, stabilizer	aminophylline	Aminophylline is a combination of theophylline and ethylenediamine	41 43 56
ethylenediamine		piperazine citrate/phosphate		4 6 65 66
formaldehyde	in plastics, textile finishes and antiperspirants	hexamethylene tetramine formaldehyde	Hexamethylene tetramine liberates formaldehyde in an acid medium	49 88
furazolidine	antimicrobial	furantoin	Accidental contact in food industry	29
gentamicin	antibiotic	sisomicin	Systematic contact dermatitis from topical eye lotion containing sisomicin	82
glycerin	vehicle ingredient	glycerol		24
halogenated hydroxyquinolines	antiseptics and antifungal drugs	halogenated hydroxyquinolines		13 36 48

(continued)

§ **17.2** *(continuation)*

Delayed-type hypersensitivity to:	Use	Substance that caused the eruption	Comment	Ref.
hydrocortisone	corticosteroid	hydrocortisone	Stimulation of the adrenal cortical hormone cortisol (= hydrocortisone) resulted in a similar skin reaction	78 107
mercurials	antiseptics	amalgam filling		30
methyl salicylate	anti-inflammatory drug	acetylsalicylic acid		25
mitomycin C	antitumour antibiotic	mitomycin C	Systemic contact dermatitis from intravesical instillation	84
neomycin	antibiotic	neomycin gentamicin		13 71 77 79
nystatin	antifungal drug	nystatin		9
oxyphenbutazone	non-steroidal anti-inflammatory drug	oxyphenbutazone		98
parabens	preservatives	parabens		1 32 76
penicillin	antibiotic	penicillin	Anaphylaxis may occur	51
peppermint oil	flavour	peppermint oil		11
pheniramine	antihistamine	diphenhydramine		14
phenylbutazone	anti-inflammatory drug	phenylbutazone	Cross-reaction to oxyphenbutazone	52
p-phenylenediamine	various	sulfonamides, procaine	Anaphylactic reactions have occurred	46
piperazine	vermifuge	hydroxyzine, buclizine	Accidental contact in pharmaceutical industry	7 21
prednisolon	corticosteroid	prednisolon		68
pristinamycin	antibiotic	pristinamycin	Anaphylaxis with stupor, vomiting and urticaria occurred [3]	3 97
procaine	local anaesthetic	procaine		20 46
promethazine	antihistamine	promethazine		47
propolis	folk medicine	propolis		99
propylene glycol	vehicle constituent	propylene glycol		19 24 55

(continued)

§ **17.2** *(continuation)*

Delayed-type hypersensitivity to:	Use	Substance that caused the eruption	Comment	Ref.
pyrazinobutazone	anti-inflammatory drug	pyrazinobutazone		106
quinine	in liquids and hair preparations	quinine		31
ribostamycin	antibiotic	neomycin		100
sorbic acid	preservative	sorbic acid		63
streptomycin	antibiotic	streptomycin	The drug was administered subcutaneously for desensitization	54
sulfanilamide	chemotherapeutic in vaginal cream	tolbutamide chlorpropamide carbutamide	Tolbutamide, chlorpropamide and carbutamide are sulfonylurea antidiabetic drugs	59 61
sulfonamide	chemotherapeutic	sulfonamides		46 50
tetramethylthiuram disulfide	rubber chemical	tetramethylthiuram disulfide	Oral provocation tests were positive. TMTD is also used as antifermentative agent in certain foods	22 60
thiomersal	antiseptic	thiomersal		37 81
		piroxicam	Systemic *photo*contact dermatitis	89
tobramycin	antibiotic	tobramycin	Systemic contact dermatitis from ocular instillation of tobra-mycin eye lotion	83
tromantadine	antiviral drug	amantadine	Possibility of systemic contact dermatitis mentioned; no case reports	17
virginiamycin	antibiotic	virginiamycin pristinamycin		34 74
vitamin B_1	vitamin	vitamin B_1	Accidental contact	26
vitamin B_{12}	treatment of pernicious anaemia	vitamin B_{12}	The patients were sensitized by the cobalt in vitamin B_{12}	16 38
vitamin C	vitamin	vitamin C		39

17.3 REFERENCES

1. Aeling, J.L. and Nuss, D.D. (1974): Systemic eczematous 'contact type' dermatitis medicamentosa caused by parabens. *Arch. Dermatol., 110*, 640.
2. Baer, R.L. and Sulzberger, M.B. (1938): Eczematous dermatitis due to chloralhydrate (following both oral administration and topical application). *J. Allergy, 9*, 519.
3. Baes, H. (1974): Allergic contact dermatitis to virginiamycin. *Dermatologica (Basel), 149*, 231.
4. Bernstein, J.E. and Lorincz, A.L. (1979): Ethylenediamine induced exfoliative erythroderma. *Arch. Dermatol., 112*, 156.
5. Binder, E. (1954): Über das hämatogene Kontaktekzem, *Archiv für Dermatol., 198*, 1.
6. Burry, J.N. (1978): Ethylenediamine sensitivity with a systemic reaction to piperazine citrate. *Contact Dermatitis, 4*, 380
7. Calas, E., Castelain, P.Y., Blanc, A. and Campana, J.M. (1975): Un nouveau cas de sensibilisation à la pipérazine. *Bull. Soc. Fr. Dermatol. Syph., 82*, 41.
8. Christianson, H.B. and Perry, H.O. (1956): Reactions to chloralhydrate. *Arch. Dermatol., 74*, 232.
9. Cronin, E. (1980): In: *Contact Dermatitis*, p. 233. Churchill Livingstone, Edinburgh.
10. Curtis, G.H. and Crawford, P.F. (1951): Cutaneous sensitivity to monoglycerol para-aminobenzoate: Cross-sensitization and bilateral eczematization. *Cleveland Clin. Quart., 18*, 35.
11. Dooms-Goossens, A., Degreef, H., Holvoet, C. and Maertens, M. (1977): Turpentine-induced hypersensitivity to peppermint oil. *Contact Dermatitis, 3*, 304.
12. Drevets, C.C and Seebohm, P.M. (1961): Dermatitis from alcohol, *J. Allergy, 32*, 277.
13. Ekelund, A.G. and Möller, H. (1969): Oral provocation in eczematous contact allergy to neomycin and hydroxyquinolones. *Acta Derm.-Venereol. (Stockh.), 49*, 422.
14. Epstein, E. (1949): Dermatitis due to antihistamine agents. *J. Invest. Dermatol., 12*, 151.
15. Fisher, A.A. (1966): Systemic eczematous 'contact-type' dermatitis medicamentosa. *Ann. Allergy, 24*, 406.
16. Fisher, A.A. (1972): Contact dermatitis: At home and abroad. *Cutis, 10*, 719.
17. Van Ketel, W.G. (1988). Systemic contact-type dermatitis by derivatives of adamantane? *Dermatosen, 36*, 23–24.
18. Fisher, A.A. (1975): Contact dermatitis due to food additives, *Cutis, 16*, 961.
19. Fisher, A.A. (1978): Propylene glycol dermatitis, *Cutis, 10*, 166.
20. Fisher, A.A. and Sturm, H.M. (1958): Procaine sensitivity. The relationship of the allergic eczematous contact-type to the urticarial-anaphylactoid variety. *Ann. Allergy, 16*, 593.
21. Fegert, S., cited by Fisher, A.A., (1973): In: *Contact Dermatitis*, 2nd Edition, p. 295. Lea and Febiger, Philadelphia.
22. Goitre, M., Bedello, P.G. and Cane, D. (1981): Allergic dermatitis and oral challenge to tetramethylthiuram disulphide. *Contact Dermatitis, 7*, 272.
23. Hannuksela, M. and Förstrom, L. (1976): Contact hypersensitivity to glycerol. *Contact Dermatitis, 2*, 291.
24. Hannuksela, M. and Förstrom, L. (1978): Reactions to peroral propyleneglycol. *Contact Dermatitis, 4*, 41.
25. Hindson, C. (1977): Contact eczema from methylsalicylate reproduced by oral aspirin (acetylsalicylic acid). *Contact Dermatitis, 3*, 348.
26. Hjorth, N. (1958): Contact dermatitis from Vitamin B1 (thiamine). Relapse after ingestion of thiamine. Cross-sensitization to co-carboxylase. *J. Invest. Dermatol., 30*, 261.
27. Hjorth, N. (1961): *Eczematous Allergy to Balsams, Allied Perfumes and Flavoring Agents*. Munkgaard, Copenhagen.
28. Hjorth, N. (1971): Allergy to balsams. *Spectrum, 8*, 97.
29. Jirásek, L. and Kalensky, J. (1975): Kontakní alergicky ekzém z krmnch smesi v zivocisné vyrobe. *Cz. Derm., 50*, 217.
30. Johnson, H.H., Schonberg, I.L. and Bach, N.F. (1951): Chronic atopic dermatitis with pronounced mercury sensitivity. Partial clearing after extraction of teeth containing mercury amalgam fillings. *Soc. Trans. A.M.A. Arch. Dermatol., 63*, 279.
31. Pevny, I. and Hutzler, D. (1988): Gruppenallergien bzw. Mehrfachreaktionen bei Patienten mit Allergie gegen Hydroxychinolin-Derivate. *Dermatosen, 36*, 91–98.
32. Kleinhans, D. and Knoth, W. (1973): On allergic contact dermatitis to virginiamycin. *Dermatologica (Basel), 146*, 320.
33. Minet, A., Frankart, M., Eggers, S. Lachapelle, J.M. and Bourlond, A. (1989): Réactions allergiques aux implants de disulfirame. *Ann. Dermatol. Venereol., 116*, 543–545.

34. Lachapelle, J.M. and Lamy, F. (1973): On allergic contact dermatitis to virginiamycin. *Dermatologica (Basel), 146*, 320.
35. Leifer, W. (1951): Contact dermatitis due to cinnamon. *Arch. Dermatol., 64*, 52.
36. Leifer, W. and Steiner, K. (1951): Studies in sensitization to halogenated hydroxyquinolines and related compounds. *J. Invest. Dermatol., 17*, 233.
37. MacKenzie, D. and Vlahcevic, Z.R. (1979): Adverse reaction to gammaglobulin due to hypersensitivity to thiomersal. *New Engl. J. Med., 290*, 749.
38. Malten, K.E. (1975): Flare reaction due to vitamin B12 in a patient with psioriasis and contact eczema. *Contact Dermatitis, 1*, 325.
39. Metz, J., Hundertmark, U. and Pevny, I. (1980): Vitamin C allergy of the delayed type. *Contact Dermatitis, 6*, 172.
40. Morris-Owen, R.M. (1963): 'Cover-Dose' management of contact sensitivity to chlorpromazine. *Br. J. Dermatol., 75*, 167.
41. Petrozzi, J.W. and Shore, R.N. (1976): Generalized exfoliative dermatitis from ethylenediamine. *Arch. Dermatol., 112*, 525.
42. Pirilä, V. (1970): Endogenic contact eczema. *Allergie Asthma, 16*, 15.
43. Provost, T.T. and Field Jillson, O. (1967): Ethylene diamine contact dermatitis. *Arch Derm., 96*, 231.
44. Roed-Petersen, J. and Hjorth, N. (1976): Contact dermatitis from antioxidants. *Br. J. Dermatol., 94*, 233.
45. Sherman, W.B. and Cooke, R.A. (1950): Dermatitis following the use of pyribenzamine and Antistine. *J. Allergy, 21*, 63.
46. Sidi, E. and Dobkevitch-Morrill, S. (1951): The injection- and ingestion test in cross-sensitization to the ParaGroup. *J. Invest. Dermatol., 16*, 299.
47. Sidi, E., Hincky, M. and Gervais, A. (1955): Allergic sensitization and photosensitization to phenergan cream. *J. Invest. Dermatol., 24*, 345.
48. Skog, E. (1975): Systemic eczematous contact-type dermatitis induced by iodochlorhydroxyquin and chloroquine phosphate. *Contact Dermatitis, 1*, 187.
49. Sulzberger, M.B. (1940): *Dermatologic Allergy*, p. 380. Charles C. thomas, Springfield, Illinois.
50. Sulzberger, M.B., Kanof, A., Baer, R.L. and Löwenberg, C. (1947): Sensitization by topical application of sulfonamides. *J. Allergy, 18*, 92.
51. Vickers, H.R. Bagratuni, L. and Alexander, S. (1958): Dermatitis caused by penicillin milk. *Lancet, 61*, 351.
52. Fernández de Corres, L., Bernaola, G., Lobera, T., Leanizbarrutia, I. and Muñoz, D. (1986): Allergy from pyrazoline derivatives. *Contact Dermatitis, 14*: 249–250.
53. Vuletic, A. (1934): Über Salvarsanüberempfindlichkeit mit akuter Salvarsan-Intoxikation infolge beruflicher Benetzungen der Finger mit Salvarsanlösungen. *Arch. Dermatol. Symph. (Berl.), 169*, 436.
54. Wilson, H.T.H. (1958): Streptomycin dermatitis in nurses. *Br. Med. J., 1*, 1378.
55. Andersen, K.E. and Storrs, F. (1982): Hautreizungen durch Propylenglykol. *Hautarzt, 33*, 12.
56. Neumann, H. (1983): Allergische und toxische Nebenwirkungen von Ethylendiamin. *Allergologie, 6*, 27.
57. Coskey, R.J. (1983): Contact dermatitis caused by diphenhydramine hydrochloride. *J. Am. Acad. Dermatol., 8*, 204.
58. Berman, B.A. and Ross, R.N. (1983): Ethylenediamine: Systemic eczematous contact-type dermatitis, *Cutis, 29*, 551.
59. Fisher, A.A. (1982): Systemic contact dermatitis from Orinase® and Diabinese® in diabetics with para-amino hypersensitivity, *Cutis, 29*, 551.
60. Goitre, M., Bedello, P.G. and Cane, D. (1981): Allergic dermatitis and oral challenge to tetramethylthiuram disulphide. *Contact Dermatitis, 7*, 273.
61. Angelini, G. and Meneghini, C.L. (1981): Oral tests in contact allergy to para-amino compounds. *Contact Dermatitis, 7*, 311.
62. Fisher, A.A. (1980): The antihistamines. *J. Am. Acad. Dermatol., 3*, 303.
63. Röckl, H. and Pevny, I. (1976): *Fortschritte der praktischen Dermatologie und Venereologie*. Springer Verlag, Berlin.
64. King, C.M. and Beck, M. (1983): Oral promethazine hydrochloride in ethylenediamine-sensitive patients. *Contact Dermatitis, 9*, 444.
65. Price, M.L. and Hall-Smith, S.P. (1984): Allergy to piperazine in a patient sensitive to ethylenediamine. *Contact Dermatitis, 10*, 120.
66. Wright, S. and Harman, R.R.M. (1983): Ethylenediamine and piperazine sensitivity. *Br. Med. J., 287*, 463.

67. Andersen, K.E., Hjorth, N. and Menné, T. (1984): The baboon syndrome: systemically induced allergic contact dermatitis. *Contact Dermatitis, 10*, 97.
68. Pambor, M. (1984): Kortikosteroid-Kontaktallergie. *Dt. Gesndh.-Wesen, 39*, 276.
69. Menné, T. and Maibach, H.I. (1987): Systemic contact allergy: reactions. *Seminars in Dermatology, 6*, 108–118.
70. van Hecke, E. and Vermander, F. (1984): Allergic contact dermatitis by oral disulfiram. *Contact Dermatitis, 10*, 254.
71. Menné, T. and Weismann, K. (1984): Hämatogenes Kontaktekzem nach oraler Gabe von Neomyzin. *Hautarzt, 35*, 319.
72. Kaaber, K., Menné, T., Tjell, J.C. and Veien, N. (1979): Antabuse® treatment of nickel dermatitis. Chelation — a new principle in the treatment of nickel dermatitis. *Contact Dermatitis, 5*, 221.
73. Menné, T. (1985): Flare-up of cobalt dermatitis from Antabuse® treatment. *Contact Dermatitis, 12*, 53.
74. Pilette, M., Claudet, J.P., Muller, C. and Lorette, G. (1990): Toxicodermie à la Pristinamycine après sensibilisation à la virginiamycine topique. *Allergie Immunol., 22*, 197.
75. Fernandez de Corres, L., Bernaola, G., Urritia, I. and Munoz, D. (1990): Allergic dermatitis from systemic treatment with corticosteroids. *Contact Dermatitis, 22*, 104–106.
76. Carradori, S., Peluso, A.M. and Faccioli, M. (1990): Systemic contact dermatitis due to parabens. *Contact Dermatitis, 22*, 238–239.
77. Guin, J.D. and Philips, D. (1989): Erythroderma from systemic contact dermatitis: a complication of systemic gentamicin in a patient with contact allergy to neomycin. *Cutis, 43*, 564–567.
78. Lauerma, A.I., Reitamo, S. and Maibach, H.I. (1991): Systemic hydrocortisone/cortisol induces allergic skin reactions in presensitized subjects. *J. Am. Acad. Dermatol., 24*, 182–185.
79. Ghadially, R. and Ramsay, C.A. (1988): Gentamicin: Systemic exposure to a contact allergen. *J. Am. Acad. Dermatol., 19*, 428–430.
80. Tomb, R.R., Lepoittevin, J.-P., Espinassouze, F., Heid, E. and Foussereau, J. (1991). Systemic contact dermatitis from pseudoephedrine. *Contact Dermatitis, 24*, 86–88.
81. Pierchalla, P., Petri, H., Rüping, K.-W. and Stary, A. (1987): Urtikarielle Reaktion nach Injektion von H.-B. Vax bei Sensibilisierung auf Thiomersal (merthiolat). *Allergologie, 10*: 97–99.
82. Katayama, I. and Nishioka, K. (1987): Systemic contact dermatitis medicamentosa induced by topical eye lotion (sisomicin) in a patient with corneal allograft. *Arch. Dermatol., 123*, 436–437.
83. Tanaki, I., Sasaki, T., Oozeki, H. et al. (1978): Clinical studies in tobramycin eye lotion. *Jpn. Rev. Clin. Opthalmol., 72*, 822–828.
84. de Groot, A.C. and Conemans, J.M.H. (1991): Systemic allergic contact dermatitis from intra-vesical instillation of the antitumor antibiotic mitomycin C. *Contact Dermatitis, 24*, 201–209.
85. Nakayama, H., Niki, F., Shona, M. et al. (1983): Mercury exanthem. *Contact Dermatitis, 9*, 411–417.
86. Nishimura, M. and Takano, Y. (1988): Systemic contact dermatitis medicamentosa occurring after intravesical dimethyl sulfoxide treatment for interstitial cystitis. *Arch. Dermatol., 124*, 182–183.
87. Veien, N.K., Hattel, T., Justesen, O. and Nørholm, N. (1985): Oral challenge with balsam of Peru. *Contact Dermatitis, 12*, 104–107.
88. Ring, J. (1986): Exacerbation of eczema by formalin-containing hepatitis B vaccine in formaldehyde-allergic patients. *Lancet, 2*: 522–533.
89. Serrano, G., Bonillo, J., Aliaga, A., Cuadra, J., Pujol, C., Pelufo, C., Cervera, P. and Miranda, M.A. (1990): Piroxicam-induced potosensitivity and contact sensitivity to thiosalicylic acid. *J. Am. Acad. Dermatol., 23*, 479–483.
90. Kaaber, K., Menné, T., Tjell, J.C. et al. (1979): Antabuse treatment of nickel dermatitis. Chelation — a new principle in the treatment of nickel dermatitis. *Contact Dermatitis, 5*: 221–228.
91. Bruynzeel, D.P., van den Hoogenband, H.M. and Koedijk, F. (1984): Purpuric vasculitis-like eruption in a patient sensitive to balsam of Peru. *Contact Dermatitis, 11*: 207–209.
92. Ekenvall, L. and Forsbeck, M. (1978): Contact eczema produced by a β-adrenergic blocking agent (alprenolol). *Contact Dermatitis, 4*, 190–194.
93. Maibach, H.I. (1987): Oral substitution in patients sensitized by transdermal clonidine treatment. *Contact Dermatitis, 16*, 1–9.
94. Meneghini, C.L., Angelini, G. (1985): Eczémas de contact allergiques et réactions par voie générale à l'allergène. *Méd. Hyg., 43*, 879–886.
95. Aquilina, C.H. and Sayag, J. (1989): Eczémas par réactogènes internes. *Ann. Dermatol. Venereol., 116*, 753–765.

17. Systemic eczematous contact-type dermatitis medicamentosa

96. Menné, T., Veien, N.K. and Maibach, H.I. (1989): Systemic contact-type dermatitis due to drugs. *Semin. Dermatol., 8*, 144–148.
97. Bernard, P., Fayol, J., Bonnafoux, A. et al. (1988): Toxicodermies après prise orale de pristinamycine. *Ann. Dermatol. Venereol., 115*, 63–66.
98. Ebner, H. (1986): Beitrag zur Kenntnis der Kontaktallergie auf nicht-steroidale Antiphlogistica und Rheumamittel. *Akt. Dermatol., 12*, 197–199.
99. Rudzki, E., Grzywa, Z. and Pomorski, Z. (1985): New data on dermatitis from propolis. *Contact Dermatitis, 13*, 198–199.
100. Puig, L.L., Abadias, M. and Alomar, A. (1989): Erythroderma due to ribostamycin. *Contact Dermatitis, 21*, 79–82.
101. Fernandez de Corrés, L., Urrutia, I., Audicana, M., Echechipia, S. and Gastaminza, G. (1991): Erythroderma after intravenous injection of methylprednisolone. *Contact Dermatitis, 25*, 68–69.
102. Goh, C.L. (1989): Cross-sensitivity to multiple topical corticosteroids. *Contact Dermatitis, 26*, 65–67.
103. English, J.S.C., Ford, G., Beck, M.H. and Rycroft, R.J.G. (1990): Allergic contact dermatitis from topical and systemic steroids. *Contact Dermatitis, 23*, 196–197.
104. Brambilla, L., Boneschi, V., Chiappino, G., Fossati, S. and Pigatto, P.D. (1989): Allergic reactions to topical desoxymethasone and oral triamcinolone. *Contact Dermatitis, 21*, 272–273.
105. Maucher, O.M., Faber, M., Knipper, H., Kirchner, S. and Schöpf, E. (1987): Kortikoidallergie. *Hautarzt, 38*, 577–582.
106. Bris, J.M.D., Montanes, M.A., Candela, M.S. and Diez, A.G. (1992): Contact sensitivity to pyrazinobutazone (Carudol®) with positive oral provocation test. *Contact Dermatitis, 26*, 355.
107. Lauerma, A.I. (1992): Contact hypersensitivity to glucocorticosteroids. *Am. J. Contact Dermatitis, 3*, 112–132.
108. Wilkinson, S.M., Smith, A.G. and English, J.S.C. (1992): Erythroderma following the intradermal injection of the corticosteroid budesonide. *Contact Dermatitis, 27*, 121–122.
109. Hayakawa, R., Ogino, Y., Aris, K., Matsunaga, K. (1992): Systemic contact dermatitis due to amlexanox. *Contact Dermatitis, 27*, 122–123.

18. Side effects of photochemotherapy

PUVA THERAPY

18.1 In photochemotherapy, therapeutic advantage is taken of the interaction of a phototoxic drug [167] and light, usually an undesirable effect, for the treatment of cutaneous disorders. Classic examples are the Goeckerman regimen for psoriasis, in which the application of tar preparations (the photosensitizer) is followed by irradiation with ultraviolet B (UVB) [28] and the treatment of vitiligo with psoralens and light. More recently, psoralen and ultraviolet A (PUVA) therapy was introduced for the treatment of various dermatoses, especially psoriasis and mycosis fungoides [226]; other indications have included pustulosis palmoplantaris [131], dyshidrotic eczema [132], urticaria pigmentosa [87], hyperkeratotic dermatitis of the palms [86], alopecia areata [136], atopic eczema [137], polymorphous light eruption [138], pityriasis lichenoides, parapsoriasis en plaques, lichen planus, disseminated cutaneous sarcoid, solar urticaria [227], lichenoid graft-versus-host disease and disseminated granuloma annulare [20].

The psoralen is usually 8-methoxypsoralen (methoxsalen), but trimethyl psoralen (trioxsalen) is also used, especially in Scandinavia. The drug is usually administered per os, but bath-water delivery of 8-MOP may be preferred in those who do not tolerate oral 8-MOP. Bath-water delivery of 8-MOP has another advantage in that the cumulative UVA dose is far less than with oral administration [234]; this may result in diminished carcinogenicity of bath PUVA compared with the oral form [93].

Side effects of PUVA therapy (For reviews, *see* [19,236])

18.2 Melski et al. [49] provided a report on a large-scale collaborative study in which 1308 patients with psoriasis were treated 2 to 3 times a week with oral 8-methoxy-psoralen (8-MOP) photochemotherapy; 41,000 courses of treatment were analyzed.

The acute side effects observed are summarized in § 18.3. The results are expressed by the authors as a percentage of treatments rather than of patients. Serious acute reactions such as phototoxicity with erythema and blistering, nausea, or pruritus, requiring discontinuation of therapy, were rare. Dizziness, depression and headache were occasional complications of the treatment. The major limiting factor is erythema; however, this is dose-related with respect to both drug and light and is therefore predictable and avoidable. Patients using trimethylpsoralen bath PUVA may acquire linear phototoxicity of parts of the body corresponding to the bath water level, due to the insolubility of trimethylpsoralen powder in water resulting in a higher concentration of the drug at water level [94].

18.3 Immediate side effects after PUVA*

Side effect	Percent of treatments	Side effect	Percent of treatments
Erythema/burns — local or diffuse		Nausea after last treatment	3.21
– any grade	9.77	– interfered with activity	0.64
– localized edema or blistering	0.24	– at least 12 hour duration	0.37
– diffuse marked red or edema	1.12	– with vomiting	0.30
– caused missed treatment	1.15	– caused missed treatment	0.08
Pruritus	14.08	Headache	2.00
– generalized	6.43	– continuous	1.25
– interfered with sleep	5.13	– interfered with activity	0.36
– for more than 3 days	5.02	– at least 24 hour duration	0.21
– interfered with activity	1.74	– caused missed treatment	0.02
– caused missed treatment	0.44		
Dizziness	1.52		
– continuous	0.74		
– interfered with activity	0.38		
– at least 8 hour duration	0.29		
– caused missed treatment	0.02		

*Side effects expressed as a percentage of treatments. Neither the major categories nor the subcategories are mutually exclusive. For example, one episode of nausea may cause a missed treatment, result in vomiting, last for more than 12 hours, and interfere with activities.

MALIGNANCIES

Cutaneous carcinogenicity

18.4 Potential hazards of PUVA therapy such as cutaneous aging, actinic damage and especially cutaneous carcinogenicity, are major concerns in the appraisal of the safety of this valuable therapeutic modality. Skin cancer in mice has been provoked by 8-MOP and ultraviolet A [22], and carcinogenicity of PUVA in man could therefore be anticipated.

One of the major difficulties in determining the oncogenic risks of PUVA in man is the long latency period that is characteristic of the generation of radiation-induced tumours. By the time of writing (1993), several long-term follow-up studies have clarified the issue, and PUVA appears to be both a promoter of squamous cell carcinoma in patients with certain risk factors as well as a primary carcinogen.

Non-melanoma skin cancers

18.5 In 1979, Stern et al. [72] were the first to report an increased incidence of non-melanoma skin cancers, especially squamous cell carcinomas, in patients treated with PUVA. The observed incidence of squamous cell carcinomas was 9.1 times higher than could be expected on the basis of age, sex and geographic location

[127]. The squamous cells occurred frequently on relatively non-exposed areas of the body, such as the trunk and legs. The frequency of squamous cell carcinomas in patients with a history of cutaneous carcinogens was significantly greater after 80 PUVA treatments, when compared with the frequency after fewer than 80 treatments. These data suggested that PUVA may act as a *promoter* of squamous cell carcinoma in human subjects previously exposed to cutaneous carcinogens, and that this effect increases with higher numbers of PUVA treatment [72,127]. Since then, several follow-up studies for the detection of non-melanoma skin cancer have been published, mostly from the USA and from Europe [38,43,65,129, 186–194,196-201,204], some from other countries [195,203]. Most of the reports from the USA described an increased incidence of squamous cell carcinoma [187,188,191]. Two of the American groups showed a substantial dose-related increase, suggesting that PUVA is also a *primary carcinogen* [187,188,191]. This was in contrast with most of the European studies, which only reported an increased incidence of squamous cell carcinomas related to previous exposure to other carcinogens such as X-ray therapy, arsenic or methotrexate and to skin cancer prior to PUVA treatment [189,190,193,204], or no increased incidence at all [192,194–197]. The different skin cancer risks found in the USA and in Europe was explained by different treatment protocols [32]. In Europe, a PUVA schedule is used which provides for fewer, but higher, single-dose treatments as compared with the schedule used in the USA. Recently, however, a Dutch group also found a dose-related increase in the incidence of squamous cell carcinomas (12-fold increased risk) [201]. A positive correlation was observed between the development of squamous cell carcinomas and the total UVA dosage, the age of the patient at the start of PUVA treatment and a history of arsenic use. The average time period between the start of PUVA and the diagnosis of the first malignant skin tumour was 6.0 years for squamous cell carcinoma. This long latency period may explain why an increased incidence of squamous cell carcinomas was not observed in several previous studies, in which the follow-up period was shorter than 6 years [201]. In accordance with studies from the USA [187–188], a trend towards an increased occurrence of skin tumours on non-exposed skin was found, suggestive of a primary carcinogenic effect of PUVA treatment. The carcinogenic potential of PUVA was also most recently confirmed in the largest epidemiological study performed thus far [205], 4799 Swedish patients were followed up for 7 years. A dose-dependent increase in the risk of squamous cell cancer of the skin was observed. Male patients who had received more than 200 treatments had over 30 times the incidence of squamous cell cancer found in the general population [205]. A site particularly susceptible to the development of squamous cell carcinomas appears to be the male genitals [200,202]. In patients exposed to high levels of PUVA, the incidence of invasive squamous-cell carcinoma was found to be 286 times that in the general population and 16 times that in patients exposed to low levels (200). The skin of the scrotum, foreskin, and glans is thin and tans poorly, and therefore a far higher proportion of incident ultraviolet radiation may reach the germinative layer there than at other sites. Therefore it is advisable to shield the genitals that are not affected by psoriasis and to limit exposure of the involved genitalia [200,202]. The risk of the development of basal cell carcinomas in patients treated with PUVA is also increased, albeit to a lesser degree. The correlation with total UVA dosage is less clear, but exposure to other carcinogenic agents such as arsenicals may increase the risk of basal cell carcinomas [191,201].

It may be concluded that PUVA can act both as a promoter of non-melanoma skin cancers in patients with risk factors (previous use of arsenic, previous cancer, previous treatment with methotrexate, X-ray therapy, skin type I) and as a primary carcinogen, especially in patients receiving high total dosage of Ultraviolet A.

In order to limit risk, it has been suggested that patients with a history of therapeutic ionizing radiation, arsenic exposure, or previous skin cancer be excluded from PUVA therapy and those with type I skin be watched closely. Male genital sites not involved with psoriasis should be carefully shielded [191].

Malignant Melanoma

18.6 Several isolated case reports of malignant melanoma arising during PUVA therapy have been documented [9,25,57,79,206]. In epidemiological studies, however, no increased incidences of malignant melanoma have been observed. No malignant potential has as yet been ascribed to PUVA-induced freckles and other pigmentation side effects (§ 18.12).

Epidermal dystrophy and actinic keratoses

18.7 Epidermal dystrophy is defined as any alteration in cell size or arrangement to a degree not seen in pretreatment control specimens from sunlight-exposed or sunlight-protected clinically uninvolved skin [113]. Epidermal dystrophy, which has histologic features resembling those seen in actinic keratoses, has been reported in association with PUVA therapy by several investigators [37,96,122, 139,140]. No such changes were found in the study of Levin et al. [92]. In a large series [122], epidermal dystrophy was a common occurrence in PUVA-treated patients. In 57% of 107 patients dystrophic changes in keratinocytes were seen, more commonly in patients previously treated with arsenic. Its incidence does not increase with prolonged PUVA therapy [96], but it has been shown that epidermal dystrophy may persist long after cessation of therapy [141].

Abel et al. [96] have noted focal dystrophy of epidermal cells in more than half of 70 patients one year or more following the onset of PUVA therapy, in clinically uninvolved skin of sunlight-protected and sunlight-exposed areas. Prior to therapy control biopsies had shown no such changes. Although it is not currently known whether this type of dystrophy is a precursor of keratosis or skin cancer, the possibility that it reflects a precancerous change should be recognized.

In 104 PUVA-treated patients returning for dermatologic follow-up after the first year of therapy, 17 (16.3%) developed actinic keratoses during the course of, or following the cessation of, treatment with PUVA [96]. As in the majority of patients multiple keratoses occurred in sun-exposed areas, it has been suggested that PUVA accelerates or promotes actinically induced lesions. However, keratoses have also been observed on non-exposed skin, suggesting a primary relationship between the development of these lesions and PUVA treatment. These 'PUVA-keratoses' show a histological resemblance to the usually highly differentiated squamous cell carcinomas seen in PUVA treated patients. Currently it is unknown whether PUVA-keratoses represent premalignant lesions [201].

In a large European study the percentage of patients developing actinic keratoses was 2.6 [190].

The development of multiple actinic keratoses inpatients with no risk factors for cutaneous (pre)malignancies has been reported in single cases [212,213].

To determine the extent of clinical actinic damage that occurred in association with exposure to oral methoxysalen photochemotherapy (PUVA), dermatologists at 16 university centres assessed the wrinkling, teleagiectasia, and altered skin markings on the buttocks and the dorsa of the hands among 1380 patients treated with PUVA. These changes are similar to those seen in skin that is chronically exposed to sunlight. After more than 5 years of prospective study, patients with psoriasis exposed to PUVA showed a significant dose-dependent increase in the prevalence of clinical actinic degeneration of the skin of the buttocks. The prevalence of moderate or severe change among those patients exposed to high doses of PUVA (more than 160 treatments) was low (11%). The degree of increased clinical actinic degeneration noted on the dorsa of the hands was significantly related to total exposure to PUVA. These findings indicate that long-term PUVA exposure is associated with an increase in clinical actinic degeneration of the skin. However, the magnitude of this increase is small and, after more than 5 years, is of limited clinical consequence to most patients [214].

Internal malignancies

18.8 There have been occasional published reports of patients developing preleukaemia [81], acute myeloid leukaemia [207], myelomonocytic leukaemia [209] and myelodysplastic syndrome [81] following PUVA therapy for psoriasis. None of these patients had preceding risk factors. One patient known to have chronic myelomonocytic leukaemia transformed to acute myeloid leukaemia during PUVA [209]. These events may all have been purely coincidental and not causally related to PUVA. In a large-scale epidemiological study among 4799 Swedish patients treated with PUVA [205], a significant increase in incidence of respiratory cancer was found in both men and women, pancreatic cancer in men, and kidney and colonic cancer in women. The increased risk of respiratory cancer may be related to smoking habits [210]. The other malignancies were not ascribed to PUVA, but an increased risk of colonic cancer among psoriatics has been reported [211]. In one patient suffering from actinic reticuloid, treated for 15 months with PUVA, non-mycosis fungoides T cell lymphoma developed. According to the authors the use of PUVA may have predisposed the patient to the development of frank malignancy [221].

THE EYES

Cataract formation

18.9 Experimental studies have clearly shown that animals treated with psoralens in high doses and exposed to ultraviolet light develop cataracts [13,148]. Therefore, the possible development of cataracts in PUVA-treated patients has always been one of the major concerns regarding the long-term safety of oral photochemotherapy.

8-MOP has been demonstrated in human lenses 12 hours after the ingestion of a single therapeutic dose [149]. From animal studies it has been shown that in the absence of photic stimuli, the 8-MOP will diffuse out of the lens within 24 hours. In the presence of photic stimuli (ambient room light as well as direct UV (360 nm) irradiation) however, there is an enhancement of lenticular fluorescence and phosphorescence. Photoaddition products (at 360 nm) can be generated with tryptophan as well as with lens proteins (*in vitro*) in the presence of 8-MOP and oxygen. Such a reaction *in vivo* would result in permanent retention of the photoproduct within the ocular lens, thus predisposing to cataract formation. Indeed, one such photoproduct has been demonstrated in material derived from patients who required cataract surgery after long-term PUVA therapy [102]. These data provide objective evidence that PUVA therapy can generate specific photoproducts within the human ocular lens. These photoproducts have been shown to be associated with experimental PUVA cataracts in rats; this evidence substantiates reports of (presumptive) PUVA cataracts.

Aside from the lens, 8-MOP can be found in other ocular tissues, including the corneal epithelium, the ciliary processes, and the retina (of young animal eyes) after intraperitoneal administration [85]. Because the *mature* ocular lens is an effective filter for UVA radiation in man there can be no photobinding of 8-MOP in the mature retina. However, UVA radiation can penetrate to the retina in aphakic and pseudophakic patients. It has also been suggested that a larger proportion of UVA can penetrate the lens of very young patients [119]. Lerman [85,119] warns that PUVA therapy in such individuals can result in increasing accumulation of photoproducts in the lens and retina; subtle retinal changes in young children on long-term PUVA might occur, which may be undetectable in standard eye examination [119].

18.10 From the inception of PUVA therapy it has repeatedly been stressed that it is essential to shield the psoralen-photosensitized eye adequately from UVA radiation in order to prevent the development of cataracts. Recommendations on eye protection have been published by a subcommittee of the Task Forces of Psoriasis and Photobiology [114]. According to these recommendations, patients must wear UVA-blocking wraparound glasses on each day of PUVA treatment, from the time of ingestion of the drug. Preferably, these glasses should also be worn on the second day. Of course, while in the PUVA chamber, the eyes must be totally covered with UVA-opaque goggles provided by the PUVA therapist. Environmental sources of UVA have been investigated [159]. With the demonstration of presumed PUVA cataracts patient compliance in wearing their UVA blocking glasses for the advised period of time is essential and this should repeatedly be stressed to the patient. Convenient compliance is much easier with the availability of clear, cosmetically acceptable UVA-blocking spectacles [150]. Unfortunately, many patients are either unwilling or unable to wear such glasses for extended periods, and this poses considerable potential risk of cataracts in PUVA-treated patients.

Clinical studies and case reports

In the study of Rönnerfält et al. [103] 46 patients with severe psoriasis maintained on long-term PUVA therapy have been followed up for 6.5 years after the initiation of treatment. Repeated ophthalmological examinations were performed; no ocular side effects attributed to the photochemotherapy were revealed during this period.

Hammershøy and Jessen [104] examined 96 patients treated with PUVA between 1975 and 1980; no patient developed cataract during the PUVA treatment period and their findings were found to correspond to those in a (control) standard population. In an American 5-year prospective study involving 1299 patients treated with PUVA for psoriasis, no significant dose-dependent increase in the risk of developing symptomatic cataracts was found [37]. However, a small increase in the risk for development of nuclear sclerosis and posterior subcapsular opacities among patients who received at least 100 PUVA treatments, compared with patients with fewer than 100 treatments (relative risk = 2.3 and 3.0, respectively), was found [37]. Several cases of cataracts presumably or probably induced by PUVA therapy have been reported [14,52,102,118,119]. From animal studies it has been reported that the anterior cortical location of punctate lens opacities is characteristic of ocular injury induced by psoralen photosensitization [13]. The first report of a presumptive PUVA cataract was reported in 1980 [14]. Kasick et al. [118] have reported bilateral punctate cortical opacities in two PUVA-treated patients who had normal eye examinations prior to therapy. Lerman [52,102,119] has reported additional cases; most of these patients had histories of inadequate ocular protection [52].

Boukes and Bruynzeel [2] investigated 340 patients treated with PUVA. In 20, cataract development was encountered during the period of investigation. In most of these, older than 50 years, the cataractic growth was attributed to ageing effects. In 3 patients, aged 28, 30 and 35 years, the occurrence of lens capacities was considered to be “at least partly due to the effect of PUVA” [2].

Careful monitoring of ocular changes is recommended not only in patients currently receiving photochemotherapy, but also in those who have discontinued PUVA treatment [118], since the latency period of symptomatic ocular abnormalities may be longer than the duration of reported studies [37,52].

With adequate eye protection, PUVA therapy is accompanied by, at most, a small risk of eye damage. The necessity of wearing adequate eye protection for at least 12 hours after psoralen ingestion should continue to be stressed to patients [19,37, 109,196].

Other ocular side effects

18.11 Of 15 patients treated with PUVA, 8 were found to have a mild form of photokeratoconjunctivitis [111]. The ocular manifestations included photophobia, conjunctivitis, keratitis and dry eyes. Tear break-up time was reduced significantly immediately after treatment in two patients, but returned to normal 8 hours later.

Keratitis may occur when patients neglect to wear their goggles. Visual field defects to PUVA therapy have been described in 3 patients [115]. One patient developed nausea and photophobia, with a central scotoma which lasted up to 20 minutes before disappearing to the left of her visual field. These episodes were dose-dependent and reproducible on challenge with an increase in psoralen dosage. Two other patients experienced nausea and tunnel vision lasting for 5 minutes and 8 hours, respectively; in one, attacks of sudden pain in one eye were concomitant. These symptoms were also dose-related [115].

THE SKIN

Pigmentary changes

18.12 The diffuse tanning following PUVA therapy indicates that stimulation of melanocytes has occurred. The prolonged nature of PUVA-induced tanning might be attributed in part to a change in the distribution of melanosomes from an aggregated to a large single, dispersed pattern in the keratinocytes. Several other forms of pigment alterations have been described in patients undergoing oral photochemotherapy [113].

PUVA lentigines

PUVA lentigines [112] appear to be the commonest long-term side effect of PUVA treatment, occurring in more than 40% of patients after 2–3 years of extensive PUVA therapy (or earlier, [161]) with more than 100 exposures and a total UVA dose of more than 1000 J/cm^2 [112,128,196]. Both sexes are said to be equally affected [112], but a male preponderance has been observed by some [161]. PUVA lentigines are always located on the shoulders and the upper back and, in most cases, also on the arms and legs. There is a direct correlation with the cumulative UVA dose and an inverse one with the degree of pigmentation. PUVA lentigines regress to some degree after discontinuation of PUVA therapy, but they remain visible for up to 2 years [112]. This eruption has been described under various names: lentigo eruptiva [51], freckles [8, 128], disseminated pigmented spots [151], stellate hyperpigmented freckling [90], PUVA-induced pigmented macules [91] and star-like hyperpigmented lentigines [153]. Histopathological findings have differed, but Rhodes et al. [91] showed that the pigmented macules are characterized by a lentiginous proliferation of functionally active melanocytes; thus the PUVA-induced macules were rather 'lentigines' than 'freckles' according to current pathologic classification. Dysplastic changes in the melanocytes have been observed both in PUVA lentigines [91,110,154] and chronically PUVA-exposed skin [110], and thus, although the significance of these pigment alterations is unknown, a close clinical and histopathological monitoring of PUVA patients for atypical melanocyte lesions has been recommended [91,154]. Until now (1993), however, no malignant transformation from PUVA lentigines has been observed.

Nevus spillus-like hyperpigmentation

Some authors have described nevus spillus-like hyperpigmentation in PUVA-treated patients [34,36,130,152]. Melanocyte numbers are reportedly normal [34,36].

Ashen-grey macules

A male patient treated with PUVA for psoriasis noticed ashen-grey macules up to 1 cm in diameter on the trunk after 130 exposures (total UVA dose 930 J/cm^2). A biopsy revealed large amounts of pigment-containing macrophages (melanophages) in the upper dermis [128]. Berlin blue staining for hemosiderin was negative. Two years after discontinuation of PUVA the macules still persisted. According to the authors, the finding of large amounts of melanophages reflects the greatly increased production of melanin in melanocytes possibly combined with inflammation and a disturbance of the epidermis-dermis junction during PUVA therapy [128].

Mottled hypo- and hyperpigmentation

Mottled hypo- and hyperpigmentation due to phototoxicity was reported in 13 of 572 patients undergoing PUVA therapy over a long period [117]. The skin in the affected parts of the body appeared dry, glistening and somewhat atrophic. In all patients mottling occurred at skin sites which had been overdosed and had exhibited erythema during the initial treatment phase. Mottling was first noted between 4 weeks and 12 months after the first PUVA exposure. DOPA-preparations revealed increased numbers of melanocytes in hyperpigmented areas, and reduced numbers in hypopigmented areas. In a number of patients the pigmentary changes proved (partially) reversible [117].

Hypo- and depigmentation

Irreversible hypopigmentation in some PUVA-treated patients has been observed [94]. Increased intracellular lipid deposits were demonstrated, which may precede degeneration of cells; thus overstimulation of melanocytes might explain the irreversible hypopigmentation. Farber et al. [113] have observed a case of extensive depigmentation, resembling vitiligo, appearing during PUVA treatment of psoriasis, and two patients in whom widespread depigmentation developed during PUVA therapy for mycosis fungoides. The depigmentation was not confined to clinically involved areas, nor was it associated with obvious phototoxicity. None of the patients had a history of vitiligo. Three more patients with vitiligo presumably due to PUVA therapy were reported by Todes-Taylor et al. [160].

Pityriasis alba-like hypopigmentation

Tegner [130] observed hypopigmentation with the clinical appearance of pityriasis alba in 5 patients after prolonged PUVA therapy. Since the clinical picture was identical in all patients, she concluded that this pigmentary change probably represented a side effect of PUVA.

18.13 Other skin disorders

Acantholytic dyskeratotic epidermal nevus

Acantholytic dyskeratotic epidermal nevus, formerly considered to be a 'forme fruste' of Darier's disease based on its similar histopathological features, is a nevoid eruption characterized by crustal and keratotic lesions in a nevoid distribution. It has a delayed onset, a negative family history, and may be provoked by hot and humid weather and sun exposure. A 79-year-old man with psoriasis developed a zosteriform acantholytic dyskeratotic epidermal nevus during PUVA therapy. The eruption was successfully treated with oral etretinate. In a subsequent course of PUVA recurrence of the nevus was prevented by covering the affected area [175].

Acne

A case of acneiform eruption induced by PUVA treatment has been described by Jones and Bleehen [40]. According to the authors, this is due to the hot and humid atmosphere in the enclosed cabinets in which patients undergoing PUVA treatment are usually irradiated. Acneiform exanthema has also been observed by Hofmann et al. [36].

Actinic lichenoid dermatitis

Actinic lichenoid dermatitis is a peculiar subtype of lichen planus with a distinct photodistribution. It occurs mostly in dark-complexioned individuals in subtropical areas. However, actinic lichenoid dermatitis has also been observed in a white woman; the lesions could be provoked by UVB irradiation [172].

Wennersten [173] described 3 caucasian patients with extensive longstanding vitiligo, who developed actinic lichenoid dermatitis during PUVA therapy with oral trimethylpsoralen. In 2 of the patients the lichenoid eruptions were confined exactly to non-responding vitiligo areas [173].

'Allergic' cutaneous vasculitis

A 67-year-old woman was being treated with PUVA therapy because of premycotic erythema of one year's standing in patches on the trunk and the extremities. After the fifth PUVA treatment purpura developed on the legs, first petechial in appearance, then progressing into a severe necrotic phase. Histopathological examination revealed a typical leukocytoclastic vasculitis. Later the patient developed proteinuria and haematuria; a kidney biopsy showed focal necrotizing glomerulonephritis. A spontaneous recovery ensued. The patient had used various drugs, but the event was most likely due to 8-MOP, as circulating antibodies to this drug could be demonstrated [4].

Atypical psoriasis of the hands

Thick, infiltrated, deep red plaques or papules developed in 13 out of 60 patients treated with PUVA on the knuckles, the dorsum of the first interphalangeal joints or the thenar eminence [165]. This apparent side effect of PUVA was dose-related. This type of lesion tends to heal with repeated PUVA treatment, but local rebound occurs afterwards. The lesions were considered to be atypical psoriasis, but no histopathology was available [165].

Bacterial infections

Bacterial infections such as folliculitis and erysipelas are said to occur infrequently during PUVA therapy [130].

Bullous eruptions

Three types of bullous eruptions due to PUVA therapy may be distinguished:

1. *Acrobullous eruption*, usually localized on the hands and/or feet. Bullae arise on normal skin; clinically and histologically they resemble bullous pemphigoid, but its characteristic immunofluorescence findings are absent [64, 105,108,143,144]. The eruption is considered to be the result of phototoxicity.
2. *Bullous pemphigoid.* Coexistence of psoriasis and bullous pemphigoid is well-documented [106,107]. It has been shown that a variety of cutaneous insults can produce the bullous lesions of pemphigoid, and a number of treatment modalities have been implicated, including dithranol, coal tar, salicylic acid and UVB [107]. Thomsen and Schmidt [77] were the first to describe bullous pemphigoid in PUVA-treated patients. In one case there was a previous diagnosis of bullous pemphigoid, albeit quiescent at the time of PUVA treatment. It was evident that the photochemotherapy caused the disease to relapse. Subsequently, several authors reported bullous pemphigoid during photochemotherapy [1,64,106,107,145,146]. Most patients develop bullous pemphigoid shortly after beginning of PUVA therapy, but delayed onset 4 weeks after discontinuance of photochemotherapy has also been reported [107]. The eruption is sometimes limited to psoriatic lesions; treatment with oral steroids and/or immunosuppressive agents has been necessary in some cases.
3. *Phytophotodermatitis-like lesions.* Three patients treated with PUVA developed linear blisters on the trunk and leg. In all cases, the surrounding skin was normal and the clinical picture resembled phytophotodermatitis [18]. Clinically and histopathologically, the condition can be differentiated from acrobullous eruptions and PUVA-induced bullous pemphigoid [36]. Phytophotodermatitis-like lesions are considered to be the result of a phototoxically-induced decrease of the dermo-epidermal adherence which, on friction, results in subepidermal blister formation [36].

In one report [147] pemphigus foliaceus (Senear-Usher) was seen to exacerbate during PUVA therapy.

Contact allergy

Several cases of contact allergy to 8-MOP have been documented [68,82]. Trimethylpsoralen has also been identified as sensitizer [68].

Discoid lupus erythematosus

There have been three case reports of the development of discoid lupus erythematodes in patients treated for vitiligo [182], polymorphous light eruption [183] and psoriasis [184].

Disseminated epidermolytic acanthoma

The term disseminated epidermolytic acanthoma (DEA) was introduced in 1973 to describe nonsystematized multiple verrucoid lesions showing histologically the characteristic features of epidermolytic hyperkeratosis. In one patient, DEA lesions developed after starting PUVA therapy and the majority of the lesions disappeared spontaneously after cessation of PUVA [177]. This circumstantial evidence suggests, according to the authors, that DEA was 'revealed' by PUVA therapy. Immunosuppressions from PUVA may have allowed the proliferation of abnormal clones in the epidermal cells [177].

Disseminated superficial actinic porokeratosis

Disseminated superficial actinic porokeratosis is a rare dominant autosomal dermatosis, of which some sporadic cases are recorded. Reymond et al. [63] have described a 67-year-old female patient with psoriasis, who developed lesions essentially localized on the anterior surface of both legs, clinically and histologically designated as superficial actinic porokeratosis; she had been treated with 8-MOP photochemotherapy, 8-MOP being administered both orally and (on the legs) topically. There was no family history of this dermatosis. The authors state that this entity might be expected as a side effect of PUVA therapy; typical lesions have been experimentally provoked with prolonged artificial UV light [11]. As a mechanism it was proposed that PUVA-induced immunosuppression may allow the proliferation of latent abnormal clones of epidermal cells, thereby producing the porokeratosis [169,170]. Disseminated superficial actinic porokeratosis has also been induced by UVB phototherapy [171].

Exacerbation of polymorphous light eruption

PUVA is effective in preventing chronic polymorphous light eruption, but during a course the dermatosis may also be provoked [157].

Exanthematous drug eruption

One case report describes a patient who developed a widespread papular and vesicular drug eruption during PUVA. A provocation with 8-MOP resulted again in this eruption. Skin prick tests and epicutaneous tests were negative [230]. A similar case was seen later [235].

Granuloma annulare

The etiology and pathogenesis of annular granuloma is as yet unknown. Dorval et al. [16] reported a case in which typical granuloma annulare developed in a psoriatic patient during PUVA treatment. The authors try (somewhat unconvincingly) to associate these findings.

Herpes simplex

Herpes simplex and other photosensitive dermatoses may be aggravated or exacerbated by PUVA therapy. A case of Kaposi's varicelliform eruption in a patient with mycosis fungoides during PUVA therapy has been documented [70].

Herpes zoster

The development of herpes zoster as a complication of PUVA therapy has been reported by Roenigk and Martin [66]. Stuttgen [109] found 8 cases of zoster occurring among 1013 patients treated with PUVA during the first 1.5 years of therapy.

Lichen planus

Lichen planus as a possible side effect of PUVA therapy was described by Dupré et al. [17]: A 62-year-old male suffering from extensive long-standing psoriasis with joint involvement was treated with photochemotherapy. At the beginning of the therapy the patient also took pyritinol tablets; previously he had received chloroquine for five years because of his rheumatism. After three PUVA treatments a lichenoid micropapular eruption developed, which was aggravated by each subsequent session until it was almost generalized; by that time erythroderma was noted, which was attributed to photosensitivity. After nine PUVA treatments the therapy was discontinued and the intake of pyritinol was stopped. Histopathology confirmed the clinical diagnosis of lichen planus. Gradually, the lichenoid skin eruption improved after discontinuation of PUVA therapy and pyritinol intake.

Lichenoid reactions and photosensitization have been noted with pyritinol before; it is not certain whether the adverse event should be attributed to pyritinol or to PUVA therapy. The authors hypothesize that pyritinol may have potentiated the effects of PUVA therapy and vice versa, therefore it would seem to be contraindicated, according to these authors, to apply PUVA therapy in patients using pyritinol.

Multiple keratoacanthomas

Two patients developed multiple keratocanthomas while receiving PUVA. Both had received excessive doses of UVA, which resulted in severe phototoxicity. As ultraviolet light may be an important factor in the induction of these lesions, since most are localized to areas exposed to ultraviolet radiation, and as two similar cases had been described previously and multiple keratoacanthomas following a severe sunburn has been reported, it was suggested that PUVA phototoxicity may have been a stimulus to provoke these multiple keratoacanthomas [215].

Neurofibromas

A 58-year-old man treated with PUVA for psoriasis developed multiple tiny red papules along scratches on the trunk and the extremities [174]. These were diagnosed histologically as neurofibromas. Until that time, the patient did not have any sign suggesting neurofibromatosis. The authors suggest that this event was *not* related to PUVA therapy, but reported the case as a causal relationship could not be excluded [174].

Photoallergic dermatitis

A case of photoallergic dermatitis to 8-MOP has been described by Plewig et al. [60]: A 36-year-old woman with psoriasis developed generalized photoallergic dermatitis to 8-MOP after 16 uneventful courses of PUVA. The diagnosis of photoallergy was confirmed by re-exposure, phototests using both topical and oral 8-MOP with a new high-intensity light apparatus for the delivery of UVA, and histological studies. Photoallergy occurred only with UVA, but not with either UVB or UVC. Three cases of photoallergy to topically applied 8-MOP were documented by Fulton and Willis [27]. Other psoralens causing photocontact allergy include 3-carbethoxypsoralen, and 4,6,4′-trimethylangelicin [68].

Photo-onycholysis

Zala et al. [84] described two patients who had developed photo-onycholysis from orally administered 8-MOP and exposure to sunlight. One of these patients had taken 8-MOP for vitiligo. the other for cosmetic reasons. Histological examination of the nail bed showed edema of the extracellular spaces and deposits of an unidentified crystalline substance. Numerous multinuclear cells were evident in the epithelium; globular keratohyaline granules were seen in some of the malpighian layer cells. An intraepithelial cyst-like degeneration was present in the upper malpighian layers. Other cases of photo-onycholysis induced by PUVA therapy have been described [10,55,62,130].

Prolonged phototoxicity

Stuttgen [109] has reported that up to 4–6 weeks after 8-MOP has been discontinued, it is possible to provoke a phototoxic reaction to sunbathing. This author has seen erythroderma-like eruptions following exposure to subtropical sun after discontinuance of PUVA-therapy.

Phototoxic reactions to drugs unrelated to methoxsalen after discontinuance of PUVA and restricted to psoriatic plaques have been observed [176].

Pustular psoriasis

Pustular transformation of previously non-pustular psoriasis was reported in 12 of 400 patients in the series described by Langner and Christophers [42]. This event, the authors postulate, can be linked with an inability of PUVA to completely suppress leukocyte chemotaxis. The development of pustular psoriasis during PUVA therapy has also been noted by Roenigk and Martin [66].

Rosacea

Rosacea may be aggravated by natural sunlight. Exacerbation of rosacea may be expected to occur from PUVA and, indeed, the author has observed several such cases (de Groot, A.C., unpublished observations). Rosacea developed in one patient who had never has this before during PUVA treatment [168].

Scleroderma-like changes

In two patients treated for vitiligo with PUVA therapy scleroderma-like skin changes were noted in vitiligo patches after 8 and 16 months of therapy; the patients had received 325.6 J/cm^2 and 683 J/cm^2, respectively. Histopathological examination revealed characteristics of both actinic elastosis and scleroderma. After cessation of therapy all findings, both clinical and histological, returned to normal [99].

Seborrhoeic dermatitis of the face

Seborrhoeic dermatitis of the face was observed in 28 of 347 patients on PUVA therapy for psoriasis [123]. Most patients had never previously noted any facial rash. The dermatitis always started after discontinuation of the PUVA therapy, the latency time ranging from a few days to a couple of weeks. When patients with induced seborrhoeic dermatitis were given a new PUVA series, the facial rash again cleared up but recurred soon after discontinuation of treatment. The author hypothesizes that PUVA treatment means both an activation and a therapy of a latent seborrhoeic dermatitis. The clinical appearance of the dermatitis would then represent a rebound phenomenon due to withdrawal of the PUVA treatment. Verhagen et al. [165] noted seborrhoeic dermatitis-like lesions on the face in 16 out of 60 patients, usually after discontinuance of PUVA therapy. These authors consider the lesions to be atypical psoriasis [165].

Systemic lupus erythematosus

Systemic lupus erythematosus (SLE) developed in a 23-year-old woman with psoriasis during PUVA therapy. She displayed a typical facial rash, hair loss, photosensitivity, arthralgia with pain on joint movements, renal and CNS involvement, splenomegaly and leukopenia. Serum antinuclear antibodies were present in high titer, and hypocomplementemia developed. Kidney and skin biopsy specimens were consistent with SLE [21]. Although the authors admit that the association of psoriasis and SLE in this case may have been coincidental, they argue that the appearance of SLE shortly after the onset of PUVA treatment suggests that ultraviolet A or photoactivated psoralen may have played a role in the development of this connective tissue disease. Other sporadic cases of autoimmune disorders with positive ANA tests have included an SLE-like syndrome [181], a (fatal) scleroderma-like syndrome [180], and, more recently, a case of subacute cutaneous lupus erythematosus with pancytopenia, antibodies to double-stranded DNA, and hypocomplimentemia [185].

Antinuclear antibodies (ANA) were studied in patients receiving PUVA therapy [7]. Ten patients out of 124 (8%), considered for PUVA had ANA prior to therapy. During PUVA treatment ANA appeared in 34 out of 100 patients. Eight patients with ANA initially were treated and in 4 of them a significant increase in ANA titre was noted. A statistically significant difference was noted, when the first and last ANA tests for each patient were compared. No such different was seen in a control group consisting of 33 patients. All PUVA patients generating ANA were evaluated clinically and with a laboratory screening. This evaluation was negative in all patients except one who developed ANA of the nucleolar staining pattern together with symptoms consistent with a collagen vascular disease [180]. The ANA titers were generally low and the staining pattern was of the homogenous type in all patients but one [7].

At 14 centres, 1023 patients had two or more ANA determinations. There was no statistically significant increase of positive ANA's following PUVA therapy [73]. These authors point out that psoralen-DNA photoproducts are antigenic and may give rise to antinuclear antibodies, which may be detected only when using a tissue substrate irradiated with UVA in the presence of psoralens. In the study of Picascia et al. [178], 269 patients received therapy for more than 3 months and had at least two antinuclear antibody (ANA) determinations. It was found that the difference between the number of significantly positive ANAs pre-PUVA therapy (4 of 269) compared with post-PUVA therapy (16 of 269) was not statistically significant. Furthermore, of the patients who did develop a significantly positive ANA, not one was found to have any symptoms, signs, or laboratory evidence of systemic lupus erythematosus. The authors therefore suggest obtaining ANAs prior to initiating PUVA therapy and obtaining follow-up ANAs only if the initial ANA is significantly positive. Patients with pre-PUVA-positive ANAs can, according to the authors, be started on PUVA therapy if there is no evidence of lupus erythematosus [178]. Other authors, however, are more cautious, and advise that patients with psoriasis who have positive ANA test results should have studies for DNA, SSA/Ro, complement, microscopic examination of haematoxylin-eosin-stained sections, and immunofluorescence prior to PUVA therapy [179].

18.14 Disorders of the nails

Nail pigmentation

Naik and Singh [54] reported on nail pigmentation that developed in four patients while on oral 8-MOP photochemotherapy for vitiligo. Although other possible causes for this phenomenon were not excluded, the authors believed this pigmentation to be attributable to 8-MOP. The same authors treated 10 psoriatic patients with PUVASOL (8-MOP and sunlight exposure) and observed hyperpigmentation of the nail plates in three. The hyperpigmentation started about one month after beginning of treatment, starting proximally and spreading distally to involve the entire nail plate [100]. After cessation of therapy the pigmentation disappeared (in one patient observed after two months). The adverse effect was ascribed to increased melanogenesis. The pigmentation may be longitudinal [44].

Psoriasis of the nails

De Groot [71] described a patient who developed a clinical picture of nail psoriasis of the hand but not the feet during PUVA treatment. This coincided with a phototoxic reaction of the skin. The patient had never had psoriasis of the nails before, and after discontinuing PUVA the nails regrew in a normal fashion. The reaction was considered to be a koebner phenomenon due to phototoxicity [71].

Subungual bleeding

Subungual bleeding due to PUVA therapy has been described by several investigators [37,130].

18.15 Disorders of the hair

Hirsutism

Whereas hypertrichosis following photochemotherapy with oral psoralens has been reported by several authors (see below), there is only one documented case of hirsutism [33]: a 31-year-old female patient with psoriasis was treated with PUVA. There were no signs of hypertrichosis or hirsutism at the beginning of the therapy. Seventy days after the first treatment (having received a total dose of 171.5 J/cm^2) the patient noticed increased hair growth on her face. Four weeks later, she had abnormal hair growth on the cheeks, chin, upper lip, lower back and buttocks, designated as hirsutism Grade III according to Baron [3]; no signs of virilization were present. Hormonal causes for hirsutism were excluded. The authors consider this to be a case of iatrogenic hirsutism caused by PUVA therapy; they hypothesize that the photosensitizing agents change the metabolism of androgens in the skin.

Hypertrichosis

Hypertrichosis as a side effect of psoralen photochemotherapy has been reported repeatedly [130,158]. Rampen [158] reported moderate to severe hypertrichosis in 15/23 (65%) of patients on PUVA therapy; especially the face and extremities were affected. Excessive hair growth started within 6–12 weeks after commencement of PUVA. According to the author the hair growth can be attributed to stimulation of keratinocytes in the hair bulb [158].

18.16 Cardiovascular effects

Cardiovascular stress

Cardiac insufficiency and severe hypertension are contraindications for PUVA treatment. In the investigation of Ciafone et al. [12], oral PUVA therapy in a treatment enclosure (mean duration 19.3 minutes) resulted in ambient temperatures of 39.2±2.1°C and skin temperatures of 38.2±1.4°C in 17 patients. In the upright position, the heart rate rose by 30.8% to 114.4±25.2 beats per minute, and the authors warned that PUVA therapy is thus associated with a definite cardiovascular stress when the box-type of therapeutic unit is used. However, Chappe et al. [98] concluded from their study that PUVA therapy is a safe method of treatment, since their patients, including those with cardiovascular disease and hypertension, tolerated the stress of PUVA therapy well. The study group of these investigators consisted of 40 patients, of which 6 had cardiovascular disease; 16 had documented hypertension. The following parameters were monitored: standing brachial artery blood pressure immediately before and after PUVA, taken in the same arm by the same observer; 12-lead electrocardiograms in 22 patients immediately before and after PUVA; heart rate and rhythm of all patients while standing in the phototherapy cabinet, using standard Holter monitoring technic (modified leads V_1 and V_5). The patients were closely observed during treatment, and any subjective symptoms were recorded. Electrocardiograms showed no significant changes after PUVA; Holter monitoring revealed no significant arrhythmias other than recorded before therapy. All patients had an increase in heart rate, the mean increase being 20 beats per minute (22%). There were no significant changes in the systolic or diastolic blood pressure. Subjective symptoms of dizziness occurred in 6 patients: in 3 of them this did not interfere with treatment but in 3 others dizziness required interruption of treatment. In these cases dizziness was ascribed to anxiety and hyperventilation (2) and influenza (1). In general, patients tolerated the stress of standing in a warm phototherapy cabinet well, and therefore PUVA therapy was considered to be a safe method (in their group) by the investigators. Nevertheless, they also state that it would be desirable to use cardiac monitoring, including electrocardiogram and arterial blood pressure, when treating patients with significant heart disease, in whom a rise in heart rate might present a significant stress.

An increase of heart rate was also the only cardiovascular finding in another study [216]. By applying adequate air-conditioning, the cardiovascular stress during PUVA therapy can be diminished [216]. There is one isolated case report of a woman with pre-existing valvular disease (mitral insufficiency) which could not be demonstrated by electrocardiogram, who developed decompensation in the cardiac function after being burnt from PUVA treatment [217].

Temporal arteritis

Temporal arteritis in a 75-year-old male developed after three weeks of photochemotherapy with oral trioxsalen and subsequent exposure to sunlight [47]. This disease has not been reported in connection with photochemotherapy in any other study and must probably be regarded as coincidental.

18.17 Respiratory system

Several cases of bronchoconstriction due to methoxsalen have been reported [218–220]. This reaction, characterized by dry coughs developing 3.5 hours after ingestion of 8-MOP, may develop in asthmatics [219], but also in patients with no history of respiratory disease [218]. UVA is not necessary for the provocation of bronchoconstriction, and fever may accompany the bronchial reaction. Prophylactic anti-asthmatic therapy may enable PUVA therapy to be continued [218]. The pathomechanism is obscure [218–220].

18.18 Liver disease

Hepatitis

The incidence of psoralen hepatotoxicity, if any, has been debated and certain literature is frequently cited [24,78]. Slight and transient elevations of liver enzymes during PUVA treatment have been reported [121], but were usually attributable to pre-existing liver injury caused by intake of alcohol or other drugs. Liver damage is not considered to be a contraindication to the use of PUVA [20].

Case reports

Until now (1993), in only two reports could hepatotoxicity be clearly attributed to PUVA therapy, or rather to oral 8-MOP. Bjellerup et al. [6] presented a case of liver damage due to 8-MOP. The reaction manifested itself by elevated serum alanine-aminotransferase and serum aspartate-aminotransferase; it was provoked by PUVA on 3 occasions. During the last such episode, the liver enzymes were elevated after a test dose of 40 mg 8-MOP, without irradiation. The liver damage seemed to be of the hepatocellular type; unfortunately, no liver biopsy was available. The authors reporting the case believe this side effect to be allergic in nature.

The other report on hepatotoxicity of PUVA was published by Pariser and Wyles [56]. A 59-year-old white nurse with long-standing psoriasis, who had a damaged liver from methotrexate, developed a toxic hepatitis while on oral 8-MOP photochemotherapy. Fever and marked elevation of the liver enzymes occurred after the fifteenth PUVA treatment; spontaneous recovery ensued within 5 days after stopping PUVA. One week later, following the next PUVA treatment, the same toxic hepatitis developed and again spontaneously resolved. Topical 8-MOP followed by UVA did *not* produce this reaction.

A third case of liver damage during PUVA therapy, rapidly deteriorating to hepatic encephalopathy, renal failure, septicemia and death may have been caused by chronic and gross alcohol abuse rather than by PUVA [223].

Tegner [130] reports liver damage in two patients, but no details are mentioned.

Reactivation of viral hepatitis during PUVA therapy has rarely been observed [222]. Small and nonspecific histological changes were found in 12 patients in whom liver biopsies were taken before and after 1 year of PUVA [224].

18.19 Renal disease

Glomerulonephritis

Dahl [15] reported an increase in serum creatinine to abnormal values in 12 of 106 patients treated with PUVA therapy. A renal biopsy showed uncharacteristic glomerulonephritis in one of them. In one case report nephrotic syndrome developed during PUVA therapy [225].

18.20 Miscellaneous

Skin pain

One of the most troublesome short-term side-effects of PUVA treatment is severe itching or skin pain [50,76,130,163], which can develop during an initial PUVA treatment as well as during maintenance treatment. In some cases, the condition is so severe that the patient cannot sleep, becomes very upset, refuses further PUVA treatment, and may even consider suicide if the itch or pain does not subside. It can be a frequent reason for dropping out of treatment, especially in the patient is not properly monitored by the doctor himself. Such severe itching or skin pain is very resistant to therapy. Several treatments have been tried. Analgesics, antihistamines, topical anaesthetics, topical steroids, and even steroids

— up to 60 mg of prednisolone daily — have had little or no effect. PUVA therapy often has to be terminated, but even then the itching of pain may still persist for weeks and sometimes even months to a year [163].

The clinical pattern is very stereotypical. All the patients have severe itching or a prickling, smarting pain "under the skin" that is compared to "stacks of needles". They have never experienced anything like it before in their lives. The "stacks of needles" occur intermittently in attacks lasting from a few minutes to several hours. They do not occur or are not very pronounced when the patient is busy and usually start when he or she has finished working and "starts watching TV". The attacks can occur at night and disturb sleep. Very typically, the itching or pain is never generalized but always confined to a specific area of clinically normal skin, frequently in the interscapular region, but it may also occur in other areas. There is no question of an overdose of UVA. Other medications seem to have no influence on it.

The attacks are not always confined to the same area but can jump from one area to another, even on the same day. They can start spontaneously, but they can be elicited by heat (at night), friction from clothing, stretching the skin, or scratching. The pain will temporarily subside or disappear during a shower or cold bath, which patients often report spontaneously.

Roelandts and Stevens [164] identified two types of skin pain: a dermatome-localized hyperalgesia and a more diffuse hyperalgesia not limited to a specific dermatome. If the hyperalgesia was felt in a specific dermatome, articular dysfunctions were found in the corresponding vertebral joints. The skin pain disappeared immediately when the articular dysfunctions were treated by means of manipulative techniques. In patients who had more diffuse hyperalgesia, there was a clear vegetative dysfunction (hyperactivity of the sympathetic nervous system): an uncomfortable emotional sensation and strong transpiration with panalgesia. These patients are usually very nervous and tend to be upset very easily. When the sympathetic nervous system is suppressed, e.g. by low-frequency electrotherapy or sympathicus blocking with lidocaine, the skin pain disappears, although usually not immediately [164].

Drug fever

Two cases of drug fever during PUVA therapy have been reported [231,232]. In one case [231] the side effect was caused by 8-MOP, in the other [232] by the combination of 8-MOP and UVA.

Perichondritis

Perichondritis of the ear has been observed, but no details were provided [237].

Immune haemolytic anaemia

Immune haemolytic anaemia during PUVA has been observed, but no details were provided [237].

Effects on Langerhans cells (LC)

ATPase-stained LC have been shown to disappear during PUVA treatment [116]. Friedmann et al. [89] have studied the effects of PUVA therapy in psoriatic patients on LC using both ATP-ase staining of epidermal biopsies obtained from suction blisters and electron microscopy on blister tops. Langerhans cells lost ATPase activity before they disappeared by ultrastructural criteria: 90% of ATPase-stained cells had disappeared after 7 treatments (2 weeks), whereas it was only after 15 treatments (5 weeks) that they were seen to be reduced on electron microscopy. Their numbers remained low throughout the course of treatment, but they had returned to normal by 3 weeks after cessation of therapy. It was shown that these effects were due to PUVA potentiated by 8-MOP. Disappearance of LC may cause or contribute to changes in delayed cutaneous hypersensitivity, which reportedly is reduced in psoriatic patients undergoing oral photochemotherapy [88] (see below).

Effects on delayed cutaneous hypersensitivity

Several investigators have shown that PUVA reduces delayed hypersensitivity to 2,4-dinitrochlorobenzene (DNCB) in patients with psoriasis [75,88,133]. The PUVA-mediated inhibition of cutaneous immune responsiveness is of short duration, being completely restored after 6 weeks [229]. PUVA suppresses both induction and expression of delayed cutaneous hypersensitivity by systemic as well as local actions, but the major effect is local inhibition of induction [88]; reduction of the numbers of Langerhans cells, which are required for the induction of contact hypersensitivity, is probably a major factor for the latter.

The pathological consequences of impairment of immunity by PUVA are uncertain. However, it has been shown that DNCB responsiveness is reduced in patients with cancer, and a possible role of impaired immunity in the cutaneous carcinogenicity of PUVA has been suggested [75]. On the other hand, Moss et al. [88] argue that treatment with conventional therapy (tar, UVB and anthralin) has also reduced DNCB responsiveness [133], and that these forms of treatment have proved safe over many years of use.

Inadequate or uncontrolled application of photochemotherapy

Fritsch [26] discussed the danger of uncontrolled use of 8-MOP. He described 2 patients who painted their skin with 8-MOP and went out into the sun. This resulted in an extensive erythematous and bullous dermatitis. A similar life-threatening phototoxic reaction was provoked by topical 8-MOP painting followed by 2 hours of solarium exposure [162]. Other accidents listed are mistakes in the dose of UV light, and accidental contact with 8-MOP, e.g. by hospital personnel, or from leaking from ruptured capsules [166].

SECOND GENERATION EFFECTS

18.21 Because PUVA therapy is mutagenic, concern exists about the potential for teratogenic effects resulting from the use of this treatment at the time of conception and during pregnancy. In a 12.8 year prospective study, the pregnancy outcomes among 1380 patients were documented. Ninety-four men reported 167 pregnancies in their partners, and 93 women reported 159 pregnancies. Two congenital malformations and two stillbirths occurred, an incidence not significantly different from that expected for the general population. These data do not ensure the safety of exposure to PUVA at the time of conception or during pregnancy, but they do suggest that if an increase in the risk of adverse fetal outcomes does exist, it is likely to be small [228].

OVERDOSAGE

18.22 Very little information on the signs and symptoms of overdosage of methoxsalen is available. A woman who took 85 tablets of 8-MOP (850 mg, 20 times the therapeutic dose) became very nauseated, vomited frequently and complained of severe dizziness. No other signs and symptoms of intoxication were noted, and the patient completely recovered in 36 hours [233].

ONCOGENIC EFFECTS OF THE GOECKERMAN REGIMEN

18.23 Tar

Coal tar ointments have been used for many decades in the treatment of various dermatoses, especially eczematous dermatitis and psoriasis. Crude coal tar, a heterogeneous mixture of 10,000 different compounds [124] of which 400 have been identified, has the known dermatological effects of being antipruritic, antibacterial, keratoplastic and photosensitizing [53].

The carcinogenic effects of coal tar, particularly of the benzpyrene constituent, have been well documented in laboratory animals [35]. Concentrations that are used clinically can cause benign as well as malignant neoplasms in animals [61]. Moreover, workers in the coal tar industry have an increased risk of developing malignancies, particularly non-melanoma skin cancers [29]. There is concern that prolonged topical application of tar preparations might induce skin cancers [239]. Also, urine extracts prepared from patients undergoing Goeckerman therapy and patients treated with topical coal tar [241] have been shown to contain (unidentified) materials, which are mutagenic in the Ames assay [125]. It has previously been established that as little as 100 μg of crude coal tar is mutagenic in this test [124].

Case studies

In a review of the world literature up to 1967, made at that time by Greither et al. [30], a total of 13 cases of skin cancer were reported, all probably induced by prolonged application of therapeutic tar preparations. The most frequent sites of the cancers were the genital areas and the adjacent skin. In nine of the cases there was a history of prolonged self-medication, ranging from 3 months to 34 years.

One case was reported in detail by Rook et al. [67], who commented on the rarity of carcinomas induced by therapeutical application of tar, as contrasted with the frequency of occupational tar cancer. In later case reports, squamous cell carcinomas after prolonged coal tar application also were located on the scrotum, which seems to be particularly susceptible [83,238]. In an epidemiologic study, the observed incidence of carcinoma in 719 tar-treated psoriatics was not increased over that expected in the general population [239].

Although several case reports have suggested an association between tar exposure and cutaneous carcinomas, no study has been able to document an increased risk of cutaneous carcinomas in patients treated with these externa. At present, therapy with tar preparations would hardly seem to endanger patients thus treated with regard to the development of skin cancers [5,61,239,240].

Other side effects

Other side effects of topical coal tar therapy include irritant dermatitis, folliculitis, tar acne, phototoxic dermatitis, and contact allergy [240].

Tar + ultraviolet light

18.24 Adequate evidence exists to support the statement that sunlight is a causal factor in human skin cancer [80,142]. Artificial light in the UVB range has been shown to induce cutaneous tumours in albino and hairless mice [31]. Ultraviolet radiation potentiates the carcinogenic effect of topical coal tar in animals [23].

The successful treatment of psoriasis by the application of crude coal tar and subsequent exposure to ultraviolet light was first reported by Goeckerman in 1925 [28]. Although the action spectrum of coal tar lies within the long-wave ultraviolet range (UVA, 400 to 320 nm), studies have shown that exposure to erythemal radiation (UVB, 320 to 280 nm) is more effective in this regimen [58]. Therefore, the 'Goeckerman regimen' commonly employed for the treatment of psoriasis, consists of topical tar preparations (1–5%), followed by short-wave (UVB) radiation. In recent years it has been postulated that the efficacy of the Goeckerman regimen can be ascribed solely to the UVB irradiation, and that topical tar has, at most, a small therapeutic benefit when used in conjunction with UVB phototherapy [242].

The question as to whether or not the Goeckerman therapy increases the risk of cutaneous carcinomas has always been a matter of dispute.

Case studies

Earlier studies have failed to document an increased risk of cutaneous carcinomas in patients treated for psoriasis with tar and artificial ultraviolet radiation [39].

Several more recent reports are of interest: Maughan et al. [48] reported on a 25-year follow-up study of 305 patients with atopic dermatitis or neurodermatitis, who had been hospitalized and treated with coal tar ointments and ultraviolet light at the Mayo Clinic from 1950 through 1954; information concerning the development of malignancies of the skin or other cancers since the initial treatment was gained either by follow-up questionnaire or telephone. Of the 305 patients with adequate follow-up, thirteen reported that skin cancer had developed; eight patients had basal cell carcinomas, one had a squamous cell carcinoma, two had an unknown variety of skin malignancy (biopsy specimens not available and therefore regarded as 'presumed skin cancers'), and two had malignant melanoma. Ten of eleven non-melanoma skin cancers were localized to sun-exposed areas. The number of patients with atopic dermatitis in whom skin cancer developed, was compared with the anticipated values of occurrence calculated from data of the Third National Cancer Survey for non-melanoma skin cancer [69]; the incidence in this study was not significantly increased. A total of 8 non-cutaneous malignancies was noted in the Mayo group, which does not differ appreciably from values reported elsewhere.

Comparison with the general population, as has been done in this study, is not ideal, but seems to be valid, since Kaaber [41] has shown that the incidence of skin cancer in patients with atopic dermatitis is similar to that in the general population.

A similar study of the long-term effects of tar and/or ultraviolet radiation on the incidence of cutaneous neoplasms in psoriatics was reported by Pittelkow et al. [59]: A 25-year follow-up of 280 psoriasis patients treated with the Goeckerman regimen, revealed 20 patients with a total of 33 skin cancers. There were 22 basal cell carcinomas, 7 squamous cell carcinomas, 3 of 'unknown variety', and 1 melanoma. The vast majority of these cancers occurred on exposed areas of the skin. Prior to initial treatment, 9% had a history of premalignant skin diseases (radiodermatitis, actinic dermatitis, and arsenical keratoses) and 70% received ionizing radiation, arsenic, methotrexate, or prolonged UV radiation. Two major risk factors were noted for the cancer patients: history of precancerous dermatitis and previous treatment with ionizing radiation. Just as in the study of Maughan et al. [48] on patients with dermatitis, there was no more cancer in this group of psoriatics treated with tar and ultraviolet light than would be expected in a normal population, considering sex, age and geographic distribution [69].

Stern et al. [74] conducted a case-control study, consisting of 59 skin cancer patients with severe psoriasis, to evaluate the effect of treatment with tar and/or artificial UV radiation on the risk of developing cutaneous carcinoma. Using 924 unmatched controls, the crude rate of skin cancer was estimated to be 2.4 fold for patients *with high exposure* to tar and ultraviolet radiation compared with those *lacking high exposure.* When using a control series of 126 patients matched for age, skin type, region of residence, sex, history of exposure to ionizing radiation, and number of PUVA treatments, a stronger association (relative rate = 4.7, 95% confidence limits = 2.2 to 10.0) was observed. The rate of cutaneous carcinoma for subjects exposed to ultraviolet radiation or tar was significantly increased *only* for patients with histories of *very high* exposure. A separate analysis of patients, who were moderately exposed to either of these agents, showed that they had insignificant increases in their risk of developing cutaneous carcinoma, suggesting a dose-response relation between exposure and risk. The male genitals may be particularly susceptible to developing UV-induced squamous cell carcinomas [200]. Although the increased risk of skin carcinoma for patients with psoriasis, who have had very high exposures to tar or ultraviolet radiation is an argument in favour of continued careful surveillance for the early detection of tumours among patients with psoriasis on long-term tar and UV light therapy [120], it is not a contraindication to the use of these agents, considering the extremely limited morbidity from skin cancer.

At present, the Goeckerman regimen may be considered as a safe therapeutic approach to psoriasis, although it must be kept in mind that patients with very high exposure to tar and/or ultraviolet light may have a slightly increased risk of developing cutaneous carcinomas [74].

18.25 REFERENCES

1. Abel, E.A. and Bennett, A. (1979): Bullous pemphigoid. Occurrence in psoriasis treated with psoralens plus long-wave ultra violet radiation. *Arch. Dermatol., 115,* 988.
2. Boukes, R.J. and Bruynzeel, D.P. (1985): Ocular findings in 340 long-term treated PUVA patients. *Photodermatol., 2,* 178–180.
3. Baron, J. (1974): Diagnostik und Therapie des Hirsutismus. *Zbl. Gynëk., 96,* 129.
4. Barrière, H., Bureau, B. and Planchon, B. (1981): Purpura par sensibilisation au 8 MOP au cours d'une puvathérapie. *Nouv. Presse Méd., 10,* 337.
5. Bickers, D.R. (1981): The carcinogenicity and mutagenicity of therapeutic coal tar; a perspective (Editorial). J. *Invest. Dermatol., 77,* 173.
6. Bjellerup, M., Bruze, M., Hansson, A., Krook, G. and Ljunggren, B. (1979): Liver injury following administration of 8-methoxypsoralen during PUVA therapy. *Acta Derm.-Venereol. (Stockh.), 59,* 371.
7. Bruze, M. and Ljunggren, B. (1985): Antinuclear antibodies appearing during PUVA therapy. *Acta. Derm.-Venereol., 65,* 31–36.
8. Bleehen, S.S. (1978): Freckles induced by PUVA treatment. *Br. J. Dermatol., 99 (Suppl. 16),* 20.
9. Kemmett, D., Reshad, H. and Baker, H. (1984): Nodular malignant melanoma and multiple squamous cell carcinomas in a patient treated by photochemotherapy for psoriasis. *Br. Med. J., 289,* 1498.
10. Briffa, D.V. and Warin, A.P. (1977): Photo-onycholysis caused by photochemotherapy. *Br. Med. J., 2,* 1150.
11. Chernosky, M.E. and Anderson, D.E. (1969): Disseminated superficial actinic porokeratosis. Clinical studies and experimental production of lesions. *Arch. Dermatol., 99,* 401.
12. Ciafone, R.A., Rhodes, A.R., Audley, M., Freedberg, I.M. and Abelmann, W.H. (1980): The cardiovascular stress of photochemotherapy (PUVA). *J. Am. Acad. Dermatol., 3,* 499.
13. Cloud, T.M., Hakim, R. and Griffin, A.C. (1961): Photosensitization of the eye with methoxsalen. II. Chronic effects. *Arch. Ophthal., 6,* 689.
14. Cyrlin, M.N., Pedvis-Leftick, A. and Sugar, W. (1980): Cataract formation in association with ultraviolet photosensitivity. *Ann. Ophthal., 12,* 786.
15. Dahl, K.B. (1979): Fotokemoterapi af psoriasis med psoralen og langbolget ultraviolet lys (PUVA). *Ugeskr. Laeg., 141,* 1975.
16. Dorval, J. C., Leroy, J. P. and Masse, R. (1979): Granulomes annulaires dissemines apres Puva therapie. *Ann. Derm. Venereol. (Pari.s). 106,* 79.
17. Dupre, A., Carrere, S., Launais, B. and Bonafe, J.L. (1980): Lichen plan avec photosensibilisation apres pyritinol et PUVA-therapie. *Ann. Derm. Venereol. (Paris), 107,* 557.
18. Roelandts, R., Loncke, J. and Degreef, H. (1985): Phytophotodermatitis-like lesions induced by PUVA. *Photodermatol., 2,* 40–43.
19. Wolff, K. (1990): Side-effcts of psoralen photochemotherapy. *Br. J. Dermatol., 122 (Suppl. 36),* 117–125.
20. Morison, W.L. (1990): Recent advances in phototherapy and photochemotherapy of skin disease. *J. Derm. Science, 1,* 141–148.
21. Eyanson, S., Greist. M.C., Brandt, K.D. and Skinner, B. (1979): Systemic lupus erythematodes. Association with psoralen-ultraviolet, a treatment of psoriasis. *Arch. Dermatol., 115,* 54.
22. Young, A.R. (1990): Cumulative effects of ultraviolet radiation on the skin, cancer and photoaging. *Semin. Dermatol., 9,* 25–31.
23. Findlay, G.M. (1928): Ultraviolet light and skin cancer. *Lancet, 2,* 1070.
24. Fitzpatrick, T.B., Imbrie, J.D. and Labby, D. (1958): Effect of methoxsalen on liver function. *J. Am. Med. Assoc., 167,* 1586.
25. Forrest, J.B. and Forrest, H.J. (1980): Case report on malignant melanoma arising during drug therapy for vitiligo. *J. Surg. Oncol., 13,* 337.
26. Fritsch, P. (1977): Gefahren unsachgemässer und unkontrollierter Anwendung von Psoralen. *Z. Hautkr., 52,* 1058.
27. Fulton. J.E. and Willis, I. (1968): Photoallergy to methoxsalen. *Arch. Dermatol., 98,* 445.
28. Goeckerman, W.H. (1925): Treatment of psoriasis. *Northw. Med. (Seattle), 24,* 229.
29. Götz, H. (1976): Tar keratosis. In: *Cancer of the Skin. Biology — Diagnosis — Management. Vol. 1,* pp. 492–523. Editors: R. Andrate, S.L. Gumport, G.L. Popkin et al. W.B. Saunders Co., Philadelphia.
30. Greither, A., Gisbertz. C. and Ippen, H. (1967): Teerbehandlung und Krebs. *Z. Haut-u. Geschlkhr., 42,* 631.

31. Griffin, A.C., Dolman, V.S., Bohlke, E.F., Bouvart, P. and Tatum, E. (1955): The effect of visible light on the carcinogenicity of ultraviolet light. *Cancer Res., 15,* 523.
32. Gibbs, N.K., Höningsmann, H. and Young, A.R. (1986): PUVA treatment strategies and cancer risk. *Lancet, i,* 150–151.
33. Heise, H., Geidel, H. and Valerius, B. (1980): Hirsutismus als seltene Komplikation der PUVA-Therapie. *Derm. Mschr., 166,* 611.
34. Helland. S. and Bang, G. (1980): Nevus spilus-like hyperpigmentation in psoriatic lesions during PUVA therapy. *Acta Derm.-Venereol. (Stockh.), 60,* 81.
35. Hirohata. T., Masuda, Y., Horie, A. and Masanori, K. (1973): Carcinogenicity of tar-containing skin drugs: animal experiment and chemical analysis. *Gann, 64,* 323.
36. Drijkoningen, M., de Wolf-Peeters, C., Roelandts, R., Loncke, J. and Desmet, V. (1986): A morphological and immunohistochemical study of phytophotodermatitis-like bullae induced by PUVA. *Photodermatol., 3,* 199–201.
37. Stern, R.S., Parris, J.A. and Fitzpatrick, T.B. (1985): Ocular findings in patients treated with PUVA. *J. Invest. Dermatol., 85,* 269–273.
38. Hönigsmann, H., Wolff, K., Gschnait, F., Brenner, W. and Jaschke, E. (1980): Keratoses and non-melanoma skin tumors in long-term photochemotherapy (PUVA). *J. Am. Acad. Dermatol., 3,* 406.
39. Jacobs, P.H., Farber, E.M. and Hall, M.L. (1977): Psoriasis and skin cancer. In: *Psoriasis. Proceedings of the Second International Symposium,* pp. 350–352. Editors: E.M. Farber, A. Cox. P. Jacobs et al. Yorke Medical Books, New Jersey.
40. Jones, C. and Bleehen, S.S. (1977): Acne induced by PUVA treatment. *Br. Med. J., 2,* 866.
41. Kaaber, K. (1976): Occurrence of malignant neoplasms in patients with atopic dermatitis. *Acta Derm.-Venereol. (Stockh.), 56,* 445.
42. Langner, A. and Christophers, E. (1977): Leukocyte chemotaxis after in vitro treatment with 8-methoxypsoralen and UVA. *Arch. Dermatol. Res., 260,* 51.
43. Lassus, A., Reunala, J., Idänpää-Heikkilä, J., Juvakoski, T. and Salo, O. (1981): PUVA treatment and skin cancer: a follow-up study. *Acta Derm.-Venereol. (Stockh.), 61,* 141.
44. McDonald, K.J.S., Hargreaves, G.K. and Ead, R.D. (1986): Longitudinal melanonychia during photochemotherapy. *Br. J. Dermatol., 114,* 395–396.
45. Lerman, S., Jocoy, M. and Borkman, R.F. (1977): Photosensitization of the lens by 8-methoxypsoralen. *Invest. Ophthal. Vis. Sci., 16,* 1065.
46. Lerman, S., Megaw, J. and Willis, I. (1980): The photoreaction of 8-MOP with tryptophan and lens proteins. *Photochem. Photobiol., 31,* 235.
47. Mahakrishnan, A. and Shesan Narayanan, G.V. (1981): Temporal arteritis following trimethoxypsoralen therapy. *Indian J. Dermatol. Venereol. Leprol., 47,* 53.
48. Maughan, W.Z., Muller, S.A., Perry. H.A., Pittelkow, M.R. and O'Brien, P.C. (1980): Incidence of skin cancers in patients with atopic dermatitis treated with coal tar. *J. Am. Acad. Derm., 3,* 612.
49. Melski, J.W., Tanenbaum, L., Parrish, J.A., Fitzpatrick, T.B., Bleich, H.L. et al. (1977): Oral methoxsalen photochemotherapy for the treatment of psoriasis: a cooperative clinical trial. *J. Invest. Dermatol., 68,* 328.
50. Miller, J. and Munro, D.D. (1980): Severe skin pain following PUVA. *Acta Derm.-Venereol. (Stockh.), 60,* 187.
51. Molin, L., Thomsen, K., Volden, G. and Groth, O. (1980): Photochemotherapy (PUVA) in the pretumour stage of mycosis fungoides: a report from the Scandinavian mycosis fungoides study group. *Acta Derm.-Venereol. (Stockh.), 61,* 47.
52. Woo, T., Wong, R.C., Wong, J.M., Anderson, T.F. and Lerman, S. (1985): Lenticular psoralen photoproducts and cataracts of a PUVA-treated psoriatic patient. *Arch. Dermatol., 121,* 1307–1308.
53. Muller, S.A. and Kierland, R.R. (1964): Crude coal tar in dermatologic therapy. *Mayo Clin. Proc., 39,* 275.
54. Naik, R.P.C. and Singh, G. (1979): Nail pigmentation due to oral 8-methoxypsoralen. *Br. J. Dermatol., 100,* 229.
55. Orlonne, J.P. and Baran, R. (1978): Photo-onycholyse induite par la photochimiothérapie orale. *Ann. Derm. Vénéréol. (Paris).* 105, 887.
56. Pariser, D.M. and Wyles, R.J. (1980): Toxic hepatitis from oral methoxsalen photochemotherapy (PUVA). *J. Am. Acad. Dermatol., 3,* 248.
57. Marx, J.L., Auerbach, R., Possick, P., Myrow, R., Gladstein, A.H. and Kopf, A.W. (1983): Malignant melanoma in situ in two patients treated with psoralens and ultraviolet A. *J. Am. Acad. Dermatol., 9,* 904–911.

58. Petrozzi, J.W., Barton, J.O., Kaidbey. K.H. and Kligman, A.M. (1978): Updating the Goeckerman regimen for psoriasis. *Br. J. Dermatol.,* 98. 437.
59. Pittelkow, M.R., Perry, H.O., Muller, S.A., Maughan, W.Z. and O'Brien, P.C. (1980): Skin cancer in patients with psoriasis treated with coal tar. *Arch. Dermatol., 117,* 465.
60. Plewig, G., Hofmann, C. and Braun-Falco, O. (1978): Photoallergic dermatitis from 8-methoxypsoralen. *Arch. Derm. Res.,* 261. 201.
61. Lin, A.N. and Moses, K. (1985): Tar revisited. *Int. J. Dermatol., 24,* 216–218.
62. Rau, R.C., Flowers, F.P. and Barrett, J.L. (1978): Photo-onycholysis secondary to psoralen use. *Arch. Dermatol., 114,* 448.
63. Reymond, J.L., Beani, J.C. and Amblard, P. (1980): Superficial actinic porokeratosis in a patient undergoing long-term PUVA therapy. *Acta Derm.-Venereol. (Stockh), 60,* 539.
64. Robinson, J.K., Baughman, R.D. and Provost, T.T. (1978): Bullous pemphigoid induced by PUVA therapy. *Br. J. Dermatol., 99,* 709.
65. Roenigk, H.H. and Caro, W.A. (1981): Skin cancer in the PUVA-48 cooperative study. *J. Am. Acad. Dermatol., 4,* 319.
66. Roenigk, H.H. and Martin, J.S. (1977): Photochemotherapy for psoriasis. *Arch. Dermatol., 113,* 1667.
67. Rook, A.J., Gresham, G.A. and Davis, R.A. (1956): Squamous epithelioma possibly induced by the therapeutic application of tar. *Br. J. Cancer, 10,* 17.
68. Takashima, A., Yamamoto, K., Kimura, S., Takakuwa, Y. and Mizuno, N. (1991): Allergic contact and photocontact dermatitis due to psoralens in patients with psoriasis treated with topical PUVA. *Br. J. Dermatol., 124,* 37–42.
69. Scotto, J., Kopf, A.W. and Urbach, F. (1974): Non-melanoma skin cancer among Caucasians in four areas of the United States. *Cancer,* 34, 1333.
70. Segal, R.J. and Watson, W. (1978): Kaposi's varicelliform eruption in mycosis fungoides. *Arch. Dermatol., 114,* 1067.
71. De Groot, A.C. (1992): Psoriasis unguium geprovoceerd door PUVA. *Ned. Tijdschr. Derm. Venereol., 2,* 252–253.
72. Stern, R.S., Thibodeau, L.A., Kleinerman, R.A., Parrish, J.A. and Fitzpatrick, T.B. (1979): Risk of cutaneous carcinoma in patients treated with oral methoxsalen photochemotherapy for psoriasis. *New Engl. J. Med., 300,* 809.
73. Stern, R.S., Morison, W.L., Thibodeau, L.A., Kleinerman, R.A., Parrish, J.A., Geer, D.E. and Fitzpatrick, T.B. (1979): Antinuclear antibodies and oral methoxsalen photochemotherapy (PUVA) for psoriasis. *Arch. Dermatol., 115,* 1320.
74. Stern, R.S., Zierler, S. and Parrish. J.A. (1980): Skin carcinoma in patients with psoriasis treated with topical tar and artificial ultraviolet radiation. *Lancet, 1,* 732.
75. Strauss, G.H., Bridges, B.A., Greaves. M., Vella Briffa, D., Hall Smith. P. and Price, M. (1980): Methoxsalen photochemotherapy. *Lancet, 2,* 1134.
76. Tegner, A. (1979): Severe skin pain after PUVA treatment. *Acta Derm.-Venereol. (Stockh.), 59,* 467.
77. Thomsen, K. and Schmidt, H. (1976): PUVA-induced bullous pemphigoid. *Br. J. Dermatol.,* 95, 568.
78. Tucker, H.H. (1959): Clinical and laboratory tolerance studies in volunteers given oral methoxsalen. *J. Invest. Dermatol., 32,* 277.
79. Binet, O., Bruley, C.L., Beltzer-Garelly, E. and Cesarini, J.P. (1985): Mélanome malin après traitement par rayons ultra-violets A et psoralène. *Press Medicale, 14,* 1842.
80. Hönigsmann, H. (1990): Phototherapy and photochemotherapy. *Semin. Dermatol., 9,* 84–90.
81. Wagner, J., Manthorpe, R., Philip, P. and Frost, F. (1978): Preleukemia (haemopoielic dysplasia) developing in a patient with psoriasis treated with 8-methoxypsoralen and ultraviolet light. *Scand. J. Haemat., 21,* 299.
82. Weissmann, I., Wagner, G. and Plewig. G. (1980): Contact allergy to 8-methoxypsoralen. *Br. J. Dermatol., 102,* 113.
83. McGarry, G.W. and Robertson, J.R. (1989): Scrotal carcinoma following prolonged use of crude coal tar ointment. *Br. J. Urology, 63,* 211.
84. Zala, L., Omar, A. and Krebs, A. (1977): Photo-onycholysis induced by 8-methoxypsoralen. *Dermatologica (Basel), 154,* 203.
85. Lerman, S., Megaw, J.M., Gardner, K.H. and Drake, L. (1983): Ocular and cutaneous manifestations of PUVA therapy — a review. *J. Toxicol.-Cut. Ocul. Toxicol., 1,* 257.
86. Mobacken, H., Rosen, K. and Swanbeck, G. (1983): Oral psoralen photochemotherapy (PUVA) of hyperkeratotic dermatitis of the palms. *Br. J. Dermatol., 109,* 205.

87. Vella Briffa, D., Eady, R.A.J., James, M.P. et al. (1983): Photochemotherapy (PUVA) in the treatment of urticaria pigmentosa. Br. J. *Dermatol., 109,* 67.
88. Moss, C., Friedmann, P.S. and Shuster. S. (1982): How does PUVA inhibit delayed cutaneous hypersensitivity? *Br. J. Dermatol., 107,* 511.
89. Friedmann, P.S., Ford, G., Ross, J. and Diffey, B.L. (1983): Reappearance of epidermal Langerhans cells after PUVA therapy. *Br. J. Dermatol., 109,* 301.
90. Miller, R.A. (1982): Psoralens and UV-A-induced stellate hyperpigmented freckling. *Arch. Dermatol., 118,* 619.
91. Rhodes, A.R., Harrist, T.J. and Momtaz, T.K. (1983): The PUVA-induced pigmented macule: A lentiginous proliferation of large, sometimes cytologically atypical, melanocytes. *J. Am. Acad. Dermatol., 9,* 47.
92. Levin, D.L., Roenigk, H.H. Jr., Caro, W.A. and Lyons, M. (1982): Histologic, immunofluorescent, and antinuclear antibody findings in PUVA-treated patients. *J. Am. Acad. Dermatol., 6,* 328.
93. Lindelöf, B., Sigurgeirsson, B., Tegner, E., Larkö, O. and Berne, B. (1992): Comparison of the carcinogenic potential of trioxsalen bath PUVA and oral methoxsalen PUVA. *Arch. Dermatol., 128,* 1341–1344.
94. George, S.A. and Ferguson, J. (1992): Unusual pattern of phototoxic burning following trimethylpsoralen (TMP) bath photochemotherapy (PUVA). *Br. J. Dermatol., 127,* 444–445.
95. Stern, R.S., Morison, W.L., Thibodeau, L.A. et al. (1979): Antinuclear antibodies and oral methoxsalen photochemotherapy (PUVA) for psoriasis. *Arch. Dermatol., 115,* 1320.
96. Abel, E.A., Cox, A.J. and Farber, E.M. (1982): Epidermal dystrophy and actinic keratoses in psoriasis patients following oral psoralen photochemotherapy (PUVA). *J. Am. Acad. Dermatol., 7,* 333.
97. Halprin, K.M., Comerford, M. and Taylor, J.R. (1982): Cancer in patients with psoriasis. *J. Am. Acad. Dermatol., 7,* 633.
98. Chappe. S.G., Roenigk, H.H. Jr., Miller, A.J. et al. (1981): The effects of photochemotherapy on the cardiovascular system. *J. Am. Acad. Dermatol., 4,* 561.
99. Thurlimann, W. and Harms, M. (1982): Sklerodermiforme Veranderungen nach PUVA-Therapie bei Vitiligo. *Dermatologica (Basel), 164,* 305.
100. Naik, R.P.C. and Parameswara, Y.R. (1982): 8-Methoxypsoralen-induced nail pigmentation. *Int. J. Dermatol., 21,* 275.
101. Fitzsimons, C.P., Long, J. and MacKie, R.M. (1983): Synergistic carcinogenic potential of methotrexate and PUVA in psoriasis (Letter). *Lancet, 1,* 235.
102. Lerman, S., Megaw, J. and Gardner, K. (1982): Psoralen-long-wave ultraviolet therapy and human cataractogenesis. *Invest. Ophthalmol. Vis. Sci., 23.* 801.
103. Ronnerfalt, L., Lydahl, E., Wennersten, G. et al. (1982): Ophthalmological study of patients undergoing long-term PUVA therapy. *Acta Derm.-Venereol. (Stockh.)., 62,* 501.
104. Hammershøy, O. and Jessen, F. (1982): A retrospective study of cataract formation in 96 patients treated with PUVA. *Acta Derm.-Venereol. (Stockh.), 62,* 444.
105. Pullmann, H., Trost, Th. and Witte, U. (1982): Akrale Blasenbildung unter PUVA-Therapie. *Z. Hautkr., 57,* 288.
106. Brun, P. and Baran, R. (1982): Pemphigoïde bulleuse induite par la photochimiothérapie du psoriasis. *Ann. Derm. Vénéréol. (Paris), 109,* 461.
107. Albergo, R.P. and Gilgor, R.S. (1982): Delayed onset of bullous pemphigoid after PUVA and sunlight treatment of psoriasis. *Cutis, 30,* 621.
108. Marsch, W.Ch. and Stüttgen, G. (1982): Ultrastruktur der 'akrobullösen Dermatose' PUVA-therapierter Psoriatiker. *Z. Hautkr., 57,* 1811.
109. Glew, W.B. and Nigra, T.P. (1984): Psoralens and ocular effects in humans. *Nat. Cancer Inst. Monogr., 66,* 235–259.
110. Abel, E.A., Reid, H., Wood, C. and Hu, C.-H. (1985): PUVA-induced melanocytic atypica: is it confined to PUVA lentigines? *J. Am. Acad. Dermatol., 13,* 761–768.
111. Backman, H.A. (1982): The effects of PUVA on the eye. *Am. J. Optom. Physiol. Optics, 59,* 86.
112. Jung, E.G. and Obert, W. (1986): The incidence of PUVA lentigines. *Photodermatol., 3,* 46–47.
113. Kietzmann, H. and Christophers, E. (1984): Pigmentary lesions after PUVA treatment. *Dermatologica, 168,* 306–308.
114. Farber, E.M., Epstein, J.H. (co-chairman), Nall, M.L. (Ed.) and 41 compilers (1982): Current status of oral PUVA therapy for psoriasis: Eye protection revisions. *J. Am. Acad. Dermatol., 6,* 851.
115. Fenton, D.A. and Wilkinson. J.D. (1983): Dose-related visual-field defects in patients receiving PUVA therapy. *Lancet, 1,* 1106.

116. Friedmann, P.S. (1981): Disappearance of epidermal Langerhans cells during PUVA therapy. *Br. J. Dermatol., 105,* 219.
117. Gschnait, F., Wolff, K., Honigsmann, H. et al. (1980): Long-term photochemotherapy: histopathological and immunofluorescence observations in 243 patients. *Br. J. Dermatol., 103,* 11.
118. Kasick, J.M., Berlin, A.J., Berfeld, W. et al. (1982): Development of cataracts with photochemotherapy. In: *Proceedings of the Third International Symposium on Psoriasis,* pp. 467–468. Editors: E.M. Farber and A.J. Cox. Grune & Stratton Inc., New York.
119. Lerman, S. (1982): Ocular phototoxicity and psoralen plus ultraviolet radiation (320–400 nm) therapy: An experimental and clinical evaluation. *J. Nat. Cancer Inst., 69,* 287.
120. Stern, R.S.,Scott, J. and Fears, T.R. (1985): Psoriasis and susceptibility to skin cancer. *J. Am. Acad. Dermatol., 12,* 67–73.
121. Hann, S.K., Park, Y.K., Im, S., Koo, S.W. and Haam, I.B. (1992): The effect on lives transaminases of phototoxic drugs used in systemic photochemotherapy. *J. Am. Acad. Dermatol., 26,* 646–648.
122. Niemi, K.M., Niemi, A.J., Juvakoski, T. et al. (1982): Epidermal dystrophy in psoriasis patients with or without PUVA and with or without previous arsenic treatment. In: *Proceedings of the Third International Symposium on Psoriasis,* pp. 449–450. Editors: E.M. Farber and A.J. Cox. Grune & Stratton Inc., New York.
123. Tegner, E. (1983): Seborrhoeic dermatitis of the face induced by PUVA treatment. *Acta Derm.-Venereol. (Stockh.), 63,* 335.
124. Comaish, J.S. (1987): The effect of tar and ultraviolet on the skin. *J. Invest.Dermatol., 88 (Suppl. 3),* 615–45.
125. Wheeler, L.A., Saperstein, M.D. and Lowe, N.J. (1981): Mutagenicity of urine from psoriatic patients undergoing treatment with coal tar and light *J. Invest. Dermatol., 77,* 181.
126. Bickers, D.R. (1981): The carcinogenicity and mutagenicity of therapeutic tar — a perspective (Editorial). *J. Invest. Dermatol., 77,* 173.
127. Stern, R.S., Parrish. J.A., Bleich, H.L. and Fitzpatrick, T.B. (1981): PUVA (psoralen and ultraviolet A) and squamous cell carcinoma in patients with psoriasis. *J. Invest Dermatol., 76,* 311.
128. Kanerva, L., Laurahanta, J., Niemi, K.M. et al. (1983): Persistent ashen-gray maculae and freckles induced by long-term PUVA treatment. *Dermatologica (Basel), 166,* 281.
129. Lobel, E., Paver, K., King, R. et al. (1981): The relationship of skin cancer to PUVA therapy in Australia. *Aust. J. Dermatol., 22,* 100.
130. Tegner, A. (1983): Observations on PUVA-treatment of psoriasis and on 5-S-cysteinyldopa after exposure to UV light. *Acta Derm.-Venereol. (Stockholm), Suppl.,* 107.
131. Murray, D., Corbett, M.F. and Warin, A.P. (1980): A controlled trial of photochemotherapy for persistent palmoplantar pustulosis. *Br. J. Dermatol. 102,* 659.
132. LeVine, M.J., Parrish, J.A. and Fitzpatrick, T.B. (1981): Oral methoxsalen photochemotherapy (PUVA) of dyshidrotic eczema. *Acta Derm.-Venereol. (Stockh.), 61,* 570.
133. Moss, C., Friedmann, P.S. and Shuster, S. (1981): Impaired contact hypersensitivity in untreated psoriasis and the effects of photochemotherapy and dithranol/UV-B. *Br. J. Dermatol., 105,* 503.
134. Stern, R.S. (1982): Carcinogenic risks of psoriasis therapy. In: *Proceedings of the Third International Symposium on Psoriasis.* Editors: E.M. Farber and A.J. Cox. Grune & Stratton Inc., New York.
135. Segal, S., Cohen. S.N., Freeman, J. et al. (1978): A caution. *Am. Acad. Pediat., 62,* 253.
136. Lassus, A., Kianto, U., Johansson, E. and Juvakoski, T. (1980): PUVA treatment for alopecia areata. *Dermatologica (Basel), 161,* 298.
137. Morison, W.L., Parrish, J.A. and Fitzpatrick, T.B. (1978): Oral psoralen photochemotherapy of atopic eczema. *Br. J. Derm., 98,* 25.
138. Gschnait. F., Honigsmann, H., Brenner, W. et al. (1978): Induction of UV-light tolerance by PUVA in patients with polymorphous light eruption. *Br. J. Derm., 99,* 293.
139. Cox, A.J. and Abel, E.A. (1979): Epidermal dystrophy: Occurrence after psoriasis therapy with psoralen and long-wave ultraviolet light. *Arch. Derm., 115,* 567.
140. Gschnait, F., Wolff, K., Hönigsmann, H. et al. (1980): Long-term photochemotherapy: Histopathological and immunofluorescence observations in 243 patients. *Br. J. Dermatol., 103,* 11.
141. Ingraham, D., Bergfeld, W., Balin, P. et al. (1982): Histopathologic changes in the skin after prolonged PUVA therapy and after discontinuance of PUVA therapy. In: *Psoriasis. Third International Symposium on Psoriasis,* pp. 457–458. Editors: E.M. Farber and A.J. Cox. Grune & Stratton Inc., New York.
142. Epstein, J.H. (1978): Photocarcinogenesis: A review. *Nat. Cancer Inst. Monogr. 50,* 13.

143. Heidbreder, G. (1980): Lokalisierte Blasen bei Fotochemotherapie — eine akrobullöse Fotodermatose. *Z. Hautkr., 55,* 84.
144. McGibbon, D.H. and Vella-Briffa, D. (1978): Histologic features of PUVA-induced bullae in psoriatic skin. *Clin. Exp. Derm., 3,* 371.
145. Crickx, B., Girouin, D., diCrescenzo, M.C. and Hewitt, J. (1979): Psoriasis et pemphigoide bulleuse. *Journées Derm. Paris,* March 1979, p. 56.
146. Gissler, K. and Lischka, G. (1978): PUVA induziertes bulloses Pemphigoid bei Psoriasis vulgaris. *Akta Derm., 4,* 47.
147. Grupper, C., Bernejo, D., Durepaire, R. and Berretti, B. (1977): Pemphigus séborrhéique de Senear-Usher compliquant un psoriasis. Rôle aggravant de la PUVA therapie. *Journées Derm. Paris,* March 9–10, p. 77.
148. Freeman. R.G. and Troll, D. (1969): Photosensitization of the eye by 8-methoxypsoralen. *J. Invest. Dermatol., 53,* 449,
149. Lerman, S. (1984): Psoralens and ocular effects in man and animals: in vivo monitoring of human ocular and cutaneous manifestations. *Nat. Cancer Inst. Monogr., 66,* 227–233.
150. Davey, J.B.,,Piffey, B.L. and Miller, J.A. (1981): Eye protection in psoralen photochemotherapy. *Br. J. Dermatol., 104,* 295.
151. Szekeres, E., Török, L. and Szucs, M. (1981): Auftreten disseminierter hyperpigmentierter Flecke unter PUVA-Behandlung. *Hautarzt, 32,* 33.
152. Skogh. M. and Moi, H. (1978): Naevus-spilus-artige Hyperpigmentierung bei Psoriasis. *Hautarzt, 29,* 607.
153. Konrad, K., Gschnait, F. and Wolff, K. (1977): Ultrastructure of poikiloderma-like pigmentary changes after repeated experimental PUVA-overdosage. *J. Cutan. Pathol., 4,* 219.
154. Kanerva, L., Niemi, K.-M. and Lauharanta, J. (1984): A semiquantitative light and electron microscopic analysis of histopathologic changes in photochemotherapy-induced freckles. *Arch. Derm. Res., 276,* 2–11.
155. Kanerva, L., Lauharanta, J., Niemi, K.-M. et al. (1982): *Fine Structure of Freckles Induced by Long Term PUVA Treatment of Psoriasis.* XI Int. Congr. Dermatology, Tokyo. Abstr. 582, pp. 408–409.
156. MacKie, R.M. and Fitzsimons, C.P. (1983): Risk of carcinogenicity in patients with psoriasis treated with methotrexate or PUVA singly or in combination. *J. Am. Acad. Dermatol., 9,* 467.
157. Leonard, F., Morel, M., Kalis, B. et al. (1991): Psoralen plus ultraviolet A in the prophylactic treatment of benign summer light eruption. *Photodermatol. Photoimmunol. Photomed., 8,* 95–98.
158. Rampen. F.H.J. (1983): Hypertrichosis in PUVA-treated patients. *Br. J. Dermatol., 109,* 657–660.
159. Morison, W.L. and Strickland, P.T. (1983): Environmental UVA radiation and eye protection during PUVA therapy. *J. Am. Acad. Dermatol., 9,* 522.
160. Todes-Taylor, N., Abel, E.A. and Cox, A.J. (1983): The occurrence of vitiligo after psoralens and ultraviolet A therapy. *J. Am. Acad. Dermatol., 9,* 526.
161. Rhodes, A.R., Stern, R.S. and Melski, J.W. (1983): The PUVA lentigo: an analysis of predisposing factors. *J. Invest. Dermatol., 81,* 459–463.
162. Lohmann, H., Buck-Gramcko, D. and El-Makawi, M. (1985): Schwere Hautverbrennung durch ein Photochemotherapeutikum. *Dermatosen, 53,* 102–103.
163. Norris, P.G., Maurice, P.D.L., Schott, G.D. and Greaves, M.W. (1987): Persistent skin pain after PUVA. *Clin Exp. Dermatol., 12,* 403–405.
164. Roelandts, R. and Stevens, A. (1990): PUVA-induced itching and skin pain. *Photodermatol. Photoimmunol. Photomed., 7,* 141–142.
165. Verhagen, A.R., van der Wiel, A.G. and Wuite, G.G. (1984): Atypical psoriasis of the face and hands after PUVA treatment. *Br. J. Dermatol., 111,* 615–518.
166. Morison, W.L. (1989): Topical phototoxicity from oral methoxsalen capsules. *Arch. Dermatol., 125,* 433.
167. Gange, R.W., and Parrish, J.A. (1984): Cutaneous phototoxicity due to psoralens. *Natl. Cancer Inst. Monogr., 66,* 117–126.
168. McFadden, J.P., Powles, A.V. and Walker, M. (1989): Rosacea induced by PUVA therapy. *Br. J. Dermatol., 121,* 413.
169. Hazen, P.G., Carney, J.F., Walker, A.E., Stewart, J.J. and Engstrom, C.W. (1985): Disseminated superficial actinic porokeratosis: appearance associated with photochemotherapy for psoriasis. *J. Am. Acad. Dermatol., 12,* 1077–1078.
170. Lederman, J.S., Sober, A.J. and Lederman, G.S. (1986): Psoralens and ultraviolet A immunosuppression and porokeratosis. *J. Am. Acad. Dermatol., 14,* 284–285.
171. Cockerell, C.J. (1991): Induction of disseminated superficial actinic porokeratosis by phototherapy for psoriasis. *J. Am. Acad. Dermatol., 24,* 301–302.

172. van der Schroeff, G.J., Schothorst, A.A. and Kanaar, P. (1983): Induction of actinic lichen planus with artificial UV sources. *Arch. Dermatol., 119*, 498–500.
173. Wennersten, G. (1986): Actinic lichenoid dermatitis induced by PUVA therapy in vitiligo patients. *Photodermatol., 3*, 247–248.
174. Nishimura, M. and Hori, Y. (1990): Late-onset neurofibromas developed in a patient with psoriasis vulgaris during PUVA treatment. *Arch. Dermatol., 126*, 541–542.
175. Van der Wegen-Keijser, M.H., Prevoo, R.L.M.H. and Bruynzeel, D.P. (1991): Acantholytic dyskeratotic epidermal naevus in a patient with guttate psoriasis on PUVA therapy. *Br. J. Dermatol., 124*, 603–655
176. Leroy, D. and Deschamps, P. (1985): Photosensitization to drugs in skin areas previously treated with PUVA therapy. *Press Med., 14*, 432.
177. Nakagawa, T., Nishimoto, M. and Takaiwa, T. (1986): Disseminated epidermolytic acanthoma revealed by PUVA. *Dermatologica, 173*, 150–153.
178. Picascia, D.D., Rothe, M., Goldberg, N.G. and Roenigk, H.H. Jr. (1987): Antinuclear antibodies during psoralens plus ultraviolet A (PUVA) therapy — are they worthwhile? *J. Am. Acad. Dermatol., 16*, 574–577.
179. Tuffanelli, D.L. (1987): Antinuclear antibodies and photosensitivity in lupus erythematosus — relevant in PUVA therapy? *J. Am. Acad. Dermatol., 16*, 614–616.
180. Bruze, M., Krook, G. and Ljunggren, B. (1984): Fatal connective tissue disease with antinuclear antibodies following PUVA therapy. *Acta Derm. Venereol., 64*, 157–160.
181. Millns, J.L., McDuffie, F.C., Muller, S.A. and Jordon, R.E. (1978): Development of photosensitivity and an SLE-like syndrome in a patient with psoriasis. *Arch. Dermatol., 114*, 1177–1181.
182. Kürkfüoğlu, N. and Sahin, S. (1991): PUVA-induced discoid lupus erythematosus in a patient with vitiligo. *J. Am. Acad. Dermatol., 24*, 515.
183. McFadden, N. (1984): PUVA-induced lupus erythematosus in a patient with polymorphous light eruption. *Photodermatol., 1*, 148–150.
184. Domke, H.F., Ludwisen, D. and Thormann, J. (1979): Discoid lupus erythematosus possibly due to photochemotherapy. *Arch. Dermatol., 115*, 642.
185 Dowdy, M.J., Nigra, T.P. and Barth, W.F. (1989): Subacute cutaneous lupus erythematosus during PUVA therapy for psoriasis: case report and review of the literature. *Arthritis and Rheumatism, 32*, 343–346.
186. Henseler, T., Hönigsmann, H., Wolff,K., Christophers, E. (1981): Oral 8-methoxypsoralen photochemotherapy of psoriasis. The European PUVA study: a cooperative study among 18 European centres. *Lancet, i*: 853–857.
187. Stern, R.S., Laird, N., Melski, J. et al. (1984): Cutaneous squamous cell carcinoma in patients treated with PUVA. *New Engl. J. Med., 310*, 1156–61
188. Stern, R.S., Lange, R. and Members of the Photochemotherapy Follow-up Study (1988): Non-melanoma skin cancer occurring in patients treated with PUVA five to ten years after first treatment. *J. Invest. Dermatol., 91*, 120–124.
189. Tanew, A., Hönigsmann, H., Ortel, B. et al. (1986): Non-melanoma skin tumors in long-term photochemotherapy treatment of psoriasis. *J. Am. Acad. Dermatol., 15*, 960–965.
190. Henseler, T., Christophers, E., Hönigsmann, H. and Wolff, K. (1987): Skin tumors in the European PUVA study. *J. Am. Acad. Dermatol., 16,* 108–116.
191. Forman, A.B., Roenigk, H.H. Jr., Caro, W.A. and Magid, M.L. (1989): Long-term follow-up of skin cancer in the PUVA-48 cooperative study. *Arch. Dermatol., 125*, 515–519.
192. Eskelinen, A., Halme, K., Lassus, A. and Idänpään-Heikkilä, J. (1985): Risk of cutaneous carcinoma in psoriatic patients treated with PUVA. *Photodermatol., 2*, 10–14.
193. Lindskov, R. (1983): Skin carcinomas and treatment with photochemotherapy (PUVA). *Acta Derm. Venereol., 63*, 223–226.
194. Ros, A., Wennersten, G. and Lagerholm, B. (1983): Long-term photochemotherapy for psoriasis: a histopathological and clinical follow-up study with special emphasis on tumour incidence and behaviour of pigmented lesions. *Acta Derm. Venereol., 63*, 215–221.
195. Torinuki, W. and Tagami, H. (1988): Incidence of skin cancer in Japanese psoriatic patients treated with either PUVA, Goeckermann regimen or both therapies. *J. Am. Acad. Dermatol., 18*, 1278–1281.
196. Cox, N.H., Jones, S.K., Dowd, D.J. et al. (1987): Cutaneous and ocular side-effects of oral photochemotherapy: results of an 8-year follow-up study. *Br. J. Dermatol., 116*, 145–152.
197. Barth, J., Meffert, H., Schiller, F. and Sonnichsen, N. (1987): Zehn Jahre PUVA-Therapie in der DDR — Analyse zum Langzeitrisiko. *Z. Klin. Med., 42*, 889–892.

198. Reshad, H., Challoner, F., Pollock, D.J. and Baker, H. (1984): Cutaneous carcinoma in psoriatic patients treated with PUVA. *Br. J. Dermatol., 110*, 299–305.
199. Chuang, T.-Y., Tse, J. and Cripps, D.J. (1989): A preliminary study on the link between PUVA and skin cancer. *Int. J. Dermatol., 28,* 438–440.
200. Stern, R.S. and Members of the Photochemotherapy Follow-up Study. (1990): Genital tumors among men with psoriasis exposed to psoralens and ultraviolet A radiation (PUVA) and ultraviolet B radiation. *N. Engl. J. Med., 322,* 1093–1097.
201. Bruynzeel, I., Bergman, W., Hartevelt, H.M. et al. (1991): "High singledose" European PUVA regimen also causes an excess of nonmelanoma skin cancer. *Br. J. Dermatol., 124,* 49–55.
202. Perkins, W., Lamont, D. and MacKie, R.M. (1990): Cutaneous malignancy in males treated with photochemotherapy. *Lancet, ii,* 1248
203. Takashima, A., Matsunami, E., Yamamoto, K., Kitajima, S. and Mizuno, N. (1990): Cutaneous carcinoma and 8-methoxypsoralen and ultraviolet A (PUVA) lentigines in Japanese patients with psoriasis treated with topical PUVA: a follow-up study of 214 patients. *Photodermatol. Photoimmunol. Photomed., 7*: 218–221.
204. Mali-Gerrits, M.G.H., Gaasbeek, D., Boezeman, J. and van de Kerkhof, P.C.M. (1991): Psoriasis therapy and the risk of skin cancers. *Clin. Exp. Dermatol., 16,* 185–189.
205. Lindelof, B., Sigugeirsson, B., Tegner, E. et al. (1991): PUVA and cancer: a large-scale epidemiological study. *Lancet, 338,* 91–93.
206. Frenk, E. (1983): Malignant melanoma in a patient with severe psoriasis treated by oral methoxsalen photochemotherapy. *Dermatologica, 167,* 152–154.
207. Hensen, N.E. (1979): Development of acute myeloid leukaemia in a patient with psoriasis treated with oral 8-methoxypsoralen and longwave ultraviolet light. *Scand. J. Haematol., 22,* 57–60.
208. Freeman, K. and Warin, A.P. (1985): Acute myelomonocytic leukaemia developing in a patient with psoriasis treated with 8-methoxypsoralen and longwave ultraviolet light. *Clin. Exp. Dermatol., 10,* 144–146.
209. Sheehan-Dare, R.A., Cotterill, J.A. and Barnard, D.L. (1989): Transformation of myelo-dysplasia to acute myeloid leukaemia during psoralen photochemotherapy (PUVA) treatment of psoriasis. *Acta Derm. Venereol, 69,* 262–264.
210. Higgins, E.M., Todd, P. and du Vivier, A.W.P. (1991): PUVA and Cancer. *Lancet, 338,* 703–704.
211. Stern, R.S. and Lange, R. (1988): Cadiovascular diseases, cancer and cause of death in patients with psoriasis: 10 years prospective experience in a cohort of 1380 patients. *J. Invest. Dermatol., 91,* 197–201.
212. Beiteke, U., Budde, J., Lentnor, A., Stary, A. and Tronnier, H. (1988): Multiple eruptive actinic keratoses and squamous cell carcinomata following PUVA therapy of more than 11 years. *Photodermatol., 5,* 274–276.
213. Westphal, H.J., Wurdel, C. and Flegel, H. (1989): Aktinische Keratosen-Folgen einer PUVA Langzeittherapie. *Dermatol. Mon. Schr., 175,* 623–627.
214. Stern, R.S., Parrish, J.A., Fitzpatrick, T.B. and Bleich, H.L. (1985): Actinic degeneration in association with long-term use of PUVA. *J. Invest. Dermatol., 84,* 135–138.
215. Sina, B. and Adrian, R.M. (1983): Multiple keratoacanthomas possibly induced by psoralens and ultraviolet A photochemotherapy. *J. Am. Acad. Dermatol., 9,* 686–688.
216. Prens, E.P. and Smeenk, G. (1983): Effect of photochemotherapy on the cardiovascular system. *Dermatologica, 167,* 208–211.
217. Mora-Morillas, I., Vazquez-Lopez, F., Sanchez-Lozano, J.L. and Garcia-Perez, A. (1987): Cardiac complications of psoralens plus ultraviolet A (PUVA) therapy. *J. Am. Acad. Dermatol., 17,* 691–692.
218. Ramsay, B. and Marks, J.M. (1988): Bronchoconstriction due to 8-methoxypsoralen. *Br. J. Dermatol., 119,* 83–86.
219. Wennersten, G. (1987): Exacerbation of bronchial asthma during photochemotherapy with 8-methoxypsoralen and UVA (PUVA). *Photodermatol., 4,* 212–213.
220. Anderson, C.D., Frödin, Th. and Skogh, M. (1987): Bronchial reactions to photochemotherapy (PUVA). *J. Am. Acad. Dermatol., 16,* 389–390.
221. Ashinoff, R., Buchness, M.R. and Lim, H.W. (1989): Lymphoma in a black patient with actinic reticuloid treated with PUVA: possible etiologic considerations. *J. Am. Acad. Dermatol., 21,* 1134–1137.
222. Chretien, P., Galmiche, J.P. and Payenneville J.M. et al. (1983): Effects of oral methoxypsoralen photochemotherapy (PUVA) on liver function and antipyrin kinetics. *Int. J. Clin. Pharm. Res., 3,* 343–347.
223. Freeman, K. and Warin, A.P. (1984): Deterioration of liver function during PUVA therapy. *Photodermatol., 1,* 147–148.

224. Nyfors, A., Dahl-Nyfors, B. and Hopwood, D. (1986): Liver biopsies from patients with psoriasis related to photochemotherapy (PUVA): findings before and after 1 year of therapy in twelve patients. *J. Am. Acad. Dermatol., 14,* 43–48.
225. Lam Thuon Mine, L.T.K., Williams, P.F. and Anderson, J.L. (1983): Nephrotic syndrome after treatment with psoralens and ultraviolet A. *Br. Med. J., 287,* 94–95.
226. Hönigsmann, H., Brenner, W., Rauschmeier, W., Konrad, K. and Wolff, K. (1984): Photochemotherapy for cutaneous T cell lymphoma. *J. Am. Acad. Dermatol., 10,* 238–245.
227. Christophers, E. and Reusch, M. (1986): PUVA responses in skin disease - the lack of known target sites. *Photodermatol., 3,* 1–3.
228. Stern, R.S. and Lange, R. (1991): Outcomes of pregnancies among women and partners of men with a history of exposure to methoxsalen photochemotherapy (PUVA) for the treatment of psoriasis. *Arch. Dermatol., 127,* 347–350.
229. White, S.I., Friedmann, P.S., Moss, C. and Simpson, J.M. (1988): Recovery of cutaneous immune responsiveness after PUVA therapy. *Br. J. Dermatol., 118,* 403–407.
230. Gisslen, P., Kalimo, K. and Larkö. (1986): Exanthematous drug reaction caused by 8-methoxypsoralen. *Photodermatol., 3,* 308–309.
231. Berg, M. (1989): Drug fever caused by 8-methoxypsoralen. *Photodermatology, 6,* 149–150.
232. Tothkasa, I. and Dobozy, A. (1985): Drug fever caused by PUVA treatment. *Acta Derm. Venereol., 65,* 557--558.
233. Ljunggren, B. and Mattiasson, I. (1986): Acute methoxsalen intoxication. *J. Am. Acad. Dermatol., 15,* 533.
234. Collins, P. and Rogers, S. (1992): Bath-water compared with oral delivery of 8-methoxypsoralen PUVA therapy for chronic plaque psoriasis. *J. Am. Acad. Dermatol., 127,* 392–395.
235. Cox, N.H. and Rogers, S. (1989): Cutaneous drug eruption caused by 8-methoxypsoralen. *Photodermatol., 6,* 96–97.
236. Jemec, G.B.E. (1990): Unusual immediate adverse effects of photochemotherapy. *J. Derm. Treatment, 1,* 275–276.
237. Pullmann, H. (1984): Nebenwirkungen und Risiken der Phototherapie. *Z. Hautkr., 59,* 1056–1063.
238. Moy, L.S., Chalet, M. and Lowe, N.J. (1986): Scrotal squamous cell carcinoma in a psoriatic patient treated with coal tar. *J. Am. Acad. Dermatol., 14,* 518–519.
239. Jones, S.K., McKie, R., Hole, D.J. and Gillis, C.R. (1985): Further evidence of the safety of tar in the management of psoriasis. *Br. J. Dermatol., 113,* 97–101.
240. Hjorth, N. and Jacobsen, M. (1983): Coal tar. *Semin. Dermatol., 2,* 281–286.
241. Sarto, F., Zordan, M. and Tomanin, R. et al. (1989): Chromosomal alterations in peripheral blood lymphocytes, urinary mutagenicity and excretion of polycyclic aromatic hydrocarbons in six psoriatic patients undergoing coal tar therapy. *Carcinogeneis, 10,* 329–334.
242. Stern, R.S. (1988): The benefits, costs and risks of topical tar preparations in the treatment of psoriasis: considerations of cost effectiveness. *Ann. Acad. Med. 17,* 473–476.

19. Side effects of systemic drugs used in dermatology

CORTICOSTEROIDS [1–9,23]

19.1 Corticosteroids are widely used in dermatology for a variety of skin disorders (Table 19.1) [2].

Table 19.1. Dermatological indications for glucocorticosteroids

Bullous dermatoses	**Neutrophilic dermatoses**
Pemphigus vulgaris/superficial forms	Pyoderma gangrenosum
Bullous pemphigoid	Sweet's syndrome
Cicatrical pemphigoid	Behcet's disease/aphthous ulcers
Herpes gestationis	
Erythema multiforme	**Dermatitis/papulosquamous**
Epidermolysis bullosa acquisita	Contact dermatitis
Linear IgA bullous dermatosis	Exfoliative erythroderma
	Lichen planus
Connective tissue diseases	
Systemic lupus erythematosus	Other dermatoses
Dermatomyositis	(Pulmonary) sarcoidosis
Mixed connective tissue disease	Sunburn
	Urticaria (severe)
Vasculitis	Androgen excess
Cutaneous	Post-herpetic neuralgia
Systemic	

Table 19.2 lists the common glucocorticoids, together with relative potency.

Table 19.2. Relative potency of corticosteroids [3]

Corticosteroid	Equivalent dose	Relative potency	
		Glucocorticoid	Mineralocorticoid
Hydrocortisone	20	1	2
Prednisone	5	4	1
Prednisolone	5	4	1
Methylprednisolone	4	5	0
Triamcinolone	4	5	0
Betamethasone	0.6	25	0
Dexamethasone	0.75	25	0

The incidence of adverse reactions depends upon the dose level, but to an even greater degree upon the duration of treatment. Brief bursts of glucocorticosteroids for 2–3 weeks are surprisingly safe and very useful in self-limiting dermatoses. The main risks arising from longer treatment with glucocorticosteroids are summarized in Table 19.3.

Table 19.3. Risks of glucocorticosteroid therapy

I	**Exogenous hypercorticism with 'Cushing's syndrome'**
a	Moon face (facial rounding)
b	Central obesity
c	Striae
d	Hirsutism
e	Acne [21]
f	Ecchymoses
g	Hypertension
h	Osteoporosis
i	Myopathy (atrophy of hip muscles)
k	Disorders of sexual function
l	Diabetes mellitus
m	Hyperlipidaemia
n	Disorders of mineral and fluid balance
II	**Endogenous hypocortisolism (atrophy of the adrenal cortex)**
a	Insufficient or lacking stress reaction
b	Withdrawal effects
c	Relapse of disease being treated

(continued)

(continuation)

III Unwanted results accompanying the desired effects on the tissue

a Increased risk of infection

b Disturbed wound healing

c Peptic ulcer risks such as bleeding and perforation

IV Untoward side effects with unknown correlations

a Mental disturbance

b Increased risk of thrombosis

c Cataracts

d Increased intraocular pressure and glaucoma

e Aseptic necrosis of bone

f Corticoid dependence (with long-term therapy)

Cardiovascular

The mineralocorticoid activity of a steroid may lead to salt and water retention and hypertension. Fluid retention can aggravate pre-existing congestive heart failure. Cardiac lesions have included ECG changes, acute myocardial infarction, myocardial hypertrophy and myopathy. Hypokalaemia may lead to arrhythmias and cardiac arrest. Sudden death and life-threatening ventricular arrhythmias have primarily occurred with pulse intravenous methylprednisolone regimens. Arteritis has occurred, especially in rheumatic patients. Accelerated atherosclerosis has been noted in patients with lupus erythematosus and rheumatoid arthritis.

Respiratory

Allergic reactions may involve respiratory impairment.

Nervous system

Large doses can cause behavioral and personality changes ranging from nervousness, insomnia, euphoria or mood swings to psychotic episodes which can include both manic and depressive states, paranoid states and acute toxic psychoses. Cerebral atrophy and organic brain syndrome have been reported. Latent epilepsy can be rendered manifest. Intracranial hypertension is seen mainly in children and young women. Presenting symptoms include headache, nausea, vomiting, and visual changes. Papilloedema is present on physical examination. This occurs primarily as a withdrawal effect.

Endocrine, metabolic

The endocrine effects of the glucocorticosteroids involve variously the pituitary–adrenal axis, the genitals, the parathyroid and the thyroid; there are also metabolic effects, primarily involving the carbohydrates.

Pituitary–adrenal axis. Elevated glucocorticoid plasma levels result after two weeks in iatrogenic Cushing's syndrome (see Table 19.3, I). Prominent features (which may occur individually or in combination) are benign intracranial hypertension, glaucoma, subcapsular cataract, pancreatitis, aseptic necrosis of the bones, panniculitis, obesity, facial rounding, psychiatric symptoms, edema and delayed wound healing. Cushing-like effects are to be expected if the function of the adrenal cortex is suppressed by daily doses of 50 mg hydrocortisone or its equivalent (12.5 mg prednisone/prednisolone). Long-term suppression of the adrenal cortex can result in a withdrawal syndrome. In many cases this is unpleasant rather than acutely dangerous; in such instances the patients may experience headache, nausea, dizziness, anorexia, weakness, emotional changes, lethargy, arthralgias, myalgias and perhaps fever. More serious consequences can ensue, however, and in some cases acute adrenocortical insufficiency after a period of glucocorticoid treatment has actually proved fatal. Post-steroid panniculitis has been observed primarily in patients with rheumatic fever.

Menstrual cycle. Disorders of menstruation occur frequently.

Testicular function. Reduced sperm count and motility and inhibition of the secretory function of the testicle have been reported.

Thyroid function. The uptake of iodine is suppressed by corticosteroids. Pathological changes in thyroid function, however, are rare.

Carbohydrate metabolism. All glucocorticosteroids increase gluconeogenesis, and blood glucose is increased 10–20%. Steroid diabetes is seen in 20% of patients treated, and normally disappears after discontinuance. Most patients developing overt diabetes have prior abnormal glucose tolerance. Diabetic ketoacidosis and hyperosmolar nonketotic coma are rare complications.

Lipid metabolism. High-dose corticosteroid therapy may induce marked hypertriglyceridaemia with milky plasma.

Weight gain is a common result both of increased appetite and of fluid retention. This weight gain may occur even with brief courses of corticosteroids. Patients receiving pharmacologic doses for more than a month generally develop, at least, mild cushingoid facies. Truncal obesity and a 'buffalo hump' are noted less frequently.

Parathyroid. Hypocalcaemia is uncommon, but has led to tetany in children.

Mineral and fluid balance

Although glucocorticosteroids have a low mineralocorticoid activity, salt and water retention may occur. Pseudohyperaldosteronism, increased calcium and phosphorus excretion, and potassium loss have been reported.

Haematological

The total leukocyte count is increased, but the number of eosinophilic leukocytes and the lymphocyte count decrease. The thrombocyte count increases. Polycytaemia is a symptom of Cushing's syndrome and anaemia is correlated to Addison's disease. An increase in haemoglobin is frequently observed. Effects on blood coagulation may lead to thrombosis. Purpura is caused by increased fragility of the capillaries.

Liver

The influence of long-term corticosteroid treatment on liver function is still unknown. Fatty liver changes have been reported. This uncommonly leads to significant symptoms or altered liver function test results. Treatment of viral hepatitis with corticosteroids has led to chronic active hepatitis.

Gastrointestinal

Minor gastrointestinal symptoms are common with brief bursts of corticosteroid therapy. There is still no absolute proof of a markedly increased risk of peptic ulcer. That there is some effect, however, seems clear [11]. Gastrointestinal haemorrhage occurs in 2.8% of patients treated, in many of which occult blood is the only finding. Pancreatitis and derangements of pancreatic secretion can appear at any time during long-term corticosteroid treatment. Necrosis of the pancreas can be lethal. Treatment of regional ileitis may lead to perforation of the ileum, lymphatic dilatation and microscopic fistulae. With treatment of ulcerative colitis there is an increased risk of toxic megacolon or colonic perforation.

Reported gastrointestinal symptoms and signs are summarized in Table 19.4.

Table 19.4. Reported gastrointestinal complications of oral glucocorticoid therapy [3]

Anorexia	Perforation (small bowel, large bowel, colon, gallbladder)
Fatty liver	Peritonitis
Haemorrhage	Rectal ulceration
Nausea	Vomiting
Oesophagitis and ulceration	Weight gain
Pancreatitis	Weight loss
Peptic ulcer disease	

Urinary system

There is an increased possibility of formation of urinary calculi because of the raised excretion of calcium and phosphate. An increase in the incidence of proteinuria in children awaits confirmation. Changes resembling diabetic nodular glomerular sclerosis have been seen in corticoid-treated nephrosis. Nocturia is fairly common during glucocorticoid treatment.

Skin and appendages

Classic cutaneous side effects of corticosteroids include: striae, ecchymoses and purpura, atrophy, and teleangiectasias [3]. Patients may develop the androgen-like signs of acne and hirsutism [3,5]. Erythroderma may occur in patients sensitized to topical corticosteroids. Perioral dermatitis is rare [13].

Leukoderma has been observed. The function of the sebaceous glands is suppressed. Infections of the skin are often caused by suppression of the immune system. Wound-healing may be impaired [4,6]. Telogen effluvium may occur with high-dose therapy even for brief durations [3].

Injection of steroids may lead to subcutaneous atrophy and lipatrophy (with leukoderma). Table 19.5 summarizes steroid-induced skin changes [3].

Table 19.5. Skin changes reported with use of oral glucocorticoids [3]

Acanthosis nigricans
Acneiform eruption [21]
Alopecia
Atrophy and thin skin
Desquamation
Erythema
Erythromelanosis
Hirsutism
Hyperpigmentation
Hypertrichosis

Eyes

The incidence of posterior subcapsular cataract in patients undergoing long-term therapy seems to be about 10%. Spontaneous regression sometimes occur, even with continued treatment. Increased intraocular pressure and glaucoma are well-known side effects. The rise in intraocular pressure may lead to blindness. Exophthalmus is uncommon. Although transient myopia may occur, long-term refraction changes are uncommon. Other reported changes include [3] ptosis and chemosis, papilloedema, scleral thinning, increased incidence of infection (herpes keratitis) and blue sclera.

Bones and joints

Of the effects of corticosteroids on the skeleton, osteoporosis is the most important clinically. Areas with high trabecular bone content, such as the spine and ribs, as well as the vertebral bodies are at greatest risk. Manifestations can include vertebral compression fractures, scoliosis resulting in respiratory embarrassment, and fractures of the long bones. Avascular aseptic necrosis of bone has often been described and preferentially involves the femoral and humeral head. Tendon rupture has rarely been observed.

Muscles

Excessive corticoid levels result in protein catabolism and hence in muscular atrophy and fibrosis. The myopathy develops gradually, without pain and symmetrically. It is characterized mainly by muscle weakness and atrophy of the hip muscles and the shoulders. The risk is especially high in children, and the myopathy normally improves over a period of months after discontinuance.

Effects on immune defence mechanisms and incidence of infection

Corticosteroids inhibit the formation of antibodies and thereby immune responses. Aggravation of existing tuberculosis and reactivation of completely quiescent cases are known. Other bacterial infections, including sepsis, have followed glucocorticoid treatment. Fungal, candidal and viral infections may be aggravated. Strongyloidiasis, amoebic dysentery and toxoplasmosis have all on some occasion been precipitated or aggravated by corticosteroids. There appears to be a minimal risk of malignancy induction by corticosteroid monotherapy, although risk of (reversible) Kaposi's sarcoma may be increased [12].

Effect on growth

The retardation of growth by long-term corticosteroid treatment in children is a known side effect of these catabolic hormones. Growth hormone excretion is diminished. As long as the epiphyses have not closed, there will be merely a delay in growth. Children treated with high-dose corticosteroids eventually attain their expected height [10].

Second-generation effects

Teratogenic effects shown in animal experiments have not been confirmed in man. Intensive corticosteroid treatment of pregnant women may, however, result in secondary insufficiency of the adrenal cortex of the newborn. Retardation of intrauterine growth has also been reported. The figures for the possibility that the risk of stillbirth may be increased are suggestive, but the relationship is not absolutely proven.

Interactions

Diphenylhydantoin, phenobarbital, isoniazid, rifampicin and other drugs inducing liver enzymes reduce the plasma half-life of corticosteroids. Oral contraceptives may prolong the serum half-life of corticosteroids. Glucocorticosteroids reduce the plasma levels of salicylates and vitamins A, C and D. The combination with anti-inflammatory drugs increases the risk of gastric ulceration. Corticosteroids potentiate potassium loss when combined with potassium-losing diuretics. They appear to increase anticoagulant requirement, and there is an increased risk of gastric bleeding. Corticosteroids may indirectly lead to digoxin toxicity resulting from hypokalaemia.

Intralesional corticosteroid therapy

Indications for intralesional corticosteroid therapy include alopecia areata, keloids, lichen ruber obtusus, acne cystica and necrobiosis lipoidica.

Systemic side effects

Systemic side effects of intralesional corticosteroid therapy are usually related to suppression of adrenal glands [14]. Severe cramps in the back, shoulders and legs immediately following intralesional injection of corticosteroids and lasting for about half an hour have been reported [15]. This side effect was attributed to injection of crystals into a small vein.

Local side effects

The local side effects of intralesional corticosteroids include:
- alopecia [19]
- amaurosis (?) [20]
- bowstring digital deformity [19]
- calcinosis cutis [18]
- carpal tunnal infection [19]
- cutaneous atrophy, sometimes with striae
- depigmentation or hypopigmentation [19]
- granulomas [22]
- linear atrophy along lymphatic vessels [19]
- local erythema, appearing after 12 hours and lasting for about 36 hours [17]
- necrosis
- septic arthritis [22]
- tendon rupture [22]

RETINOIDS [24–27]

19.2 Retinoids are naturally occurring compounds and synthetic derivatives of retinol (Vitamin A) that exhibit vitamin A activity. The first compound of this class that was subjected to intensive research was vitamin A itself, which is essential for normal epithelial differentiation and keratinisation. When vitamin A was used in the treatment of disorders of keratinisation, it was soon recognised that there was an unfavourable ratio between its moderate clinical effects on the one hand and its frequent side effects on the other hand. The synthesis of less toxic retinoid derivatives led firstly to tretinoin (all-*trans*-retinoic acid). Although this compound soon established a place for itself in topical therapy, its systemic use did not reveal significant advantages over vitamin A. During the past 10 years, more than 1500 new retinoids have been synthesized. A therapeutically useful 'first generation' retinoid (Table 19.6) was isotretinoin (13-*cis*-retinoic acid) which showed excellent results in the treatment of severe nodular and cystic acne, the first time an oral medication had produced long-term remissions in this condition.

When the first aromatic compound, etretinate, a synthetic retinoid of the 'second generation', was developed, a real breakthrough in the treatment of severe psoriasis and other dermatoses, including various genokeratoses, was achieved. The favourable ratio between therapeutic efficacy and side effects resulted in widespread clinical use of this compound. Of particular importance with etretinate is its very long elimination half-life (6 months to 1 year). This was notably troublesome for women of childbearing age, as retinoids are teratogens. After cessation of etretinate, contraception had to be maintained for another 2 years to avoid malformations. In 1989, etretinate was replaced with acitretin, its main metabolite, because this compound, which is equally effective, has a much shorter half-life of elimination of approximately 50 hours [28]. Polyaromatic retinoids, such as the arotinoids, represent the 'third generation' of synthetic retinoids (Table 19.6). These are at, at the time of writing, still under investigation.

Table 19.6. Classification of retinoids

First generation
Tretinoin (all-*trans*-retinoic acid)
Isotretinoin (13-*cis*-retinoic acid)
Second generation (aromatic compounds)
Etretinate (Tigason)
Acitretin (Neotigason)
Ro 12-7554 (chlorinated)
Third generation (polyaromatic compounds)
Arotinoid (Ro 15-0778)
Arotinoid ethylester (Ro 13-6298)
Arotinoid carboxylic acid (Ro 13-7410)
Arotinoid sulfone (Ro 15-1570)

The natural and synthetic retinoids exert a variety of biological activities. The retinoids mainly influence proliferation and differentiation, particularly in keratinizing epithelia; in addition, they may modify immune reactions, exert marked effects on inflammatory processes and, last but not least, they markedly suppress the activity of sebaceous glands. The various synthetic retinoids show considerable differences in their spectrum of biological actions. This also applies to their side effects: the various retinoids show similar toxicity spectra, but they differ in the extent to which they affect various body systems [24].

VITAMIN A (RETINOL)

19.3 Although not entirely abated, oral vitamin A has been largely replaced by other retinoids with a higher therapeutic activity and less toxicity. Nevertheless, it is important to note symptoms and signs of acute and chronic vitamin A intoxication, as the spectrum of adverse effects from retinoids will resemble those of vitamin A intoxication. Tables 19.7 and 19.8 list the clinical and laboratory findings in acute and chronic vitamin A intoxication. These are arranged in order of decreasing frequency [29]. In *acute* vitamin A intoxication symptoms of the central nervous system are more prominent, with gastrointestinal symptoms on the second place. In *chronic* vitamin A intoxication cutaneous problems are most prominent, followed by abnormalities of the mucous membranes and pain and tenderness of the bones. For an exhaustive list of chronic hypervitaminosis A symptoms and signs see Ref. 30.

Table 19.7. Findings in acute vitamin A intoxication arranged in order of decreasing frequency [29]

Clinical findings
Increased cerebrospinal fluid pressure
– infants and children: pseudotumour cerebri and cranial hyperostosis
– adolescents and adults: headache
Anorexia, nausea, vomiting
Scaling of the skin, dry mucous membranes, cheilitis, hair loss
Fatigue, lassitude, vertigo, somnolence
Haemorrhages: formation of petechiae, epistaxis
Edema
Tenderness of the long bones
Hepatomegaly and splenomegaly
Laboratory findings
Vitamin A plasma levels increased
Calcium increased
Alkaline phosphatase, ASAT and ALAT increased

Table 19.8. Findings in chronic vitamin A intoxication arranged in order of decreasing frequency [29,30]

Clinical findings
Scaling skin, erythema, pruritus, disturbed hair growth
Dry mucous membranes, cheilitis, angular stomatitis, gingivitis, glossitis
Pain and tenderness of the bones; restricted movement
Occipital headache
Hyperirritability; sleep disturbance
Papillary edema; diplopia
Anorexia and loss of weight
Hepatomegaly [143], sometimes with splenomegaly
Edema and swelling
Fatigue, lassitude, occasionally somnolence
Haemorrhages, epistaxis, increased menstrual bleeding
Laboratory findings
Radiologically detectable bone changes in children
Increased serum alkaline phosphatase, hypercalcaemia
Increased cerebrospinal fluid pressure

TRETINOIN (all-*trans*-retinoic acid)

19.4 Tretinoin is no longer used as an oral drug, as it has been shown to be less effective and more toxic than other retinoids. Tretinoin is however widely used as a topical agent for the treatment of acne, ichthyosis, and, since 1990, actinically damaged skin. In the investigation of Stuttgen [31] 30 patients were given 50–100 mg/day of oral tretinoin for 4 weeks. Increases in ASAT, ALAT and alkaline phosphatase were each noted in 1 patient (of 11 investigated). Adverse reactions to tretinoin in these patients included:

Cheilitis	80%
Headache	80%
Xerosis/inflammation	50%
Lethargy, fatigue	43%
Dry mucous membranes	30%
Visual disturbances	30%
Anorexia	30%
Nausea, vomiting	30%
Pruritus	23%
Epistaxis, petechiae	17%
Eye bulb pressure increased	11%
Thinning of hair	10%
Psychological changes	10%

ISOTRETINOIN (13-*cis*-retinoic acid) [24–26,32–35]

19.5 Although isotretinoin (Accutane®, Roaccutane®) may be useful for the treatment of keratinizing disorders, its main indication is for severe nodulocystic acne. The exact mechanism of action of isotretinoin is not fully understood, but appears to include inhibition of sebaceous gland function and follicular keratinization. Isotretinoin reduces the size of sebaceous glands and inhibits sebum production. In large doses isotretinoin reduces the concentration of *P. acnes* on the surface of the skin. The reduction of the bacterial flora probably does not result from a direct effect of the drug on the bacteria, but from a drug-induced reduction in sebum production. In patients with cystic acne prolonged remissions frequently occur following discontinuance of isotretinoin. The pharmacokinetics or this oral retinoid have been reviewed [24,36].

Adverse reaction pattern

One or more side effects from isotretinoin can be expected to occur in almost every patient. They are, in general, somewhat predictable, resembling in type, though not in incidence, those of the parent compound's syndrome of chronic hypervitaminosis A. The frequency and severity of adverse reactions are generally dose-related, with more pronounced effects occurring at dosages greater than 1 mg/kg/day. Adverse effects usually subside with a reduction of dosage, and are reversible following discontinuance of therapy.

Cutaneous and mucous membranes symptoms (up to 90%) are by far the most noticeable side effects. Up to 50% of patients treated with isotretinoin experience conjunctivitis and irritation of the eyes.

Nervous system

Lethargy, fatigue, headache, insomnia [35], paresthesias [37], dizziness [34,37], decreased hearing [34], oculogyric crisis [34], epileptic insult (rare, [146]), pseudotumour cerebri [38]. Pseudotumour cerebri is characterized by headaches, vertigo, nausea, and visual disturbances such as spells of diminished vision and transient diplopia. Acute depression will develop in approximately 1% of patients [39]. Symptoms in 7 patients were as follows:

Symptoms	No. of patients
Fatigue (increased sleep, loss of energy)	5
Irritability	4
Decreased concentration	4
Sadness	4
Crying spells	3
Loss of motivation (school, social contacts)	3
Forgetfulness	2
Suicidal ideation	1
Angedonia	1
Abnormal dreams	1
Fear of going insane	1

Respiratory

Respiratory infections [37]. Of 10 patients treated with isotretinoin for systemic sclerosis, 1 developed eosinophilic pleural effusion, and two had asymptomatic deterioration in pulmonary function tests [40,41]. Forced expiratory flow was found to be decreased in patients with acne treated with isotretinoin [42]. The manufacturers have on record in the USA several pulmonary adverse effects occurring during isotretinoin therapy, including worsening of asthma, recurrent pneumothorax, pleural effusion, interstitial fibrosis, pulmonary granuloma and deterioration in lung function test [42]. Exercise-induced bronchoconstriction was probably caused by isotretinoin in one patient [43]. Pneumonia has also been reported as a possible side effect [44].

Cardiovascular

Palpitations [37], tachycardia [37].

Endocrine, metabolic

Hypertriglyceridaemia occurs in about 25% of patients. It is advised to monitor blood lipid concentrations, although the necessity of this has recently been questioned [45]. Decreases in serum high-density lipoprotein (HDL), and increases in serum cholesterol and low-density lipoprotein cholesterol are also frequently observed [46]. These effects are reversible upon discontinuance of therapy. Patients with increased tendency to develop hypertriglyceridaemia include those with diabetes mellitus, obesity, increased alcohol intake, and family history. The consequences of hypertriglyceridaemia are not well understood, but it has been suggested that it may increase the patient's cardiovascular risk status [46–49]. Eruptive xanthomas were described in an obese patient with Darier's disease [50]. Pancreatitis associated with isotretinoin-induced hypertriglyceridaemia has been reported in a patient who was also receiving estrogen replacement therapy [51]. Increases in fasting serum glucose concentrations have been reported [37]. Thyroxine concentrations and free thyroxine index have sometimes fallen during treatment, but remained within the reference range [48]. Thyrotoxicosis developed in one patient while on isotretinoin [52]. Menstrual irregularities associated with isotretinoin are not uncommon, symptoms generally being of a 'late' or 'skipped' menstrual period [53]. Menorrhagia has rarely been reported [54]. Adrenal androgen levels in men are not affected by isotretinoin [55], but serum testosterone and 24-h urinary excretion of several steroids were found to be reduced in women [56]. Hypercalcaemia has been reported in patients treated with high doses of isotretinoin (>1.6 mg/kg/day) [57]. In the usual dose of <1.3 mg/kg/day, however, serum calcium is unaffected by isotretinoin [58]. Unilateral breast discharge was provoked by isotretinoin on 2 occasions in one female patient [59]. Increased sweating has been reported to the manufacturer [37].

Mineral and fluid balance

Edema [37].

Haematological

Increased erythrocyte sedimentation rate (40%), decreased haemoglobin concentration and haematocrit, decreased erythrocyte counts, decrease in the number of leukocytes, especially neutrophil counts [60], leukopenia [61,62], increased platelet counts (10–20%) and, rarely, thrombocytopenia [63]. Hyperuricaemia occurs in less than 10% of patients [37].

Liver

Minimal transient increases in serum concentrations of alkaline phosphatase, ASAT and ALAT occur in 10% of patients.

Gastrointestinal

Gastrointestinal symptoms occur in 20% of patients treated with isotretinoin. Side effects have included: anorexia, nausea, vomiting, increased appetite, thirst, weight loss, gastrointestinal bleeding, acute haemorrhagic pancreatitis (1 case). It is unresolved whether isotretinoin may rarely trigger or intensify bowel disease [64,65], but 1 patient experienced proctosigmoiditis clearly caused by isotretinoin [66]. Two out of 10 patients treated with isotretinoin for Barrett's esophagus developed esophageal ulceration [67].

Urinary system

Proteinuria, haematuria, nonspecific urogenital findings [37]. Abnormalities in urinary protein [47], inflammation of the urethral meatus (rare) [68], nephrolithiasis [34].

Skin and appendages

The nature and frequency of mucocutaneous side effects of isotretinoin and etretinate are summarized in Table 19.9.

Table 19.9. Incidence of mucocutaneous side effects or oral retinoids during clinical use [24]

Side effect	Etretinate 0.25–1 mg/kg/day (%)	Isotretinoin	
		0.5 mg/kg (%)	1 mg/kg (%)
Cheilitis/dry lips	75–100	75	95
Dry mouth	25	20	30
Dry nose	25	35	50
Epistaxis	5	25	25
Facial dermatitis	5	30	50
Palmoplantar desquamation	40	10	20
Desquamation of the skin	30	10	20
Thinning of skin	50	15	25
Skin fragility	25	15	20
Xerosis	20	30	50
Retinoid dermatitis	5	5	5
Hair loss (varying degrees; sometimes permanent [33])	50	10	20
Conjunctivitis	5	30	30
Itching/pruritus	15	25	25

Other reported disorders of skin and appendages have included:
Skin and mucous membranes [110]
- acne fulminans (ulcerating cystic acne, fever, myalgias and arthralgias) [69–72]; erythema nodosum was seen in two patients with acne fulminans precipitated by isotretinoin [73]
- bleeding of the gums [37]
- bruising [37]
- delayed wound healing and keloid formation after argon laser treatment or dermabrasion [74]

- dissemination of herpes simplex [75]
- eruptive pyogenic granulomas [69,72]
- erythema nodosum [34,73]
- expression of psoriasis as a Koebner's phenomenon [76]
- facial calcified cysts [34]
- fixed drug eruption [34]
- flare-up of cystic acne
- hirsutism [37]
- hypo/hyperpigmentation [34,37]
- immune complex vasculitis [77,78]; in one case, vasculitis developed 6 weeks after discontinuation of treatment [79], which makes the association rather dubious [80]
- nummular dermatitis (frequent) [254]
- paronychia [81]
- periungual granulation tissue [34,110]
- phototoxicity (infrequent) [82,83]
- pityriasis rosea-like dermatitis [84]
- retinoid dermatitis mimicking progression in mycosis fungoides [85]
- skin infections with staphylococcus aureus [86]; in one patient with stable aortic insufficiency, endocarditis caused by Staphylococcus aureus developed [87]
- urticaria [34]
- Wegener's granulomatosis [78]
- worsening of steatocystoma multiplex [88]

Appendages
- brittle nails
- curly hair [89]
- onycholysis [34]
- pili torti [90]

Bones [91–93]

Chronic hypervitaminosis A is associated with skeletal abnormalities, resulting from accelerated bone and cartilage resorption and new bone formation [30,94]:
- demineralization of long bones and spine
- thinning of long bones
- cortical hyperostoses
- premature closure of the epiphyses
- periostitis
- periosteal calcification
- calcification of ligaments
- scoliosis

Bone or joint pain, generalized muscle ache, and stiffness occur in 15% of patients receiving isotretinoin. Pain in the chest has been reported [37].

Coincident with the long-term use of the synthetic retinoids, a spectrum of retinoid-associated bone and soft tissue abnormalities has evolved (Table 19.10 [91–93,95]).

Table 19.10. Skeletal abnormalities associated with isotretinoin therapy (adapted from [92])

Long term therapy	*Short-term therapy*
Diffuse idiopathic skeletal hyperostosis (DISH)	Skeletal aches and pains (16%) [101]
Premature epiphyseal closure [96,97]	Achilles tendonitis [145]
Ossifications of tendons and ligamentous insertions [97,98]	Acute arthritis [102,103]
Reduced bone density/osteoporosis [97,99]	Nasal bone osteophytosis [104]
Ossification of the posterior longitudinal ligament [100]	Osteoma cutis [105]
	Tietze's syndrome [106]

Initially, patients treated with long-term, high-dose isotretinoin had premature epiphyseal closure [96], skeletal hyperostoses and anterior spinal-ligament calcification similar to those seen in diffuse idiopathic skeletal hyperostosis [101,107]. More recently, lower-dose, short term isotretinoin therapy [108,109] has been associated with smaller, asymptomatic skeletal hyperostoses, which may occur even at very low doses [91]. Although the calcifications that have been reported after isotretinoin have mainly involved the spine, some patients have had extraspinal involvement as well [101,108]. Extraspinal tendon and ligament calcification has been reported [97,98].

The earliest hyperostoses occur in the spine and feet, and they become most prominent with time. Most appendicular hyperostoses occur later, are smaller, and frequently are asymmetric or unilateral [111]. These changes are occasionally associated with pain or significant impairment in function or both, but more often they occur without accompanying symptoms [112]. With long-term therapy, most patients will develop hyperostoses; usually they have no clinical significance [113,114].

With rare exceptions [115], published laboratory tests concerning bone metabolism have been in normal ranges and they are therefore not useful for the detection of pathologic, retinoid-induced calcification disorders. Bone-scintigraphic examinations are considered to be a suitable method for early screening for bone changes [116]. Routine X-ray screening at intervals during treatment is not recommended in patients without symptoms [117].

Retinoids seem to amplify and accelerate physiological and pathophysiological remodelling of the bones, thereby producing a varied range of lesions, which are characteristic for the age and the individual constitution of the patient treated [93]. Dense metaphyseal bands and growth arrest possibly due to isotretinoin has been reported in one child [118].

Eyes [119–122]

Ocular findings are among the most frequent side effects in patients taking isotretinoin, the most common being blepharoconjunctivitis [123]. Isotretinoin probably causes a decrease in tear-film breakup-time [124]. In a review article [119], 237 cases of adverse ocular reactions possibly associated with isotretinoin were evaluated:

Adverse effects	No. of patients
Eyelids	
Blepharoconjunctivitis or meibomianitis	88
Photodermatitis	6
Cornea	
Corneal opacities [125]	12
Dry eyes	47
Contact-lens intolerance [126]	19
Optic nerve	
Papilloedema or pseudotumour cerebri	18
Optic neuritis (?)	3
Congenital abnormalities	
Microphthalmos	5
Orbital hypertelorism	2
Optic nerve hypoplasia	4
Cortical blindness	1
Others	
Blurred vision	39
Myopia [127]	5
Decreased dark adaptation	3
Ocular inflammation (?) (uveitis, scleritis, retinitis, opthalmitis, iritis)	7

Ocular side effects are generally benign in nature and reversible upon discontinuation of isotretinoin. However, papilloedema necessitates discontinuation of the drug. Corneal opacities should be monitored closely. In one patient with the KID syndrome, isotretinoin may have exacerbated the corneal pannus formation [128]. In one case report [129] the development of anterior subcapsular cataract was ascribed to isotretinoin. Decreased night vision and dark adaptation are not rare [130–132].

Muscles

Muscle aches occur in 15% of patients. Elevated CPK has been reported, especially in patients who exercise heavily [133–134]. Elevated CPK levels are not associated with myalgias [135], and although isotretinoin seems to potentiate CPK abnormalities [134], the major determinant of the CPK values appears to be the patients exercise level [135]. In only 2 patients who had muscle pain was muscle damage confirmed by electromyographic evidence and histological and ultrastructural findings [136]. Rhabdomyolysis has been reported once [35].

Second-generation effects [137–140]

Isotretinoin causes malformations in 25% of pregnant women when administered in the first trimester at any therapeutic dosage [147]. Women of childbearing age should be instructed to use an effective form of contraception during isotretinoin therapy and at least one menstrual cycle after discontinuance [141]. The embryotoxicity of the drug has also manifested itself in increased abortion rates and a higher incidence of stillbirths in young women treated for acne [24]. Major malformations have included [24,137–139]:

Central nervous system	Cleft palate
Meningo/myelo/encephalocele	Agenesis/stenosis of the ear canal
Microcephaly	Nasal bridge defects
Hydrocephaly	Hypertelorism
Aqueduct stenosis	Small mouth
Posterior fossa cyst	Syndactyly
Cortical blindness	Aphalangia
Optic nerve hypoplasia	Hip and joint displacement
Cerebellar vermis absent	
Heterotopic neural tissue on leptomeningae	**Mesenchyma**
Corticospinal tract displaced	Incomplete/complete transposition of great vessels
	Various ventricular septum defects
Bone and craniofacial region	Interrupted aortic arch
Microtia/anotia	Renal abnormalities
Micrognathia	Abnormalities of the thymus
	Incomplete lung lobulation

Overdosage

For possible signs and symptoms of overdosage see Tables 19.7 and 19.8. No significant abnormalities have been reported in 2 patients with acute isotretinoin poisoning [142]. In another patient, ingestion of 800 mg isotretinoin resulted in headache, hallucinations and vertebral pain which lasted for 36 hours [32]. The manufacturer states that overdosage has been associated with transient headache, vomiting, facial flushing, cheilosis, abdominal pain, headache, dizziness and ataxia [37].

Drug interactions

Combination with tetracyclines increases the risk of pseudotumour cerebri. The concomitant medication of phenytoin or barbiturates should be avoided, since altered serum concentrations of either medication may occur [24].

ETRETINATE [24–26,148–150,172]

19.6 Until 1989, etretinate (Tigason®, Tegison®) was widely used for the treatment of psoriasis and other disorders of keratinization. It was then replaced by its main metabolite acitretin (etretin, Neo-Tigason), because of its short half-life of elimination of approximately 50 hours [28]. The reader is advised also to consult the section on isotretinoin and retinol.

Adverse reaction pattern

The adverse reaction pattern resembles that of retinol and isotretinoin. The most frequent side effects are mucocutaneous: cheilitis/dry lips, thinning of skin, hair loss, palmoplantar desquamation, desquamation of the skin, skin fragility and dry nose ([24], see under isotretinoin).

Nervous system

Sweating (either diffuse or at palms and soles), thirst, headache, drowsiness, fatigue, pseudotumour cerebri [151,152], shivering [149], hypaesthesia, paraesthesia, lethargy [153], dizziness [153], fever [150], rigors [154], amnesia [154], delirium [150], flu-like symptoms [154].

Respiratory

Dyspnea, coughing, increased sputum, dysphonia, pharyngitis [154].

Cardiovascular

One case of myocardial infarction may have been related to etretinate [154]. Other cardiovascular effects reported (which may bear no relationship to etretinate therapy) include [154]: edema, cardiovascular thrombotic or obstructive events, atrial fibrillation, chest pain, coagulation disorder, phlebitis, postural hypotension, syncope.

Endocrine, metabolic [49,253]

Changes in serum lipids during etretinate are very similar to those described with isotretinoin. Mean levels of both triglyceride and cholesterol are increased. The largest increase in triglyceride mass is in the VLDL fraction, with smaller increases in LDL-triglyceride and no change in HDL-triglyceride. The HDL-cholesterol levels are slightly reduced [49]. The changes are apparent as early as 2 weeks after starting etretinate, and have usually reached their maximum by 8 weeks. Levels of both triglyceride and cholesterol return to normal after 4 weeks of stopping etretinate. Long-term administration of etretinate may be associated with increased atherogenesis and consequently increased risk of ischemic heart disease [49]. See also under isotretinoin.

Erectile dysfunction [155,156], dysmenorrhoea and loss of libido [155] have been reported rarely. Etretinate is associated with a reduction in glucose levels in response to a glucose load [157].

Mineral and fluid balance

Generalized edema [158,159].

Renal

Impaired renal function has been described in one patient [160]. Oedema without renal dysfunction has been described several times [161]. Kidney stones [154].

Haematological

Monocytosis [162], leukopenia (?), allergic eosinophilia [163], thrombocytopenia [164].

Liver [165,166]

A transient, slight elevation of ASAT, ALAT and/or serum bilirubin may occur in some patients on etretinate therapy [162], which is reversible upon cessation of therapy and usually has no clinical implications. Nevertheless, in approximately 4% treatment is stopped because of concern over the status of the liver [167].

Although prospective studies of liver biopsies of patients treated with etretinate have shown reassuring results [168–171], several well-documented cases of hepatitis caused by etretinate have been reported [173,257]; in some cases, other hepatotoxic factors may have played a role [174]. Alcoholics and patients who have previously received methotrexate are at greater risk of developing liver injury. Although most cases of etretinate-associated hepatitis are reversible, some patients may go on to develop chronic active hepatitis [175] and several deaths from hepatitis have occurred [154]. Cholestatic jaundice has been described [176]. Hepatosplenomegaly with lymphadenopathy, disappearing after cessation of etretinate, has been observed in one patient reported to the British Committee on Safety of Medicines.

Gastrointestinal

Anorexia, loss of or increased appetite, vomiting, stomach pain, nausea [150]. Other gastrointestinal symptoms reported (which may bear no relationship to etretinate) include [154]: constipation, diarrhoea, melena, flatulence, weight loss, oral ulcers, taste perversion and tooth caries.

Urinary system

Urethritis [149]. Dysuria, polyuria, urinary retention [154].

Skin and appendages

The nature and frequency of the most common mucocutaneous side effects of etretinate are summarized in Table 19.9 (under isotretinoin). For mechanisms of etretinate alopecia, see Ref. [177]. Other reported disorders of skin and appendages have included:

Skin and mucous membranes
Abnormal skin odor [154]
Bullous eruption [154]
Bullous pemphigoid [248]
Cystic and comedonal acne [178,179]
Erythema multiforme [180]
Erythroderma [181]
Exacerbation of porokeratosis [182]
Exacerbation of scabies [183]
Hirsutism [154]
Immune complex vasculitis [77]
Infections with Staphylococcus aureus [184]
Mucosal erosions, sore tongue [150]
Oedema without renal dysfunction [161]
Papular/pustular eruption of the palms and soles [185]
Paronychia [186]
Petechiae at the extremities
Phototoxicity (infrequent) [82,83,187]
Prurigo nodularis [188]
Pyogenic granulomata [186,189]
Retinoid dermatitis mimicking mycosis fungoides
Rosacea-like eruption [190]
Skin fragility with blistering and erosions [191,192]
Striae atroficae [193]
Toxic epidermal necrolysis [250]
Urticaria [154]
Vulvitis [194]
Appendages
Alopecia areata (?)
Kinking of the hair [195–196]
Nails disorders [197]:
- Beau's lines [198]
- chronic paronychia
- excess granulation tissue
- fragility (splitting)
- increased growth
- onychomadesis
- onycholysis
- onychorrhexis
- shedding
- transverse leuconychia

Oiliness of the hair
Pili torti [90]

Bones [92,172]

Etretinate has been used in Europe for over 10 years to treat disorders of keratinization and psoriasis. A substantial number of patients with inherited disorders of keratinization treated with etretinate have been children, and as the treatment controls rather than cures the condition, therapy is usually of long term duration and may be envisaged as life long therapy. The skeleton of this group of patients is still growing with developing and maturing epiphyseal plates, and therefore particularly vulnerable to fundamental damage by any alteration in bone metabolism. Psoriatic patients receiving etretinate tend to be older and age-related degenerative changes in the skeleton may have already occurred. Any possible change would thus have to be interpreted in the light of these normal changes, which is of special relevance to those studies in which baseline X-ray photographs were not performed.

Bone changes in children
Several case reports have described bone changes such as calcification of the interosseal membrane of the forearm [199], premature epiphyseal closure [200–

202], although one report was doubted: [203], and slender long bones [201,202] (Table 19.11). Nineteen children and adolescents on long-term treatment with etretinate were examined for bone changes with 99m technetium methylene diphosphonate whole body bone scans, and no significant bone abnormalities were detected [204]. In 42 children treated over an 11-year period, no evidence of skeletal toxicity was found [251]. Of 10 children investigated radiographically in another study, however, bone abnormalities were found in 8: periostal thickening ($n = 6$), periostal bone resorption ($n = 2$), osteoporosis ($n = 2$), disk narrowing ($n = 3$) and slender long bones ($n = 1$). The children's physical growth and laboratory investigations were normal. Unfortunately, only 1 child had a skeletal survey prior to starting etretinate [205].

Bone changes in adults

The assessment of skeletal changes in adults due to etretinate has to be made against a background of possible degenerative changes. These include arthritis conditions, both those associated with and distinct from the skin disorder, and primary metabolic bone disease. Following the initial anecdotal reports there have now been several well controlled studies on the effect of long term etretinate treatment on the adult skeleton. In several studies, no bone abnormalities were found attributable to etretinate [116,117,258]. In more recent investigations however, nearly 50% of the patients developed bone changes [206,207]. Two areas are most commonly involved in this process; the vertebrae and extraspinal ligaments [92]. Abnormalities of the vertebrae (osteophytes, bony bridges, changes resembling DISH (Diffuse Idiopathic Skeletal Hyperostosis)) are found in nearly all reported studies [206,208]. Extraspinal tendon and ligament calcification occurs not infrequently [208]. The most common sites of involvement are the ankles, the pelvis and the knees. As with isotretinoin, the bone and extraosseous changes due to etretinate are often asymptomatic and the severity of changes is minor [207], although concern has been raised that spinal hyperostosis and calcification of spinal ligaments may lead to spinal cord compression [209]. With rare exceptions [206] published laboratory tests concerning bone metabolism have been in normal ranges. The results of bone scintigraphy for detecting hyperostosis has been disappointing, and annual lateral thoracic spine radiographs with additional views of symptomatic areas are recommended [206]. The bone changes with etretinate generally occur after a longer treatment period than with isotretinoin.

Table 19.11. Skeletal abnormalities associated with etretinate therapy [92,207]

Children:	cortical bone resorption
	disc narrowing
	ossification of interosseal membranes of forearm [199]
	osteoporosis [202,210]
	periostal thickening [210]
	premature epiphyseal closure [200]
	skeletal pain
	slender long bones [201] with increased curvatures [202]

Adults:	bridging of vertebral bodies [211]
	calcification of the anterior spinal ligament [211]
	'DISH'-like changes [211,212]
	disk degeneration [207]
	extraspinal ligament and tendon calcification [208,211]
	periarticular bone formation of both hips, ligamenta teres and insertion of the psoas muscle onto the femur [212]
	ossification of the interosseous membrane of the forearm [213,214]
	osteophytes on vertebral bodies
	osteoporosis [207]
	periosteal thickening [207]
	slender long bones [207]
	spinal hyperostoses [215,216]

Gout has been linked to etretinate [154].

Muscles

Elevated CPK levels have been reported rarely [217]. See also under isotretinoin. Muscle pain is a frequent side effect of retinoids, but objective evidence of muscle damage has only once been recorded [218]. Electromyographic studies have shown that etretinate may cause subclinical muscle damage [219]. A single case report has described increased muscle tone during etretinate therapy [220].

Eyes

Etretinate has many of the same ocular side effects of isotretinoin. The incidence of the most frequent reaction, conjunctivitis (eye irritation) may be lower with etretinate [121]. Possible retinotoxicity [221] with impaired colour vision [222–224] has rarely been described, but has remained unconfirmed [225]. Other ophthalmic effects include corneal erosions, abrasion, irregularity and punctate staining. Corneal opacities, decreased visual acuity and blurred vision, posterior subcapsular cataract, iritis, blot retinal haemorrhage, scotoma, and photophobia [154].

Ears

Earache [226], excessive cerumen production [227], ototis externa [149].

Miscellaneous

Two patients have developed malignant lymphomas while taking etretinate [228]. Other cases of malignancies during etretinate therapy have been reported [229,249], but the relation of tumour development to retinoid therapy is tenuous.

Second-generation effects

Etretinate is teratogenic and women of childbearing age should receive adequate contraception when using etretinate and for at least 2 years after cessation of therapy. Etretinate may be detected in serum more than 2 years after discontinuing etretinate, especially in overweight women [230]. Embryopathy has been observed in an infant conceived one year after termination of maternal etretinate [231]. The spectrum of defects associated with exposure to etrctinate corresponds to that of hypervitaminosis A [232], but it is probably less teratogenic than isotretinoin [255,256]. See for further information under isotretinoin.

Interactions

See under isotretinoin. In one patient, etretinate may have reduced the therapeutic effect of warfarin [233].

ACITRETIN (ETRETIN, NEO-TIGASON®)

19.7 Acitretin is the main acid derivative and metabolite of etretinate (Tigason®, Tegison®). Thus, the adverse reaction pattern is virtually identical to that of etretinate (see above). Acitretin, which replaced etretinate in 1989, has a profound pharmacokinetic advantage over etretinate, because it is eliminated more rapidly from the body, its half-life of elimination being only approximately 50 hours [28]. This was considered to be especially advantageous for women of childbearing age. Whereas with etretinate in view of the teratogenicity of the retinoids contraception had to be continued for up to 2 years after discontinuation, this period could be shortened to 2 months [234]. However, currently the manufacturer advises avoiding pregnancy after stopping acitretin also for 2 years [235], as etretinate has been found in patients treated with acitretin [236].

Adverse reaction pattern

The spectrum of adverse events seen in clinical trials is typical for hypervitaminosis A and is similar to that reported with the use of other retinoids.

Table 19.12 shows the frequency of acitretin side effects in 518 patients, and compares them with etretinate and placebo [237].

Table 19.12. Adverse events recorded during clinical trials (percentages)

	Acitretin (n = 518)	Etretinate (n = 69)	Placebo (n = 54)
Mucous membranes			
Dry lips/cheilitis	82	85	22
Dry mouth	30	36	4
Stomatitis/gingivitis	6	3	
Dry nose/rhinitis sicca	34	42	4
Epistaxis	2		
Dry eyes/conjunctivitis	17	14	9

(continued)

(continuation)

	Acitretin (n = 518)	Etretinate (n = 69)	Placebo (n = 54)
Skin and Appendages			
Dry skin	30	36	17
Scaling (palms/soles)	26	19	
Scaling (elsewhere)	28	19	9
Hair loss	20	19	4
Pruritus	16	20	15
Nail changes	10	16	2
Skin atrophy/fragility	5	10	
(Retinoid) dermatitis	9	12	2
Various eruptions	9	14	4
Others			
Fatigue/asthenia	5		
Chills/increased sweating	9	1	4
Headache	5	3	7
Dysesthesia	4	6	
Dizziness	1	1	
Arthralgia/myalgia	7	3	9
Nausea	2	1	4
Gastrointestinal disturbances	3	4	9
Vision abnormalities	1	1	
Earache/otitis	1	2	

The most frequently reported adverse events are those affecting the mucocutaneous system, which account for approximately 90% of the total number of side effects [237]. Acitretin tends to give more discomfort than etretinate with regard to hair loss and peeling of the palms and soles [238]. Serum lipid changes resemble those of etretinate and isotretinoin [239]. Serum transaminases rise in approximately 20% of patients, but toxic hepatitis has been observed infrequently [239,240,252].

Other reported side effects have included:

Nervous system

Somnolence [241], insomnia [241], pain [243], depression [243].

Endocrine, metabolic

Diminution of libido [241]. Glucose should be monitored more carefully in diabetic patients [234].

Haematological

Thrombocytopenia [244].

Urinary system

Haematuria [242], dysuria [245].

Skin and appendages

Abnormal hair texture [243], granulation tissue [246], purpura [245], generalized edema [234].

Ears

Ear congestion [242].

Miscellaneous

Rhinorrhea [242].

ANTIBIOTICS

THE PENICILLINS [259–262,265]

19.8 The penicillins are used in dermatology for the treatment of gonorrhoea, syphilis, erysipelas and other infections caused by Streptococcus pyogenes and Staphylococcus aureus, rosacea, and Gram-negative folliculitis. Penicillin is a suitable treatment for erysipeloid and is an alternative to tetracycline for the early stages of Lyme disease. Suspected or proven staphylococcal infections that are due to beta-lactamase-producing strains are treated with penicillinase-resistant isoxazolyl penicillins (oxacillin, cloxacillin, dicloxacillin, flucloxacillin). Rosacea and gram-negative folliculitis respond best to the aminopenicillin ampicillin [259].

Adverse reactions pattern

The majority of adverse reactions to penicillins are hypersensitivity reactions, ranging in severity from a mild rash to anaphylaxis, and, rarely, death. The oral route of administration is much less likely to cause serious reactions than the parenteral route. In addition to immunoglobulin-E-mediated hypersensitivity, penicillins have been associated with delayed hypersensitivity, cytotoxic antibody responses, and immune complex disease.

Hypersensitivity to penicillins [262]

Allergy to any one of the penicillin preparations indicates to the clinician that an allergy to all other penicillin preparations, and in some cases also to the related cephalosporins, must be assumed.

A list of reaction types based upon the classification of Gell and Coombs is shown below. It may be impossible to proof that any of these 4 mechanisms is responsible for individual observations. Mixed type reactions occur frequently.

Type I reactions
Anaphylactic shock
Allergic bronchial asthma
Allergic rhinitis
Urticaria and angio-edema

Type II reactions
Haemolytic anaemia
Agranulocytosis, leukopenia and thrombocytopenia (which might be toxic)

Type III reactions
Serum sickness syndrome
Drug fever
Allergic vasculitis
Arthus phenomenon

Type IV reaction
Allergic dermatitis from locally applied, ingested, injected or inhaled allergens

Classification of reaction type not possible
Macular and maculopapular exanthemas (often type IV allergy)
Erythema multiforme-like eruptions
Vesicular and bullous exanthemas
Exfoliative dermatitis
Toxic epidermal necrolysis (Lyell)
Vascular purpura
Coagulopathy due to an acquired inhibition of Factor VIII
Fixed drug eruptions
Transient eosinophilic pulmonary infiltrate
Hepatitis and active chronic (lupoid) hepatitis
Allergic (interstitial) nephropathy
Encephalitis and benign intracranial hypertension
Polyradiculitis (neuritis)
Development of a positive LE-cell phenomenon
Pancytopenia
So-called 'leukaemoid reactions'

Central nervous system

Administration of higher doses of penicillin, in the order of several 10 million units daily, may produce myoclonic jerks, hyperreflexia, seizures or coma. Also occasionally drowsiness and hallucinations occur. Myasthenia gravis may be worsened by ampicillin and amoxicillin.

Cardiovascular system

Anaphylactic shock may take a lethal course even after oral administration. The incidence of anaphylactic shock is between 0.015% and 0.04% of all penicillin-treated patients, with death occurring in 0.002%. Occlusion and thrombosis following penicillin injection into arteries is rare.

Respiratory system

Allergic bronchial asthma may occur as a consequence of penicillin allergy. Transient eosinophilic pulmonary infiltrate is rare but has been observed with penicillin hypersensitivity.

Haematological

An immunologically induced haemolytic anaemia is rare. Microangiopathic haemolysis and thrombocytopenia related to penicillins have also been described. Penicillin can probably also cause a haemolytic uraemic syndrome. Agranulocytosis has been observed mainly with isoxazolyl-penicillins. Pancytopenia has been observed rarely. The appearance of a bleeding disorder due to an acquired inhibition of factor VIII is an extremely rare situation.

Gastrointestinal tract

Gastrointestinal disturbances include diarrhoea (rarely of the acute haemorrhagic type), nausea, vomiting, and antibiotic-induced pseudomembranous colitis.

Liver

Hepatic and intrahepatic cholestasis have been observed with various penicillin preparations. Hepatitis and active chronic (lupoid) hepatitis, probably as a hypersensitivity reaction, is only very rarely seen.

Mineral and fluid balance

Potassium and sodium Penicillin G are capable of significantly altering the electrolyte balance when administered in very high doses. Penicillin, and more especially carbenicillin, ticarcillin and nafcillin, induce urinary potassium loss.

Urinary system

Allergic nephropathy or interstitial nephritis have been seen with various penicillins. Fever and haematuria are the dominating symptoms. Exanthema, eosinophilia in the blood and signs of non-oliguric renal failure may be but are not always present. With the combination of methicillin and gentamicin, renal failure may be of toxic origin. Haemorrhagic cystitis has been observed with methicillin and carbenicillin.

Skin and appendages

In penicillin allergy, skin manifestations, primarily generalized urticaria, angioedema and maculopapular eruptions predominate. Less frequently, erythema multiforme-like rashes, erythema nodosum-like eruptions, purpuric lesions, exfoliative dermatitis and toxic epidermal necrolysis as well as fixed drug eruptions may be encountered. Ampicillin and amoxicillin have a higher incidence of cutaneous reactions than the other penicillins. These drugs cause a nonallergic maculopapular eruption in 5–10% of patients. The risk is increased in patients receiving allopurinol and in those with infectious mononucleosis, AIDS, renal failure, or chronic lymphatic leukaemia. A localized pustular eruption [263] and severe pustular psoriasis in a patient with psoriasis vulgaris [264] have been described.

Genital system

Antibiotic-induced candida vaginitis may result from the use of the penicillins.

Miscellaneous

Local reactions
Intramuscular injection of high doses of depot preparations may lead to painful swelling. Repeated intramuscular injection of the thighs of newborns and infants may cause severe and widespread muscular contractures of the quadriceps femoris.

Serum sickness syndrome
The diagnosis of serum sickness syndrome should be limited to patients with at least 3 of the classical symptoms of real serum sickness: fever, exanthema, arthritis, lymphadenitis and leukopenia.

Jarisch–Herxheimer reaction
Two to twelve hours after administration of the first dose of penicillin in the treatment of syphilis some patients develop fever with shaking chills. This is often accompanied by an aggravation of the syphilitic symptoms. Influenza-like symptoms with headache and joint pains, and in some cases jaundice, can be observed. A flare-up of cutaneous lesions, a sudden aneurysmal dilatation of the aortic arch, an acute coronary occlusion, convulsions or an acute reduction of vision in cases with optic neuritis may occur.

Embolic-toxic reactions to penicillin depot preparations
Procaine penicillin, antihistamine penicillin, benzathine penicillin and possibly other depot penicillins, may lead to toxic embolic reactions following accidental intravascular injection.The symptoms comprise fear of death, confusion, acoustic and visual hallucinations, and possibly palpitations and cyanosis. Generalized seizures and twitching of the extremities have also been observed, especially in children. As a rule the symptoms diminish and disappear within several minutes to an hour.

Interactions

Administration of allopurinol concurrently with ampicillin may increase the risk of ampicillin-induced skin rash. Concomitant use of bacteriostatic antibiotics such as erythromycin and tetracycline, with penicillin may reduce the bactericidal effects of the penicillins. The use of beta-blockers may increase the risk and severity of anaphylactic reactions. It is unsettled whether penicillins may reduce the efficacy of oral contraceptives. Probenecid prolongs blood levels of penicillin by blocking its renal tubular secretion. If penicillins are given in higher doses by the intravenous route, aminoglycosides may be inactivated.

TETRACYCLINES [259,262,266,267,279,281]

19.9 The tetracycline antibiotics were the first broad-spectrum antibiotics effective against a broad range of gram-positive and gram-negative organisms. The first-generation tetracyclines (chlortetracycline, oxytetracycline, tetracycline hydrochloride, demethylchlortetracycline) were introduced in the 1950s. The second generation tetracyclines (doxycycline, minocycline) were semi-synthetic congeners with longer half-lives, enhanced bacterial activity, and lower toxicity. In dermatology, the main indications for tetracyclines are acne, rosacea, perioral dermatitis, chlamydial infections, and the cutaneous manifestations of Lyme disease [259].

Central nervous system

Benign intracranial hypertension has been reported with tetracycline and minocycline [276]. Minocycline administration may cause dizziness, vertigo, and ataxia, especially in women. As an exception, vertigo accompanied by visual disturbances, including hallucinations and scotoma or 'double vision' was observed. The symptoms begin soon after the patient starts taking the drug, are dose-related, and are reversible when therapy is discontinued.

Cardiovascular system

Exceptional patients with anaphylactic shock have been described.

Respiratory system

Minocycline and tetracycline have caused neutrophilic and eosinophilic alveolitis [280]. Asthmatic reactions, sometimes accompanied with urticaria, have been observed infrequently.

Haematological

Haematologic changes occurring with tetracycline preparations are extremely rare. However, in individual cases haemolytic anaemia [283], neutropenia and/or slight leukopenia, thrombocytopenia and aplastic anaemia have all been described. Disseminated intravascular coagulation in association with hepatorenal failure has been reported once.

Gastrointestinal tract

Tetracyclines can cause a wide variety of adverse reactions on the gastrointestinal tract: epigastric burning, abdominal discomfort, nausea, vomiting, esophagitis, and esophageal ulceration. Diarrhoea can result from irritation of the bowel mucosa or from bacterial superinfection. Pseudomembranous colitis due to *Clostridium difficile* has been reported with tetracycline. Overgrowth of *Candida albicans* may occur in the oral mucosa, vagina, and bowel. Stomatitis, black hairy tongue and rashes in and around the mouth have been described, but especially in review articles. The number of original observations may be small [262]. One case report suggested metallic taste as a side effect of tetracycline [282]. Tetracycline has been implicated as a cause of pancreatitis. There are also reports of fulminating staphylococcus enteritis.

Liver

Hepatotoxicity has been reported in patients receiving high dosages of intravenous tetracycline. It was promoted by pregnancy, liver disease, malnutrition and renal insufficiency. The 'tetracycline-associated fatty liver' with severe hepatic insufficiency has become a rarity since the use of lower doses of tetracycline.

Endocrine, metabolic

Tetracyclines may increase urea in the serum without an increase of the creatinine level, of metabolic origin.

Urinary system [279]

There are 3 separate effects on the kidney. A Fanconi-type syndrome of renal tubular acidosis and proteinuria is associated with the use of degraded tetracyclines. Nephrogenic diabetes insipidus is dose-related, and is most frequently due to demethylchlortetracycline. Tetracyclines (with the exception of doxycycline) exacerbate azotemia in patients with pre-existing renal disease. There is an isolated report of acute interstitial nephritis with a high dose of minocycline.

Skin and appendages

Skin rashes from tetracyclines are infrequent, but a variety of cutaneous reactions to tetracyclines have been reported, including morbilliform rashes, erythema multiforme [278], erythema nodosum [280], exfoliative erythroderma [284], toxic epidermal necrolysis [285], an acneiform eruption, gram-negative folliculitis, urticaria and anaphylaxis. More common are phototoxic dermatitis and photo-onycholysis, which are seen especially with doxycycline and demethylchlortetracycline. It has not been reported with minocycline. Fixed drug eruptions have been caused by both tetracycline and minocycline. There are several reports of the possible precipitation of an SLE-like syndrome by oxytetracycline. There are reports of fluorescent yellow lunules with tetracycline hydrochloride therapy. Long-term administration of minocycline has been associated with the rare occurrence of abnormal pigmentation. At least two types of minocycline-induced pigmentation can be distinguished on the basis of clinical and histologic features. The first type consists of dark bluish-black macules arising in areas of inflammation, such as acne scars and venous ectasias treated with sclerotherapy [267]. This type shows staining properties of hemosiderin histologically. The second type is characterized by a more generalized brown or blue-grey pigmentation, with accentuation on sun-exposed skin. In addition to cutaneous [275] and mucous membrane [269] pigmentation, minocycline has also been associated with greyish discoloration of the teeth [268,269], black thyroid glands, discoloration of the bones [273], the nails [272], the eyes [274], blood and lymphatic vessels [271] and black galactorrhoea [270].

Musculoskeletal system

Tetracyclines are deposited in bone. This probably has no pathological implications.

Genital system

Candida albicans infections of the vulva and vagina appear more frequently in pregnant women, with the use of oral contraceptives and in diabetes mellitus.

Special senses

Eyes

Acute transitory myopia may be caused by tetracycline.

Second-generation effects

Tetracyclines stain growing bone and teeth during enamel deposition, and should not be used after the first 14 weeks of pregnancy or in children. Congenital cataracts have been observed in human fetuses of women treated with oral tetracycline hydrochloride during the first 8–12 weeks of pregnancy. The fetal corneas and lenses showed a yellow discoloration. There is little evidence to suggest teratogenicity.

Interactions

A variety of drugs, foods, and some dairy products may interfere with the gastrointestinal absorption of tetracycline; they include liquid antacids, cimetidine, iron salts, and sodium bicarbonate. The serum half-life of doxycycline is decreased by drugs such as barbiturates, phenytoin and carbamazepine, and increased by cimetidine and ketoconazole. It is inadvisable to give tetracyclines with nephrotoxic drugs such as gentamicin or diuretics [279]. The general anaesthetic methoxyflurane has been reported to cause renal failure in patients receiving tetracycline. Tetracyclines may increase the serum levels of digoxin and may increase or decrease lithium levels. Tetracyclines may decrease insulin requirements and may increase the hypothrombinaemic effects of concurrent anticoagulants. Bacteriostatic drugs such as tetracycline may interfere with the bactericidal action of penicillins. Warnings should always be given about the use of outdated or poorly stored tetracycline, as degraded tetracycline may cause a Fanconi-type syndrome of renal tubular acidosis and proteinuria, lactic acidosis and a condition simulating lupus erythematosus. An interaction with oral contraceptives leading to increased risk of unwanted pregnancy has not convincingly been demonstrated [277].

ERYTHROMYCIN [259,265,290]

19.10 Erythromycin has been used for 40 years. Four oral preparations of this macrolide antibiotic are available: erythromycin base, stearate, estolate, and ethylsuccinate. The free base is the form that has antimicrobial activity, and the other three forms are hydrolyzed to the active base in the body. Erythromycin is used in dermatology for the treatment of acne, rosacea and perioral dermatitis, of skin and soft tissue infections with Staphylococcus aureus and Streptococcus pyogenes, for Chlamydia trachomatis urethritis, and acne. It is an alternative choice of treatment of syphilis and gonorrhoea in penicillin-allergic patients.

Adverse reaction pattern

Erythromycin is a very safe antibiotic, virtually the only serious side effect being cholestatic jaundice, especially from its estolate ester. The most common adverse reactions are dose-related gastro-intestinal disturbances: nausea, vomiting, epigastric distress, and diarrhoea.

Central nervous system

There have been a few reports in which erythromycin therapy has been associated with complications such as confusion, paranoia, visual hallucinations, fear, lack of control and nightmares.

Cardiovascular system

Intravenous infusions of 1 g doses of erythromycin tend to produce thrombophlebitis.

Gastrointestinal tract

The most common adverse reactions associated with erythromycin are dose-related gastrointestinal disturbances: nausea, vomiting, epigastric distress, diarrhoea, and rectal irritation. Their incidence may range from 5–30%, depending on the dose. Pseudomembranous colitis caused by overgrowth of Clostridium difficile has been reported, as has pancreatitis.

Liver

Administration as base or salt may be followed in 0–10% of cases by apparently benign increases in the SGOT and the SGPT. Erythromycin (especially the estolate esther) may cause cholestatic jaundice, especially in pregnant women. The clinical presentation includes fever, abdominal pain, nausea, vomiting, eosinophilia, and elevated serum bilirubin and serum transaminases.

Urinary system

Acute renal insufficiency has been observed in a patient with Henoch–Schoenlein syndrome. Another case presented as interstitial nephritis with acute renal failure.

Skin and appendages

Reports of skin eruptions are rare, including a few patients with fixed drug eruption, urticarial reactions, a maculopapular rash, and toxic epidermal necrolysis [288].

Special senses

Ears
Rare instances of hearing loss, usually but not always [287] reversible, after the use of high doses of the drug have been reported, particularly in elderly patients with renal insufficiency and with intravenous administration [286].

Miscellaneous

A myasthenia-like clinical picture has been documented by electromyography.

Interactions [289]

Erythromycin, being bacteriostatic, may inhibit the bactericidal action of simultaneously administered penicillins or cephalosporins. Erythromycin use may result in alterations of hepatic cytochrome P-450 enzymes systems responsible for drug metabolism. This may result in delayed clearance of other drugs. Drugs that interact with erythromycin include theophylline, cyclosporine, carbamazepine [289], warfarin, digitalis, ergotamine, and methylprednisolone.

CEPHALOSPORINS [259,262,265]

19.11 Since the introduction of cephalothin in 1962, numerous other broad-spectrum antibiotics of this class have been released. The parenteral cephalosporins are generally divided into first-, second-, and third-generation agents. The first generation possesses excellent coverage for Staphylococcal infections, in addition to their efficacy in treating gram-negative organisms such as *Escherichia coli* or *Proteus*. The second- and third-generation are generally more active against certain gram-negatives and anaerobes. The orally administered (most employed in dermatology) cephalosporins include cephalexin, cephradine, cephadroxil, cephaclor and cephixime. These are used for the treatment of skin infections caused by *S. aureus* and group-A beta-haemolytic streptococci. The parenteral agent cephtriaxone is effective in uncomplicated gonorrhoea. Preliminary studies indicate that cephtriaxone may be more effective than penicillin in the treatment of late Lyme borreliosis.

In this section, adverse effects that have only occurred from parenteral administration of cephalosporins not usually given in dermatology, are *not* mentioned.

Central nervous system

With the orally administered cephalexin reversible toxic psychosis, headache and dizziness have rarely been reported.

Cardiovascular system

Anaphylactic shock from hypersensitivity reactions may occur. Intravenous administration may lead to thrombophlebitis.

Respiratory system

Bronchospasm from hypersensitivity reactions may occur.

Haematological

Immune haemolytic anaemia, intravascular haemolysis, agranulocytosis, leukopenia, pancytopenia, and allergic thrombocytopenia, are all very rare. Eosinophilia, at times accompanied by pruritus and maculopapular exanthema, has been repeatedly described.

Gastrointestinal tract

Gastro-intestinal disturbances, such as nausea and/or vomiting, may occur but are usually mild and transient. The incidence of diarrhoea is also low at 0.7–5%. Antibiotic colitis and pseudomembranous colitis as a complication has rarely been recorded. Stomatitis with or without candidiasis was described in association with cephalexin therapy, but is probably not specific for any particular cephalosporin preparation. The frequent incidence of vulvovaginitis and pruritus ani has been a disturbing factor in several reports. In some patients, *Candida albicans* infection was proven.

Liver

Mildly elevated liver enzyme levels have been shown to occur in a few patients during treatment with various cephalosporins, but the causal relationship has not been ascertained. Immune-mediated cholestasis has occurred after oral cephadroxil.

Urinary system

Acute renal insufficiency has been observed during treatment with cephaloridine and less frequently with cephalotin. Cephalotin and cephaloridine nephrotoxicity may produce acute interstitial nephritis. More frequently, however, it will result in uraemia with oliguria as an expression of acute tubular necrosis. Nephrotoxicity occurs mainly in patients with pre-existing renal disease or those simultaneously treated with other nephrotoxic drugs (aminoglycosides, polymyxine).

Skin and appendages

The most common adverse systemic effects are hypersensitivity reactions, such as maculopapular rash. Immediate hypersensitivity reactions such as anaphylaxis, urticaria and bronchospasm occur less frequently. Cephalosporins are contraindicated for patients who have either a history of allergy to these drugs or a history of anaphylaxis or severe immediate reactions to penicillins. Penicillin-allergic patients may exhibit cross-allergenicity to cephalosporins at a rate of 5–10%. Patients who have only a history of a nonurticarial, penicillin-induced drug eruption can generally safely tolerate the cephalosporins. If their reaction is of the immediate-type (urticaria, angio-edema, or anaphylaxis), however, cephalosporins should not be used. Some cases of erythema multiforme (Stevens–Johnson) have been caused by cephalosporins. One case of cephadroxil-induced pemphigus vulgaris was described with improvement after withdrawal of the preparation. On administration of ampicillin an exacerbation was observed [291].

Second-generation effects

No relevant human data are available concerning possible teratogenic effects.

Interactions

Bacteriostatic agents may interfere with the bactericidal action of cephalosporins. Concurrent administration of probenecid increases and prolongs plasma levels of the cephalosporins. The combination of cephalosporins with other potentially nephrotoxic drugs (especially aminoglycosides and polymyxin) must be undertaken with caution. Administration of cephadroxil and cephalexin with cholestyramine causes interference in the absorption of the antibiotic.

METRONIDAZOLE [259,265,292,296]

19.12 Metronidazole is the first of the nitroimidazole group of antibiotics. It is used for the treatment of urethritis and vaginitis caused by Trichomonas vaginalis and Gardnerella vaginalis, and of rosacea (usually topical treatment).

Central nervous system

The most serious adverse reactions are neurological symptoms and include peripheral neuropathy, ataxia, headache, dizziness, convulsions and, rarely, psychosis and encephalopathy. These effects usually occur after prolonged administration with high doses or in patients with hepatic failure. Use of the drug for longer than 3 months should be avoided because of the risk of sensory peripheral neuropathy. Fever has been cited a side effect [295].

Cardiovascular system

Thrombophlebitis occurs in 6% following parenteral administration. Flushing has been cited as a side effect [295].

Respiratory system

Pneumonitis has been observed in a single case [294].

Haematological

Transient and mild blood disorders, mainly leukopenia and neutropenia, have been reported. Agranulocytosis and aplastic anaemia are very rare. Metronidazole may be linked to some cases of haemolytic-uraemic syndrome in children.

Gastrointestinal tract

The most common side effects, occurring in 5–10% of patients are gastrointestinal symptoms such as anorexia, metallic taste, nausea, abdominal pains, vomiting and diarrhoea. Pseudomembranous colitis has been reported, as has pancreatitis. Glossitis and stomatitis has been noted occasionally [295]. Black hairy tongue is commonly seen [295].

Liver

Elevated serum liver enzyme levels have been observed in 1 patient following intravenous infusion.

Urinary system

The urine of patients on metronidazole may be red-brown because of the presence of an azo metabolite of the drug.

Skin and appendages

Pruritus and rashes have been reported, including erythematous eruptions, urticaria, fixed drug eruptions [295] and pityriasis rosea-like eruptions [296].

Musculoskeletal system

Joint pain has been cited as a side effect [295].

Special senses

Eyes
Acute transient myopia has been observed in a single case [293].

Miscellaneous

Various animal studies have shown carcinogenic effects of metronidazole, other animal studies have been negative. Although there is no evidence of carcinogenicity in humans thus far, the question is not settled.

Second-generation effects

Although no direct evidence of teratogenicity exists, it is prudent to avoid use of metronidazole during pregnancy, especially during the first trimester, and also to avoid breast-feeding by a mother receiving metronidazole or related compounds.

Interactions

Drug interactions with metronidazole include a disulfiram-like reaction that occurs in 10%–25% of patients who consume ethanol while taking the drug. Alcoholics may experience an acute psychotic state. Metronidazole increases the hypoprothrombinaemic effect of warfarin. Simultaneous administration of cimetidine prolongs the half-life of metronidazole. Conversely, a shorter half-life results from concurrent administration of phenobarbital and phenytoin. Metronidazole can promote renal retention of lithium and, occasionally, can induce lithium intoxication [297].

ANTIFUNGAL DRUGS

GRISEOFULVIN [265,298,299,302,310]

19.13 Griseofulvin is a fungistatic drug which has been used since 1959 in the treatment of fungal infections of the skin and the nails. It is ineffective against Candida albicans and Pityrosporum species. Nowadays, its use has largely been abandoned in favour of the more effective, fungicidal and safer antimycotics itraconazole and terbinafine. Nevertheless, it has been a very useful drug for three decades for the treatment of superficial fungal infections caused by dermatophytes.

Adverse reaction pattern

General and toxic reactions
Gastrointestinal upset (often mild), headache and central nervous system disturbances which can be severe enough to enforce discontinuation of treatment are the main side effects.

Hypersensitivity reactions
Hypersensitivity reactions, mainly in the form of skin reactions, are not uncommon, but are rarely severe. A serum-sickness-like illness has been reported in rare instances, as has angioedema.

Nervous system

Headaches occur in about 50% of patients, and can be severe. Drowsiness, dizziness, fatigue, lethargy, confusion and depression as well as irritability have been reported. Impaired coordination and unsteadiness while walking during the confused state have been reported in some cases. The psychic symptoms can be very disturbing and are aggravated by alcohol intake. Peripheral neuropathy may occur [311].

Haematological

Leukopenia, neutropenia, monocytosis and punctate basophilia have all been reported, but there is no evidence that griseofulvin causes serious blood disorders.

Gastrointestinal tract

Anorexia, a feeling of fullness in the stomach and mild nausea are quite common during treatment, as is mild diarrhoea. Black hairy tongue, glossodynia, angular stomatitis, dry mouth and taste disturbances have been described.

Liver

Reports of hepatitis and cholestasis do appear, but these events have never been shown to have a causal relationship with griseofulvin. Griseofulvin interferes with porphyrin metabolism, and acute intermittent porphyria is an absolute contra-indication.

Endocrine, metabolic

An estrogen-type effect has been reported in children affecting the genitals and the breasts.

Urinary system

Proteinuria (rare), non-specific sediment abnormalities.

Skin and appendages

Dermatological side effects have included pruritus, urticaria [306], cold urticaria, photosensitivity eruptions [309], lichen planus, erythema multiforme [305], vesicular and morbilliform rashes, serum-sickness-like reactions, and angio-edema. Fixed drug eruptions [307], Stevens–Johnson syndrome, toxic epidermal necrolysis [309], anhidrosis [312] and cutaneous vasculitis have been described in case-histories. There are a few reports of cases in which lupus erythematosus was unmasked or exacerbated [300,304].

Special senses

Eyes
Blurred vision [310].

Miscellaneous

Epistaxis.

Second-generation effects

Embryotoxicity and mutagenicity have in the past been demonstrated in animal experiments. Clinical findings neither support nor refute a possible influence on the human fetus, although an association with conjoined twins and an increased risk of spontaneous abortions has been suggested [303].

Interactions

The effect of warfarin-type anticoagulants may be inhibited. Phenobarbital may decrease absorption of griseofulvin. Griseofulvin may affect the enzymes involved in steroid metabolism, and a role as a cause of contraceptive failure is very likely [301].

KETOCONAZOLE [265,299,298,313,325]

19.14 Ketoconazole is one of the imidazole antimycotics and the first orally effective antimycotic agent of broad spectrum. Its major draw-back has been its potential to cause hepatotoxicity [315]. Newer antifungals, which are equally or even more effective and have a more favourable side effects profile such as terbinafine and itraconazole, are likely to replace ketoconazole in the near future.

Adverse reaction pattern

General and toxic reactions. Gastrointestinal complaints ranging from anorexia, nausea and gastralgia to constipation are the most frequently occurring side effects. Hepatotoxicity, ranging from mild disturbances of liver function tests to clinical hepatitis and even fulminating hepatic necrosis has been reported. Pruritus and exanthemas have been reported but do not cause major problems. *Hypersensitivity reactions* are rare. Anaphylaxis with angioedema has been described.

Central nervous system

Headache, dizziness, nervousness and somnolence have been reported in less than 1% of patients treated.

Gastrointestinal tract

Nausea, mild gastrointestinal symptoms and vomiting occur in 3–10% of cases. Diarrhoea has been reported. Such symptoms can usually be avoided by taking ketoconazole immediately before meals.

Liver

Transient mild abnormalities in liver function tests are not unusual, occurring in up to 12%. In March, 1982, the manufacturer cited 22 cases of hepatitis and liver toxicity in a warning letter to all physicians. Cases of liver damage of varying severity ranging from mild toxic hepatitis to acute hepatic necrosis have been reported since, with several fatalities [315]. In cases of hepatotoxicity, the incidence of which has been estimated to be 0.1–1%, there usually is a fairly acute onset. Ketoconazole-induced hepatotoxicity is believed to be due to metabolic idiosyncrasy in susceptible persons. Predisposing factors are a history of idiosyncrasy for other drugs, prior hepatic reactions and a history of alcoholism. Women over 40 years old on chronic therapy are also at risk. Close monitoring of the patient and his liver function tests is advisable. The risk of hepatotoxicity is minimal when treatment duration is less than 2 weeks.

Endocrine, metabolic

Ketoconazole at high doses (600–800 mg/day) is a potent inhibitor of testicular and adrenal steroid synthesis and gynaecomastia has been observed repeatedly. Libido may be reduced and impotence has occurred. Patients taking high doses should be considered at risk for symptomatic adrenal insufficiency [320]. Menstrual irregularities occur only with higher doses (400–800 mg/day). One case of hyponatraemia has been reported [317]. Ketoconazole is an inhibitor of cholesterol production [318]. Hypoglycaemia was (not very convincingly) ascribed to ketoconazole in one case-report [319]. Hypothyroidism in a father and son may have been unrelated to ketoconazole [321,322].

Urinary system

An increase in frequency of micturation has been reported in one article.

Skin and appendages

Pruritus and occasional rashes (including one reported case of exfoliative erythroderma) may occur. The incidence seems to be about 3%. Urticaria, angioedema and anaphylaxis have rarely occurred. Lichenoid reactions of the oral mucosa have been observed [314]. Alopecia occurs with higher doses (800 mg/day). One (inadequately diagnosed) case of phototoxicity has been reported [323]. Fixed drug eruption is rare [324].

Musculoskeletal system

Myalgia occurs occasionally in patients treated with 800 mg/day.

Interactions

Concomitant use of antiacids and of cimetidine and similar preparations may impair resorption. Ketoconazole may enhance the anticoagulant effects of coumarin-like drugs, decrease the concentration of rifampicin and isoniazid (INH) and increase the serum levels of cyclosporin. A disulfiram-like reaction with alcohol has been recorded repeatedly. Combined administration of ketoconazole and phenytoin may alter the metabolism of one or both drugs and monitoring of serum levels of both drugs is recommended. Enhanced side effects from methylprednisolone may be expected if used in combination with ketoconazole. Ketoconazole may reduce theophylline blood levels. In one report, 7 of 147 women taking low-dose oral contraceptives experienced break-through bleeding within 2 to 5 days of starting a 5-day course of 400 mg ketoconazole daily. Although intermenstrual bleeding may be a sign of a decrease in the effectiveness of oral contraceptives [316], to date no pregnancies ascribed to the interaction between ketoconazole and oral contraceptives have been reported.

Further information on (possible) drug interactions involving ketoconazole is given in Table 19.13 [326]:

Table 19.13. Drug interactions involving ketoconazole

Drugs that should not be used concurrently with ketoconazole or should be used judiciously with it:

- Cyclosporin
- Hepatotoxic drugs
- Isoniazid
- Rifampicin
- Warfarin and other coumarin anticoagulants

Drugs that may affect the absorption of ketoconazole:

- Antacids
- Antimuscarinic agents
- Antisecretory drugs (omeprazole)
- H_2-receptor antagonists (cimetidine)

Drugs that have the potential to interact with ketoconazole (or have been shown to interact with it) but the clinical significance of which interaction remains to be qualified:

- Chlordiazepoxide
- Ethanol
- Methylprednisolone and other glucocorticoids
- Phenytoin
- Other drugs metabolised by hepatic mixed-function oxidases

TERBINAFINE [265,327,331,332,336]

19.15 Terbinafine is an allylamine antifungal agent which appears to act by preventing fungal ergosterol biosynthesis via specific and selective inhibition of fungal squalene epoxidase. In standard *in vitro* susceptibility tests terbinafine has demonstrated activity against a wide range of dermatophyte, filamentous, dimorphic and dematiaceous fungi, as well as yeasts. Terbinafine shows primarily fungicidal activity against dermatophytes, but is only fungistatic against Candida albicans. Clinical trials have demonstrated that terbinafine, administered either orally (250 or 500 mg/day) or as a 1% topical cream (twice daily), is extremely effective in the treatment of dermatophyte infections of the skin, producing mycological cure in approximately 90% of patients with tinea corporis/cruris and tinea pedis, with an associated clinical cure in approximately 80% of cases. Oral terbinafine has also achieved similar rates of cure in dermatophyte fingernail and toenail infections after 3 to 12 months' treatment. Oral terbinafine is less effective against candida albicans and ineffective against pityriasis versicolor, but these infections do respond to the topical formulation of terbinafine.

Adverse reaction pattern

General and toxic reactions. Adverse effects occur in approximately 10% of patients receiving oral terbinafine [335], consisting mostly of gastrointestinal (6%) or cutaneous (2%) symptoms, central nervous symptoms such as headache and vertigo [333,334] or nonspecific effects such as tiredness or malaise (similar to placebo-treated patients).

Hypersensitivity reactions. Cutaneous reactions such as pruritus and rash (including urticaria) occur in 2% of patients treated with terbinafine.

Central nervous system

Central nervous system symptoms such as headache and vertigo occur in 1% [333,334]

Gastrointestinal tract

The gastrointestinal side effects (6%), including fullness, dyspepsia, nausea, and diarrhoea occur usually in the first weeks of treatment, and are mild and transient. Some of these reactions may be the result of the drug's delaying effect on gastric emptying, and may cause particular discomfort in patients with hiatus hernia or peptic ulcer. Loss of taste has been ascribed to terbinafine [337].

Liver

Monitoring of liver function in 1350 terbinafine-treated patients did not reveal any hepatocellular toxicity [328], although occasional transient elevations in liver enzymes have been reported [329,333].

Skin and appendages

The cutaneous reactions are (allergic) drug eruptions (including urticaria) and itching [327], occurring in 2% of patients treated.

Interactions

Elimination of terbinafine is increased by cimetidine and decreased by rifampicine [330].

ITRACONAZOLE [265,338,339,348]

19.16

Itraconazole is a new dioxolane triazole derivative that appears to have most of the antifungal spectrum of ketoconazole and, thus far, few of the potential hepatic and endocrine side effects. In onychomycosis, short courses of therapy (4 months) may be sufficient, as the drug reaches all portions of the nail within one month, presumably because itraconazole penetrates the nail not only via the nail matrix (as is the case with griseofulvin and ketoconazole), but also via the nail bed [345]. Therapeutic itraconazole concentrations are found in the nail plate for up to six months after treatment [347].

Adverse reaction pattern

General and toxic reactions. Adverse reactions are reported in 8% of itraconazole-treated patients. Gastro-intestinal disorders (abdominal pain, nausea, dyspepsia, diarrhoea, vomiting) and headache are the most common complaints. There seems to be no relation between the occurrence of adverse effects and the dosage. *Hypersensitivity reactions*. Rashes have been observed occasionally [340], including urticaria, angio-edema and a case of Stevens–Johnson syndrome [349].

Central nervous system

After gastrointestinal reactions, headache is the most common adverse event. Dizziness has been observed occasionally [339]. Fatigue was reported by 4 of 75 patients treated for coccidioidomycosis, and nervousness in one [343].

Gastrointestinal tract

Gastro-intestinal disorders (abdominal pain, nausea, dyspepsia, diarrhoea, vomiting) are the most common complaints. Dry mouth has rarely been reported [342].

Liver

Increased transaminase levels and bilirubin have been observed occasionally [342,343] as has an increased alkaline phosphatase level [343]. Monitoring serum liver enzymes in patients who receive (long-term) therapy with itraconazole has been advised [346].

Endocrine, metabolic

Increased triglyceride levels have been observed in 8 of 75 (11%) patients treated for coccidioidomycosis [342]; the relevance of this finding to possible itraconazole toxicity is uncertain because serum samples were not uniformly obtained in the fasting state. Impotence/decreased libido was reported in 3 of 75 patients treated for coccidioidomycosis, and gynaecomastia in one [342]. Hypercalcaemia has been observed once [343].

Urinary system

One case of hypokalaemia associated with edema and elevations in blood pressure developed in a patient treated with itraconazole for phaeohyphomycosis [341]; it was also reported in other studies [342,343]. Polyuria has been observed [342].

Skin and appendages

Rashes have been observed occasionally [340,342].

Interactions

Low serum levels of itraconazole have been observed in epileptics taking phenobarbitone and phenytoin [344]. The concurrent administration of rifampicin may result either in increased or decreased itraconazole levels. Itraconazole increases the blood concentrations of cyclosporine and terfenadine. Possibly, interactions may occur with digoxine and warfarin [349].

CYTOSTATICS AND IMMUNOSUPPRESSANTS

METHOTREXATE [265,350–352,367,371]

19.17 Methotrexate is a folic acid antagonist used in dermatology for the treatment of severe, refractory psoriasis and mycosis fungoides. It is also used for other conditions, including bullous disorders, selected collagen vascular disorders, proliferative conditions such as pityriasis rubra pilaris and miscellaneous unrelated diseases such as sarcoidosis and lymphomatoid papulosis [350]. An important nondermatologic indication is for the treatment of rheumatoid arthritis [371]. For methotrexate monitoring guidelines see Refs. [350] and [351]. In cancer chemotherapy, side effects may occur from high doses intravenous and intrathecal administration of methotrexate, which are not seen with the far lower doses employed for treatment of psoriasis. These side effects are not always mentioned here.

Central nervous system

Neurotoxicity is mainly seen with the intrathecal administration of methotrexate (not discussed here). Headache, chills, fatigue, and dizziness are reported occasionally. Fever to 102°F during the first few days after high-dose methotrexate infusion without signs of infection has been observed.

Respiratory system

In rare instances, pulmonary toxicity such as acute pneumonitis can occur. This pulmonary toxicity is idiosyncratic, can occur with extremely small doses of methotrexate, and can be life-threatening if the methotrexate is not stopped. In addition, some patients develop a more gradual pulmonary toxicity that is manifest by pulmonary fibrosis on chest X-ray [363].

Haematological

Myelosuppression [368], specifically leukopenia, is the dose-limiting toxicity for methotrexate. The incidence is approximately 20% in those receiving high-doses; patients with nephrotoxicity are particularly at risk. Frequent blood counts are important monitors for bone marrow toxicity. Increased susceptibility to infection secondary to leukopenia may develop.

Gastrointestinal tract

Nausea, abdominal pain and anorexia are commonly encountered. Diarrhoea, vomiting, enteritis and pharyngitis are less frequently observed. Mucositis with pain, erythema, burning sensation and sometimes ulcerations is seen in 6–20% of cases treated with high-doses methotrexate. MTX-induced loss of taste acuity is a rare idiosyncratic reaction which is probably centrally mediated and is amendable to correction by folic acid administration [376].

Liver

Hepatotoxicity is the most significant problem with long-term methotrexate. Elevation of hepatic transaminases occurs in 20% or more immediately after oral methotrexate dosing but generally resolves within 1–3 weeks. Although liver function tests may be abnormal in the presence of liver toxicity, they are frequently normal. Therefore, it is necessary to examine the histologic appearance of the liver during long-term therapy with liver biopsies, although the risk of significant hepatic toxicity in the absence of clinical signs and with normal enzyme levels is said to be small [375]. The data on the risk of methotrexate-induced cirrhosis have varied widely with reported frequencies ranging from 0 to 25%. Risk factors include alcoholism, underlying liver disease and obesity, diabetes mellitus, renal insufficiency or concomitant use of medications that lead to higher or more sustained methotrexate levels. It appears that the risk of liver damage is low for patients whose cumulative dosage is below 1.5 gram. The clinical course of the cirrhosis is often nonaggressive [373,374].

Endocrine, metabolic

Menstrual dysfunction has been mentioned as a side effect of methotrexate [372]. Impotence has rarely been observed.

Urinary system

High-dose therapy may lead to renal toxicity secondary to precipitation of methotrexate in the renal tubules. Glomerular filtration rate falls in the majority of patients in a rapid dose-related fashion. In the absence of manifestations of systemic toxicity, this generally returns to baseline in 7–10 days. Renal damage attributable to the doses of methotrexate used in psoriasis treatment are rare [369].

Skin and appendages [386]

Cutaneous reactions to methotrexate are said to be uncommon [350], although erythematous, patchy, macular eruptions have been observed in 15% of patients given high-doses for malignancies [368]. Methotrexate is felt to be potentially phototoxic. It may cause an unusual reaction in which either a recent sunburn is 'recalled' [354] or previously irradiated skin [360] will develop a toxic reaction with the administration of the drug. Other reported cutaneous eruptions from methotrexate include papular eruptions, exfoliative dermatitis, acute paronychia [355], bullous eruption with onycholysis [356], urticaria with anaphylaxis [357], (dose-related) cutaneous necrosis of normal [358] and psoriatic [359] skin, and capillaritis [368]. Alopecia occurs in 6% of patients given low-dose methotrexate. Hyperpigmentation of the nails may be seen [377].

Musculoskeletal system

One child who had been taking daily methotrexate for 255 days developed bony osteoporosis and severe scoliosis.

Special senses

Eyes
Ocular irritation is seen frequently [351], conjunctivitis rarely.

Miscellaneous

There is no evidence that methotrexate increases the risk of developing a subsequent malignancy. Isolated case reports of squamous cell carcinoma are unconvincing [361].

Second-generation effects

Methotrexate is a potent teratogen and abortifaciens. Previously treated patients do not have an increased risk of fetal abnormalities in subsequent pregnancies. Men should be counselled with regard to a possible, reversible oligospermia.

Interactions

Drugs that may increase the potential for methotrexate toxicity include the following [351,353]:

Mechanism	Drugs
Decrease renal elimination of MTX	Nephrotoxins Salicylates [358] Non-steroidal anti-inflammatory drugs
Pharmacologic enhancement of MTX toxic effects	Trimethoprim-sulfamethoxazole [366] Ethanol Phenylbutazone
Reduced tubular secretion	Salicylates [358] Sulfonamides Probenecid Cephalothin Penicillins Colchicine Cisplatin [366] *p*-Aminobenzoic acid [366] Phenylbutazone [366]
Displacement of MTX from plasma protein binding	Salicylates [358] Probenecid Barbiturates Chloramphenicol [366] *p*-Aminobenzoic acid [366] Phenylbutazone [366] Phenytoin [366] Sulfonamides [366] Tetracyclines [366] Tranquillizers [366]
Intracellular accumulation of MTX	Probenecid Dipyridamole
Hepatotoxicity	Retinoids [364]

AZATHIOPRINE [265,372,378–380]

19.18 Azathioprine is a derivative of the cytostatic drug 6-mercaptopurine. Azathioprine is primarily used for immunosuppression, rather than for cancer chemotherapy. Nondermatological uses include renal transplantation and rheumatoid arthritis. In dermatology it is used for various forms of vasculitis, bullous dermatoses, neutrophilic dermatoses (Behçet disease, pyoderma gangrenosum), connective tissue diseases, severe eczematous (photo)dermatitis, pityriasis rubra pilaris, psoriasis and sarcoidosis. Azathioprine is usually given together with corticosteroids for its steroid-sparing effect.

Central nervous system

Fever occurs in less than 1%. Polyneuropathy causing muscle weakness has been quoted [381].

Cardiovascular system

Azathioprine has been blamed for causing atrial fibrillation. Shock from hypersensitivity reactions has been observed [381].

Respiratory system

Interstitial pneumonitis has been quoted as a side effect of azathioprine [381]. Reversible alveolitis has been recorded once.

Haematological

The bone marrow suppression effects of azathioprine are dose-related and may occur late in the therapeutic course. Most common is leukopenia. Thrombocytopenia and macrocytic anaemia occur less commonly. Macrocytosis is observed frequently in renal transplant patients.

Gastrointestinal tract

Nausea and vomiting occur early in therapy in at least 10% of patients. Diarrhoea and steatorrhoea occur uncommonly. Oral ulcerations and pancreatitis have been reported.

Liver

Hepatotoxicity occurs in less than 1% of nontransplantation patients receiving azathioprine and is generally reversible. Cases of cholestatic jaundice, portal fibrosis, and hepatocellular necrosis have been observed [379,381].

Skin and appendages

Morbilliform rashes and alopecia occur in less than 1%. Disseminated superficial porokeratosis [382] and porokeratosis of Mibelli have rarely been attributed to azathioprine.

Musculoskeletal system

Muscle wasting and arthralgia occur in less than 1%.

Miscellaneous

Azathioprine entails increased risk of non-Hodgkin lymphomas and cutaneous squamous cell carcinoma; the greatest risk is to transplantation patients. The briefest duration with the lowest dose possible is the goal for any immunosuppressive agent. Opportunistic infections should always be considered in the treatment of any therapeutically immunosuppressed patient. Overall, these opportunistic fungal, bacterial, viral, and parasitic infections are relatively uncommon in nontransplantation patients.

Second-generation effects

Chronic high doses may reduce fertility in either sex. Teratogenicity has been reported primarily in patients receiving combined therapy with prednisone and not azathioprine alone. However, usage of azathioprine in pregnancy is contraindicated, as premature delivery and low birth-weight are more common, and babies born to mothers receiving azathioprine for renal transplantation often have haematologic abnormalities, reduced immunoglobulin levels, and are more prone to septicaemia and other infections.

Interactions

Allopurinol inhibits the metabolism of azathioprine. Other concomitant immunosuppressive drugs may accentuate bone marrow depression, infection, or subsequent neoplasia. The neuromuscular blockade of succinylcholine is accentuated by azathioprine. In contrast, neuromuscular blockade induced by D-tubocurarine and pancuronium is antagonized by azathioprine.

CYCLOSPORIN A [384,396,398,400,407,409]

19.19 Cyclosporin A is a potent immunosuppressant, blocking the activity of T-lymphocytes [414]. The management of patients who have received transplants of kidneys, livers, heart and lungs, pancreas, bone marrow and small bowel relies heavily on the use of cyclosporin to prevent graft rejection. Disorders with an immunological basis, such as rheumatoid arthritis, Sjögren's syndrome, Crohn's disease, systemic sclerosis, Grave's ophthalmopathy, Behçet's disease, and aplastic anaemia also respond to cyclosporin administration. In dermatology, cyclosporin is used to treat severe refractory cases of psoriasis [385,418] and a variety of other dermatoses (Table 19.14). Cyclosporin is an important agent with multisystem toxicity, which requires careful and regular dermatological, physical and laboratory examinations [386].

Table 19.14. Dermatologic uses of cyclosporin [407,408]

Papulosquamous	**Neoplastic**
Psoriasis	Sezary's syndrome
Lichen planus	Mycosis fungoides
Acrodermatitis continua	Multicentric reticulohistiocytosis
Pityriasis rubra pilaris	
	Dermatitis
Bullous dermatoses	Atopic dermatitis
Pemphigus	Allergic contact dermatitis
Pemphigoid	
Epidermolysis bullosa acquisita	**Alopecia**
	Alopecia areata
Connective tissue diseases	Male pattern alopecia
Dermato/polymyositis	
Lupus erythematosus	**Other dermatoses**
Sjögren's syndrome	Allografts/xenografts
Scleroderma	Ichthyosis
	Persistent light reaction
Neutrophilic dermatoses	Erythema nodosum leprosum
Behçet's disease	Panniculitis
Pyoderma gangrenosum [415]	Sarcoidosis
	Toxic epidermal necrolysis

Adverse reaction pattern

Many adverse reactions to cyclosporin are reversible and occur within the first few weeks of starting therapy. In particular, paraesthesia, hypertrichosis, gingival hyperplasia and gastrointestinal disorders may occur, but are generally transient and require rarely discontinuation of therapy [400].

Among the most important effects are those involving the kidneys (nephrotoxicity) and the systemic vasculature (hypertension) [402]. There is a risk of tumour development in many organ systems [384]. Pre-existing renal and/or liver disease seem to predispose to toxic side effects of cyclosporin. The side effects are dose-dependent: in dermatology, far lower doses are used that in transplantation medicine. Thus, some side effects mentioned below, seen in patients treated with high-dose cyclosporin for transplantation, may not or in a lower frequency occur in psoriasis patients treated with low-dose cyclosporin.

Nervous system

Neurological side effects can be troublesome and serious, with an incidence of about 10%. Most presentations involve the central nervous system with seizures, cerebellar disorders, neuropathies and a variety of other problems (Table 19.15). Generalized major motor seizures occur in 1% of cases.

Table 19.15. Neurological side effects of cyclosporin [387]

Common	Uncommon
Tremor	Encephalopathy
Irritability	Cerebellar disorders
Confusion	Spinal cord syndromes
Neuropathies	Expressive aphasia
Seizures	Amnesia
Visual hallucinations	Mania
Fatigue [396]	Depression [407]
Headache [400]	

Respiratory

Respiratory distress syndrome [384].

Cardiovascular [402]

Cardiac side effects include a 'benign' myocardial fibrosis and a report of a pericardial effusion [384]. Systemic hypertension, usually affecting both systolic and diastolic pressures, develops in 85% of patients, usually within a few weeks of beginning cyclosporin treatment. This adverse effect is caused by vasoconstriction and vessel damage from cyclosporin rather than by nephrotoxicity.

A flushing sensation of the trunk or mouth shortly after ingestion of cyclosporin may occur, especially around the time of peak cyclosporin levels. Peripheral edema occurs in >1% of patients [400]. Raynaud's phenomenon has been reported [407].

Endocrine, metabolic

Glucose intolerance may occur, and the incidence of fasting hyperglycaemia on cyclosporin is about 8%. Hyperchloraemic metabolic acidosis occurs frequently. Hypercholesterolaemia and hypertriglyceridaemia are well-known complications of cyclosporine therapy [400,409,416,422]. Gynaecomastia has been reported once [406], as have benign breast fibroadenomas and breast tenderness.

Mineral and fluid balance

Hyperkalaemia and hypomagnesaemia have been reported. Hyperuricaemia is probably the result of reduced renal excretion of urate, and gouty attacks have been observed [400].

Haematological

Haematological effects of cyclosporin appear to include coagulation defects, intravascular coagulation in the renal vessels, and an association with thrombosis (mainly a feature of renal allografts). Myelosuppression does not usually occur, although anaemia, thrombocytopenia and granulocytopenia have been described [400]. An elevated sedimentation rate may be observed [396].

Liver

Hepatic dysfunction, with hyperbilirubinaemia (up to 50%, Ref. [409]), raised alkaline phosphatase and occasionally elevated transaminase levels being noted, usually occurs within the first few weeks of treatment with cyclosporin in a minority of patients [400].

Gastrointestinal

Gastrointestinal disturbances (nausea, vomiting, dyspepsia, abdominal pain, diarrhoea and weight loss) occur in 5–10% [384,396,400]. Upper gastrointestinal bleeding has occurred [407].

Urinary system [401,402,411]

Nephrotoxicity is the major problem seen in patients receiving cyclosporin. Cyclosporin nephrotoxicity is clinically characterized by fluid retention and dependent edema, increasing serum creatinine and urea concentrations, reduced creatinine clearance, and sometimes a hyperchloraemic, hyperkalaemic, metabolic acidosis. Tubular proteinuria is uncommon. The incidence of azotemia in the first 6 months of therapy ranges from 45 to 100%, increasing with the duration of exposure. However, the renal dysfunction is not usually progressive [384]. In psoriasis, patients treated with low-dose cyclosporin also frequently develop alterations in renal function [403]. Slight but significant increase in interstitial fibrous tissue, negatively correlating with creatinine clearance, was found in kidney biopsy specimens. The clinical relevance is unknown [404].

Skin and appendages [388,392]

Skin lesions occur in the majority of patients, principally affecting the pilosebaceous unit [388]. The most common problem is hypertrichosis which occurs in 40% of patients. Epidermal cysts, pilar keratoses, folliculitis and sebaceous hyperplasia [421] are also commonly present. Cutaneous lesions can occur from a variety of viral infections. The risk of squamous cell carcinomas is highly increased [389,390], especially in patients with other risk factors including PUVA and methotrexate [417]. The development of malignant melanoma [412] during cyclosporine treatment may have been coincidental [413]. Amelanosis has been reported for skin and optic fundi. Prurigo [393], eruptive benign keratoses [405] and pigmentation [394] have been described, as have benign lymphocytic infiltrates of the face and chest [397]. Gingival hyperplasia occurs in 5% of psoriasis patients [392,400].

Musculoskeletal system

Muscular weakness has rarely been reported [396]. Myalgia, back pain and muscle cramps are not uncommon [399,400] and arthralgia has been observed [407].

There appear to be 2 patterns of cyclosporin-associated muscular disorder. The first is myopathy without evidence of rhabdomyolysis developing in transplant patients. Electromyograms are normal or show changes compatible with myopathy or mild sensory motor neuropathy. Biopsy reveals toxic or non-specific myopathy; muscle enzymes are normal. These changes appear to be dose-dependent. The second type consists of rhabdomyolysis. This type of disorder seems to result primarily from interactions with other drugs, notable lovastatin and colchicine [420].

Eyes

Toxic retinopathy has been reported once. An embolism in a branch of the retinal artery has also been described. Loss of visual acuity occasionally occurs in association with other neurotoxicity.

Ears

Hearing loss has been reported [407].

Malignancy and infection

Both malignancy, particularly of the skin and lymphoreticular system (Table 19.16), and opportunistic infections, particularly cytomegaly virus, herpes simplex and zoster, and Pneumocystis carinii, can develop whilst patients are treated with cyclosporin. Lymphomas occur especially in transplant patients who are virtually all taking much higher doses of cyclosporin and conventional immunosuppressive therapy compared with those used in dermatology. The development of lymphoma is a function of the depth of immunosuppression. Otherwise healthy patients treated for relatively short periods with low-dose cyclosporine without any other immunosuppressive therapy, should have an incidence of lymphoma (and other malignancies?) closer to that of the general population [396,400].

Table 19.16. Cyclosporin malignancy rates as a risk ratio of expected rates [391]

Kaposi's sarcoma	>×100	Small intestine	×6.3
Microgliomas	>×100	Cervix invasive	×6.2
CNS tumours	>×100	Liver	×5.9
Parathyroid	>×100	Pharynx	×4.4
Vulva-vagina	×34	Bladder	×4.3
non-Hodgkin lymphoma	×9.9	Oesophagus	×4.2
Leukaemia	×9.5	Pleura	×4.0
Kidney	×6.9		

Miscellaneous

Sinusitis has been reported [407].

Second-generation effects

Pregnancy remains a major exclusion criterion for treatment with cyclosporine, although the experience of 107 transplant recipients suggests that there is no conclusive evidence of a teratogenic effect in man [410].

Overdosage

Acute poisoning with cyclosporin has been described with symptoms of altered taste, a variety of sensory changes, flushing of the face, swelling of feet and a sensation of increased abdominal girth, gum bleeding and stomach upset. These symptoms seem to be reversible if detected early.

Drug interactions [384,407,409]

An important cause of side effects of cyclosporin results from drug interactions. Any drugs with known nephrotoxic side effects or drugs which are known to act on the cytochrome P-450 system should be avoided or used with great caution. Drugs enhancing cyclosporin-induced nephrotoxicity are summarized in Table 19.17.

Table 19.17. Drugs enhancing cyclosporin-induced nephrotoxicity

Acyclovir
Aminoglycosides
Amphotericin B
Captopril
Cephalosporins
Etoposide
Furosemide
Indomethacin
Ketoconazole
Mannitol
Melphalan
Non-steroidal anti-inflammatory drugs [386]
Sulfonamides/trimethoprim
Vancomycin

Other drugs alter cyclosporin concentrations (Table 19.18).

Table 19.18. Drug interactions with cyclosporin manifesting as alterations in blood concentrations of cyclosporin [384,407,409]

Drugs that increase blood cyclosporin levels	Drugs that decrease blood cyclosporin levels
Acyclovir	Carbamazepine
Amphotericin B	Cilastatin
Cephalosporins	Isoniazid [396]
Cimetidine [395]	Phenobarbitone
Danazol	Phenytoin
Diltiazem	Rifampicin
Doxycycline	Sulfadimidine/trimethoprim
Erythromycin	Valproate
Furosemide	
Ketoconazole	
Methotrexate [419]	
Nicardipine	
Norfloxacin	
Steroids (androgenic, corticosteroids, oral contraceptives)	
Thiazide diuretics	
Verapamil	
Warfarin	

Patients receiving concomitant immunosuppressive or radiation therapy (including PUVA and UVL) should not receive cyclosporin because of the risk of (skin) malignancy [386]. Digitalis toxicity may result from interaction of digoxin with cyclosporine, and the combination with lovastatin and colchicine has resulted in rhabdomyolysis [409,420].

ANTIHISTAMINES [265,423–429,442,444]

19.20 Since their introduction in the early 1940s, antihistamines have become very popular, and are used in almost all medical disciplines. Many antihistamine preparations, both topical and oral, can be bought over-the-counter. The 'classical' antihistamines antagonize only a subset of histamine receptors, subsequently called H_1-histamine receptors. In 1972, the existence of gastric H_2-histamine receptors was discovered when scientists generated compounds chemically related to the structure of histamine, producing agents that antagonized H_2-receptors (cimetidine, ranitidine) [427].

The major side effect limiting the successful use of classical H_1-antihistamines has been sedation. Recently, H_1-antihistamines have been developed that possess a much lower incidence of central nervous system side effects [424,425]. Examples are terfenadine, loratadine and astemizole.

THE CLASSICAL H_1-ANTIHISTAMINES

19.21 The classical antihistamines have been classified on the basis of their chemical structure. The ethylamine moiety forms the nucleus of each compound; substitutions at various positions produce six major categories:

Category	Example
Ethanolamines	Diphenhydramine hydrochloride
Alkylamines	Chlorpheniramine maleate
Piperazines	Hydroxyzine hydrochloride
Piperidines	Cyproheptadine hydrochloride
Phenothiazines	Trimeprazine tartrate
Ethylenediamines	Tripelennamine hydrochloride

The main indications for H_1-antihistamines are urticaria (including physical urticarias, symptomatic dermographism) and angio-edema. They are also used for symptomatic mastocytosis and flushing reactions, in which histamine plays an important role. In addition, the antihistamines are widely used for the treatment of pruritus and pruritic dermatoses (including atopic dermatitis), in which the beneficial effect may be caused by their sedative effect rather than their antihistaminic activity, as histamine usually plays a minor role in the pathophysiology of these diseases.

The lipophilic nature of the classical H_1-antihistamines allows for wide tissue distribution and passage through the blood-brain barrier, through the placenta and into breast milk. As a result, a variety of potential side effects and complications may be anticipated.

Central nervous system

CNS depression (drowsiness, sedation) is the most common side effect. Gradual tolerance usually develops. Sedation is often significant with ethanolamines, phenothiazines and ethylenediamines. Stimulatory side effects are occasionally noted, especially in children [446] and the elderly: nervousness, irritability, insomnia, tremor, and nightmares. In adults, electroencephalogram alterations have been reported along with rare instances of seizures. Individual case-reports of oral and facial dyskinesias have been reported with antihistamine-decongestant combinations. Acute dystonia has been reported with diphenhydramine. Autonomic side effects relate primarily to the degree of anticholinergic activity and include dryness of mucous membranes, urinary retention, blurred vision, and nasal stuffiness. Toxic psychosis developed in a patient treated with cyproheptadine. Fever is an occasional complication.

Cardiovascular system

Tachycardia, extrasystoles and hypertension have been incidentally reported with various antihistamines. Some of these compounds (e.g. cinnarizine) have been found to improve peripheral blood flow. Anaphylactic reactions have been described.

Respiratory system

Nasal stuffiness and tightness of the chest in some patients may be caused by antihistamines with high anticholinergic activity.

Haematological

Severe haematologic reactions are very rare. Chlorpheniramine has been associated with pancytopenia, agranulocytosis, thrombocytopenia, and aplastic anaemia. There are rare reports of blood dyscrasias such as agranulocytosis and haemolytic anaemia with other antihistamines [430].

Gastrointestinal tract

Occasional gastrointestinal side effects include nausea, vomiting, anorexia, epigastric distress, constipation, and diarrhoea. It has been reported that antihistamines can provoke release of catecholamines from a phaeochromocytoma.

Liver

Repeated reports of liver function changes may be due to nothing more than coincidence. Occasionally, however, cholestatic jaundice seems to have occurred.

Endocrine, metabolic

Cyproheptadine has been associated with weight gain. Occasional reports of antihistamine-induced hypoglycaemia may well reflect mere coincidence.

Urinary system

Urinary retention may be caused by antihistamines with a high anticholinergic activity.

Skin and appendages

Dry mucous membranes may be caused by antihistamines with a high anticholinergic activity. Aspirin-sensitive patients may develop urticaria from certain dyes present in antihistamine tablets, e.g. tartrazine. Dimenhydrinate has caused a fixed drug eruption [445]. Mebhydrolin caused exanthema in 2 patients [447].

Special senses

Eyes
Blurred vision may be caused by antihistamines with a high degree of anticholinergic activity. Theoretically, this activity could result in exacerbation of narrow-angle glaucoma.

Dimenhydrinate was found to affect colour discrimination, night vision, reaction time and stereopsis. It is likely that other antihistamines have similar effects.

Second-generation effects

Despite widespread use of over-the-counter and prescription H_1-antihistamines, there is a paucity of cogent evidence linking these drugs with congenital defects. Possible occasional associations with individual congenital defects have been noted but whether these were fortuitous or drug-related is unknown. The use of H_1-blockers for the treatment of hyperemesis gravidarum is associated with an increased risk of cleft palate, but hyperemesis *sec* is also. Judicious use of chlorpheniramine and diphenhydramine would be allowed in pregnancy [423]. Information regarding H_1-antihistamine use during breast-feeding is controversial. The American Academy of Pediatrics feels that diphenhydramine and trimeprazine are compatible with breast feeding. However, case reports of CNS toxicity in nursing infants have been reported with maternal intake of clemastine. Cyproheptadine is stated by the manufacturer to inhibit lactation.

Interactions

The CNS depressant and anticholinergic effects of classical H_1-antihistamines may be additive with other drugs that possess similar effects (hypnotics, sedatives, narcotic analgesics, neuroleptics, anticholinergics, phenothiazines, tricyclic antidepressives). Alcohol increases the impairment of performance skills induced by antihistamines. Antihistamines are best avoided by patients taking monoamine oxidase inhibitors. Antihistamines are said to antagonize the effectiveness of steroids, diphenylhydantoin, oral anticoagulants, phenylbutazone, griseofulvine, and other drugs metabolized by liver enzymes [426]. A possible toxic interaction between cyproheptadine and phenelzine has been reported.

THE LESS SEDATING ANTIHISTAMINES

19.22 The discovery of oral H_1-antihistamines with poor CNS penetration provides for a more specific action at peripheral H_1-receptors. Terfenadine, astemizole and loratadine are usually referred to as 'non-sedating'. However, these drugs can cause sedation, albeit at a frequency generally approaching the incidence seen with placebo. An additional improvement is their relative lack of activity at receptor sites other than H_1-receptors. Unwanted effects, such as anticholinergic effects, are therefore encountered less frequently than with classical antihistamines. Also, tolerance to therapeutic effects after chronic administration has not been detected in most clinical studies.

The main indication for these antihistamines is chronic idiopathic urticaria. Because these drugs are virtually devoid of sedating activity, they are of no value for the treatment of other pruritic dermatoses in which histamine plays no or a minor role.

Central nervous system

Sedation is rarely a problem. These antihistamines interfere less with performance skills than the classical H_1-antihistamines. Headache occurs very infrequently.

Cardiovascular system

Torsade de pointes, a form of polymorphic ventricular tachycardia that is associated with prolongation of the QT interval, is observed with terfenadine overdose, and may occur from an interaction with ketoconazole and erythromycine [443]. Ventricular tachycardia, ventricular fibrillation and other arrhythmias may also be observed from high terfenadine plasma levels. Atrioventricular blockade and torsade de pointes have also been caused by astemizole. A quinidine-like effect on the myocardium with convulsions has been reported in a patient with terfenadine toxicity.

Respiratory system

Terfenadine may occasionally precipitate or worsen asthma.

Gastrointestinal tract

Nausea and diarrhoea occur very infrequently.

Liver

Mild to moderate elevations of serum transaminase levels may occur occasionally. Hepatitis has rarely been reported [435].

Endocrine, metabolic

Increased appetite and weight gain have been associated with astemizole use.

Skin and appendages

Stricker and coauthors cited 108 cases of dermatologic reactions with terfenadine reported in Europe [431]. Reactions included photosensitivity [432], urticaria, maculopapular eruptions, erythema, and peeling of the skin of the hands and feet. Six cases of alopecia have been associated with terbinafine [433]. Psoriasis may be severely exacerbated during terfenadine treatment [434]. Dry mouth occurs very infrequently.

Second-generation effects

Because of limited data in humans, the less sedating antihistamines are best avoided by pregnant women and in nursing mothers.

Interactions

No significant drug interactions have been definitely correlated with these antihistamines, but coadministration of ketoconazole and erythromycin may increase terfenadine plasma levels [443]. They do not enhance the CNS effects of ethanol and diazepam.

H_2-ANTIHISTAMINES [427,436,438,441]

19.23 H_2-antihistamines (cimetidine, ranitidine) are used mainly for the treatment of gastrointestinal diseases, such as duodenal ulcer and gastric ulcer; hypersecretory states, such as Zollinger–Ellison syndrome; and mastocytosis. The potential role of H_2-antihistamines in dermatology has been studied most extensively with cimetidine [427,436]. A main dermatologic indication for cimetidine is in the treatment of chronic idiopathic urticaria refractory to H_1-antihistamines alone.

Cimetidine has an immune enhancing effect by inhibiting suppressor T-cell activity, and has been used for the treatment of herpes simplex, herpes zoster, metastatic malignant melanoma and mycosis fungoides. It has also antiandrogenic activity, which may explain its reported success in treating female androgenic alopecia and hirsutism [437].

The overall frequency of adverse effects associated with H_2-antihistamines is <3%. Associated side effects are variable in presentation, and all are apparently reversible upon discontinuation.

Central nervous system

Dizziness, somnolence, and headache may occur. Rapidly reversible mental confusional states, such as disorientation and agitation, are sometimes seen in patients who received high-dosage therapy, have diminished renal or hepatic function, are elderly, or are hospitalized with other underlying medical conditions. Extrapyramidal and cerebellar disturbances have been postulated but not proven.

Cardiovascular system

Reports of significant cardiovascular complications are uncommon [438], but may occur with high dose intravenous use and in high-risk patients. Rapid intravenous administration (which is not done in dermatology) has been reported to cause sinus arrest, arrhythmias, bradycardia, severe hypotension, and shock. Chest pain and cardiac arrest have been observed with ranitidine.

Respiratory system

Bronchospasm is occasionally reported. Central nervous effects can rarely lead to respiratory depression. A case of interstitial lung disease may have been caused by cimetidine.

Haematological

Agranulocytosis, thrombocytopenia and neutropenia have rarely been described.

Gastrointestinal tract

Diarrhoea and constipation occasionally occur. A case of pancreatitis possibly associated with cimetidine and one possibly with ranitidine have been reported.

Liver

Occasional transient elevations in serum transaminase levels, which often disappear despite continued therapy, may be observed. Individual cases of hepatotoxicity have been reported [439,448]. Significant hepatotoxicity appears to be uncommon, idiosyncratic, not dosage-related, and structure-specific.

Endocrine, metabolic

Occasional side effects with cimetidine from its antiandrogenic activity have included loss of libido, impotence (also with ranitidine), gynaecomastia, reduced sperm count, and galactorrhoea. Cimetidine may derange severe diabetes. Modest increases in serum high-density lipoproteins have occasionally been noted. A 40% reduction in serum cortisol has been found with active doses of cimetidine but not with ranitidine.

Urinary system

Slight elevations of serum creatinine levels regularly occur with cimetidine use. These are not reflective of renal toxicity, and do not require discontinuation. Rarely, cases of acute interstitial nephritis have been reported.

Skin and appendages

Cutaneous side effects appear to be uncommon. Cimetidine has been reported to cause dryness of the skin, asteatotic dermatitis, urticaria, angioedema, exfoliative dermatitis, erythema multiforme major, and urticarial vasculitis. Cimetidine has caused alopecia [440]. Hypersensitivity reactions to ranitidine have several times resulted in anaphylaxis.

Musculoskeletal system

A small proportion of patients develop troublesome myalgia when treated with cimetidine. It may be associated with arthritis and joint effusion, but this is highly unusual. There have been incidental reports of polymyositis and of a form of myopathy, probably of motor neuron origin.

Special senses

Eyes
Increased ocular pressure with ocular pain and blurred vision was seen with both cimetidine and ranitidine in a patient with chronic glaucoma.

Second-generation effects

Because data on these drugs' effects in humans are lacking, the use of H_2-antihistamines during pregnancy and in women nursing infants is best avoided.

Interactions [438,441,442]

The large number of interactions described are mainly attributable to the binding of cimetidine to hepatic mixed-function oxidase and hence to inhibition of drug metabolism. In addition, cimetidine can also inhibit the renal excretion of drugs.

Both effects are of modest degree, and the long list of drugs for which interference is demonstrable (Table 19.19) is out of all proportion compared with the list of those for which interference is of clinical significance.

Table 19.19. Groups of drugs interacting with cimetidine [442]

Group	Drug	Effect
Anaesthetics	succinylcholine	delayed recovery*
Antiarrhythmics	lidocaine	toxic levels in volunteers
	procainamide	increased plasma levels
	quinidine	increased plasma levels
Anticoagulants	warfarin	enhanced activity*
Antidiabetics	gliclazide	increased level
Anticonvulsants	phenytoin	raised steady-state levels*
Antidepressants	imipramine	retarded metabolism
Antiinflammatory	indomethacin	retarded metabolism
Antimitotics	fluorouracil	increased levels
Cardiovascular drugs	propranolol	enhanced activity
	nifedipine	increased plasma levels
	diltiazem	increased plasma levels
	verapamil	increased plasma levels
Diuretics	furosemide	increased plasma-curve area
Immunosuppressants	cyclosporine	increased plasma levels*
Respiratory drugs	theophylline	toxic levels reached*

*Effects likely or proven to be of clinical importance.

Interactions with ranitidine include increased plasma concentrations of nifedipine and metoprolol. In addition, the clearance of valproate sodium and carbamazepine may be modestly decreased, and diltiazem and midazolam bioavailability may be increased. All effects are small and are unlikely to be clinically significant. Generally speaking, any interaction described with one H_2-blocker should be anticipated with all others until the contrary has been firmly proven.

ANTIMALARIALS [265,292,449–451,462]

19.24 The antimalarial drugs used for dermatological diseases are quinacrine, chloroquine, and hydroxychloroquine. They were developed in that order as alternatives to quinine in the prophylaxis and suppressive treatment of *Plasmodium* malaria.

Non-dermatological indications for their use are malaria and rheumatoid arthritis. In dermatology, the 'antimalarials' are used mainly for lupus erythematosus and photosensitivity dermatoses (polymorphous light eruption, porphyria cutanea tarda, dermatomyositis, and solar urticaria). Other diseases in which antimalarials have been demonstrated to be occasionally or anecdotally effective include: granulomatous dermatoses (sarcoidosis, Miescher's granuloma, generalized granuloma annulare), lymphocytic infiltrates (lymphocytoma cutis, lymphocytic infiltrate of Jessner), and miscellaneous conditions (reticular erythematous mucinosis syndrome, lichen sclerosus et atrophicus, epidermolysis bullosa, atopic dermatitis, urticarial vasculitis, localized scleroderma, idiopathic panniculitis).

The mechanism or mechanisms of action of the drugs in malaria, or any skin diseases (except perhaps for porphyria cutanea tarda, in which it increases urinary uroporphyrin excretion), are not precisely known: they have sunscreen effects, and may have anti-inflammatory and immunomodulatory effects.

An impressive list of possible side effects has been published [450,451] and almost any organ system can be affected. All the adverse reactions can occur with any of the three antimalarials, with the exceptions that quinacrine therapy produces a yellowish stain of the skin and the sclera in about a third of patients after months of therapy, and that quinacrine is *not* toxic to the retina.

Central nervous system

Infrequent central nervous system effects that occur in susceptible patients or with doses higher than recommended include restlessness, nervousness, vertigo, tinnitus, excitement, confusion, headache, seizures, myasthenia, neuromyopathy, neuritis, myopathy, and toxic psychosis [452]. The neuromyopathy is characterized by the insidious onset of slowly progressive weakness, starting in the lower limbs. A spastic pyramidal tract syndrome of the lower limbs in young children was reported in relation to chloroquine.

Cardiovascular system

Acute intoxication is associated with cardiac arrest. Rarely, heart block and congestive heart failure have been reported.

Respiratory system

Respiratory arrest may occur with gross overdosage.

Haematological

Rare but fatal bone marrow toxicity has been reported, including anaemia, neutropenia and agranulocytosis, and rarely thrombocytopenia. Chloroquine has been associated with haemolysis in glucose-6-phosphate dehydrogenase deficiency.

Gastrointestinal tract

Gastrointestinal side effects such as nausea, vomiting and diarrhoea are the most common reasons for early decreases in dosage or discontinuation of treatment. Approximately 10% is unable to tolerate chloroquine. Stomatitis occasionally with buccal ulceration has been mentioned. Stomach ulcers have been observed.

Liver

Slight liver function abnormalities have rarely been observed.

Skin and appendages

A bluish-grey to black hyperpigmentation may occur in 10–30% of patients treated for 4 months or longer with any of the drugs. The pigmentation typically affects the shins, the face, the palate, and the nail beds. Progressive bleaching of the hair roots of the scalp, the face and the body may appear in as many as 10% of the patients taking chloroquine [453]. Both processes are reversible. The incidence of pruritus and "dermatitis" has been reported to be 10–20% [454]. The rashes included urticaria, morbilliform, eczematous, lichenoid, exfoliative dermatitis, erythroderma [457], and erythema annulare centrifugum patterns [455]. The frequency with which antimalarials exacerbate preexisting psoriasis (also of the pustular type, Ref. [464]) is controversial [456,457]. Photosensitivity and photoallergic dermatitis have been seen particularly during long-term therapy with high doses [292]. Anaphylaxis has been described once [292].

Musculoskeletal system

The myopathy described is often in fact a neuromyopathy. Myasthenia gravis-like reactions have been observed.

Special senses

Eyes [459,460]
The antimalarials can cause several ocular adverse effects, but it is the inherent retinal toxicity of chloro- and hydroxychloroquine that is most worrying. Chloroquine has an affinity for melanin-containing tissues and accumulates in the eye (iris, choroid, pigmented epithelium of the cornea). Here it persists for years after cessation of therapy. The incidence of true retinopathy is low: only about 300 cases have been described in the world's literature [449]. The classic picture of chloroquine retinopathy consists of granular or stippled hyperpigmentation of the macula, surrounded by a clear zone of depigmentation and then by another ring of pigmentation. This 'bull's-eye' lesion represents an advanced stage of retinopathy with a more serious field deficit (absolute scotomas) and possible progression of the scotoma and loss in visual acuity even after the drug is discontinued (for up to 7 years!). However, long-term daily dosages of 3.5 mg/kg of chloroquine or 6.5 mg/kg of hydroxychloroquine lie below the threshold at which retinal toxicity may be anticipated [461].

Neuromuscular effects of antimalarials that affect the eye include a bilateral abducens muscle paralysis and ciliary body dysfunction. The abducens paralysis causes diplopia. Ciliary body dysfunction results in disturbances of accommodation. Both effects are dose-related and reversible [451].

Corneal reactions are an acute congestive reaction that leads to corneal edema and blurred vision, and corneal deposition of antimalarials, which may either be asymptomatic or lead to blurred vision, especially the perception of coloured halos around lights, notably at night. Bilateral edema of the optic nerve has been reported once.

Ears

Ototoxicity (tinnitus, deafness, cochlear vestibular dysfunction) has been reported infrequently, but may be more common from chloroquine phosphate *injections*.

Second-generation effects

Chloroquine readily crosses the placenta and has been reported to result in cochlear damage and sensorineural hearing loss in the newborn. However, there have been many clinical observations of full-term and uncomplicated pregnancies and deliveries without apparent damage to either mother or child in rheumatic patients treated with chloroquine.

Interactions

Digoxin levels may be elevated by antimalarials. Chloroquine and hydroxychloroquine should not be administered concurrently because of the additive retinotoxic potential. The concurrent administration of probenecid increases the risk of retinotoxicity. Interactions with antibiotics have been observed, which may be either synergistic or antagonistic [292].

Overdosage

Fatal reactions from irreversible cardiac arrest have been reported after accidental or intentional overdosage with chloroquine. The particular sensitivity of very young children (aged 1–3 years) to only 1 gram has been emphasized, but was challenged by Rasmussen who stated that adults exhibit a similar sensitivity when compared on a mg/kg basis [458]. Cardiovascular collapse, cardiac and/or respiratory collapse, and convulsions have been described. Rapid onset of headache, drowsiness, deranged vision, vomiting and diarrhoea is followed by arrhythmias.

MISCELLANEOUS DRUGS

ACYCLOVIR [265,465,466,469]

19.25 The advent of acyclovir in the beginning of the 1980s greatly enhanced the management and outcome of herpes virus infections and paved the way for further promising antiviral agents. Although newer drugs such as ganciclovir, foscarnet and deoxyacyclovir are in experimental use, acyclovir, which is available for topical use, as tablets and for intravenous injections, remains the first-line agent for therapy of herpes virus infections [480]. Acyclovir is an ideal antiviral agent in that it essentially destroys only virally infected cells, leaving normal cells intact.

Adverse reactions pattern

General and toxic reactions. In general, acyclovir is a remarkably safe antiviral agent. In most studies, no significant toxic effects were noted. Toxic effects from overdosage have not occurred with oral acyclovir; however, renal and neurologic sequelae have developed with parenteral doses.

Hypersensitivity reactions. Occasional rashes and urticaria have been caused by acyclovir. Drug-induced fever is uncommon [468].

Central nervous system [467]

Encephalopathic changes such as lethargy, tremors, confusion and seizures are observed in 1% of patients treated with intravenous therapy. Coma has rarely been associated with acyclovir [473]. Psychiatric symptoms have been observed [469,472,475]. Headaches are common, and seen mostly with chronic suppressive therapy (13%) and less so with short-term therapy. Vertigo and fatigue are rarely reported. Drug-induced fever (with or without central nervous system symptoms) is uncommon [468]. Neurotoxicity from oral acyclovir can be expected only in patients on haemodialysis [470] who have very high serum concentrations of acyclovir.

Cardiovascular system

Recurrent tachycardia was observed in an infant each time he used acyclovir [466].

Haematological

Haematological disorders, including leukopenia, are extremely rare.

Gastrointestinal tract

Nausea or vomiting (8%) and diarrhoea (9%) are encountered frequently with oral administration but rarely with parenteral use [471]. Anorexia is rarely reported.

Liver

Elevated liver enzymes have occasionally been observed, but a relationship with acyclovir was not clearly demonstrated.

Urinary system

Impaired renal function has been reported in 10% of patients who receive rapid (less than 10 minutes) intravenous infusions and in 5% of patients who receive slow (over 1 hour) intravenous infusion of acyclovir. Acyclovir precipitates in the renal tubules, which leads to an obstructive nephropathy when high doses are given rapidly intravenously. Elevated blood urea nitrogen or serum creatinine returns to pretreatment levels with appropriate dosage adjustment, discontinuation of the drug, or correction of fluid and electrolyte abnormalities. In rare cases, however, acute renal failure occurs [466]. Oral acyclovir has not been associated with renal dysfunction. Frequent urination was observed in 4% of 157 patients treated with oral acyclovir [476].

Skin and appendages

Cutaneous side effects include occasional rashes and urticaria (less than 1%), in one reported case associated with vasculitis. Parenteral acyclovir is frequently associated with inflammation or phlebitis at infiltrated intravenous sites, and rarely with vesicles [474].

Special senses

Eyes
Local application of 3% ophthalmic ointment may cause mild transient stinging. Diffuse, superficial, punctate and non-progressive keratopathy may develop. This quickly resolves as soon as the drug is omitted [478]. In one patient suffering from herpes zoster and treated with acyclovir, progressive bilateral amaurosis developed. Autopsy revealed a possibly drug-related necrotizing vasculitis of the left optic nerve at the chiasm [479].

Risk situations

Parenteral acyclovir should be used with caution in patients who have had neurologic reactions to cytotoxic drugs.

Second-generation effects

Acyclovir does not impair fertility. It has not been shown to be teratogenic in animals or in humans, but data to consider acyclovir safe for use in pregnancy are lacking [477].

Interactions

Concomitant use of probenecid will decrease urinary excretion of acyclovir.

Overdosage

No toxic effects from overdosage have been observed.

DAPSONE [265,481,482,484,486,487]

19.26 Dapsone (diaminodiphenylsulfone, DDS) has antimicrobial activity against leprosy and other infectious diseases and remains the mainstay for the treatment of leprosy today. In addition, the drug has been shown to have anti-inflammatory activity comparable with that of corticosteroids and indomethacin. Many of the cutaneous diseases that are responsive to dapsone are thought to be autoimmune in nature, or, in particular, to be diseases in which polymorphonuclear leukocytes have a prominent pathophysiological role.

Dapsone is the treatment of choice for leprosy and dermatitis herpetiformis. Other dermatologic uses include bullous diseases, the vasculitides, neutrophilic dermatoses (pyoderma gangrenosum, Sweet's syndrome, Behçet's disease/aphthous ulcers), infectious diseases (actinomycotic mycetoma, chloroquine-resistant malaria, cutaneous leishmaniasis, *pneumocystis carinii* pneumonia in Aids) and miscellaneous disorders (pustular psoriasis, panniculitis, relapsing polychondritis, granuloma annulare).

Central nervous system [488]

Headache, fatigue and dizziness may be observed. Dapsone may cause axon damage, which results in a peripheral neuropathy that affects motor nerves much more frequently than sensory nerves [487]. Patients should be monitored for the development of weakness, loss of sensation, and paraesthesias. Psychosis may also occur, especially in patients with a prior or concurrent history of mental disturbances [488].

Cardiovascular system

Tachycardia may occur with hypersensitivity reactions. Signs of heart failure with edema, ascites and severe hypoalbuminaemia have been described in the treatment of dermatitis herpetiformis.

Respiratory system

Shortness of breath has been recorded.

Haematological

Haematologic effects of dapsone include haemolysis, methaemoglobinaemia, (delayed) sulfhaemoglobinaemia, leukopenia, and in rare cases, agranulocytosis [482,484]. Haemolysis and methaemoglobinaemia are dosage-related, and the former occurs in patients with or without glucose-6-phosphatase dehydrogenase deficiency, although it is much more severe in patients with a deficiency of this enzyme. Haemolysis and the resulting anaemia may be severe in patients treated with 200–300 mg/day of dapsone. Methaemoglobinaemia may produce obvious cyanosis in some patients, but it is usually clinically significant only in patients with cardiovascular disease. A rare but dreaded complication of dapsone is agranulocytosis [484]. The typical syndrome includes fever, sore throat with necrotic white pharyngeal pseudomembranes, pyoderma or cellulitis, and occasionally a morbilliform rash. Death, when it occurs, is due to bacterial sepsis. Associated conditions have included a reversible monoclonal IgD gammopathy, pseudoleukaemia, and reversible aplastic anaemia.

Gastrointestinal tract

Nausea and vomiting are rarely serious.

Liver

Toxic hepatitis and cholestatic jaundice may occur (see under "Miscellaneous" below).

Urinary system

Very rare instances of renal papillary necrosis and the nephrotic syndrome have been described. Renal failure is possible in severe haemolytic conditions.

Skin and appendages

Cutaneous hypersensitivity reactions are uncommon. Reactions include itching, morbilliform exanthemas, erythema multiforme, erythema nodosum (leprosum), and toxic epidermal necrolysis [482]. Rare reactions are photodermatitis [489] and pustular and acneiform eruptions [490].

Special senses

Eyes

There are 2 case reports of visual impairment associated with dapsone. One patient who took an overdose had blurred vision and reduced visual acuity.

Miscellaneous

An unusual but potentially fatal infectious mononucleosis-like syndrome is known as the Dapsone Hypersensitivity Syndrome [483]. The syndrome is characterized by fever, malaise, and lymphadenopathy. A maculopapular (morbilliform) eruption initially presents after 5–6 weeks of treatment and frequently progresses to exfoliative erythroderma. Hepatomegaly with jaundice accompanies the rash. Laboratory findings include abnormal liver function tests either on a hepatocellular basis or cholestatic. Eosinophilia and an increased number of atypical lymphocytes are generally present. Several cases have been fatal, the cause of death being severe hepatitis with liver failure.

Second-generation effects

Dapsone has been used safely during pregnancy by many patients with leprosy, but use of the drug by pregnant women has not been studied adequately for clinicians to assume that it is completely safe for the foetus. Dapsone is distributed into breast milk and should be avoided by nursing women whenever possible.

Interactions

Probenecid may reduce renal excretion of dapsone. Serum levels may be lower in patients also taking rifampicine.

Overdosage

Methaemoglobinaemia, anaemia, and vomiting occurs in poisoning. Restlessness may progress from excitement to coma.

Transient blurring of vision, followed by full recovery, has often been noted with acute dapsone poisoning.

FUMARIC ACID [491–493,501]

19.27 During the past few years, fumaric acid therapy for psoriasis has gained interest among Dutch and German patients. This treatment was empirically devised by the German chemist Schweckendiek and further developed by the German physician Schäfer. Fumaric acid therapy is based on the following principles: 1. oral treatment with monoethyl and dimethyl esters of fumaric acid; 2. topical treatment with monoethylfumarate, and: 3. a diet that forbids the consumption of nuts, spices, wines, and distilled products of wine. In a few controlled studies, fumaric acid therapy has proven useful for the treatment of psoriasis [502], but side effects, which are frequent and sometimes severe (especially nephrotoxicity [498–501]), are an important drawback [491–493].

Adverse reaction pattern

General and toxic reactions. The most frequent adverse reactions are flushing, gastrointestinal side effects (gastric and oesophageal pain, nausea, vomiting, diarrhoea), and fatigue. Renal insufficiency may develop. Although the pattern of side effects for the various esters of fumaric acid is similar, the frequency of individual reactions differs.

Central nervous system

Fatigue is common, as is general malaise. Dizziness has been reported [493], as has headache [491].

Cardiovascular system

Flushing of the face and the upper arms develops in more than 50% of patients, appearing 10–15 minutes after intake and lasting for half an hour, but sometimes up to 8 hours. The flushes are dependent on the individual, the fumarate in question, and the dosage. With enteric-coated tablets, flushes usually appear after 3–4 hours. Edema has been cited as a side effect of fumaric acid derivatives [499].

Haematological

Eosinophilia and lymphopenia, resulting from a decrease in T-suppressor lymphocytes [492,494] are quite common. Leukopenia has also been observed [492,501].

Gastrointestinal tract

Gastric and oesophageal pain, nausea, vomiting and diarrhoea are common. The use of enteric-coated tablets may diminish these side effects. Worsening of peptic ulcers and stomach perforation have been observed [501]. Metallic taste has been cited as side effect of fumarates [499].

Liver

A transient rise in liver function tests is not uncommon.

Endocrine, metabolic

Isolated cases of hypoglycaemia from fumarates have been cited [499].

Urinary system

Topical application of monoethylfumarate ointment 3% caused proteinuria in 3 of 6 patients with extensive psoriasis [495]. Proteinuria from systemic use of fumarates has also been observed [493]. Several cases of significant nephrotoxicity have been reported [498–501). Both acute tubular necrosis and tubulo-interstitial reactions can develop, which may sometimes be only partially reversible [498]. Other investigators found no signs of nephrotoxicity even after long-term oral application [496].

Skin and appendages

Contact with fumaric acid derivatives may cause (nonallergic) erythematous rashes in virtually all patients [492]. Oral intake has uncommonly caused a rash [492,501]. Toxic dermatitis from 3% monoethylfumarate ointment has been reported [497].

ACKNOWLEDGEMENT

For this chapter, the authors have drawn heavily upon:
Wolverton, S.E. and Wilkins, J.K. (Eds.), *Systemic Drugs used in Skin Diseases.* Saunders, Philadelphia, 1991.
Meyler's Side Effects of Drugs (11th Edition), and *The Side Effects of Drugs, Annuals 12–15*, Edited by M.N.G. Dukes, L. Bealy and J.K. Aronson. Elsevier, Amsterdam, 1988–1991.

19.28 REFERENCES

1. von Eickstedt, K.-W., Elsasser, W. (1988): Corticotrophins and Corticosteroids. In: *Meyler's Side Effects of Drugs, 11th Edition*, pp. 812–27. Editor: M.N.G. Dukes. Elsevier Science Publishers, Amsterdam.
2. Wolverton, S.E. (1991): Glucocorticosteroids. In: *Systemic Drugs for Skin Diseases*, pp. 86–124. Editors: S.E. Wolverton and J.K. Wilkin. Saunders, Philadelphia.
3. Gallant, C. and Kenny, P. (1986): Oral glucocorticoids and their complications: A review. *J. Am. Acad. Dermatol., 14*, 161–177.
4. Truhan, A.P. and Ahmend, A.R. (1989): Corticosteroids: A review with emphasis on complications of prolonged systemic therapy. *Ann. Allergy, 62*, 375–391.
5. Seale, J.P. and Compton, M.R. (1986): Side effects of corticosteroid agents. *Med. J. Austral., 144*, 139–142.
6. Davis, G.F. (1986): Adverse effects of corticosteroids. II. Systemic. Clin Dermatol., 4, 161–169.
7. Lester, R.S. (1989): Corticosteroids. Clin. Dermatol., 7, 80–97.
8. Spark, R.F. (1987): Systemic Corticosteroids. In: *Dermatology in General Medicine*, pp. 2564–2570. Editors: T.B. Fitzpatrick et al. Lippincott, Philadelphia.
9. Glick, M. (1989): Glucocorticosteroid replacement therapy: A literature review and suggested replacement therapy. *Oral Surg. Oral Med. Oral Pathol., 67*, 614–620.
10. Lucky, A.W. (1984): Principles of the use of glucocorticosteroids in the growing child. *Pediatr. Dermatol., 1*, 226–235.
11. Messer, J., Reitman, D., Sacks, H.S. et al. (1983): Association of adrenocorticosteroid therapy and peptic ulcer disease. *New Engl. J. Med., 309*, 21–24.
12. Scaparro, E., Borghi, S. and Rebora, A. (1984): Kaposi's sarcoma after immunosuppressive therapy for bullous pemphigoid. *Dermatologica, 169,* 156–159.
13. Adams, S.J., Davison, A.M., Cunliffe, W.J. and Giles, G.R. (1982): Perioral dermatitis in renal transplant recipients maintained on corticosteroids and immunosuppressive therapy. *Br. J. Dermatol., 106*, 589.
14. Potter, R.A. (1971): Intralesional triamcinolone and adrenal suppression in acne vulgaris. *J. Invest. Dermatol., 57*, 364.
15. Shelmire, D. (1968): Reaction to triamcinolone. *Cutis, 4*, 71.
16. Rimbaud, P., Meynadier, J., Gilhou, J.J. and Meynadier, J. (1974): Complications dermatologiques locales secondaires aux injections cortisonées. *Nouv. Presse Med., 3*, 665.
17. Francon, F. (1968): Accidents cutanes et souscutanes par le Tedarol en injections locales. *Med. Hyg. (Geneve), 26*, 480.
18. Baden, H.P. and Bonaz, L.C. (1967): Calcinosis cutis following intralesional injection of triamcinolone hexacetonide. *Arch. Dermatol., 96,* 689.
19. Friedman, S.J., Butler D.F. and Pittelkow, M.R. (1988): Perilesional linear atrophy and hypopigmentation after intralesional corticosteroid therapy. *J. Am. Acad. Dermatol., 19*, 537–541.

20. Baran, M.L.R. (1964): Le risque d'amaurose au cours du traitement local des alopecies par corticotherapie injectable. *Bull. Soc. Fr. Derm. Syph., 71*, 25.
21. Hurwitz, R.M. (1989): Steroid acne. *J. Am. Acad. Dermatol., 21,* 1179–1181.
22. Fjellner, B., Herczka, O. and Wennersten, G. (1983): Complications in the intralesional injection of triamcinolone acetonide by jet injector (Dermojet). *Acta Derm. Venereol., 63*, 456–457.
23. Dukes, M.N.G., Beeley, L. and Aronson, J.K., eds. (1988–1991): *Side Effects of Drugs, Annuals 12–15.* Elsevier, Amsterdam.
24. Orfanos, C.E., Ehlert, R. and Gollnick, H. (1987): The retinoids. A review of their clinical pharmacology and therapeutic use. *Drugs, 34*, 459–503.
25. Lowe, N.J. and David, M. (1988): New retinoids for dermatologic diseases. Uses and toxicity. *Dermatologic Clinics, 6*, 539–552.
26. David, M., Hodak, E. and Lowe N.J. (1988): Adverse effects of retinoids. *Med. Toxicol., 3*, 273–288.
27. Halioua, B. and Saurat, J.-H. (1990): Risk:benefit ratio in the treatment of psoriasis with systemic retinoids. *Br. J. Dermatol., 122 (Suppl. 36),* 135–150.
28. Brindley, C.J. (1989): Overview of recent clinical pharmacokinetic studies with acitretin (Ro 10-1670, etretin). *Dermatologica, 178*, 79–87.
29. Korner, W.F. and Vollm, J. (1975): New aspects of the tolerance of retinol in humans. *Int. J. Vit. Nutrit. Res., 45*, 363–372.
30. Silverman, A.K., Ellis, C.N. and Voorhees, J.J. (1987): Hypervitaminosis A syndrome: a paradigm of retinoid side effects. *J. Am. Acad. Dermatol., 16*, 1027–1039.
31. Stuttgen, G. (1975): Oral vitamin A acid therapy. *Acta Derm. Venereol., 55 (Suppl. 74)*, 174–179.
32. Lindemayer, H. (1986): Isotretinoin intoxication in attempted suicide. *Acta Derm. Venereol., 66*, 452–453.
33. Shalita, A.R., Armstrong, R.B., Leyden, J.J., Pochi, P.E. and Strauss, J.S. (1988): Isotretinoin revisited. *Cutis, 42*, 1–19.
34. Bigby, M. and Stern, R.S. (1988): Adverse reactions to isotretinoin. A report from the Adverse Drug Reaction Reporting System. *J. Am. Acad. Dermatol., 18*, 543–552.
35. Harms, M. (1989): *Systemic isotretinoin (Roaccutan).* Editiones Roche, Basel.
36. Vahlquist, A. and Rollman, O. (1987): Clinical pharmacology of 3 generations of retinoids. *Dermatologica, 175 (Suppl. 1)*, 20–27.
37. Accutane Package Insert (1992): Nutley, New Yersey.
38. Roytman, M., Frumkin, A. and Bohm, T.G. (1988): Pseudotumor cerebri caused by isotretinoin. *Cutis, 42*, 399–400.
39. Scheinman, P.L., Peck, G.L., Rubinow, D.R., DiGiovanna, J.J., Abangan, D.L. and Ravin, P.D. (1990): Acute depression from isotretinoin. *J. Am. Acad. Dermatol., 22*, 1112–1114.
40. Bunker, C.B., Sheron, N., Maurice, P.D.L, Kocjan, G., Johnson, N.M.C. and Dowd, P.M. (1989): Isotretinoin and eosinophilic pleural effusion. *Lancet, i*, 435–436.
41. Bunker, C.B., Maurice, P.D.L., Little, S., Johnson, N.McI. and Dowd, P.M. (1991): Isotretinoin and lung function in systemic sclerosis. *Clin. Exp. Dermatol., 16*, 11–13.
42. Bunker, C.B., Tomlinson, M.C., Johnson, N.McI. and Dowd, P.M. (1991): Isotretinoin and the lung. *Br. J. Dermatol., 125 (Suppl. 38)*, 29.
43. Fisher, D.A. (1985): Exercise-induced bronchoconstriction related to isotretinoin therapy. *J. Am. Acad. Dermatol., 13*, 524.
44. Stone, S.P. (1983): Accutane problems. *The Schoch Letter, 33*, 107.
45. Barth, J.H., MacDonald-Hull, S.P., Mark, J., Jones, R.G. and Cunliffe, W.J. (1992): Isotretinoin therapy for acne vulgaris: routine monitoring of plasma lipids and liver function tests is not necessary. *Br. J. Dermatol., 127 (Suppl. 40)*, 30.
46. Melnik, B.C., Bros, U. and Plewig, G. (1987): Evaluation of the atherogenic risk of isotretinoin-induced and etretinate-induced alterations of lipoprotein cholesterol metabolism. *J. Invest. Dermatol., 88 (Suppl. 3),* 39s–43s.
47. Marsden, J. (1986): Hyperlipidaemia due to isotretinoin and etretinate: possible mechanisms and consequences. *Br. J. Dermatol., 114,* 401–407.
48. Bershad, S., Rubinstein, A., Paterniti, J.R. et al. (1985): Changes in plasma lipoproteins during isotretinoin therapy for acne. *New Engl. J. Med., 313*, 981–985.
49. Marsden, J.R. (1989): Lipid metabolism and retinoid therapy. *Pharmac. Ther., 40*, 55–65.
50. Dicken, C.H. and Connolly, S.M. (1980): Eruptive xanthomas associated with isotretinoin. *Arch. Dermatol., 116*, 951–953.

51. Authors unknown (1987): Pancreatitis associated with isotretinoin-induced hypertriglyceridemia. *Ann. Int. Med., 107*, 63.
52. Minuk, E. and Jackson, R. (1986): Thyrotoxicosis developing while on isotretinoin. *J. Am. Acad. Dermatol., 15*, 120.
53. Cox, N.H. (1988): Amenorrhoea during treatment with isotretinoin. *Br. J. Dermatol., 118*, 857–858.
54. Christmas, T. (1988): Roaccutane and menorrhagia. *J. Am. Acad. Dermatol., 18*, 576–577.
55. Matsuoka, L.Y., Wortsman, J., Lifrak, E.T., Parker, L.N. and Mehta, R.J. (1989): Effect of isotretinoin in acne is not mediated by adrenal androgens. *J. Am. Acad. Dermatol., 20*, 128–129.
56. Rademaker, M., Wallace, M., Cunliffe, W. and Simpson, N.B. (1991): Isotretinoin treatment alters steroid metabolism in women with acne. *Br. J. Dermatol., 124*, 361–364.
57. Valentic, J.P., Elias, A.N. and Weinstein, G.D. (1983): Hypercalcemia associated with oral isotretinoin in the treatment of severe acne. *JAMA, 250*, 1899–1900.
58. Duncan, W.E., Guill, M. and Aton, J. (1986): Serum calcium concentrations during treatment with isotretinoin. *J. Am. Acad. Dermatol., 14*, 1096.
59. Larsen, G.K. (1985): Iatrogenic breast discharge with isotretinoin. *Arch. Dermatol., 121*, 450–451.
60. Michaelsson, G., Vahlquist, A., Mobacken, H., et al. (1986): Changes in laboratory variables induced by isotretinoin treatment of acne. *Acta Derm. Venereol., 66*, 144–148.
61. Landi, F.L., Gatti, M. and Pompili, A. (1989): Leucopenia e/o trombocitopenia in quattro casi di acne cistica trattati con isotretinoina a basso dosaggio. *Chron. Derm., 20*, 591–594.
62. Friedman, S.J. (1987): Leukopenia and neutropenia associated with isotretinoin therapy. *Arch. Dermatol., 123*, 293–294.
63. Johnson, T.M. and Rapini, R.P. (1987): Isotretinoin-induced thrombocytopenia. *J. Am. Acad. Dermatol., 17*, 838–839.
64. Brodin, M.B. (1986): Inflammatory bowel disease and isotretinoin. *J. Am. Acad. Dermatol., 14*, 843.
65. Schleicher, S.M. (1986): Inflammatory bowel disease and isotretinoin (Reply). *J. Am. Acad. Dermatol., 14*, 843.
66. Martin, P., Manley, P.N., Depew, W.T. and Blakeman, J.M. (1987): Isotretinoin-associated proctosigmoiditis. *Gastroenterology, 93*, 606–609.
67. Fennerty, B., Sampliner, R. and Garewal, H. (1989): Esophageal ulceration associated with 13-cis-retinoic acid therapy in patients with Barrett's esophagus. *Gastrointest. Endoscopy, 35*, 442–443.
68. Shalita, A.R., Cunningham, W.J., Leyden, J.J. et al. (1983): Isotretinoin treatment of acne and related disorders: An update. *J. Am. Acad. Dermatol., 9*, 629–635.
69. Blanc, D., Zultak, M., Wendling, D. and Lonchampt, F. (1988): Eruptive pyogenic granulomas and acne fulminans in two siblings treated with isotretinoin. *Dermatologica, 177*, 16–18.
70. Hagler, J., Hodak, E., David, M. and Sandbank M. (1992): Facial pyogenic granuloma-like lesions under isotretinoin therapy. *Int. J. Dermatol., 31*, 199–200.
71. Joly, P., Prost, C., Gaudemar, M. and Revuz, J. (1991). Acne fulminans declenchée par la prise d'isotretinoine. *Ann. Derm. Venereol., 118*, 369–372.
72. Konrad, E., Rahmed, B. and Rassner G. (1991): Acne fulminans bei Isotretinoin-Behandlung. *Akt. Dermatol., 17*, 182–3.
73. Kellett, J.K., Beck, M.H. and Chalmers, R.J.G. (1985): Erythema nodosum and circulating immune complexes in acne fulminans after treatment with isotretinoin. *Br. Med. J., 290*, 820.
74. Zachariae, H. (1988): Delayed wound healing and keloid formation following argon laser treatment or dermabrasion during isotretinoin treatment. *Br. J. Dermatol., 118*, 703–706.
75. Joly, P., Bagot, M., Chosidow, O., Tribout, C. and Revuz J. (1990): Herpes dissemine declenche par l'isotretinoine chez un atopique. *Ann. Derm. Venereol., 117*, 860–861.
76. Davis, T.L. and Hayes, T.J. (1987): Isotretinoin-induced psoriasis: a case of Koebner's phenomenon. *J. Assoc. Milit. Dermatol., 13*, 23–26.
77. Dwyer, J.M., Taylor Thompson, B., LaBraico, J. et al. (1989): Vasculitis and retinoids. *Lancet, ii*, 494–496.
78. Epstein, E.H, McNutt, N.S., Beallo, R. et al. (1987): Severe vasculitis during isotretinoin therapy. *Arch. Dermatol., 123*, 1123–1125.
79. Reynolds, P., Fawcett, H., Waldram, R. and Prouse, P. (1989): Delayed onset of vasculitis following isotretinoin. *Lancet, ii*, 1216.
80. Aractingi, S., Lassoued, K. and Dubertret, L. (1990): Post-isotretinoin vasculitis. *Lancet, i*, 362.
81. Voorhees, J.J. and Orfanos, C.E. (1981): Oral retinoids. *Arch. Dermatol., 117*, 418–422.

82. Ferguson, J. and Johnson, B.E. (1989): Retinoid associated phototoxicity and photosensitivity. *Pharmac. Ther., 40*, 123–135.
83. Ferguson, J. and Johnson, B.E. (1984): Photosensitivity due to retinoids: clinical and laboratory studies. *Br. J. Dermatol., 115*, 275–283.
84. Helfman, R.J., Brickman, M. and Fahey, J. (1984): Isotretinoin dermatitis simulating acute pityriasis rosea. *Cutis*, 33, 297–299.
85. Molin, L., Thomsen, K., Volden, G. and Lange Wantzin, G. (1985): Retinoid dermatitis mimicking progression in mycosis fungoides: a report from the Scandinavian mycosis fungoides group. *Acta Derm. Venereol., 65*, 69–70.
86. Williams, R.E.A., Doherty, V.R., Perkins, W., Aitchison, T.C. and Mackie, R.M. (1992): Staphylococcus aureus and intranasal mupirocin in patients receiving isotretinoin for acne. *Br. J. Dermatol., 26*, 362–366.
87. Graham, M.L., Corey, R., Califf, R. and Phillips, H. (1986): Isotretinoin and Staphylococcus aureus infection. *Arch. Dermatol., 122*, 815–817.
88. Rosen, B.L. and Brodkin, R.H. (1986): Isotretinoin in the treatment of steatocystoma multiplex: a possible adverse reaction. *Cutis, 37*, 115–116.
89. Bunker, C.B., Maurice, P.D.L. and Dowd, P.M. (1990: Isotretinoin and curly hair. *Clin. Exp. Dermatol., 15*, 143–145.
90. Hays, S.B. and Camisa, C. (1985): Acquired pili torti in two patients treated with synthetic retinoids. *Cutis, 35*, 466–468.
91. Tangrea, J.A., Kilcoyne, R.F., Taylor, P.R. et al. (1992): Skeletal hyperostosis in patients receiving chronic, very-low-dose isotretinoin. *Arch. Dermatol., 128*, 921–925.
92. White, S.I., MacKie, R.M. (1989): Bone changes associated with oral retinoid therapy. *Pharmac. Ther., 40*, 137–144.
93. Zelger, B., Frank, R., Kemmler, G. and Fritsch, P. (1990): Retinoid-bedingte Veranderungen am Knochenbandapparat. *Hauarzt, 41*, 537–544.
94. De Groot, A.C. and Nater, J.P. (1988): Dermatologic drugs and cosmetics. In: *Side Effects of Drugs, Annual 12*, pp. 127–141. Editors: M.N.G. Dukes and L. Beeley. Elsevier Science Publishers, Amsterdam.
95. Melnik, B. and Plewig, G. (1987): Unerwunschte Knochenveranderungen unter systemischer Behandlung mit synthetischen Retinoiden. Hautarzt, 38, 193–197.
96. Nilstone, L.M., McGuire, J. and Ablow, R.C. (1982): Premature epiphyseal closure in a child receiving oral 13-cis-retinoic acid. *J. Am. Acad. Dermatol., 7*, 663–665.
97. Lawson, J.K. and McGuire, J. (1987): The spectrum of skeletal changes associated with long term administration of 13-cis-retinoic acid. *Skeletal Radiol., 16*, 91–97.
98. DiGiovanna, J.J., Helfgott, R.K., Gerber, L.H. and Peck, G.L. (1986): Extraspinal tendon and ligament calcification associated with long term therapy with etretinate. *New Engl. J. Med., 315*, 1177–1182.
99. McGuire, J. and Lawson, J.P. (1987): Skeletal changes associated with chronic isotretinoin and etretinate therapy. *Dermatologica, 175 (Suppl. 1),* 169–181.
100. Pennes, D.R., Martel, W. and Ellis, C.N. (1985): Retinoid induced ossification of the posterior longitudinal ligament. *Skelet. Radiol., 14,* 191–193.
101. Pittsley, R.A. and Yoder, F.W. (1983): Retinoid hyperostosis: skeletal toxicity associated with long-term administration of 13-cis-retinoic acid for refractory ichthyosis. *New Engl. J. Med., 308*, 1012–1016.
102. Camisa, C. (1986): Acute arthritis during isotretinoin therapy for acne. *J. Am. Acad. Dermatol., 15*, 1061–1062.
103. Matsuoka, L.Y., Wortsman, J. and Pepper, J.J. (1984): Acute arthritis during isotretinoin treatment for acne. *Arch. Int. Med., 144*, 1870–1871.
104. Novick, N.L., Lawson, W. and Schwartz, I.S. (1984): Bilateral nasal bone osteophytosis associated with short-term oral isotretinoin therapy for cystic acne vulgaris. *Am. J. Med., 77*, 736–739.
105. Brodkin, R.H. and Abbey, A.A. (1985): Osteoma cutis: a case of probable exacerbation following treatment of severe acne with isotretinoin. *Dermatologica, 170*, 210–212.
106. Grob, J.J. and Bonerandi, J.J. (1986): Syndrome de Tietze au cours d'un traitement par l'isotretinoine. *Ann. Derm. Venereol., 113*, 359.
107. Gerber, L.H., Helfgott, R.K., Gross, E.G. et al. (1984): Vertebral abnormalities associated with synthetic retinoid use. *J. Am. Acad. Dermatol., 10*, 817–823.
108. Ellis, C.N., Madison, K.C., Pennes, D.R., Martel, W. and Voorhees, J.J. (1984): Isotretinoin therapy is associated with early radiographic changes. *J. Am. Acad. Dermatol., 10*, 1024–1029.

109. Kilkoyne, R.F., Cope, R., Cunningham, W. et al. (1986): Minimal spinal hyperostosis with low-dose isotretinoin therapy. *Invest. Radiol., 21*, 41–44.
110. Shalita, A.R. (1987): Mucocutaneous and systemic toxicity of retinoids: Monitoring and management. *Dermatologica (Suppl. 1)*, 151–157.
111. Pennes, D.R., Martel, W., Ellis, C.N. and Voorhees, J.J. (1988): Evolution of skeletal hyperostoses caused by 13-cis-retinoic acid therapy. *Am. J. Radiol., 151*, 967–973.
112. Archer, C.B., Elias, P.M., Lowe, N.J. and Griffith, W.A.D. (1989): Extensive spinal hyperostosis in a patient receiving isotretinoin — progression after 4 years of etretinate therapy. *Clin. Exp. Dermatol., 14*, 319–321.
113. Ellis, C.N., Pennes, D.R., Hermann, B.A., Blauvelt, A., Martel, W. and Voorhees, J.J. (1988): Long-term radiographic follow-up after isotretinoin therapy. *J. Am. Acad. Dermatol., 18*, 1252–1261.
114. Carey, B.M., Parkin, G.J.S., Cunliffe, W.J. and Pritlove, J. (1988): Skeletal toxicity with isotretinoin therapy: a clinico-radiological evaluation. *Br. J. Dermatol., 119*, 609–614.
115. Haustein, U.F. and Heilmann, S.T. (1987): Knochenveranderungen unter Langzeittherapie mit Etretinat (Tigason®). *Z. Hautkr., 62*, 395–400.
116. Torok, L., Galuska, L., Kasa, M. and Kadar, L. (1989): Bone-scintigraphic examinations in patients treated with retinoids: a prospective study. *Br. J. Dermatol., 120*, 31–36.
117. Kilcoyne, R.F. (1988): Effects of retinoids in bone. *J. Am. Acad. Dermatol., 19*, 212–216.
118. Marini, J.C., Hill, S. and Zasloff, M.A. (1988): Dense metaphyseal bands and growth arrest associated with isotretinoin therapy. *Am. J. Dis. Childh., 142*, 316–318.
119. Fraunfelder, F.T., LaBraico, J.M. and Meyer, S.M. (1985): Adverse ocular reactions possibly associated with isotretinoin. *Am. J. Ophthalmol., 100*, 534–540.
120. Lebowitz, M.A. and Berson, D.S. (1988): Ocular effects of oral retinoids. *J. Am. Acad. Dermatol., 19*, 209–211.
121. Gold, J.A., Shupack, J.L. and Nemec, M.A. (1989): Ocular side effects of the retinoids. *Int. J. Dermatol., 28*, 218–225.
122. Lebowitz, M.A. and Berson, D.S. (1988): Ocular effects of oral retinoids. J. Am. Acad. Dermatol., 19, 209–211.
123. Milson, J., Jones, D.H., King, K. and Cunliffe, W.J. (1982): Ophthalmological side effects of 13-cis-retinoic acid therapy for acne vulgaris. *Br. J. Dermatol., 107*, 491–494.
124. Ensink, B.W. and van Voorst Vader, P.C. (1983): Opthalmologic side-effects of 13-cis-retinoic therapy. *Br. J. Dermatol., 108*, 627–628.
125. Weiss, J., Degnan, M., Leupold, R. and Lumpkin, L.R. (1981): Bilateral corneal opacities. Occurrence in a patient treated with oral isotretinoin. *Arch. Dermatol., 117*, 182–183.
126. Layton, A.M. and Cunliffe, W.J. (1990): Ocular problems in contact lens wearers and non-contact lens wearers on isotretinoin — practical guidelines. *J. Derm. Treatm., 1*, 247–249.
127. Palestine, A.G. (1984): Transient acute myopia resulting from isotretinoin (Accutane) therapy. Ann. Ophthalmol., 16, 660–661.
128. Hazen, P.G., Carney, J.M., Langston, R.H.S. and Meisler, D.M. (1986): Corneal effect of isotretinoin: possible exacerbation of corneal neovascularization in a patient with the keratitis, ichthyosis, deafness ("KID") syndrome. *J. Am. Acad. Dermatol., 14*, 141–142.
129. Herman, D.C. and Dyer, J.A. (1987): Anterior subcapsular cataracts as a possible adverse ocular reaction to isotretinoin. *Am. J. Ophthalmol., 103*, 236–237.
130. Denman, S., Weleber, R., Hanifin, J.M., Cunningham, W. and Phipps, R. (1986): Abnormal night vision and altered dark adaptometry in patients treated with isotretinoin for acne. *J. Am. Acad. Dermatol., 14*, 692–693.
131. Weleber, R.G., Denman, S.T., Hanifin, J.M. and Cunningham, W.J. (1986): Abnormal retinal function associated with isotretinoin therapy for acne. *Arch. Ophthalmol., 104*, 831–837.
132. Grattan, C.E.H., Brown, R.D., Cowan, M.A. and Ryatt, K.S. (1987): Retinoids and the eye — reduced rod function with isotretinoin. *Br. J. Dermatol., 117 (suppl. 32)*, 23.
133. McBurney, E.I. and Rosen, D.A. (1985): Elevated CPK and isotretinoin. *J. Am. Acad. Dermatol., 12*, 582–583.
134. Chen, D. and Rofsky, H.E. (1985): Elevated CPK and isotretinoin. *J. Am. Acad. Dermatol., 12*, 583–585.
135. Tillman, D.M., White, S.I. and Aitchison, T.C. (1990): Isotretinoin, creatinine kinase and exercise. *Br. J. Dermatol., 123*, 22–23.
136. Hodak, E., Gadoth, N., David, M. and Sandbank, M. (1986): Muscle damage induced by isotretinoin. *Br.*

Med. J., 293, 425–426.

137. Public Affairs Committee and the Council of the Teratology Society (1991): Recommendations for isotretinoin use in women of childbearing potential. *Teratology, 44*, 1–6.
138. Lammer, E.J., Chen, D.T., Hoar, R.M. et al. (1985): Retinoic acid embryopathy. *New Engl. J. Med., 313*, 837–841.
139. Lammer, E.J., Hayes, A.M., Schunior, A. and Holmes, L.B. (1988): Unusually high risk for adverse outcomes of pregnancy following fetal isotretinoin exposure. *Am. J. Hum. Genet., 43*, A58.
140. Willhite, C.C., Hill, R.M. and Irving, D.W. (1986): Isotretinoin-induced craniofacial malformations in humans and hamsters. *J. Craniofacial Genet. Developm. Biol., suppl. 2*: 193–209.
141. Dai, W.S., Hsu, M.-A. and Itri, L.M. (1989): Safety of pregnancy after discontinuation of isotretinoin. *Arch. Dermatol., 125*, 362–365.
142. Hepburn, N.C. (1990): Deliberate self-poisoning with isotretinoin. *Br. J. Dermatol., 122*, 840–841.
143. Geubel, A.P., de Galocsy, C., Alves, N., Rahier, J. and Dive, C. (1991): Liver damage caused by therapeutic vitamin A administration: estimate of dose-related toxicity in 41 cases. *Gastroenterol., 100*, 1701–1709.
144. Bottomley, W.W. and Cunliffe, W.J. (1992): Median nail dystrophy associated with isotretinoin therapy. *Br. J. Dermatol., 127*, 447–448.
145. Bottomley, W.W. and Cunliffe, W.J. (1992): Acute Achilles tendonitis following oral isotretinoin therapy for acne vulgaris. *Clin. Exp. Dermatol., 17*, 250–251.
146. Masson, C. and Szern, A. (1991): Isotretinoine, cause possible dew crise d'epilepsie. *La Presse Médicale, 20*, 2264–2265.
147. Dai, W.S., LaBraico, J.M. and Stern, R.S. (1992): Epidemiology of isotretinoin exposure during pregnancy. *J. Am. Acad. Dermatol., 26*, 599–606.
148. Yoh, E.H. and Pochi, P.E. (1987): Side effects and long-term toxicity of synthetic retinoids. *Arch. Dermatol., 123*, 1375–1378.
149. Jager K. (1988): Nebenwirkungen der Etretinat-therapie. *Dermatol. Monatsschr., 174*, 449–461.
150. Landow, R.K. (1988): Etretinate. A clinician's view. *Dermatologic Clinics, 6*, 553–560.
151. Bonnetblanc, J.M., Hugon, J. and Dumas, M. (1983): Intracranial hypertension with etretinate. *Lancet, ii*, 974.
152. Viraben, R., Mathien, C. and Fontan, B. (1985): Benign intracranial hypertension during etretinate therapy for mycosis fungoides. *J. Am. Acad. Dermatol., 13*, 515–517.
153. Cunningham, W. (1985): Safety profile of etretinate. *Semin. Dermatol., 4*, 303–305.
154. Tegison package insert. Nutley, New Jersey, 1989.
155. Halkier-Sorensen, L. (1987): Menstrual changes in a patient treated with etretinate. *Lancet, ii*, 636.
156. Reynolds, O.D. (1991): Erectile dysfunction in etretinate treatment. *Arch. Dermatol., 127*, 425–426.
157. Ellis, C.N., Kang, S., Vinik, A.I., Grekin, R.C., Cunningham, W.J. and Voorhees, J.J. (1987): Glucose and insulin responses are improved in patients with psoriasis during therapy with etretinate. *Arch. Dermatol., 123*, 471–475.
158. Laurahanta, J. (1982): Oedema, a rare adverse reaction to etretinate (Tigason). *Br. J. Dermatol., 106*, 251.
159. Noulopoulou-Karakitsou, K., Mavrikakis, M. and Anastasiou-Nana, M. (1981): An unusual adverse reaction to RO 10-9359. *Br. J. Dermatol., 104*, 709.
160. Horber, F.F., Zimmermann, A. and Frey, F.J. (1984): Impaired renal function with hypercalcaemia associated with etretinate. *Lancet, ii*, 1093.
161. Allan, S. and Christmas, T. (1988): Severe edema associated with etretinate. *J. Am. Acad. Dermatol., 19*, 140.
162. Orgfanos, C.E., Mahrle, G., Goerz, G. et al. (1979): Laboratory investigations in patients with generalized psoriasis under oral retinoid therapy. *Dermatologica, 159*, 62–68.
163. Bedello, P.G., De Paoli, M.A. and Molinero, A. (1987): Case of eosinophilia induced by etretinate. *Arch. Dermatol., 123*, 863.
164. Naldi, L., Rozzoni, M., Finazzi, G., Pini, P., Marchesi, L. and Cainelli, T. (1991): Etretinate therapy and thrombocytopenia. *Br. J. Dermatol., 124*, 395.
165. Roenigk, H.H. Jr. (1989): Liver toxicity of retinoid therapy. *Pharmac. Ther., 40*, 145–55.
166. Roenigk, H.H. Jr. (1988): Liver toxicity of retinoid therapy. *J. Am. Acad. Dermatol., 19*, 199–208.
167. Thirumoorthy, T. and Shupack, J.L. (1988): Adverse hepatic reactions associated with etretinate in patients with psoriasis — analysis of 22 cases. *Ann. Acad. Med., 17*, 477–481.
168. Roenigk, H.H. Jr., Gibstine, C., Glazer, S., Sparberg, M.S. and Yokoo, H. (1985): Serial liver biopsies in psoriatic patients receiving long-term etretinate. *Br. J. Dermatol., 112*, 77–81.

169. Glazer, S.D., Roenigk, H.H. Jr., Yokoo, H., Sparberg, M.S. and Paravicini, U. (1984): Ultrastructural survey and tissue analysis of human livers after 6 months course of etretinate. *J. Am. Acad. Dermatol., 10*, 632–638.
170. Camuto, P., Shupack, J., Orbuch, P. and Sidhu, G. (1987): Long term effects of etretinate on the liver in psoriasis. *Am. J. Pathol., 11*, 30–37.
171. Foged, E., Bjerring, P., Kragballe, K., Sogaard, H. and Zachariae, H. (1984): Histologic changes in the liver during etretinate treatment. *J. Am. Acad. Dermatol., 11*, 580–583.
172. Ellis, C.N. and Voorhees, J.J. (1987): Etretinate therapy. *J. Am. Acad. Dermatol., 16*, 267–291.
173. Kamm, M.A., Davies, D.J. and Breen, K.J. (1988): Acute hepatitis due to etretinate. *J. Gastroenterol. Hepatol., 3*, 663–666.
174. Beck, H.T. and Foged, E.K. (1983): Toxic hepatitis due to combination therapy with methotrexate and etretinate in psoriasis. *Dermatologica, 167*, 94–96.
175. Weiss, V.C., Layden, T., Spinowitz, A., et al. (1985): Chronic active hepatitis associated with etretinate therapy. *Br. J. Dermatol., 112*, 591–597.
176. Gavish, D., Katz, M., Gotteher, A. et al. (1985): Cholestatic jaundice, an unusual side effect of etretinate. *J. Am. Acad. Dermatol., 13*, 669–670.
177. Berth-Jones, J., Shuttleworth, D. and Hutchinson, P.E. (1990): A study of etretinate alopecia. *Br. J. Dermatol., 122*, 751–755.
178. Lowe, L. and Herbert, A.A. (1989): Cystic and comedonal acne: a side effect of etretinate therapy. *Int. J. Dermatol., 28*, 482.
179. Menter, A. and Boyd, A. (1988): Cystic acne in psoriatic patients undergoing etretinate therapy. *J. Am. Acad. Dermatol., 18,* 751–752.
180. David, M., Sandbank, M. and Lowe, N.J. (1989): Erythema multiforme-like eruptions associated with etretinate therapy. *Clin. Exp. Dermatol., 14*, 230–232.
181. Levin, J. and Almeyda, J. (1985): Erythroderma due to etretinate. *Br. J. Dermatol., 112*, 373.
182. Knobler, R.M. and Neumann, R.A. (1990): Exacerbation of porokeratosis during etretinate therapy. *Acta Derm. Venereol., 70,* 319–320.
183. Zlotogorski, A. and Leibovici, V. (1987): Does etretinate exacerbate scabies? *Br. J. Dermatol., 116,* 882.
184. James, W.D. (1986): Staphylococcus aureus and etretinate. *Arch. Dermatol., 122*, 976–977.
185. David, M., Ginzburg, A., Hodak, E. and Feuerman, E.J. (1986): Palmoplantar eruption associated with etretinate therapy. *Acta Derm. Venereol., 66,* 87–89.
186. Sahre, E.-M. and Hubner, U. (1988): Paronychien und uberschiessende Granulationen als Tigason-Nebenwirkung. *Akt. Dermatol., 14*, 254–256.
187. Collins, M.R.L., James, W.D. and Rodman, O.G. (1986): Etretinate photosensitivity. *J. Am. Acad. Dermatol., 14,* 274.
188. Boer, J. and Smeenk, G. (1987): Nodular prurigo-like eruptions induced by etretinate. *Br. J. Dermatol., 116*, 271–274.
189. Katayama, H., Okabe, N., Kano, T. and Yaoita, H. (1990): Granulation tissue that developed after a minor trauma in a psoriatic patient on long-term etretinate therapy. *J. Dermatol., 17*, 187–190.
190. Crivellato, E. (1982): A rosacea-like eruption induced by Tigason (RO 10-9359) treatment. *Acta Derm. Venereol., 62*, 450–451.
191. Ramsay, B., Bloxham, C., Eldred, A., Munro, C. and Marks, J. (1989): Blistering, erosions and scarring in a patient on etretinate. *Br. J. Dermatol., 121*, 397–400.
192. Shelley, E.D. and Shelley, W.B. (1990): Inframammary, intertriginous, and decubital erosions due to etretinate. *Cutis, 45*, 111–112.
193. Bordier, C., Flechet, M.-L., Thomine, E. and Lauret, Ph. (1984): Rupture de vergetures au cours d'un psoriasis pustuleux traite par etretinate (Tigason). *Ann. Derm. Venereol., 111*, 929–931.
194. Thomson, J. (1987): Etretinate and vulvitis. *Retinoids Today and Tomorrow, 5*, 49.
195. Archer, C.B., Cerio, R. and Griffith, W.A.D. (1987): Etretinate and acquired kinking of the hair. Clin. Exp. Dermatol., 12, 238–239.
196. Mortimer, P.S. (1985): Unruly hair. *Br. J. Dermatol., 113*, 467–473.
197. Baran, R. (1986): Etretinate and the nails (study of 130 cases): possible mechanisms and some side-effects. *Clin. Exp. Dermatol., 11*, 148–152.
198. Garioch, J. and Simpson, N.B. (1989): Etretinate and severe nail plate dystrophies. *Clin. Exp. Dermatol., 14*, 261.
199. Sillevis Smitt, J.H. and De Mari, F. (1984): A serious side-effect of etretinate (Tigason). *Clin. Exp.*

Dermatol., 9, 554–556.
200. Prendiville, J., Bingham, E.A. and Burrows, D. (1986): Premature epiphyseal closure — a complication of etretinate in children. *J. Am. Acad. Dermatol., 15*, 1259–1262.
201. Burrows, D. (1984): Ichthyosiform erythroderma treated with etretinate. *Br. J. Dermatol., 111 (suppl. 226)*, 76.
202. Cuny, J.F., Schmutz, J.L., Terver, M.N. et al. (1989): Effets rhumatologiques de l'etretinate. *Ann. Derm. Venereol., 116*, 95–102.
203. Glover, M.T. and Atherton, D.J. (1987): Etretinate and premature epiphyseal closure in children. *J. Am. Acad. Dermatol., 17*, 853–854.
204. Glover, M.T., Peters, A.M. and Atherton, D.J. (1987): Surveillance for skeletal toxicity of children treated with etretinate. *Br. J. Dermatol., 116*, 609–614.
205. Halkier-Sorensen, L., Laurberg, G. and Andresen, J. (1987): Bone changes in children on long-term treatment with etretinate. *J. Am. Acad. Dermatol., 16*, 999–1006.
206. Wilson, D.J., Kay, V., Charig, M., Hughes, D.G. and Creasy, T.S. (1988): Skeletal hyperostosis and extraosseous calcification in patients receiving long-term etretinate (Tigason). *Br. J. Dermatol., 119*, 597–607.
207. Halkier-Sorensen, L. and Andresen, J. (1989): A retrospective study of bone changes in adults treated with etretinate. *J. Am. Acad. Dermatol., 20*, 83–87.
208. DiGiovanni, J.J., Helfgott, R.K., Gerber, L.H. and Peck, G.L. (1986): Extraspinal tendon and ligament calcification associated with long-term therapy with etretinate. *New Engl. J. Med., 315*, 1177–1182.
209. Tfelt-Hansen, P., Knudsen, B. and Petersen, E. (1989): Spinal cord compression after long-term etretinate. *Lancet, ii*, 325–326.
210. Cointin, M., Sommelet-Olive, D., Cuny, J.F. and Bretagne, M.C. (1990): Complications osseuses de l'intoxication chronique par l'etretinate chez l'enfant. *Ann. Pediatr. (Paris), 37*, 458–460.
211. Melnik, B., Gluck, S., Jungblut, R.M. and Goerz, G. (1987): Retrospective radiographic study of skeletal changes after long-term etretinate therapy. *Br. J. Dermatol., 116*, 207–212.
212. Cerio, R., Wells, R.S. and MacDonald, D.M. (1987): Calcifying arthropathy of the hips and diffuse hyperostosis associated with etretinate. *Clin. Exp. Dermatol., 12*, 129–131.
213. Zabarino, Ph., Krause, E., Gary-Bobo, A., Dandurand, M., Sany, J. and Guilhou, J.J. (1989): Ossification de la membrane inter-osseuse antibrachiale sous etretinate. *Ann. Derm. Venereol., 116*, 123–126.
214. Dodd, H.J., Dootson, G. and Sarkany, I. (1988): Ossification in the interosseous membrane of the forearm after etretinate treatment for psoriasis. *Br. J. Dermatol., 119 (suppl. 33)*, 105–106.
215. Papasavvas, G.K., Bhalla, A.K. and Logan, R.A. (1987): Vertebral hyperostosis associated with etretinate therapy. *Clin. Exp. Dermatol., 12*, 202–203.
216. Grimm, J. and Baumann, U. (1989): Skelettveranderungen unter Langzeitbehandlung mit oralen synthetischen Retinoiden. *Akt. Dermatol., 15*, 133–137.
217. Jacyk, W.K. (1986): Elevated creatinine phosphokinase levels associated with the use of etretinate. *J. Am. Acad. Dermatol., 15*, 710.
218. Hodak, E., David, M., Gadoth, N. and Sandbank, M. (1987): Etretinate-induced skeletal muscle damage. *Br. J. Dermatol., 116*, 623–626.
219. David, M., Hodak, E., Sandbank, M. and Gadoth, N. (1988): Electromyographic abnormalities in patients undergoing long-term therapy with etretinate. *J. Am. Acad. Dermatol., 19*, 273–275.
220. Ellis, C.N., Gilbert, M., Cohen, K.A. et al. (1986): Increased muscle tone during etretinate therapy. *J. Am. Acad. Dermatol., 14*, 907–909.
221. Calissendorff, B.M. (1989): Retinale Veranderungen — Degeneration oder Nebenwirkung durch Etretinat (Tigason®)-Therapie? *Klin. Mbl. Augenheilk., 194*, 187–189.
222. Weber, U., Goerz, G., Michaelis, L. and Melnik, B. (1988): Retinale Funktionsstorungen unter Langzeittherapie mit dem Retinoid Etretinat. *Klin. Mbl. Augenheilk., 192*, 706–711.
223. Weber, U., Melnik, B., Goerz, G. et al. (1988): Abnormal retinal function associated with long-term etretinate? *Lancet, i*, 235–236.
224. Brown, R.D. and Grattan, C. (1988): Etretinate and vision. *Lancet, i*, 585–586.
225. Pitts, J.F., Mackie, R.M., Dutton, G.N., McClure, E.A. and Allan, D. (1991): Etretinate and visual function: a 1-year follow-up study. *Br. J. Dermatol., 125*, 53–55.
226. Juhlin, L. (1983):)Ear ache during etretinate treatment. *Acta Derm. Venereol., 63*, 181.
227. Kramer, M. (1982): Excessive cerumen production due to the aromatic retinoid Tigason in a patient with Darier's disease. *Acta Derm. Venereol., 62*, 267–268.

228. Woll, P.J., Kostrzewski, A. and Glen-Bott, A.M. Lymphoma in patients taking etretinate. *Lancet, ii*, 563–564.
229. Harrison, P.V. (1987): Retinoids and malignancy. *Lancet, ii*, 801.
230. DiGiovanni, J.J., Zech, L.A., Ruddel, M.E., Gantt, G. and Peck, G.L. (1989): Etretinate. Persistent serum levels after long-term therapy. *Arch. Dermatol., 125*, 246–251.
231. Lammer, E.J. (1988): Embryopathy in infant conceived one year after termination of maternal etretinate. *Lancet, ii*, 1080–1081.
232. Happle, R., Traupe, H., Bounameaux, Y., Fisch, T. (1984): Teratogene Wirkung von Etretinat beim Menschen. *Deutsche Med. Wschrift., 39*, 1476–1480.
233. Ostlere, L.S., Langtry, J.A.A., Jones, S. and Staughton, R.C.D. (1991): Reduced therapeutic effect of warfarin caused by etretinate. *Br. J. Dermatol., 124*, 505–510.
234. Neotigason (acitretin). Active metabolite of Tigason (etretinate). Rapid elimination, no tissue accumulation. F. Hoffmann-La Roche Ltd., Basel, 1989.
235. Neotigason package insert. Hoffmann-La Roche, Basel, 1992.
236. Wiegand, U.W., Busslinger, A.A. and Jensen, B.K. (1991): The pharmacokinetics of acitretin: an update. Data presented at the 2nd Congress of the European Academy of Dermatology and Venereology, Athens, 12 October 1991 (supplement to *Retinoids Today and Tomorrow, 26*).
237. Geiger, J.-M. and Czarnetzki, B.M. (1988): Acitretin (Ro 10-1670, etretin): Overall evaluation of clinical studies. *Dermatologica, 176*, 182–190.
238. Bjerke, J.R. and Geiger, J.-M. (1989): Acitretin versus etretinate in severe psoriasis. A double-blind randomized Nordic multicenter study in 168 patients. *Acta Derm. Venereol., 146*, 206–207.
239. Vahlquist, C., Selinus, I., Vessby, B. (1988): Serum lipid changes during acitretin (etretin) treatment of psoriasis and palmo-plantar pustulosis. *Acta Derm. Venereol., 68*, 300–305.
240. Kragballe, K., Jansen, C.T., Geiger, J.-M. et al. (1989): A double-blind comparison of acitretin and etretinate in the treatment of severe psoriasis. *Acta Derm. Venereol., 69*, 35–40.
241. Ledo, A., Martin, M., Geiger, J.-M. and Marron, J.M. (1988): Acitretin (Ro 10-1670) in the treatment of severe psoriasis. *Int. J. Dermatol., 27*, 656–660.
242. Olsen, E.A., Weed, W.W., Meyer, C.J. and Cobo, C.L. (1989): A double-blind, placebo-controlled trial of acitretin for the treatment of psoriasis. *J. Am. Acad. Dermatol., 21*, 681–686.
243. Murray, H.E., Anhalt, A.W., Lessard, R. et al. (1991): A 12-month treatment of severe psoriasis with acitretin: results of a Canadian open multicenter study. *J. Am. Acad. Dermatol., 24*, 598–602.
244. Saurat, J.-H., Geiger, J.-M., Amblard, P. et al. (1988): Randomized double-blind multicenter study comparing acitretin-PUVA, etretinate-PUVA and placebo-PUVA in the treatment of severe psoriasis. *Dermatologica, 177*, 218–224.
245. Lassus, A. and Geiger, J.-M. (1988): Acitretin and etretinate in the treatment of palmoplantar pustulosis: a double-blind comparative trial. *Br. J. Dermatol., 119*, 755–759.
246. Goldfarb, M.T., Ellis, C.N., Gupta, A.K. et al. (1988): Acitretin improves psoriasis in a dose-dependent fashion. *J. Am. Acad. Dermatol., 18*, 655–662.
247. Halter, U. (1991): Der Fall aus der Praxis (224). *Schweiz Rundschau Med. (PRAXIS), 80*, 883–884.
248. Puiatto, P., Veglio, S., Cellini, P. and Maiocco, I. (1991): Pemfigoide bolloso indotto da etretinato. *G. Ital. Derm. Venereol., 126*, 319–321.
249. Vilkon, P., Fiche, M., Mangars, Y. et al. (1991): Sarcomne parosteale du radius apparu lors d'un traitement par etretinate. *Rev. Rhumatisme, 58*, 825–827.
250. McIvor, A. (1992): Fatal toxic epidermal necrolysis associated with etretinate. *Br. Med. J., 304*, 548.
251. Paige, D.G., Judge, M.R., Shaw, D.G., Atherton, D.J. and Harper, J.I. (1992): Bone changes and their significance in children with ichthyosis on long-term etretinate therapy. *Br. J. Dermatol., 127*, 387–391.
252. van Ditzhuyzen, Th.J.M., van Haelst, U.J.G.M., van Dooren-Greebe, R.J., van de Kerkhof, P.C.M. and Yap, S.H. (1990): Severe hepatotoxic reaction with progression to cirrhosis after use of a novel retinoid (acitretin). *J. Hepatol., 11*, 185–188.
253. Melnik, B. and Plewig, G. (1986): Retinoide und Lipidstoffwechsel. *Hautarzt, 37*, 304–311.
254. Bettoli, V., Tosti, A. and Varotti, C. (1987): Nummular eczema during isotretinoin treatment. *J. Am. Acad. Dermatol., 16*, 617.
255. Chalmers, R.J.G. (1992): Retinoid therapy: a real hazard for the developing embryo. Br. J. Obstet. Gynecol., 99, 276–278.
256. Mitchell, A.A. (1992): Oral retinoids. What should the prescriber know about their teratogenic hazards among women of child-bearing potential? *Drug Safety, 7*, 79–85.

257. Green, C. and Lakshmipathi, T. (1991): A case of hepatitis related to etretinate therapy and hepatitis B vaccine. *Dermatologica, 182*, 119–120.
258. Gilbert, M., Ellis, C.N. and Voorhees, J.J. (1986): Lack of skeletal radiographic changes during short-term etretinate therapy for psoriasis. *Dermatologica, 172*, 160–163.
259. Bruce, S. and Wolf, J.E. Jr. (1991): Antibacterial agents. In: S.E. Wolverton and J.K. Wilkin (Editors). *Systemic Drugs for Skin Diseases*. Chapter 3, pp. 47–85. Saunders, Philadelphia.
260. Reboldi, A.C. and Delbene, V.E. (1988): Oral antibiotic therapy of dermatologic conditions. *Dermatol. Clinics, 6*, 497–520.
261. Feingold, D.S. and Wagner, R.F. (1986): Antibacterial therapy. *J. Am. Acad. Dermatol., 14*, 535–548.
262. Hoigne, R., Keller, H. and Sonntag, R. (1986): Penicillins, cephalosporins and tetracyclines. In: M.N.G. Dukes (Editor). *Meyler's Side Effects of Drugs, 11th Edition*. Chapter 26, pp. 501–542. Elsevier, Amsterdam.
263. Shuttleworth, D. (1989): A localized, recurrent pustular eruption following amoxycillin administration. *Clin. Exp. Dermatol., 14*, 367–368.
264. Katz, M., Seidenbaum, M. and Weinrauch, L. (1987): Penicillin-induced generalized pustular psoriasis. *J. Am. Acad. Dermatol., 17*, 918–920.
265. Dukes, M.N.G., Beeley, L. and Aronson, J.K. (Eds.) (1988–1991): *Side Effects of Drugs, Annuals 12–15*. Elsevier, Amsterdam.
266. Fellner, M.J., Ledesina, G.N. and Miller, A.D. (1986): Adverse reactions to antibiotics other than penicillin. *Clin. Dermatol., 4*, 142–148.
267. Leffel, D.J. (1991): Minocycline hydrochloride hyperpigmentation complicating treatment of venous ectasia of the extremities. *J. Am. Acad. Dermatol., 24*, 501.
268. Rosen, T. and Hoffmann, T.J. (1989): Minocycline-induced discoloration of the permanent teeth. *J. Am. Acad. Dermatol., 21*, 569.
269. Berger, R.S., Mandel, E.B., Hayes, T.J. and Grimwood, R.R. (1989): Minocycline staining of the oral cavity. *J. Am. Acad. Dermatol., 21,* 1300–1301.
270. Basler, R.S.W. and Lynch, P.J. (1985): Black galactorrhea as a consequence of minocycline and phenothiazine therapy. *Arch. Dermatol., 121*, 417–418.
271. Prigent, F., Cavelier-Balloy, B., Tollenaere, C. and Civatte, J. (1986): Pigmentation cutanee induite par la minocycline: deux cas. *Ann. Derm. Venereol., 113*, 227–233.
272. Gordon, G., Sparano, B.M. and Iatropoulos, M.J. (1985): Hyperpigmentation of the skin associated with minocycline therapy. *Arch. Dermatol., 121*, 618–623.
273. Wolfe, I.D. and Reichmister, J. (1984): Minocycline hyperpigmentation: skin, tooth, nail, and bone involvement. *Cutis, 33*, 457–458.
274. Angeloni, V.L., Salasche, S.J. and Ortiz, R. (1987): Nail, skin, and scleral pigmentation induced by minocycline. *Cutis, 40*, 229–233.
275. Okada, N., Moriya, K., Nishida, K. et al. (1989): Skin pigmentation associated with minocycline therapy. *Br. J. Dermatol., 121*, 247–254.
276. Delaney, R.A. and Narayanaswamy, T.R. (1990): Pseudo-tumor cerebri and acne. *Military Medicine, 155*, 511.
277. Fleischer, A.B. Jr. and Resnick, S.D. (1989): The effects of antibiotics on the efficacy of oral contraceptives: A controversy revisited. *Arch. Dermatol., 125*, 1562–1564.
278. Lewis-Jones, M.S., Evans, S. and Thompson, C.M. (1988): Erythema multiforme occurring in association with lupus erythematosus during therapy with doxycycline. *Clin. Exp. Dermatol., 13*, 245–247.
279. Wright, A.L. and Colver, G.B. (1988): Tetracyclines — how safe are they? *Clin. Exp. Dermatol., 13*, 57–61.
280. Bridges, A.J., Graziano, F.M., Calhoun, W. and Reizner, G.T. (1990): Hyperpigmentation, neutrophilic alveolitis, and erythema nodosum resulting from minocycline. *J. Am. Acad. Dermatol., 22*, 259–262.
281. Reisner, R.M. (1983): Antibiotic and antiinflammatory therapy of acne. *Dermatologic Clinics, 1*, 385–397.
282. Magnasco, L.D. and Magnasco, A.J. (1985): Metallic taste associated with tetracycline therapy. *Clin. Pharm., 4*, 455–456.
283. Simpson, M.B., Pryzbylik, J., Innis, B. and Denham, M.A. (1985): Hemolytic anemia after tetracycline therapy. *New Engl. J. Med., 312*, 40–42.
284. Davies, M.G. and Kersey, P.J.W. (1989): Acute hepatitis and exfoliative dermatitis associated with minocycline. *Br. Med. J., 298*, 1523–1524.
285. Tatnall, F.M., Dodd, H.J. and Sarkany, I. (1985): Elevated serum amylase in a case of toxic epidermal necrolysis. *Br. J. Dermatol., 113*, 629–630.

286. Boyd, I. (1991): Erythromycin-induced hearing loss. *Lancet, 337*, 113.
287. Dylewski, J. (1988): Irreversible sensorineural hearing loss due to erythromycin. *Can. Med. Assoc. J., 139*, 230–231.
288. Kofoed, M.L. and Oxholm, A. (1985): Toxic epidermal necrolysis due to erythromycin. *Contact Dermatitis, 13*, 273.
289. Zitelli, B.J., Howrie, D.L., Altman, H. and Maroon T.J. (1987): Erythromycin-induced drug interactions. *Clin. Pediatr. 26*, 117–119.
290. Keller, H. and Follath, F. (1988): Miscellaneous antibiotics. In: M.N.G. Dukes (Editor). *Meyler's Side Effects of Drugs, 11th Edition*. Chapter 27, pp. 543–566. Elsevier, Amsterdam.
291. Wilson, J.P., Koren, J.F., Daniel, R.C. et al. (1986): Cefadroxil-induced ampicillin-exacerbated pemphigus vulgaris: case report and review of the literature. *Drug Intell. Clin. Pharm., 20*, 219–223.
292. Tester-Dalderup, C.B.M. (1988): Antiprotozoal drugs. In: M.N.G. Dukes (Editor). *Meyler's Side Effects of Drugs, 11th Edition*. Chapter 29, pp. 581–602. Elsevier, Amsterdam.
293. Grinbaum, A., Ashkenazi, I., Avni, I. and Blumenthal, M. (1992): Transient myopia following metronidazole treatment for trichomonas vaginalis. *JAMA, 267*, 511–512.
294. Kristenson, M. and Fryden, A. (1988): Pneumonitis caused by metronidazol. *JAMA, 260*, 184.
295. Shelley, W.B. and Shelley, E.D. (1987): Fixed drug eruption due to metronidazole. *Cutis, 39*, 393–394.
296. McEvoy, G.K. (1987): Metronidazole. *Drug Information, 87*, 408–413.
297. Teicher, M.H., Altesman, R.I., Cole, J.O. and Schatzberg, A.F. (1987): Possible nephrotoxic interaction of lithium and metronidazole. *JAMA, 24*, 3365–3366.
298. Millikan, L.E. and Shrum, J.P. (1991): Antifungal agents. In: S.E. Wolverton and J.K. Wilkin (Editors). *Systemic Drugs for Skin Diseases*. Chapter 3, pp. 47–85. Saunders, Philadelphia.
299. Tester-Dalderup, C.B.M. (1988): Antifungal drugs. In: M.N.G. Dukes (Editor). *Meyler's Side Effects of Drugs, 11th Edition*. Chapter 29, pp. 567–580. Elsevier Science Publishers, Amsterdam.
300. Madhok, R., Zoma, A. and Capell, H. (1985): Fatal exacerbation of systemic lupus erythematosus after treatment with griseofulvin. *Br. Med. J., 291*, 249–251.
301. Van Dijke, C.P.H. and Weber, J.C.P. (1984): Interaction between oral contraceptives and griseofulvine. *Br. Med. J., 288*, 1125–1127.
302. Lesher, J.L. and Smith, J.G. Jr. (1987): Antifungal agents in dermatology. *J. Am. Acad. Dermatol., 17*, 383–394.
303. Rosa, F.W., Hernandez, C. and Carlo, W.A. (1987): Griseofulvin teratology, including two thoracopagus conjoined twins. *Lancet, i*, 171.
304. Miyagawa, S., Okuchi, T., Shiomi, Y. and Sakamoto, K. (1989): Subacute cutaneous lupus erythematosus lesions precipitated by griseofulvin. *J. Am. Acad. Dermatol., 21*, 343–346.
305. Rustin, M.H.A., Bunker, C.B., Dowd, P.M. and Robinson, T.W.E. (1989): Erythema multiforme due to griseofulvin. *Br. J. Dermatol., 120*, 455–458.
306. Feinstein, A., Sofer, E., Trau, H. and Schewach-Millet, M. (1984): Urticaria and fixed drug eruption in a patient treated with griseofulvin. *J. Am. Acad. Dermatol., 10*, 915–917.
307. Boudghene-Stambouli, O. and Merad-Boudia, A. (1989): Fixed drug eruption induced by griseofulvin. *Dermatologica, 179*, 92–93.
308. Kawabe, Y., Mizuno, N., Miwa, N. and Sakakibara, S. (1988): Photosensitivity induced by griseofulvin. *Photodermatol., 5*, 272–274.
309. Mion, G., Verdon, R., Le Gulluche, Y., Carsin, H., Garcia, A. and Guilbaud, J. (1989): Fatal toxic epidermal necrolysis after griseofulvin. *Lancet, ii*, 1331.
310. Becker, L.E. (1984): Griseofulvin. *Dermatologic Clinics, 2*, 115–118.
311. Lecky, B.R.F. (1990): Griseofulvin-induced neuropathy. *Lancet, i*, 230–231.
312. Duvanel, T. (1986): Ongles jaunes, anidrose acquise et griseofulvine. *Ann. Dermatol. Venereol., 113*, 471–472.
313. Jones, H.E. (Editor) (1987): *Ketoconazole Today. A Review of Clinical Experience*. ADIS Press Ltd., Manchester.
314. Markitziu, A., Katz, J. and Pisanty, S. (1986): Lichenoid lesions of the oral mucosa associated with ketoconazole. *Mykosen, 29*, 317–322.
315. Knight, T.E., Shikuma, C.Y. and Knight, J. (1991): Ketoconazole-induced fulminant hepatitis necessitating liver transplantation. *J. Am. Acad. Dermatol., 25*, 398–400.
316. Stockley, I.H. (1991): Use of griseofulvin. *J. Am. Acad. Dermatol., 24*, 665.
317. Pillans, P.I., Cowan, P. and Whitelaw, D. (1985): Hyponatraemia and confusion in a patient taking ketoconazole. *Lancet, i*, 821–822.

318. Kraemer, F.B. and Pont, A. (1986): Inhibition of cholesterol synthesis by ketoconazole. *Am. J. Med., 80*, 616–622.
319. Lobo, B.L., Miwa, L.J. and Jungnickel, P.W. (1988): Possible ketoconazole-induced hypoglycemia. *Drug Intell. Clin. Pharm., 22*, 632.
320. Best, T.R., Jenkins, J.K., Murphy, F.Y. et al. (1987): Persistent adrenal insufficiency secondary to low-dose ketoconazole therapy. *Am. J. Med., 82*, 676–680.
321. Kitching, N.K. (1986): Hypothyroidism after treatment with ketoconazole. *Br. Med. J., 293*, 993–994.
322. Tanner, A.R. (1987): Hypothyroidism after treatment with ketoconazole. *Br. Med. J., 294*, 125.
323. Mohamed, K.N. (1988): Severe photodermatitis during ketoconazole therapy. *Clin. Exp. Dermatol., 13*, 54–55.
324. Bharije, S.C. and Belhai, M.S. (1988): Ketoconazole-induced fixed drug eruption. *Int. J. Dermatol., 27*, 278.
325. van Tyle, J.H. (1984): Ketoconazole. Mechanism of action, spectrum of activity, pharmacokinetics, drug interactions, adverse reactions and therapeutic use. *Pharmacotherapy, 4*, 343–373.
326. Dhondt, A., de Doncker, P. and Cauwenbergh, G. *Focus on Ketoconazole*. Janssen Research Foundation, Beerse, Belgium. Report no. N 80575.
327. Balfour, J.A. and Faulds, D. (1992): Terbinafine. A review of its pharmacodynamic and pharmacokinetic properties, and therapeutic potential in superficial mycoses. *Drugs*, 43, 259–284.
328. Savin, R. (1989): Succesful treatment of chronic tinea pedis (mocassin type) with terbinafine (Lamisil). *Clin. Exp. Dermatol., 14*, 116–119.
329. Goodfield, M.J.D. (1992): Short-duration therapy with terbinafine for dermatophyte onychomycosis: a multicentre trial. *Br. J. Dermatol., 126 (suppl. 39)*, 33–35.
330. Jensen, J.C. (1990): Pharmacokinetics of Lamisil in humans. *J. Dermatol Treatm., 1 (suppl. 2)*, 15–18.
331. Hay, R.J. and Stratigos, J.D. (Eds.) (1992): Therapeutic potential of terbinafine (Lamisil) in dermatomycoses. Proceedings of a symposium. *Br. J. Dermatol., 126, suppl. 39.*
332. Smith, E.B. (Ed.) (1990): Terbinafine: a new topically and systemically effective allylamine antifungal. Proceedings of a symposium. *J. Am. Acad. Dermatol., 23*, 775–812.
333. Schroeff, J.G. van der, Cirkel, P.K.S., Crijns, M.B. et al. (1992): A randomized treatment duration-finding study of terbinafine in onychomycosis. *Br. J. Dermatol., 126 (suppl. 39)*, 36–39.
334. Baudraz-Rosselet, F., Rasoki, T., Wili, P.B. and Kenzelmann, R. (1992): Treatment of onychomycosis with terbinafine. *Br. J. Dermatol., 126 (suppl. 39)*, 40–46.
335. Villars V.V. and Jones, T.C. (1992): Special features of the clinical use of oral terbinafine in the treatment of fungal diseases. *Br. J. Dermatol., 126 (suppl. 39)*, 61–62.
336. Marks, R, Finlay, A.Y. and O'Sullivan, D.P., eds. (1990):The allylamines: a new class of antimycotic agents. *J. Dermatol. Treatm., 1, suppl. 2.*
337. Juhlin, G. (1992): Loss of taste and terbinafine. *Lancet, 339*, 1483.
338. Millikan, L.E. and Shrum, J.P. (1991): Antifungal agents. In: S.E. Wolverton and J.K. Wilkin(Editors). *Systemic Drugs for Skin Diseases*. Chapter 3, pp. 25–46. Saunders, Philadelphia
339. Alcantara, R. and Garibay, J.M. (1988): Itraconazole therapy in dermatomycosis and vaginal candidiasis: efficacy and adverse effects profile in a large multicenter study. *Adv. Ther., 5*, 326–334.
340. Saul, A. and Bonifaz, A. (1990): Itraconazole in common dermatophyte infections of the skin: Fixed treatment schedules. *J. Am. Acad. Dermatol., 23*, 554–558.
341. Sharkey, P.K., Graybill, J.R., Rinaldi, M.G., et al. (1990): Itraconazole treatment of phaeohyphomycosis. *J. Am. Acad. Dermatol., 23*, 577–586.
342. Tucker, R.M., Denning, D.W., Arathoon, E.G., Rinaldi, M.G. and Stevens, D.A. (1990): Itraconazole therapy for nonmeningeal coccidioidomycosis: clinical and laboratory observations. *J. Am. Acad. Dermatol., 23*, 593–601.
343. Dupont, B. (1990): Itraconazole therapy in aspergillosis: study in 49 patients. *J. Am. Acad. Dermatol., 23*, 607–614.
344. Hay, R.J., Clayton, Y.M., Moore, M.K. and Midgely, G. (1988): An evaluation of itraconazole in the management of onychomycosis. *Br. J. Dermatol., 119*, 359–366.
345. Matthieu, L., de Doncker, P., Cauwenbergh, G., et al. (1991): Itraconazole penetrates the nail via the nail matrix and the nail bed — an investigation in onychomycosis. *Clin. Exp. Dermatol., 16*, 374–376.
346. Lavrijsen, A.P.M., Balmus, K.J., Nugteren-Huying, W.M., Roldaan, A.C., van 't Wout, J.W. and Stricker, B.H.Ch. (1992): Hepatic injury associated with itraconazole. *Lancet, 340*, 252.
347. Willemsen, M., de Doncker, P., Willems, J. et al. (1992): Posttreatment itraconazole levels in the nail. *J.*

Am. Acad. Dermatol., 26, 731–735.
348. De Beule, K., Lubin, G. and Cauwenbergh, G. (1991): Safety aspects of itraconazole therapy in vaginal candidosis, dermatomycosis and onychomycosis. A review. *Curr. Ther. Res., 49*, 814–822.
349. Trisproral data sheet. Janssen Pharmaceutica, Tilburg, July 1992.
350. Callen, J.P. and Kulp-Shorten, C.A. (1991): Methotrexate. In: S.E. Wolverton and J.K. Wilkin (Editors). *Systemic Drugs for Skin Diseases.* Chapter 6, pp. 152–166. Saunders, Philadelphia.
351. Roenigk, H.H., Auerbach, R., Maibach, H.I. et al. (1988): Methotrexate in psoriasis: Revised guidelines. *J. Am. Acad. Dermatol., 19*, 145–156.
352. Lester, R.S. (1989): Methotrexate. Clin. Dermatol., 7, 128–35.
353. Evans, W.E and Christensen, M.L. (1985): Interactions with methotrexate. *J. Rheumatol., 12 (suppl. 12)*, 15–20.
354. Westwick, T.J., Sherertz, E.F., McCarley, D. and Flowers, F.P. (1987): Delayed reactivation of sunburn by methotrexate: sparing of chronically sun-exposed skin. *Cutis, 39*, 49–51.
355. Wantzin, G.L. and Thomsen, K. (1983): Acute paronychia after high-dose methotrexate therapy. *Arch. Dermatol., 119*, 623–624.
356. Chang, J.C. (1987): Acute bullous dermatosis and onycholysis due to high-dose methotrexate and leucovorin calcium. *Arch. Dermatol., 123*, 990–992.
357. Huber, A. (1990): Anaphylaktoide Reaktion auf das Zytostatikum Methotrexat. *Allergologie, 13*, 33–34.
358. Harrison, P.V. (1987): Methotrexate-induced epidermal necrosis. *Br. J. Dermatol., 116*, 867–869.
359. Kaplan, D.L. and Olsen, E.A. (1988): Erosion of psoriatic plaques after chronic methotrexate administration. *Int. J. Dermatol., 27*, 59–62.
360. Logan, R.A., McFadden, J.P. and Eady, R.A.J. (1988): Reactivation of cutaneous radionecrosis associated with methotrexate therapy for psoriasis. *Clin. Exp. Dermatol., 13*, 350–352.
361. Baack, B.R. and Burgdorf, W.H.C. (1991): Chemotherapy-induced acral erythema. *J. Am. Acad. Dermatol., 24*, 457–461.
362. Jensen, D.B., Albrektsen, S.B. and Krag, C. (1989): Development of metastatic skin cancer during methotrexate therapy for psoriasis. *Acta Derm. Venereol., 69*, 274–275.
363. Phillips, T.J., Hugh Jones, D. and Baker, H. (1987): Pulmonary complications following methotrexate therapy. *J. Am. Acad. Dermatol., 16*, 373–375.
364. Harrison, P.V., Peat, M., James, R. and Orrell, D. (1987): Methotrexate and retinoids in combination for psoriasis. *Lancet, 2*, 512.
365. Burton, J.L. (1991): Drug interactions with methotrexate. *Br. J. Dermatol., 124*, 300–301.
366. Groenendal, H. and Rampen, F.H.J. (1990): Methotrexate and trimethoprim-sulphamethoxazole — potentially hazardous combination. *Clin. Exp. Dermatol., 15*, 358–360.
367. Olsen, E.A. (1991): The pharmacology of methotrexate. *J. Am. Acad. Dermatol., 25*, 306–318.
368. Shupack, J.L. and Webster, G.F. (1988): Pancytopenia following low-dose oral methotrexate therapy for psoriasis. *J. Am. Med. Assoc., 259*, 3594–6.
369. Zachariae, H., Hansen, H.E., Sogaard, H. et al. (1990): Kidney biopsies in methotrexate-treated psoriatics. *Dermatologica, 181*, 373–376.
370. Bronner, A.K. and Hood, A.F. (1983): Cutaneous complications of chemotherapeutic agents. *J. Am. Acad. Dermatol., 9*, 645–663.
371. Wilke, W.S. and Mackenzie, A.H. (1986): Methotrexate therapy in rheumatoid arthritis. Current status. *Drugs, 32*, 103–113.
372. McDonald, C.J. (1985): Cytotoxic agents for use in dermatology. I. *J. Am. Acad. Dermatol., 12*, 753–775.
373. Zachariae, H. and Sogaard, H. (1987): Methotrexate-induced liver cirrhosis. A follow-up. *Dermatologica, 175*, 178–182.
374. Newman, M., Auerbach, R., Feiner, H. et al. (1989): The role of liver biopsies in psoriatic patients receiving long-term methotrexate treatment. *Arch. Dermatol., 125*, 1218–1224.
375. O'Connor, G.T., Olmstead, E.M., Zug, K. et al. (1989): Detection of hepatotoxicity associated with methotrexate therapy for psoriasis. *Arch. Dermatol., 125*, 1209–1217.
376. Duhra, P. and Foulds, I.S. (1988): Methotrexate-induced impairment of tast acuity. *Clin. Exp. Dermatol., 13*, 126–127.
377. Daniel, C.R. III and Scher, R.K. (1984): Nail changes secondary to systemic drugs or ingestants. *J. Am. Acad. Dermatol., 10*, 250–258.
378. Rapini, R.P., Jordon, R.E. and Wolverton, S.E. (1991): Cytotoxic agents. In: S.E. Wolverton and J.K. Wilkin (Editors). *Systemic Drugs for Skin Diseases.* Chapter 5, 125–151. Saunders, Philadelphia.

379. Folb, P.I. (1988): Cytostatic and immunosuppressive drugs. In: *Meyler's Side Effects of Drugs, 11th Edition*. Chapter 47, pp. 928–960. Elsevier, Amsterdam.
380. Younger, I.R., Harris, D.W.S. and Colver, C.B. (1991): Azathioprine in dermatology. *J. Am. Acad. Dermatol., 25*, 281–286.
381. Saway, P.A., Heck, L.W., Bonner, J.R. et al. (1988): Azathioprine hypersensitivity. *Am. J. Med., 84*, 960–964.
382. Neumann, R.A., Knobler, R.M., Metze, D. et al. (1988): Disseminated superficial actinic porokeratosis and immunosuppression. *Br. J. Dermatol., 119*, 375–380.
383. Lawson, D.H., Lovatt, G.E., Gurton, C.S. and Hennings, R.C. (1984): Adverse effects of azathioprine. *Adverse Drug Reactions & Acute Poisoning Reviews, 3*, 161–173.
384. Scott, J.P. and Higenbottam, T.W. (1988): Adverse reactions and interactions of cyclosporin. *Medical Toxicology, 3*, 107–127.
385. Bos, J.D., van Joost, Th., Powles, A.V., Meinardi, M.M.H.M., Heule, F. and Fry, L. (1989): Use of cyclosporin in psoriasis. *Lancet, ii*, 1500–1502.
386. Mihatsch, M.J. and Wolff, K. (1992): Consensus conference on cyclosporin A for psoriasis February 1992. *Br. J. Dermatol., 126*, 621–623.
387. Rubin, A.M. and Kang, H. (1987): Cerebral blindness and encephalopathy with cyclosporin A toxicity. *Neurology, 37*, 1072–1076.
388. Bencini, P.L., Montagnino, G., Sala, F. et al. (1986): Cyclosporin-induced cutaneous lesions in 67 renal transplant recipients. *Dermatologica, 172*, 24–30.
389. Bos, J.D. and Meinardi, M.M.H.M. (1989): Two distinct squamous cell carcinomas in a psoriasis patient receiving low-dose cyclosporine maintenance therapy. *J. Am. Acad. Dermatol., 21*, 1305–1306.
390. Bouwes Bavinck, J.N., Vermeer, B.J., van der Woude, F.J. et al. (1991): Relation between skin cancer and HLA antigens in renal-transplant recipients. *New Engl. J. Med., 325*, 843–848.
391. Sheil, A.G.R., Flavel, S., Disry, A.P.S., Mathew, T.U. and Hall, B.M. (1987): Cancer incidence in renal transplantation patients treated with azathioprine or cyclosporine. *Transplantation Proceedings, 19*, 2214–2216.
392. Thivolet, J. and Kanitakis, J. (1991): La ciclosporine A en dermatologie. *La Presse Médicale, 20*, 2249–2255.
393. Frosch, P.J., Ruder, H., Stiefel, A., Hehls, O. and Bersch, A. (1988): Gingivalhyperplasie und Seropapeln unter Ciclosporinbehandlung. *Hautarzt, 39*, 611–616.
394. Brady, A. and Wing, A. (1989): Hyperpigmentation due to ciclosporin. *Nephrol. Dial. Transpl., 4*, 309–310.
395. Kolansky, G. (1989): Cyclosporine: pharmacokinetics, administration, and efficacy in organ transplantation and other applications. *Hosp. Formul., 24*, 583–597.
396. Gupta, A.K., Brown, M.D., Ellis, C.N. et al. (1989): Cyclosporine in dermatology. *J. Am. Acad. Dermatol., 21*, 1245–12156.
397. Gupta, A.K., Cooper, K.D., Ellis, C.N. et al. (1990): Lymphocytic infiltrates of the skin in association with cyclosporine therapy. *J. Am. Acad. Dermatol., 23*, 1137–1141.
398. Mihatsch, M.J. and Wolff, K. (Eds) (1990): Risk/benefit ratio of Cyclosporin A (Sandimmun) in psoriasis. *Br. J. Dermatol., 122, suppl. 36.*
399. Meinardi, M.M.H.M., de Rie, M.A. and Bos, J.D. (1990): Oral cyclosporin A in the treatment of psoriasis: an overview of studies performed in the Netherlands. *Br. J. Dermatol., 122 (suppl. 36)*, 27–31.
400. Krupp, P. and Monka, C. (1990): Side-effect profile of cyclosporin A in patients treated for psoriasis. *Br. J. Dermatol., 122 (suppl. 36)*, 47–56.
401. Mason, J. (1990): Renal side-effects of cyclosporin A. *Br. J. Dermatol., 122 (suppl. 36)*, 71–77.
402. Feutren, G., Abeywickrama, K., Friend, D. and von Graffenried, B. (1990): Renal function and blood pressure in psoriatic patients treated with cyclosporin A. *Br. J. Dermatol., 122 (suppl. 36)*, 57–69.
403. Margolis, D.J., Guzzo, C., Johnson, J. and Lazarus, G.S. (1992): Alterations in renal function in psoriasis patients treated with cyclosporine, 5 mg/kg/day. *J. Am. Acad. Dermatol., 26*, 195–197.
404. Zachariae, H., Hansen, H.E., Kragballe, K. and Olsen, S. (1992): Morphologic renal changes during cyclosporine treatment of psoriasis. *J. Am. Acad. Dermatol., 26*, 415–419.
405. Ross, M., Goodman, M.M., Barr, R.J. and Liao, S.Y. (1992): Multiple eruptive benign keratoses associated with cyclosporine therapy for psoriasis. *J. Am. Acad. Dermatol., 26*, 128–129.
406. van Joost, Th., Bos, J.D., Heule, F. and Meinardi, M.M.H.M. (1988): Low-dose cyclosporin A in severe psoriasis. A double-blind study. *Br. J. Dermatol., 118*, 183–190.

407. Gurenther, L. (1991): Cyclosporine. In: S.E. Wolverton and J.K. Wilkin (Editors). *Systemic Drugs for Skin Diseases*. Chapter 7, pp. 167–186. Saunders, Philadelphia.
408. Ho, V.C., Lui, H. and McLean, D.I. (1990): Cyclosporine in nonpsoriatic dermatoses. *J. Am. Acad. Dermatol., 23*, 1248–1259.
409. Fradin, M.S., Ellis, C.N. and Voorhees, J.J. (1990): Management of patients and side effects during cyclosporine therapy for cutaneous disorders. *J. Am. Acad. Dermatol., 23*, 1265–1275.
410. Krupp, P., Cheang, A. and Monka, C. (1989): *Present Experience of Sandimmune in Pregnancy*. Sandoz Ltd, Landon.
411. Bennett, W.M. (1990): Renal effects of cyclosporine. *J. Am. Acad. Dermatol., 23*, 1280–1287.
412. Merot, Y., Miescher, P.A., Balsiger, F. et al. (1990): Cutaneous malignant melanomas occurring under cyclosporin A therapy: a report of two cases. *Br. J. Dermatol., 123*, 237–239.
413. Arellano, F. and Krupp, P.F. (1991): Cutaneous malignant melanoma occurring after cyclosporin A therapy. *Br. J. Dermatol., 124*, 611.
414. Griffiths, C.E.M. and Voorhees, J.J. (1990); Cyclosporine A in the treatment of psoriasis: a clinical and mechanistic perspective. *J. Invest. Dermatol., 95*, 53S–55S.
415. Soria, C., Allegue, F., Martin, M. and Ledo, A. (1991): Treatment of pyoderma gangrenosum with cyclosporine A. *Clin. Exp. Dermatol., 16*, 392–394.
416. Grossmann, R.M., Delaney, R.J., Brinton, E.A., Carter, D.M. and Gottlieb, A.B. (1991): Hypertriglyceridemia in patients with psoriasis treated with cyclosporine. *J. Am. Acad. Dermatol., 25*, 648–651.
417. Bouwes Bavinck, J.N., Van der Woude, F.J., Vandenbroucke, J.P., Wolterbeek, R., Meyboom, R.H. and Vermeer, B.J. (1991): Cyclosporine for treatment of psoriasis. *New Engl. J. Med., 324*, 1894.
418. Ellis, C.N., Fradin, M.S., Messana, J.M. et al. (1991): Cyclosporine for plaque-type psoriasis. Results of a multidose, double-blind trial. *New Engl. J. Med., 324*, 277–284.
419. Korstanje, M.J., Van Breda Vriesman, C.J.P. and Van de Staak, W.J.B.M. (1990): Cyclosporine and methotrexate: a dangerous combination. *J. Am. Acad. Dermatol., 23*, 320–321.
420. Arellano, F. and Krupp, P. (1991): Muscular disorders associated with cyclosporin. *Lancet, 337*, 915.
421. Pakula, A. and Garden, J. (1992): Sebaceous hyperplasia and basal cell carcinoma in a renal transplant patient receiving cyclosporine. *J. Am. Acad. Dermatol., 26*, 139–140.
422. Stiller, M.J., Pak, G.H., Kenny, C. et al. (1992): Elevation of fasting serum lipids in patients treated with low-dose cyclosporine for severe plaque-type psoriasis. *J. Am. Acad. Dermatol., 27*, 434–438.
423. Del Rosso, J.Q. (1991): Antihistamines. In: S.E. Wolverton and J.K. Wilkin (Editors). *Systemic Drugs for Skin Diseases*. Chapter 12, pp. 285–326. Saunders, Philadelphia.
424. Drouin, M.A. (1985): H1 antihistamines. Perspective on the use of the conventional and new agents. *Ann. Allergy, 55*, 747–752.
425. Woodward, J.K. (1988): Pharmacology and toxicology of nonclassical antihistamines. *Cutis, 42*, 5–9.
426. Flowers, F.P., Araujo, O.E. and Nieves, C.H. (1986): Antihistamines. *Int. J. Dermatol., 25*, 224–231.
427. Aram, H. (1987): Cimetidine in dermatology. *Int. J. Dermatol., 26*, 161–166.
428. Monroe, E.W. (1987): Treatment of urticaria: Drug management. *Semin. Dermatol., 6*, 342–347.
429. Monroe, E.W. (1988): Chronic urticaria: Review of nonsedating H1 antihistamines in treatment. *J. Am. Acad. Dermatol., 19*, 842–849.
430. Schuller, D.E. and Turkewitz, D. (1986): Adverse effects of antihistamines. *Postgrad. Med., 79*, 75–86.
431. Stricker, B.H., van Dijcke, C.P.H., Isaacs, A.J. and Lindquist, M. (1986): Skin reactions to terfenadine. *Br. Med. J., 293*, 536.
432. Fenton, D. and Signy, M. (1986): Photosensitivity associated with terfenadine. *Br. Med. J., 293*, 823.
433. Jones, S.K. and Morley, W.N. (1985): Terfenadine causing hair loss. *Br. Med. J., 291*, 940.
434. Harrison, P.V. and Stones, R.N. (1988): Severe exacerbation of psoriasis due to terbinafine. *Clin. Exp. Dermatol., 13*, 275–277.
435. Larrey, D., Palazzo, L. and Benhamou, J.P. (1985): Terfenadine and hepatitis. *Ann. Intern. Med., 103*, 634–636.
436. Landow, R.K. (1987): Myth or magic: The role of cimetidine in dermatology. *Semin. Dermatol., 6*, 43–47.
437. Aram, H. (1987): Treatment of female androgenetic alopecia with cimetidine. *Int. J. Dermatol., 26*, 128–130.
438. Freston, J.W. (1982): Cimetidine: Adverse reactions and patterns of use. *Ann. Intern. Med., 97*, 728–734.
439. Souza Lima, M.A. (1986): Ranitidine and hepatic injury. *Ann. Intern. Med., 105*, 140.
440. Brodin, M.B. (1987): Drug-related alopecia. *Dermatol. Clinics, 5*, 571-9.
441. Thomas, J.M. and Misiewicz, G. (1984): Histamine H2-receptor antagonists in the short- and long-term

treatment of duodenal ulcer. *Clin. Gastroenterol., 13*, 501–541.
442. Lunde, I. (1988): Antihistamines (H1-receptor antagonists). In: *Meyler's Side Effects of Drugs, 11th Edition*. Chapter 16, pp. 316–320.Elsevier, Amsterdam.
443. Monahan, B.P., Ferguson, C.L., Killeavy, E.S. et al. (1990): Torsades de pointes occurring in association with terfenadine use. JAMA, 264, 2788–2790.
444. Christensen, O.B. and Maibach, H.I. (1983): Antihistamines in dermatology. *Semin. Dermatol., 2*, 270–280.
445. Hogan, D.J. and Rooney, M.E. (1989): Fixed drug eruption due to dimenhydrinate. *J. Am. Acad. Dermatol., 20*, 503–504.
446. Dollberg, S., Hurvitz, H., Kerem, E., Navon, P. and Branski, D. (1989): Hallucinations and hyperthermia after promethazine ingestion. *Acta Paediatr. Scand., 78*, 131–132.
447. Wagner, G., Mahlmann, E.G. and Stadtler, E. (1989): Arzneimittelexantheme nach Mebhydrolin (Omeril). *Akt. Dermatol., 15*, 288–289.
448. Boyd, P.T., Lepre, F. and Dickey, J.D. (1989): Chronic active hepatitis associated with cimetidine. *Br. Med. J., 298*, 324.
449. Camisa, C. (1991): Antimalarials. In: S.E. Wolverton and J.K. Wilkin (Editors). *Systemic Drugs for Skin Diseases*. Chapter 11, pp. 265–284. Saunders, Philadelphia.
450. Lo, J.S., Berg, R.E. and Tomecki, K.J. (1989): Treatment of discoid lupus erythematosus. *Int. J. Dermatol., 28*, 497–507.
451. Weiss, J.S. (1991): Antimalarial medications in dermatology. A review. *Dermatologic Clinics, 9*, 377–385.
452. Ward, W.Q., Walter-Ryan, W.G. and Shehi, G.M. (1985): Toxic psychosis: a complication of antimalarial therapy. *J. Am. Acad. Dermatol., 12*, 863–865.
453. Dupré, A., Ortonne, J.-P., Viraben, R. and Arfeux, F. (1985): Chloroquine-induced hypopigmentation of hair and freckles. *Arch. Dermatol., 121*, 1164–1166.
454. Wintroub, B.U. and Stern, R. (1985): Cutaneous drug reactions: pathogenesis and clinical classification. *J. Am. Acad. Dermatol., 13*, 167–179.
455. Hudson, L.D. (1985): Erythema annulare centrifugum: an unusual case due to hydroxychloroquine sulfate. *Cutis, 36*, 129–130.
456. Abel, E.A., DiCicco, L.M., Orenberg, E.K. et al. (1986): Drugs in exacerbation of psoriasis. *J. Am. Acad. Dermatol., 15*, 1007–1022.
457. Slagel, C.A. and James, W.D. (1985): Plaquenil-induced erythroderma. *J. Am. Acad. Dermatol., 12*, 857–862.
458. Rasmussen, J.E. (1983): Antimalarials — Are they safe to use in children? *Pediatr. Dermatol., 1*, 89–91.
459. Olansky, A.J. (1982): Antimalarials and ophthalmologic safety. *J. Am. Acad. Dermatol., 6*, 19–23.
460. Portznoy, J.Z. and Callen, J.P. (1983): Ophthalmologic aspects of chloroquine and hydroxychloroquine therapy. *Int. J. Dermatol., 22*, 273–278.
461. Easterbrook, M. (1988): Ocular effects and safety of antimalarial agents. *Am. J. Med., 85 (4A)*, 23–29.
462. Willoughby, J.S. and Shear, N.H. (1988): Antimalarials. *Clin. Dermatol., 7*, 60–68.
463. Isaacson, D., Elgart, M. and Turner, M.L. (1982): Antimalarials in dermatology. *Int. J. Dermatol., 21*, 379–395.
464. Friedman, S.J. (1987): Pustular psoriasis associated with hydroxychloroquine. *J. Am. Acad. Dermatol., 16*, 1256–1257.
465. Berman, B. and Kilmer, S.L. (1991): Antiviral agents. In: S.E. Wolverton and J.K. Wilkin (Editors). *Systemic Drugs for Skin Diseases.* Chapter 1, pp. 1–24. Saunders, Philadelphia.
466. Arndt, K.A. (1988): Adverse reactions to acyclovir: topical, oral, and intravenous. *J. Am. Acad. Dermatol., 18*, 188–190.
467. Cohen, S.M.Z., Minkove, J.A., Zebley, J.W. III and Mulholland, J.H. (1984): Severe but reversible neurotoxicity from acyclovir. *Ann. Intern. Med. 100*, 920–924.
468. Shea, B.F., Harbison, M.A., Sesin, G.P., Benotti, P.N. and Hammer, S.M. (1987): Acyclovir-associated fever. *Pharmacotherapy 7*, 45–46.
469. Dorsky, D.I. and Crumpacker, C.S. (1987): Drugs five years later: Acyclovir. *Ann. Intern. Med., 107*, 859–874.
470. Swan, S.K. and Bennett, W.M. (1989): Oral acyclovir and neurotoxicity. *Ann. Intern. Med., 111*, 188.
471. Lisby, S.M., Nahata, M.C. and Powell, D.A. (1986): Nausea and vomiting possibly associated with intravenous acyclovir. *Drug Intell. Clin. Pharm., 20*, 371–373.
472. Jones, P.G. and Beier-Hanratty, S.A. (1986): Acyclovir: neurologic and renal toxicity. *Ann. Intern. Med., 104*, 892.

473. Spiegel, D.M. and Lau, K. (1986): Acute renal failure and coma secondary to acyclovir therapy. *JAMA, 255*, 1882–1883.
474. Sylvester, R.K., Ogden, W.B., Draxler, C.A. and Lewis, F.B. (1986): Vesicular eruption. A local complication of concentrated acyclovir infusions. *JAMA, 255*, 385–386.
475. Bataille, P., Devos, P., Noel, J.L. and Dautrevaux, C. (1985): Psychiatric side-effects with acyclovir. *Lancet, ii*, 724.
476. Goldberg, L.H., Kaufman, R., Conant, M.A. et al. (1986): Oral acyclovir for episodic treatment of recurrent genital herpes. *J. Am. Acad. Dermatol., 15*, 256–264.
477. Leen, C.L.S., Mandal, B.K. and Ellis, M.E. (1987): Acyclovir and pregnancy. *Br. Med. J., 294*, 308.
478. Richards, D.M., Carmine, A.A., Brogden, R.N. et al. (1983): Acyclovir: a review. *Drugs, 26*, 378–385.
479. Von Schulthess, G.K. and Sauter, Ch. (1981): Acyclovir and herpes zoster. *New Engl. J. Med., 305*, 1349–1351.
480. Whitley, R.J. and Gmann, J.W. Jr. (1992): Acyclovir: a decade later. *New Engl. J. Med., 327*, 782–789.
481. Greer, K.E. (1991): Dapsone and sulfapyridine. In: S.E. Wolverton and J.K. Wilkin (Editors). *Systemic Drugs for Skin Diseases*. Chapter 10, pp. 247–2-64. Saunders, Philadelphia.
482. Uetrecht, J. (1989): Dapsone and sulfapyridine. *Clin. Dermatol., 7*, 111–120.
483. Smith, W.C. (1988): Are hypersensitivity reactions to dapsone becoming more frequent? *Lepr. Rev., 59*, 53–58.
484. Hornsten, P., Keisu, M. and Wiholm, B.-E. (1990): The incidence of agranulocytosis during treatment of dermatitis herpetiformis with dapsone as reported in Sweden, 1972 through 1988. *Arch. Dermatol., 126*, 919–922.
485. Wozel, G. (1989): The story of sulfones in tropical medicine and dermatology. *Int. J. Dermatol., 28*, 17–21.
486. Lang, P.G. Jr. (1979): Sulfones and sulfonamides in dermatology today. *J. Am. Acad. Dermatol., 1*, 479–92.
487. Ahrens, E.M., Meckler, R.J. and Callen, J.P. (1986): Dapsone-induced peripheral neuropathy. *Int. J. Dermatol., 25*, 314–316.
488. Daneshmend, T.K. (1984): The neurotoxicity of dapsone. *Adv. Drug React. Ac. Pois. Rev., 3*, 43–58.
489. Joseph, M.S. (1987): Photodermatitis provoked by dapsone: a case report. *Lepr. Rev., 58*, 425–428.
490. Joseph, M.S. and Charoen, W.S. (1987): Problems encountered in treating one leprosy patient in a developing country: a case report. *Lepr. Rev., 58*, 165–171.
491. Nugteren-Huying, W.M., Van der Schroeff, J.G., Hermans, J. and Suurmond, D. (1990): Fumaric acid therapy for psoriasis: A randomized, double-blind, placebo-controlled study. *J. Am. Acad. Dermatol., 22*, 311–312, also published in *Ned. Tijdschr. Geneeskd. 1990, 134*, 2387–2391.
492. Nieboer, C., de Hoop, D., van Loenen, A.C., Langendijk, P.N.J. and van Dijk, E. (1989): Systemic therapy with fumaric acid derivatives: new possibilities in the treatment of psoriasis. *J. Am. Acad. Dermatol., 20*, 601–608.
493. van Dijk, E. (1985): Fumaarzuur voor de behandeling van patienten met psoriasis. *Ned. Tijdschr. Geneeskd., 129*, 485–487.
494. Kunst, L. (1985): Psoriasis behandeling. *Ned. Tijdschr. Geneeskd., 127*, 16–24.
495. Dubiel, W. and Happle, R. (1972): Behandlungsversuch mit Fumarsaure monoäthylester bei Psoriasis vulgaris. *Z. Haut-Geschlkr., 42*, 545–550.
496. Bayard, W., Hunziker, Th., Krebs, A., Speiser, P. and Joshi, R. (1987): Perorale Langzeitbehandlung der Psoriasis mit Fumarsaurederivaten. *Hautarzt, 38*, 279–285.
497. Haberland, A.K., Engst, R., Jessberger, B., Schober, C. and Borelli, S. (1991): Fumarsaure und Fumarsaureester. Antipsoriatika der Zukunft? *Z. Hautkr., 66*, 162–167.
498. Roodnat, J.I., Christiaans, Nugteren-Huying, W.M. et al. (1989): Akute Niereninsuffizienz bei der Behandlung der Psoriasis mit Fumarsaure-Estern. *Schweiz. Med. Wschr., 119*, 826–830.
499. Stuhlinger, W., Innerebner, M. and Aberer, W. (1990): Nephrotoxische Wirkung einer Therapie mit Fumarsaureestern bei Psoriasis. *Dtsch. Med. Wschr., 115*, 1712–1715.
500. Dalhoff, K., Faerber, P., Arnholdt, H., Sack, K. and Strubelt, O. (1990): Akutes Nierenversagen unter Psoriasistherapie mit Fumarsaure- derivaten. *Dtsch. Med. Wschr., 115*, 1014–1017.
501. Van Loenen, A.C., Langendijk, P.N.J. and Nieboer, C. (1989): Fumaarzuurtherapie: van fictie tot werkelijkheid? *Pharm. Weekbl., 124*, 894–900.
502. Kolbach, D. and Nieboer, C. (1992): Fumaric acid therapy in psoriasis: results and side effects of 2 years of treatment. *J. Am. Acad. Dermatol., 27*, 769–771.

20. Other therapeutic modalities

DERMAL IMPLANTS

20.1 For centuries physicians have attempted to augment skin by injecting a variety of agents into the dermis and subcutaneous tissue. Local and systemic toxicity has limited the use of most substances. Since the introduction of injectable collagen (Zyderm I) in 1976 and its FDA approval in 1981, however, more than 500,000 patients have safely received intradermal injections for soft tissue augmentation. These implants are used to correct dermal defects caused by aging (wrinkles), acne scars or trauma. Intense interest in long-lasting agents has resulted in the development of new products such as glutaraldehyde cross-linked bovine collagen implant (Zyplast) and gelatin matrix implant (Fibrel), and the reconsideration of older agents such as silicone.

Collagen

Bovine dermal collagen is solubilized, purified, and reconstituted in a neutral solution into an injectable form. The collagen fibrils are harvested and resuspended in phosphate-buffered saline containing 0.3% lidocaine. Zyderm I and II are prepared in an identical manner and differ in the final collagen concentration; I is 35 mg/ml and II is 65 mg/ml. Zyplast Implant is prepared in a similar manner except that glutaraldehyde is added during processing.

Adverse clinical reactions can be divided into local test site reactions, treatment site reactions, and systemic toxicity [1].

Local test site reactions

Approximately 5% of patients who receive a Zyderm I skin test will experience a test site reaction, characterized by erythema, induration, and occasional pruritus; 70% of these reactions occur within the first 72 hours, an additional 10% in 7 days, and the remainder within 4 weeks. Positive test site reactions are transient and last an average of 4 months. A local hypersensitivity reaction at the skin test or treatment site is a reliable predictor of systemic hypersensitivity reactions. IgG antibodies to bovine collagen are found in the serum of patients with test-site hypersensitivity reactions. The antibody response is species-specific to bovine collagen and does not cross-react with other animal or human collagens.

Treatment site reactions

Of patients with a non-reactive skin test result 1% to 4% will have an adverse treatment site reaction after their first Zyderm I treatment. These adverse reactions are identical to those caused by a skin test. Zyplast implant may cause fewer hypersensitivity reactions. Recurrent intermittent swelling at the treatment site is a rare adverse reaction, which is accompanied by erythema and induration, and may last up to 3 years. This recurrent swelling occasionally can be initiated by exercise, ingestion of alcohol, menses, stress, caffeine, high dose vitamin C, or other causes of vasodilation [4].

Overcorrection is a common problem, especially for inexperienced physicians. An area of superficial necrosis will rarely occur at the treatment site; the frequency is estimated to be 9 in 10,000 cases [2]. This complication, which is seen especially in the treatment of glabellar contour defects, is not associated with anticollagen antibodies, and is limited to the treatment site. Mechanical obstruction of superficial vessels is the presumed cause of the necrosis, and healing may be accompanied by scarring and pigmentary change. Occasionally, bruising occurs because of mechanical damage to the superficial vessels. This superficial ecchymosis usually resolves within 7 days and rarely causes pigmentary change.

Another rare complication (4 in 10,000 cases) is abscess formation [2]. Abscess formation has been reported after the first exposure to collagen implant, as well as after multiple exposures. These reactions vary, from a small fluctuant or draining papule or nodule at the injection site, which may or may not be erythematous, to severe fluctuance with significant swelling, erythema, and induration of the surrounding tissue. The abscess, which is considered to be the result of a hypersensitivity reaction, is different from a 'routine' hypersensitivity reaction to collagen implants that may be erythematous but not fluctuant [2].

Systemic reactions

In one instance an embolus of collagen entered the ophthalmic artery. This single case report of partial vision loss is the only documented systemic complication associated with bovine collagen implants. Although numerous complaints of arthralgias, malaise and headache have been investigated, no reproducible, statistically significant systemic complication has been documented. Eight cases of rheumatologic disease have been reported in more than 350,000 patients treated with injectable collagen. These are well within the prevalence range of the general population and may be considered unrelated to treatment [3]. In addition, in patients with scleroderma, rheumatoid arthritis and lupus erythematosus, antibody levels to bovine collagen were not statistically significant from those in the normal population [5].

Gelatin Matrix Implant [1,6]

Gelatin matrix implant (Fibrel), is a combination of gelatin powder and ε-aminocaproic acid reconstituted with a mixture of 0.9% sodium chloride for injection and the patients plasma in a 1:1 ratio. Few patients have been treated, and further clinical data are required. Of 321 patients [6], 1.9% had a positive skin test. In the treatment group whose initial skin tests were negative, 8% had treatment site reactions characterized by transient erythema, swelling and nodules, lasting for 2 weeks to several months [6]. No significant systemic side effects were noted.

Silicone

For soft tissue augmentation, silicone liquid, dimethylpolysiloxane, is used [1]. Injection of pure medical-grade silicone in small amounts, less than 1 ml per session, carries little risk. Treatment site reactions include erythema, ecchymosis, hyperpigmentation, texture problems, and excessive elevation [7].

Systemic embolisation from injection of liquid silicone in ophthalmic and meningeal vessels has resulted in blindness, loss of neurologic function, and death [1, 8]. Other rarely reported side effects include acute pneumonitis and respiratory distress syndrome, acute arthritis and renal failure, and erysipelas-like reaction and lymphatic obstruction from migration of silicone. The association of scleroderma and previous silicone augmentation mammaplasthy has been suggested [1].

Past problems are related primarily to the use of an impure product, excessive volumes, or inappropriate location, for example, the breasts [1].

LASER THERAPY

20.2 Lasers were first described in 1960. The name itself is an acronym for Light Amplification by Stimulated Emission of Radiation. Laser light is man-made, nonionizing radiation that has the properties of monochromaticity, coherence, and collimation. Monochromaticity permits the use of specific wavelengths that will allow selective optical absorption and consequent localized tissue damage. Coherence both in time and in space implies a uniformity of wave pattern.

Collimation indicates that the light may be propagated over a long distance with little beam spreading, which permits focusing to a small spot size. All laser machines have three elements: the laser medium, power supply, and mirrors. The medium may be solid (ruby, neodynium), liquid (dye), or gas (argon). In dermatology, usually argon lasers or CO_2 lasers are used. The argon laser has been found to be useful in the therapy of many cutaneous vascular lesions. Argon gas emits blue-green light that is strongly absorbed by the red-purple colour of oxygenated and/or reduced haemoglobin molecules. Absorbed light energy is transformed into heat that destroys endothelial cells and blood vessels without substantially altering epidermis or surrounding dermis. Other indications for laser therapy include tattoos and a variety of benign tumours of the skin including verrucae vulgares, planae and condylomata acuminata.

Adverse effects of laser therapy include atrophic or hypertrophic scarring, depression of the skin surface related to atrophy or loss of the dermal area previously filled by vascular spaces, and hyper- of hypopigmentation [9]. Hypertrophic scarring is the most frequent complication, possibly occurring in some 5% of patients treated. Other side effects of the argon and CO_2 laser mentioned by dermatologists and plastic surgeons in a survey include [10] infection, pain, intraoperative or postoperative haemorrhage, unintentional burns, and delayed wound healing. No procedure-related deaths, ocular damage, or secondary malignant neoplasms were reported [1]).

CHEMICAL FACE PEELS [11–15]

20.3 Chemical peeling is the application of a caustic chemical onto the skin to produce a controlled partial-thickness injury. The agent, usually a solution of phenol or trichloroacetic acid, removes varying amounts of the epidermis and, depending on the strength, affects dermal collagen. Wound repair consists of epidermal regeneration by migration from adnexa and replacement of new dermal connective tissue, resulting in a 'rejuvenation' of the skin. The result is a softening of rhytides, removal of actinic keratoses and lentigines, decrease in solar elastosis, and overall tightening and improvement of skin texture.

The risk of complications from peels (Table 20.1) increases proportionately with the depth of the wound. Superficial peels carry the lowest risk of adverse reactions, and these reactions are usually pigmentary in nature. Medium-depth peels can cause pigmentary changes and scarring. Deep peels with phenol are associated with the aforementioned risks and systemic reactions, notably cardiotoxicity. Trichloroacetic acid is not significantly absorbed and therefore does not produce systemic complications.

Table 20.1. Possible complications of chemical peeling [11–15]

Systemic	cardiac
	renal (theoretically, not reported)
	hepatic (theoretically, not reported)
	haematological
Cutaneous	*pigmentary*
	depigmentation (bleaching)
	hypopigmentation
	hyperpigmentation
	uneven pigmentation (streaking, mottled, blotchy)
	lines of demarcation
	accentuation of nevi
	erythema
	persistent flushing
	scarring
	keloid
	hypertrophic
	atrophic
	full-thickness skin necrosis
	structural: ectropion
	eclabium

(continued)

(continuation)

Infectious	*bacterial*
	staphylococcus
	streptococcus
	pseudomonas
	toxic shock syndrome
	viral
	herpes simplex activation
	verrucae
Miscellaneous	milia
	pruritus
	increase in pore size
	increase in amount of teleangiectasia
	laryngeal edema
	temperature sensitivity
	neuropsychiatric: depression
	destabilisation of compensated psyche

By far the most common local complication is the potential for abnormal pigmentation. The most profound and detrimental complications are systemic, which may occur with phenol. Theoretically, hepatorenal complications induced by phenol can arise. More common and significant is the striking and immediate cardiotoxicity. Cardiac arrhythmias that have been reported include premature ventricular contractions, ventricular bigeminy, ventricular tachycardia, and paroxysmal atrial tachycardia. Neither a normal preoperative electrocardiogram nor a negative cardiac history preclude the development of cardiac toxicity, nor is there a direct correlation with the patient's age, sex, administration of oxygen, or serum phenol levels [16]. The risk is greater, however, when more than a third of the face is peeled within 15 minutes. None of the cardiac changes have occurred when 50% or more of the face was peeled over a 60-minute period [11].

CRYOTHERAPY [17]

20.4 A place for cryosurgery has been firmly established in the armamentarium of many physicians, and for dermatologists it may be the treatment of choice for a variety of benign and malignant skin lesions, notably warts, actinic keratoses, seborrhoeic keratoses and superficial malignancies.

In competent hands, cryosurgery, and more specifically, liquid nitrogen (N_2) therapy, has proved to be a safe and effective therapy. Its complications can be divided into reactions of the immediate and acute type, short-term reactions, and long-term complications [17].

Reactions of the immediate and acute type

Many of the immediate and acute reactions may be considered 'normal'. Pain generally subsides within minutes after the thaw. Deeper freezing on the forehead and temples may produce a migraine or vascular type of pain lasting for hours. Urtication and edema occur within minutes of freezing and exudation within 12 to 24 hours. Haemorrhage occurring after freezing is rare. A very rare complication is nitrogen gas insufflation of subcutaneous tissue, which occurs only with the spray method. Histamine shock has been observed in a patient with cold urticaria. Cold-sensitive patients (cryoglobulinaemia, cryofibrinogenemia, cold urticaria, Raynaud's disease and collagen vascular disease) should not be treated with cryosurgery. Not infrequently, syncopal episodes occur in patients receiving N_2 therapy for warts, secondary to a vasovagal reaction. Febrile systemic toxic reactions are very rare. Cardiac arrest in a person treated with N_2 applications for actinic keratoses of the lips and forehead has been reported [18].

Short-term reactions

Haemorrhage is unusual in postoperative cryosurgical wounds. Post-operative infections are uncommon but may be seen in slow-healing wounds with a thick crust. Granuloma pyogenicum may develop in healing cryosurgical wounds. Paraesthesia of the fingers may occur in physicians from repeated contact with the nitrogen-cooled nozzle of a cryosurgical unit [23].

Long-term complications

Pseudoepitheliomatous hyperplasia, which may be confused with a recurrence of a treated malignancy, is self-limited. Milia formation is more commonly seen after a deeper freeze. Onychodystrophies from the treatment of periungual warts are usually reversible [21]. The most serious long-term complication of cryosurgery is nerve damage [19], which may occur especially at the sides of the fingers. Few cases of nerve damage have been reported, and (virtually) all appear to have been temporary [20]). Sensory loss, although mild, is regularly found following cryosurgery [22]. Pigmentary changes occur much more commonly in blacks and other deeply pigmented individuals. Tissue defects occur most commonly when treating skin cancer and include atrophy, cartilage defects, permanent alopecia, ectropion, notching of the eyelids and the ala nasi, and loss of eyelashes. Delayed healing in cryosurgical wounds may result in hypertrophic scar formation.

20.5 REFERENCES

1. Clark, D.P., Hanke, C.W. and Swanson, N.A. (1989): Dermal implants: safety of products injected for soft tissue augmentation. *J. Am. Acad. Dermatol., 21*, 992–998.
2. Hanke, C.W., Higley, H.R., Jolivette, D.M., Swanson, N.A. and Stegman, S.J. (1991): Abscess formation and local necrosis after treatment with Zyderm or Zyplast Collagen Implant. *J. Am. Acad. Dermatol., 25*, 319–326.
3. DeLustro, F., Fries, J., Kang, A., et al. (1988): Immunity to injectable collagen and autoimmune disease; a summary of current understanding. *J. Dermatol. Surg. Oncol., 14 (suppl)*, 57–65.

4. Elson, M.L. (1988): Clinical assessment of Zyplast Implant: A year of experience for soft tissue contour correction. *J. Am. Acad. Dermatol., 18*, 707–13.
5. McCoy, J.P., Waldinger, T.P., Cohen, K.A., et al. (1987): Connective tissue disease and bovine collagen implants. *J. Am. Acad. Dermatol., 16*, 315–318.
6. Ruiz-Espara, J., Bailin, M. and Bailin, P.L. (1987): Treatment of depressed cutaneous scars with gelatin matrix implants: a multicenter study. *J. Am. Acad. Dermatol., 16*, 1155–1162
7. Webster, R.C., Fuleihan, N.S., Hamdan, U.S. et al. (1986): Injectable silicone: report of 17,000 facial treatments since 1962. *Am. J. Cosmetic Surg.*, 3, 41–48.
8. Ellenbogen, R. and Rubin, L. (1975): Injectable fluid silicone therapy: human morbidity and mortality. *JAMA, 234*, 308.
9. Arndt, K.A. (1982): Argon laser therapy of small cutaneous vascular lesions. *Arch. Dermatol., 118*, 220–224.
10. Olbricht, S.M., Stern, R.S., Tang, S.V., Noe, J.M. and Arndt, K.A. (1987): Complications of cutaneous laser surgery. A survey. *Arch. Dermatol., 123*, 345–349.
11. Matarasso, S.L. and Glogau, R.G. (1991): Chemical Face Peels. In: *Cosmetics and Cosmetic Surgery in Dermatology*, pp. 131–150. (Dermatologic Clinics). Editor: M.N. O'Donoghue. Saunders, Philadelphia.
12. Brody, H.J. (1989): Complications of chemical peeling. *J. Dermatol. Surg. Oncol., 15*, 1010–1019.
13. Collins, P.S. (1989): Trichloroacetic acid peels revisited. *J. Dermatol. Surg. Oncol., 15*, 933–940.
14. Collins, P.S. (1987): The chemical peel. *Clin Dermatol., 5*, 57–74.
15. Stegman, S.J., Tromovitch, T.A. and Glogau, R.G. (1989): Chemical Peels. In: *Cosmetic Dermatologic Surgery*. pp. 35–58. Editor: S.J. Stegman. Year Book Medical Publishers, Chicago.
16. Beeson, W.H. (1987): The importance of cardiac monitoring in superficial and deep chemical peeling. *J. Dermatol. Surg. Oncol., 13,* 949–950.
17. Elton, R.F. (1983): Complications of cutaneous cryosurgery. *J. Am. Acad. Dermatol.*, 8, 513–519.
18. Goldstein, N. (1979): Cardiac arrest following application of liquid nitrogen. *J. Dermatol. Surg. Oncol., 5*, 602.
19 Millns, J.L. (1980): Neurological complications of cryosurgery. *J. Dermatol. Surg. Oncol., 6*, 207–213.
20. Zacarian, S.A. (1983): Neuropathy after cryosurgery. *J. Am. Acad. Dermatol., 8*, 422.
21. Baran, R. (1985): Brachytelephalangie revelée à l'occasion de dystrophies ungeales induites par cryothérapie. *Ann. Dermatol. Venereol., 112*, 365–367.
22. Faber, W.R., Naafs, B. and Sillevis Smitt, J.H. (1987): Sensory loss following cryosurgery of skin lesions. *Br. J. Dermatol., 117*, 343–347.
23. Heidenheim, M. and Jemec, G.B.E. (1991): Side effects of cryotherapy. *J. Am. Acad. Dermatol., 24*, 653.

21. Cosmetics: Introduction

COSMETICS: WHAT THEY ARE AND WHAT THEY DO

21.1 A 'cosmetic product' means any substance or preparation intended for placing in contact with the various external parts of the human body (epidermis, hair system, nails, lips and external genital organs) or with the teeth and the mucous membranes of the oral cavity with a view exclusively or principally to cleaning them, perfuming them or protecting them in order to keep them in good conditions, change their appearance or correct body odours (Cosmetic Directive 76/768/EEC, Article 1). The products to be considered as cosmetic products within the meaning of this definition are shown in the following illustrative list by category:

- Creams, emulsions, lotions, gels and oils for the skin (hands, face, feet, etc.)
- Face masks (with the exception of peeling products)
- Tinted bases (liquids, pastes, powders)
- Make-up powders, after-bath powders, hygienic powders, etc.
- Toilet soaps, deodorant soaps, etc.
- Perfumes, toilet waters and eau de Cologne
- Bath and shower preparations (salts, foams, oils, gels, etc.)
- Depilatories
- Deodorants and antiperspirants
- Hair care products:
  - hair tints and bleaches
  - products for waving, straightening and fixing
  - setting products
  - cleansing products (lotions, powders, shampoos)
  - conditioning products (lotions, creams, oils)
  - hairdressing products (lotions, lacquers, brilliantines)
- Shaving products (creams, foams, lotions, etc.)
- Products for making up and removing make-up from the face and the eyes
- Products intended for application to the lips
- Products for care of the teeth and the mouth
- Products for nail care and make-up
- Products for external intimate hygiene
- Sunbathing products
- Products for tanning without sun
- Skin-whitening products
- Anti-wrinkle products

In the USA a slightly different definition is used, which defines cosmetics as "articles intended to be applied to the human body for cleansing, beautifying, promoting attractiveness, or altering the appearance *without affecting the body's structure or function*" (Federal Food, Drug and Cosmetics (FD&C) Act). This means that sun tanning preparations intended to protect against sunburn, anti-caries toothpastes, anti-dandruff shampoos and antiperspirants that are also deodorants are not considered cosmetics in the USA. Instead they are classified as OTC (over the counter) drugs, for which more stringent rules apply.

Cosmetics have been used for millennia to embellish the physical, mental, and spiritual well being of mankind. These products are used with one or more of the following purposes:
- for the daily care and hygiene of the body (soap, shampoo, toothpaste, moisturising and cleansing cream)
- to enhance attractiveness (make-up, hair colour, permanent wave, setting and styling gel, nail lacquer)
- to obtain a pleasant smell (deodorant, perfume, aftershave, mouth-freshener)
- for protection (sunbathing products)
- for the masking of skin defects, e.g. vitiligo, wine spots

Recent studies have indicated that cosmetics can bring substantial psychological benefits [1].

COSMETICS: THE EXTENT OF THEIR USAGE

21.2 Cosmetic products are used by everyone. In 1974, a consumer panel of 10,050 family units (35,490 persons) located throughout the USA was interviewed on personal cosmetic usage pattern (Westat Report [2]). The results are shown in Table 21.1.

Table 21.1. Number of panel members using at least one cosmetic brand at least once during September 1974 by product category (Westat Report [2])

Product category	Number of panel members	% (n = 35,490)
Soap	30,819	87%
Toothpaste/polish/whitener	29,163	82%
Shampoo	28,287	80%
Deodorant/antiperspirant	21,703	61%
Talcum/bath powder/spray	15,925	45%
Mouthwash/breath freshener	16,983	48%
Hand/body lotion	15,347	43%
Colognes	12,117	34%
Cream rinse/conditioner	9,544	27%
Lipstick	9,517	27%
Bath bubble/oil/capsule	9,203	26%

(continued)

Table 21.1 *(continuation)*

Product category	Number of panel members	% (n = 35,490)
Hair spray/lacquer	8,763	25%
Aftershave	8,709	25%
Shave cream	8,237	23%
Nail polish	7,666	22%
Foot powder/spray	7,518	21%
Polish remover	7,267	20%
Facial skin cream/cleaner	7,100	20%
Face powder/blusher/rouge	6,828	19%
Mascara	6,623	19%
Eye shadow	6,272	18%
Suntan/sunscreen	6,449	18%
Foundation/base/lightener	5,902	17%
Moisturiser/lotion	6,128	17%
Hair dressing	5,008	14%
Eyebrow pencil	4,426	12%
Cleanser/make-up remover	3,968	11%
Skin freshener/adstringent	3,799	11%
Night cream	3,774	11%
Setting/waving gel/solution	3,307	9%
Eyeliner	3,190	9%
Hair colour/bleach	2,943	8%
Hardener/extender	2,881	8%
Cuticle remover/softener	2,898	8%
Feminine hygiene deodorant	2,168	6%
Douche	1,958	6%
Nail undercoat/base coat	2,094	6%
Eye cream	1,438	4%
Home permanent	1,466	4%
Depilatory	1,133	3%
Beard softener	615	2%
Hair relaxer/straightener	132	<1%

The product categories used by the largest number of consumers were soap (87%), toothpaste/polish/whitener (82%), shampoo (80%), deodorant/antiperspirant (61%), mouthwash/breath freshener (48%), talcum/bath powder/spray (45%) and hand/body lotion (43%). The cosmetic categories used by the smallest number of consumers were hair relaxer/straightener (<1%), beard softener (2%), depilatory (3%), eye cream (4%) and home permanent (4%).

We have conducted a survey on cosmetic usage pattern in 811 (regular) female clients of beauticians [3]. The results are shown in Table 21.2. Obviously this group of consumers is a very attractive target population to the cosmetic industry. Toothpaste, shampoo, facial cream/lotion and perfume/toilet water were used by more than 90% of the 811 women. Between 80 and 90% of the clients interviewed used deodorant/antiperspirant, eye shadow, lipstick, soap, and body lotion. Mascara, facial tonic/milk, facial mask, bath/shower foam, hand lotion/cream, and nail lacquer were used by 70–80% of these women [3].

Table 21.2. Cosmetic usage pattern in 811 female clients of beauticians [3]

Product category	No. of clients using products of this category	%
Shampoo	798	98%
Toothpaste	781	96%
Facial cream/lotion	753	93%
Perfume/toilet water	741	91%
Lipstick	703	87%
Soap	705	87%
Body lotion	662	82%
Deodorant/antiperspirant	669	82%
Eye shadow	667	82%
Facial mask	640	79%
Facial tonic/milk	629	78%
Hand lotion/cream	598	74%
Mascara	600	74%
Bath/shower foam	583	72%
Nail lacquer	570	70%
Rouge	558	69%
Nail lacquer remover	562	69%
Cream rinse	496	61%
Hair conditioner	447	55%
Liquid make-up	435	54%
Make-up remover	427	53%
Permanent (hairdresser)	430	53%
Eye pencil	418	52%
Hair lacquer	413	51%
Eye cosmetics remover	391	48%
Bath oil	310	38%
Depilatory cream	262	32%

(continued)

Table 21.2 *(continuation)*

Product category	No. of clients using products of this category	%
Brow pencil	256	32%
Hair dye/bleach	241	30%
Facial powder	205	25%
Colour shampoo	195	24%
Eye cream	193	24%
Mouth freshener	177	22%
Eyeliner	151	19%
Camouflage stick	158	19%
Bath salt	137	17%
Nail hardener (conditioner)	121	15%
Body powder	114	14%
Foot powder	100	12%
Dry shampoo	60	7%
Permanent (at home)	45	6%
Artificial nail	33	4%

Vast sums of money are involved in cosmetics and toiletry products. In the USA, the value of 1991 sales for the six major categories had an estimated value of $5.1 billion, hair care; $3.9 billion, fragrances; $1.8 billion, skin care; $1.6 billion, deodorants and antiperspirants; $1.2 billion, dentifrices; and $1.9 billion for other cosmetics, including mouthwashes, sun care items and shaving preparations [4].

In 1991, the sales (at factory prices) by the members of the Dutch Cosmetics Association amounted to 1.402 billion Dutch guilders (approximately $0.75 billion), an increase of 9.6% over 1990. This represents approximately 80% of the entire Dutch market. The shares of the various product categories are shown in Table 21.3.

Table 21.3. 1991 Sales of the members of the Dutch Cosmetics Association. Shares of various products categories and % increase over 1990

Product category	Sales 1991 (millions)	% of Total	% Increase
Hair care products	335	23.89	8.8
Perfumes, colognes	123	8.77	15.0
Products for oral hygiene	140	9.99	9.4
Baby products	35	2.50	0.0

(continued)

Table 21.3 *(continuation)*

Product category	Sales 1991 (millions)	% of Total	% Increase
Skin care products	237	16.90	12.9
Beautifying cosmetics	123	8.77	7.0
Bath cosmetics and deodorants	198	14.12	5.9
Men's cosmetics	138	9.84	15.0
Soap (luxury products)	33	2.35	0.0
Others, including sun cosmetics	40	2.85	11.1
Total	1402	100	9.6

Until recently, marketing efforts have been directed mainly at women. At present, there is an increase in the usage of cosmetic products by men.

THE INGREDIENTS OF COSMETICS

21.3 Cosmetics are complex mixtures of chemical compounds. About 8,000 vehicle raw materials and fragrance ingredients are available to the cosmetic chemist. Although the rational approach to formulation is fairly logical and simple, the abundance of available ingredients has created endless variety in cosmetic formulations. An illustrative example is moisturising cream:

Moisturising cream	
Lipid	500
Surfactant; emulsifier	1000
Polyol; humectant	20
Thickener	30
Moisturising agent	50
Antioxidant	40
Preservative	150
Colour	500
Fragrance	3500
Total	5790

Thus, nearly 6000 ingredients are available to a chemist wanting to formulate a moisturising cream. The substances used in cosmetic products may (arbitrarily) be divided into six functional classes (and subclasses):

1. *Antimicrobials and antioxidants* (§ 27.5)
   - antioxidants and chelating agents
   - antimicrobials: acids (salts), esters, alcohols, amides
   - formaldehyde and donor compounds
   - mercurials
   - phenols, halogenated phenols, organohalogen compounds
   - cationic compounds
   - miscellaneous

2. *Fragrance materials* (§ 30.7). This is the largest group of cosmetic ingredients, consisting of thousands of fragrances of natural origin and synthetic materials. The Research Institute for Fragrance Materials (RIFM) has investigated over 800 fragrance materials for their sensitising potential (§ 30.7).

3. *Colours* (§ 30.10). Colours are classified as follows:

Dyes	*Colour index numbers*
Nitroso	10000–10299
Nitro	10300–10999
Azo	
Monoazo	11000–19999
Disazo	20000–29999
Trisazo	30000–34999
Polyazo	35000–36999
Azoic	37000–39999
Stilbene	40000–40799
Carotenoid	40800–40999
Diphenylmethane	41000–41999
Triarylmethane	42000–44999
Xanthene	45000–45999
Acridine	46000–46999
Quinoline	47000–47999
Methine and Polymethine	48000–48999
Thiazole	49000–49399
Indamine and Indophenol	49400–49999
Azine	50000–50999
Oxazine	51000–51999
Thiazine	52000–52999
Sulfur	53000–54999
Lactone	55000–55999
Aminoketone	56000–56999
Hydroxyketone	57000–57999
Anthraquinone	58000–72999
Indigoid	73000–73999
Phthalocyanine	74000–74999
Natural organic colouring matters	75000–75999
Oxidation bases	76000–76999
Inorganic colouring matters	77000–77999

4. *Sunscreens* (§ 30.13)
   - PABA-derivatives
   - anthranilates
   - salicylates
   - cinnamates
   - benzophenones
   - dibenzoyl methanes
   - camphoric UV-absorbers
   - miscellaneous

5. *Lipids and surfactants* (§ 30.15)
   - lipids
   - anionic surfactants
   - cationic surfactants
   - non-ionic surfactants
   - amphoteric surfactants
   - amines, aminoalkanols
   - polyols (polyalcohols)

6. *Miscellaneous cosmetic ingredients* (§ 30.16 and 30.17)
   These include a variety of cosmetic ingredients which may be divided into the following (functional) classes

   acidic agents
   adhesive aids
   adsorbents
   adstringents
   aerosol propellants
   alcohol denaturants
   alkaline agents
   amino acids
   antiperspirants
   antiseborrhoeic agents
   buffering salts
   counterirritants
   depilating agents
   hair waving agents
   humectants
   natural ingredients
   oxidising agents
   perfume carriers
   plasticisers
   polymers
   powder fillers
   skin abrasives
   skin healing agents
   solvents
   suspending agents
   sweeteners
   thickeners
   vitamins

THE FREQUENCY OF USAGE OF COSMETIC INGREDIENTS

21.4 No data exist on the frequency of usage of the various ingredients in cosmetics and toiletries in the EC. In the USA, the Food and Drug Administration had approximately 20,000 cosmetic formulas of wholesale products on file in 1992. The 100 ingredients found most frequently to be present in these formulas (fragrances and flavors not included) are listed in Table 21.4, together with the numbers of products containing them. It should be appreciated that these data are collected in a program in which the industry submits their formulas voluntarily, and that the list may not completely reflect the actual situation in the USA. Furthermore, ingredients used by cosmetic chemists/companies in the USA and EC may differ considerably. Nevertheless, most ingredients on this list will probably also be in the 'top 100' in the EC.

Table 21.4. The 100 most frequently used ingredients in ± 20000 cosmetic formulas on file with FDA (February 1992); number of products containing the ingredients [6]

No. of products	Ingredient	Function
13014	water	solvent
7573	methylparaben	preservative
6234	propylparaben	preservative
4896	propylene glycol	solvent
3446	titanium dioxide	color; pigment
3377	triethanolamine	amine
2882	cetyl alcohol	lipid
2605	alcohol, denatured	solvent
2603	glycerin	polyol
2579	stearic acid	lipid
2489	iron oxides	color; pigment
2195	talc	color; bulking agent
2118	imidazolidinyl urea	preservative
2073	citric acid	acidic agent
2025	FD&C Yellow No. 5	color
1894	glyceryl stearate	lipid
1706	FD&C Blue No. 1	color
1568	dimethicone	lipid
1469	mica	color
1368	isopropyl myristate	lipid, solvent
1329	butylparaben	preservative
1316	hydrolyzed animal protein	protein derivative
1246	ultramarines (red, blue, pink, green, violet)	color
1152	carnauba	lipid
1105	isopropyl alcohol	solvent
1069	allantoin	skin healing agent
1029	castor oil	lipid
1025	panthenol	vitamin
1021	lanolin	lipid
1006	FD&C Red No. 4	color

(continued)

Table 21.4 *(continuation)*

No. of products	Ingredient	Function
974	D&C Red No. 7 calcium lake	color
948	ammonium hydroxide	alkaline agent
904	ethylparaben	preservative
894	carbomer 940	viscosity increasing agent
885	quaternium-15	preservative
871	sodium chloride	salt
866	candelilla wax	lipid
864	oleic acid	lipid
843	polysorbate 20	nonionic emulsifier
819	zinc stearate	anti caking agent
811	stearyl alcohol	lipid
799	resorcinol	hair dye
796	kaolin	absorbent
788	magnesium aluminum silicate	suspending agent
773	trisodium EDTA	chelating agent
771	DMDM hydantoin	preservative
767	D&C Red No. 33	color
766	ozokerite	lipid
761	*p*-phenylenediamine	hair dye
756	lanolin oil	lipid
748	lauramide DEA	non-ionic surfactant
746	disodium EDTA	chelating agent
740	hydroxyethyl ethylcellulose	viscosity increasing agent
728	carbomer 934	viscosity increasing agent
724	EDTA	chelating agent
719	FD&C Yellow No. 6	color
718	cyclomethicone	lipid
711	cocamide DEA	nonionic emulsifier
689	bismuth oxychloride	color
685	phenoxyethanol	preservative
676	paraffin	lipid
672	*p*-aminophenol	hair color
666	tocopherol	anti-oxidant
647	methylchloroisothiazolinone	preservative
644	D&C Red No. 6 barium lake	color

(continued)

Table 21.4 *(continuation)*

No. of products	Ingredient	Function
631	methylisothiazolinone	preservative
627	lecithin	skin conditioner; emulsifier
624	sodium sulfite	anti-oxidant
618	isopropyl palmitate	lipid
606	octyldodecanol	lipid
598	isopropyl lanolate	lipid
569	carmine	color
551	m-aminophenol	hair dye
551	squalane	lipid
550	sodium laureth sulfate	anionic detergent
544	D&C Yellow No. 10	color
539	silica	powder flow aid
525	sodium borate	alkaline agent
524	sorbitol	humectant, polyol
522	acetylated lanolin alcohol	lipid
522	xanthan gum	viscosity increasing agent
521	cocamidopropyl betaine	amphoteric surfactant
519	lanolin alcohol	lipid
513	octyl palmitate	lipid
505	manganese violet	color
487	isobutane	aerosol propellant
474	polysorbate 60	nonionic emulsifier
470	menthol	fragrance
468	microcrystalline wax	lipid
464	carbomer 941	viscosity increasing agent
460	benzophenone-2	sunscreen
460	dimethicone copolyol	lipid
458	propane	aerosol propellant
457	sweet almond oil	lipid
454	PVP	film former
447	diazolidinyl urea	preservative
437	oleyl alcohol	lipid
428	nonoxynol-4	nonionic surfactant
426	camphor	fragrance
421	aminomethyl propanol	aminoalkanol

LEGISLATION

European Community

21.5 Directive 76/768 EEC of the European Council and its subsequent amendments lay down the requirements for cosmetic products traded in the EC and form the basis of the legislation of cosmetic products in the EC member states. The Directive consists of a general part, which gives definitions and general regulations and seven annexes, concerned with detailing the definition and with restrictions to specific groups of ingredients.

Directive EC 76/768 defines cosmetics as "any substance or preparation intended for placing into contact with the various external parts of the human body (epidermis, hair system, nails, lips and external genital organs) or with the teeth and the mucous membranes of the oral cavity with a view exclusively or principally to cleaning them or protecting them in order to keep them in good condition, change their appearance or correct body odours." The definition is elaborated by providing an illustrative list of the product categories which are considered to fall under this definition in Annex I (see § 21.1). Cosmetic products may not be marketed within the EC when "they are liable to cause damage to human health when they are applied under normal conditions of use" (Article 2), or "when they do not conform to the provisions of the Directive and its Annexes" (Article 3). Besides Annex 1, six additional Annexes restrict the application of ingredients of different categories (Articles 3, 4 and 5). An overview of these Annexes is given in Table 21.5.

Table 21.5. Overview of Annexes to Directive 76/768 EC (up to the 12th Commission Directive (1990))

Annex	Concerned with	Restrictions	Example entries	No. of entries
I	illustrative list by category of cosmetic products		creams, perfumes, depilatories	
II	list of substances which cosmetics must not contain	use prohibited	ephedrine and its salts; bithionol; tretinoin; etc.	394
III	list of substances which cosmetics must not contain, except subject to restrictions and conditions laid down	limitations with respect to concentration and site of application; labelling requirements	thioglycollic acid (permanent waves); fluorides (tooth pastes), resorcinol (hair dyes), etc.	59
IV	list of coloring agents which can be contained in cosmetics	limitations on site of application, concentration and purity; labelling requirements	CI 14815; CI 15880; caramel; etc.	164

(continued)

Table 21.5 *(continuation)*

Annex	Concerned with	Restrictions	Example entries	No. of entries
V	list of compounds which are exempted from the Directive		strontium and its compounds with a number of exceptions; etc.	3
VI	list of preservatives which can be contained in cosmetics	limitations on concentration, site of application; labelling requirements	parabens; DMDM hydantoin; methyl-isothiazolinone and methylchloroisothia-zolinone; etc.	52
VI	list of UV filters which can be contained in cosmetics	limitations on concentration, labelling requirements	isopropyldibenzoyl-methane; homosalate; oxybenzone; etc.	122

Annex V lists a few substances which are excepted from the scope of the Directive and for which the member states may take their own measures. Its significance is weaning, and the European legislation with respect to cosmetic products may theoretically be considered to be harmonized. In practice, not all member states have implemented the Directive and its amendments completely, and trade barriers seem to increase rather than to be breaking down.

Further regulations in the Directive comprise general labelling requirements, i.e. name and address of manufacturer, contents, batch code, etc., must be listed (Article 6).

At present, ingredient labelling of cosmetic products is not compulsive in the EC, a situation that greatly obstructs effective dermatological investigation of cosmetic side effects. This situation will probably change quickly, as ingredient labelling is part of the proposed 11th amendment of the Directive, which is expected to be effected in 1995. Meanwhile the Directive provides a possibility of obtaining the necessary information for a dermatological investigation in Article 6, which allows a member state to "require, for purposes of prompt and appropriate medical treatment in the event of difficulties, that adequate and sufficient information regarding substances contained in cosmetic products is made available to the competent authority, which shall ensure that this information is used only for the purposes of such treatment". Many manufacturers are cooperative and will help the dermatologist without intervention of the competent authority, but this Article may be of value as a last resort.

When implemented, the 11th Amendment will add a number of additional requirements. They are concerned with, among other things, decreasing the use of animals for safety testing and ascertaining higher standards of production. It will also make the keeping of records of a product's side effects by its manufacturer compulsive. In addition a list will be compiled of cosmetic ingredients used in the production of cosmetic products marketed in the EC. This table will list the chemical name of the ingredient and CAS, EINECS and Color Index numbers. At present, it appears that the nomenclature to be chosen will, with few exceptions, conform to the CTFA nomenclature — the accepted standard nomenclature for cosmetic ingredients in the USA.

USA

21.6 Cosmetics marketed in the United States must comply with the provisions of the Federal Food, Drug and Cosmetic (FD&C) Act, the Fair Packaging and Labeling (FP&L) Act and the regulations published by the FDA (Food and Drug Administration) under authority of these laws.

The FD&C Act defines cosmetics as "articles intended to be applied to the human body for cleansing, beautifying, promoting attractiveness, or altering the appearance without affecting the body's structure or functions". Soap — making no label claim other than cleansing of the human body — is exempted, but skin creams, lotions, perfumes, lipsticks, fingernail polishes, eye and facial make-up preparations, shampoos, permanent waves, hair colors, tooth pastes, deodorants, etc. are considered cosmetics under this definition.

In contrast to European legislation, under US law cosmetic products can also be considered drugs at the same time if they are intended to treat or prevent disease, or affect the structure or the functions of the human body. Such products must comply both with the cosmetics regulations and the drug regulations in the FD&A Law. The latter requirements are obviously more extensive. Examples are: anti-caries toothpastes, anti-dandruff shampoos, hormone creams, sun-protection cosmetics, antiperspirants/deodorants. Such products will generally be OTC (over-the-counter) drugs.

Cosmetics may not be introduced when *adulterated* or *misbranded.* A cosmetic is *adulterated* when:
- it contains a substance or its container is composed of a substance which may make the product harmful to customers under customary conditions of use;
- it contains filth;
- it is manufactured or held under unsanitary conditions whereby it may have become harmful to the user or contaminated with filth;
- it contains a non-permitted, or in some instances non-certified, color; hair dyes bearing the proper labelling exempted.

Cosmetics are *misbranded* when:
- their labelling is false or misleading;
- the labelling required by the FD&C act is missing;
- the container is made or filled in a deceptive manner.

Manufacturers may, on their own responsibility, use essentially any raw material as an ingredient, with a few exceptions. Only FDA approved colors are allowed under certain FDA specified limitations. A number of substances are prohibited in cosmetics: bithionol, halogenated salicylanilides (for their potential as photosensitizers), chloroform, vinyl chloride, methylene chloride, and AETT. Restrictions exist on the use of hexachlorophene, chlorofluorocarbon propellants and zirconium complexes.

Labelling must comply with the regulations published by the FDA under authority of the FD&C Act and the FP&L Act (Fair Packaging and Labelling Act). For cosmetics whose safety has not been substantiated, a warning statement to this effect must appear on the label. Labelling must also include the name and address of the manufacturer, warning statements when required, directions for use and a list of the ingredients.

Ingredient declaration must declare the ingredients in descending order of predominance. Color additives and ingredients present at one percent or less may be declared without regard for predominance. The ingredients must be declared by the names accepted or adopted by regulation; in practice, with exceptions, CTFA nomenclature is used.

21.7 REFERENCES

1. Graham, J.A. (1988): Cosmetic therapy for aging skin. *J. Soc. Cosm. Chem., 39* , 43–51.
2. Westat Inc. (1975): *An Investigation of Consumers' Perceptions of Adverse Reactions to Cosmetic Products.* National Technical Information Service, US Department of Commerce.
3. De Groot, A.C., Beverdam, E.G.A., Tjong Ayong, C., Coenraads, P.J. and Nater, J.P. (1988): The role of contact allergy in the spectrum of adverse effects caused by cosmetics and toiletries. *Contact Dermatitis, 19*, 195–201.
4. The Rose sheet, 1993, Jan. 11, pp. 3–4
5. *Annual Report* (1992): Nederlandse Cosmetica Vereniging, Nieuwegein, The Netherlands.
6. Food and Drug Administration (1992): Washington DC, USA. Data provided by Dr. J.A. Wenninger and A.L. Halper.
7. *Cosmetic Bench Reference 1990* (1990): Allured Publishing Corporation, Wheaton, IL.

22. The spectrum of side effects of cosmetics

22.1 Cosmetics have often been denigrated as insignificant and frivolous. Also, many dermatologists believed that these products did more harm than good. An illustrative discussion took place in a meeting of the American Medical Association in the year 1925, in connection with a presentation on cosmetic side effects [1].

Dr. Harold N. Cole, Cleveland: It is well for our members to keep this before the profession and before the public. I hope the American Medical Association will see that this matter is circularized through the newspapers again. In that way we shall do much toward letting the *senseless women* know what they are doing in using dyes in their hair, rouge and other cosmetics.

Dr. Lulu Hunt Peters, New York: I am one of the senseless women who have been addicted to powder and rouge for some years, but I have never had a dermatitis. I wonder whether the percentage is not rather small.

It should be appreciated that, in those days, some hazardous materials were used in cosmetic products, such as lead carbonate, bismuth and mercurials. Nowadays, serious adverse reactions to cosmetics are infrequent. However, side effects do occur and are by no means rare (Chapter 23). Unwanted effects of cosmetics can be classified as follows:

1. Irritation (objective and/or subjective)
2. Contact allergy
3. Photosensitivity
4. Contact urticaria
5. Acne/folliculitis
6. Colour changes of the skin and appendages
7. Other local side effects
8. Systemic side effects

IRRITATION

22.2 *Subjective irritation* may be defined as chemically induced burning, stinging, itching, or other skin discomfort *without* visible, obvious signs of inflammation [2]. It is estimated that between 1 and 10% of all cosmetic users note and often complain of this discomfort, primarily on the face [2]. *Objective irritation* is defined as non-immunologically mediated inflammation of the skin. Its signs are usually mild erythema and scaling, but frank dermatitis may occur. Irritation may be observed with cosmetic products containing detergents such as soap, shampoo, and bath/shower foam. The humid climate in, and anatomical occlusion of, the axillae favour irritant responses to deodorants and antiperspirants [3]. Surfactants and emulsifiers present in moisturising or emollient creams may cause irritation, especially when applied to facial skin. Daily application of eye make-up cosmetics and removal with cleansing products often irritate the sensitive skin of the eyelids.

CONTACT ALLERGY

22.3 Allergic reactions to cosmetic products are often unrecognised, both by the patient and by the physician. Several factors are involved:

(a) Frequently patients have used the causative cosmetics for many years; the development of skin problems from such products conflicts with the consumer's perception of allergy, which is based on the assumption that a *new* cosmetic has to be introduced.

(b) Cosmetic allergy is sometimes manifested by mild reactions only, e.g. itching, erythema and scaling of the eyelids.

(c) Cosmetic dermatitis may sometimes be noticed, but wrongly interpreted. Psoriasis of the face may be exacerbated by cosmetic dermatitis [4]; dermatitis caused by emollient creams interpreted as worsening of dry skin or atopic dermatitis for which it was applied; and contact allergy to sunscreens as failure of the product to adequately protect the skin against the sun's rays. The literature on cosmetic allergy is surveyed in Chapters 26–29.

PHOTOSENSITIVITY (see Chapter 6)

22.4 Contact photosensitivity (CPS) implies chemical photosensitivity resulting from UV-induced excitation of a chemical applied to the skin. Traditionally, CPS has been divided into phototoxic and photoallergic reactions; however, in practice, it is often difficult to categorise the individual photochemical reaction in vivo.

Phototoxic reactions may be experienced by an individual, provided that the ultraviolet light contains the appropriate wave-lengths to activate the compound, and that the UV dose and the concentration of the photoreactive chemical are high enough. For photoallergic reactions, which are rare compared with both contact allergic and phototoxic reactions, a sensitisation period is required. The reactions are usually delayed, becoming manifest days or weeks after the UV exposure. A major problem with photoallergy is that the patients often remain photosensitive for many years, even when contact with the offending chemical is meticulously avoided ('persistent light reactions') [5].

With the exception of the epidemic caused by halogenated salicylanilides in the 1960s [6], photosensitivity has accounted for only a small proportion of cosmetic-related side effects. In a study from the USA [7], photoallergy and phototoxicity were responsible for only 9 reactions in 713 patients investigated for cosmetic dermatitis. Currently, musk ambrette, a fragrance in some aftershaves, has been reported as a major cause of cosmetic photosensitivity reactions [8].

Cosmetics and ingredients of cosmetics and topical drugs which have caused photosensitivity reactions are listed in § 6.5.

CONTACT URTICARIA (see Chapter 7)

22.5 On the basis of the action mechanisms involved, contact urticaria (nowadays also called 'immediate contact reactions') can be divided into non-immunological and immunological reactions. On a clinical basis, the following division has been suggested [9]:

Cutaneous reactions only
Stage 1: Localised urticaria
Dermatitis/dermatosis
Non-specific symptoms (e.g. itching, tingling, burning)

Stage 2: Generalised urticaria

Extracutaneous reactions
Stage 3: Bronchial asthma
Rhinoconjunctivitis
Otolaryngeal symptoms
Gastrointestinal symptoms

Stage 4: Anaphylactoid reactions

Contact urticaria is infrequently described as a cause of cosmetic-related adverse reactions. However, many cases of 'irritation' (itching, burning, tingling) may actually represent contact urticarial responses, especially non-immunological contact urticaria from sorbic acid, benzoates and cinnamic aldehyde. Cosmetic products that have been reported to induce contact urticaria are listed in Table 22.1. Cosmetics and ingredients of cosmetics and topical drugs that have caused contact urticarial reactions are listed in Table 7.5

Table 22.1. Cosmetics which have caused contact urticaria

bath oil
deodorant
diaper rash ointment
fixation fluid for permanent wave
hair bleach
hair conditioner
hair dye
hair spray
nail varnish
permanent wave fluid
rouge
shampoo (egg-containing)
tooth paste
perfumes

ACNE/FOLLICULITIS (see Chapter 9)

22.6 For follicular eruptions caused by cosmetic products the term *acne cosmetica* has been coined [10]. They consist mainly of closed comedones. Blackheads are scarce, sometimes papulo-pustules may be seen over the cheeks and the chin. The eruption is seen in adult women and is attributed to the comedogenic properties of cosmetics, mainly facial creams. It must be appreciated that cosmetics are weakly comedogenic. Daily use, year after year, may induce acne in predisposed subjects. Assays on the rabbit ear have identified a number of cosmetic ingredients to be potentially comedogenic. These are listed in § 9.2.

COLOUR CHANGES OF THE SKIN AND APPENDAGES (see Chapter 10)

22.7 Most colour changes as a result of contact with cosmetic products are intentional. However, cosmetics sometimes cause discoloration of the skin, nails or hair as an unwanted effect. With some exceptions (dihydroxyacetone, glutaraldehyde, monobenzone, resorcinol) such side effects are rare. Section 10.1 lists cosmetics and ingredients of cosmetics and topical drugs that have been reported to cause discoloration as a side effect.

OTHER LOCAL SIDE EFFECTS

22.8 A variety of other local effects has rarely been reported from cosmetic products. Overuse of soap on the female external genitals may cause dysuria. Excessive use of bubble baths may also lead to urinary tract irritation, especially in children. Cetrimonium bromide in shampoo may cause irreversible matting of scalp hair (Bird's nest hair). Selenium sulphide shampoo has been blamed for irreversible hair loss. The hair strengthener Ineral has caused nail dystrophy with onycholysis. Formaldehyde, phenolformaldehyde resin and toluenesulphonamide/formaldehyde resin in cosmetic nail products have caused a variety of nail abnormalities including paronychia, subungual hyperkeratosis, subungual haemorrhages, leukonychia, and onycholysis. Ochronosis and colloid milia have been caused by topical application of hydroquinone for whitening of the skin. Chlorhexidine in mouthwashes has caused disturbance of taste sensations (also with hexetidine mouthwash), ulceration of the oral mucosa, and reversible swelling of the parotid glands. Conjunctival pigmentation may be a consequence of applying eyeliner to the conjunctival side of the eyelid. Corneal ulcers have been associated with mascaras contaminated with Pseudonomas.

Details can be found in Chapters 26–29.

SYSTEMIC SIDE EFFECTS

22.9 Systemic reactions from percutaneous absorption of cosmetic ingredients are rare. Some reported serious adverse effects have been due to formulation errors (hexachlorophene) or inappropriate use (henna and *p*-phenylenediamine).

Systemic side effects of cosmetics and ingredients of cosmetics and topical drugs are discussed in Chapter 16.

22.10 REFERENCES

1. Miller, H.E. and Taussig, L.R. (1925): Cosmetics. *JAMA, 84*, 1999–2002.
2. Maibach, H.I. and Engasser, P.G. (1986): Dermatitis due to cosmetics. In: *Contact Dermatitis, 3rd Edition*, pp. 368–404. Editor: A.A. Fisher. Lea and Febiger, Philadelphia.
3. Consumers' Association (1976): *Which? Deodorants*, April.
4. De Groot, A.C. and Liem, D.H. (1983): Facial psoriasis caused by contact allergy to linalool and hydroxycitronellal in an aftershave. *Contact Dermatitis, 9*, 230–232.
5. Wennersten, G., Thune, P., Jansén, C.T. and Brodthagen, H. (1986): Photocontact dermatitis: Current status with emphasis on allergic contact photosensitivity (CPS) occurrence, allergens, and practical phototesting. *Semin. Dermatol., 5*, 277–289.
6. Wilkinson, D.S. (1961): Photodermatitis due to tetrachlorosalicylanilide. *Br. J. Dermatol., 73*, 213–219.
7. Adams, R.M. and Maibach, H.I. (1985): A five-year study of cosmetic reactions. *J. Am. Acad. Dermatol., 13*, 1062–1069.
8. Wojnarowska, F. and Calnan, C.D. (1986): Contact and photocontact allergy to musk ambrette. *Br. J. Dermatol., 114*, 667–675.
9. Von Krogh, G. and Maibach, H.I. (1981): The contact urticaria syndrome — an updated review. *J. Am. Acad. Dermatol., 5*, 328–342.
10. Kligman, A.M. and Mills, O.H. (1972): Acne cosmetica. *Arch. Dermatol., 106*, 843–846.
11. Fisher, A.A. (1986): Acne venerata in black skin. *Cutis, 37*, 24–26.

23. The frequency of adverse reactions to cosmetics and the products involved

FREQUENCY OF ADVERSE REACTIONS TO COSMETICS IN THE GENERAL POPULATION

The frequency of adverse reactions to cosmetics in the general population has been investigated in only a few studies [1–3]. These are discussed below.

UK Consumers' Association [1]

23.1 In 1978 the UK Consumers' Association performed a study aimed at determining the incidence of adverse reactions of the skin to cosmetics and toiletry products in the adult population of the United Kingdom. The research was carried out in three stages:

Stage I. Omnibus survey
A commercial market research omnibus survey was used to contact a representative sample of the population. The total number of people interviewed was 11,062. All were asked if they had experienced any kind of 'allergy' or 'reaction' as a result of using a cosmetic or toiletry product in the 12 months before the interview.

Stage II. Postal follow-up survey
A more detailed questionnaire was sent to each person who claimed (in Stage I) to have experienced an allergic reaction and who had agreed to provide further information. This questionnaire sought details of the product involved, the nature, severity and duration of the reaction and action taken by the person.

Stage III. Second follow-up survey
A sample was drawn which was designed to be representative of one particular parliamentary constituency; 1297 people were selected and 1022 were actually interviewed. All the people in the sample were interviewed with the basic questionnaire used in Stage I of the study. Those people who claimed to have had an adverse reaction were asked to fill in the Stage II questionnaire and were invited to participate in a patch testing programme. They were patch tested with their suspected products, and at least 25 cosmetic allergens.

Results

In the omnibus survey (Stage I), 1321 individuals (12%) of the adult population (16 years and older) interviewed claimed to have experienced some sort of adverse reaction of the skin to cosmetic or toiletry products in the preceding 12 months. In the second follow-up survey (Stage III), 8% of the sample apparently had had an adverse reaction within the preceding 12 months. The differences between the results of the 2 investigations were attributed to selection procedures. Of the 85 people who claimed adverse reactions in Stage III, 44 attended the patch test clinic. The results are shown in Table 23.1.

Table 23.1. Results of patch testing in the study of the UK Consumers Association

	No. of people	% of total sample	% of claimants	% of those patch tested
Patch tested	44	4.3	52	100
Total with positive reaction	34	3.3	40	77
Contact allergy	11	1.1	13	25
Irritant reaction	23	2.3	27	52
Not a cosmetic problem	10	1.0	12	23

In 34 of the 44 patients patch tested (77%), a positive reaction "of some kind" to cosmetics or cosmetic ingredients was found. In 11 patients (25%) the cosmetic-related side effects were considered to have been caused by contact allergy. In 23 patients (52%) irritation was considered to be the cause. In the other 10 patients (23%) the reactions were considered not to have been a cosmetic problem.

The cosmetic products held responsible for the perceived adverse reactions are summarised in Table 23.2

Table 23.2. Cosmetic categories causing side effects

	% of all respondents claiming an adverse reaction		
Category	Stage I	Stage II	Stage III
Soap	25	12	18
Deodorant/antiperspirant	18	25	14
Moisturising/skin cream	11	7	14
Eye make-up	13	14	12
Aftershave	9	5	6
Shampoo	8	3	7
Lipstick	7	3	6
Hair dye	3	2	4
Perfume	9	5	2

In each case the 4 products mentioned most frequently as causing an adverse reaction were the same: soap, deodorant, moisturising/skin cream and eye make-up.

Comment
This study shows that in any year approximately 10% of the adult population may suffer from cosmetic-related side effects. However, the conclusions of the patch testing programme are invalidated by an obvious misinterpretation of patch test results. If a patient had an irritant patch test reaction to a cosmetic/ingredient, the side effect experienced was interpreted as having been caused by irritation. If a patient did not react to the suspected products or the other allergens tested, it was concluded that the patient had *not* suffered from a genuine reaction to cosmetics. These data raise serious doubts about the expertise with which the study was conducted; consequently, no valid conclusions can be drawn from it.

Westat Report [3]

23.2 In 1974, a consumer panel of 10,050 family units (35,490 persons), located throughout the USA, was recruited to: (a) provide personal medical information; (b) participate in the collection of information on individual family members' use of cosmetics; and (c) participate in a system for the reporting of self-perceived adverse reactions from the use of cosmetics. The participants were instructed to report on cosmetic usage patterns and perceived injuries during a 3-month period. These adverse reactions were assessed by project dermatologists concerning their relationship to cosmetics and the severity of the reactions. In the period of 3 months, 701 reactions were reported by the participants. The dermatologists considered 589 of these (84%) genuine reactions to cosmetic products: 505 (86%) were graded as "mild", 63 (11%) as "moderate" and 13 (2%) as "severe". Most reactions were caused by deodorant/antiperspirant (28%), followed by soap (16%), skin care products (10%), eye cosmetics (7%), hair spray (6%), and shampoo and bath cosmetics (both 5%). It was stressed that the findings should not be generalised beyond the study population.

Dutch Study [2]

23.3 In 1985, 1,609 inhabitants of the community of Sellingen (in the north of The Netherlands), born between 1921 and 1951 (838 men, 771 women, aged 33–64 years, average age 47.5 years), were asked the following question: "Have you experienced side effects of cosmetics or toiletries in the preceding 5 years?". Of the 1609 subjects who were interviewed, 196 (12.2%) claimed to have suffered from side effects of cosmetics or toiletries in the preceding 5 years: 124 women (63%) and 72 men (37%). The percentages of men and women having experienced adverse reactions were 8.6% and 16.1%, respectively. The most frequently reported subjective symptom was itching (71%), followed by a feeling of dryness (63%), burning of the skin (50%) and prickling sensations (44%). Twenty-three subjects (12%) had had no visible skin changes. The others described their skin eruptions as redness, "spots", blisters, scales and chaps. Some complained of burning and watery eyes, and 3 patients had experienced shortness of breath (1 caused by perfume, 2 by their wives' hair lacquer). 1 patient had ascribed swelling of lymph nodes to the use of deodorant; another patient repeatedly started to sneeze when using an aftershave spray; and a third patient claimed that perfumes made her dizzy and nauseated. The products that were blamed for the adverse reactions are summarised in Table 23.3. Women ascribed most reactions to soap, facial cream, deodorant, shampoo and eye shadow. Among men soap also ranked first, followed by aftershave, deodorant and shower foam.

Table 23.3. Cosmetics to which side effects were attributed.

Women (n = 124)			Men (n = 72)		
Cosmetic	Number	(%)	Cosmetic	Number	(%)
soap	51	41%	soap	35	49%
facial cream	41	33%	aftershave	16	22%
deodorant	31	25%	deodorant	14	19%
shampoo	20	16%	shower foam	9	12%
eye shadow	14	11%	massage oil	2	3%
bath/shower foam	9	7%	(wife's) hair lacquer	2	3%
facial make-up	8	6%	shaving soap	1	1%
perfumes	8	6%			
mascara	5	4%			
depilatory cream	3	2%			
other*	18	15%			

*Product categories implicated by 1 or 2 women only.
N.B. The number of products exceeds the number of patients, as many mentioned more than 1 product.

The localisations of the side effects are summarised in Table 23.4. In both the men and the women, most reactions were localised on the face, the hands and in the axillae. In women, the face was far more frequently involved (60%) than in men (33%).

Table 23.4. Localisations of skin changes/complaints

Women (n = 124)			Men (n = 72)		
Localisation	Number	(%)	Localisation	Number	(%)
face	75	60%	face	24	33%
hands	24	19%	hands	15	21%
axillae	22	18%	axillae	10	14%
"all-over"	12	10%	arms	8	11%
neck	8	6%	legs	8	11%
groin/genitals	7	6%	head	4	6%
head	5	4%	"all-over"	4	6%
lips	5	4%	back	4	6%
arms	5	4%	other*	10	14%
legs	4	3%			
chest	4	3%			
back	4	3%			
other*	6	5%			

*These localisations were mentioned only 1–3 times.

23.4 Due to different methods used, comparisons between the 3 studies in the general population discussed above are difficult to make. Nevertheless, it seems justifiable to draw some (tentative) conclusions:

- Side effects of cosmetics and toiletries are by no means rare.
- Most reactions are mild, but nevertheless, 30% of the patients in the Dutch study consulted a physician [2].
- Product categories causing most reactions in women are: soap, deodorant, (facial) creams, shampoo, eye cosmetics and shower foam. In men most reactions are caused by: soap, aftershave, deodorant and shower foam.
- Women report side effects nearly twice as frequently as men; this difference is largely due to products applied to the face.
- The majority of adverse effects are caused by irritation; contact allergic reactions constitute a minority (see § 23.5). Atopic individuals may be at greater risk of developing side effects from cosmetics and toiletries caused by irritation.

FREQUENCY OF ADVERSE REACTIONS TO COSMETICS IN PATIENTS SEEN BY DERMATOLOGISTS

23.5 Reports of adverse cosmetic events in patients seen by the dermatologist usually refer to contact allergic reactions.

USA [6]

70 patients with allergic cosmetic dermatitis were investigated [6]. The total number of patients tested in the study period was not specified. The products involved are shown in Table 23.5. Most reactions were caused by skin care products (44%), followed by fragrance products (12%), hair colours (8%), deodorants/antiperspirants (8%) and eye make-up (7%).

Sweden [7]

35 patients with allergic cosmetic dermatitis were investigated [7]. This represented 0.05% (?) of the number of patients seen during the period of the investigation. The products involved are shown in Table 23.5. Most reactions were caused by eye make-up products (23%), followed by deodorants/antiperspirants (17%), skin care products (14%), hair colours (9%), and fragrance products (9%).

Spain [8]

195 patients with allergic cosmetic dermatitis were investigated [8]. This represented 0.3% of the total number of patients seen and 3.5% of the number of patients patch tested during the period of investigation. The products involved are shown in Table 23.5. Most reactions were caused by nail cosmetics (23%), followed by skin care products (19%), fragrance products (18%), facial make-up (10%), and shaving cosmetics (5%).

Table 23.5. Products involved in allergic cosmetic dermatitis

Product categories	USA [6] patients: 70 products: 73			Sweden [7] patients: 35 products: 35			Spain [8] patients: 195 products: 210			France [9] patients: 91 products: 96			USA [10] patients: 578 products: 600			Netherlands [5] patients: 49 products: 60			Netherlands [12] patients: 119 products: 131		
	No.	%	rank	No.	%	rank	No.	%	rank	No.	%	rank	No.	%	rank	No.	%	rank	No.	%	rank
Skin care products	32	44	1	5	14	3	39	19	2	30	31	1	175	29	1	27	45	1	67	51	1
Nail cosmetics	1	1	9	2	6	7	49	23	1	20	21	2	53	9	4	5	8	3	16	12	2
Hair colours	6	8	3	3	9	4	10	5	6	10	10	3	45	8	5	2	3	8			
Deodorants/anti-perspirants	6	8	4	6	17	2	10	5	7	8	8	5	?*			4	7	4	6	5	5
Fragrance products	9	12	2	3	9	5	38	18	3	4	4	6	43	7	6	3	5	7	10	8	3
Shaving preparations	3	4	7	3	9	6	11	5	5	1	1	9	21	4	7	6	10	2	3	2	7
Eye make-up products	5	7	5	8	23	1	9	4	8	10	10	4	18	3	8	4	7	5	3	2	8
Facial make-up products	5	7	6	1	3	9	21	10	4				61	10	3	1	2	9	1	1	9
Other hair products	2	3	8	2	6	8	2	1	9	3	3	7	98	16	2	4	7	6	7	5	4
Lip cosmetics							1	<1	10	3	3	8				1	2	10	5	4	6
Other products	4	5		2	6		20	10		7	7		86	14		3	5		13	10	

*Possibly included in "personal cleanliness products" ($n = 36$).

France [9]

91 patients with allergic cosmetic dermatitis were investigated [9]. This represented 4% of the patients patch tested during the period of investigation. The products involved are shown in Table 23.5. Most reactions were caused by skin care products (31%), followed by nail cosmetics (21%), hair colours (10%), eye make-up products (10%), and deodorants/antiperspirants (8%).

USA [10]

578 patients with allergic cosmetic dermatitis were investigated [10]. This represented 0.2% of the number of patients seen, and 4.4% of the number of patients patch tested during the period of the investigation. The products involved are shown in Table 23.5. Most reactions were caused by skin care products (29%), followed by hair products (colours excluded) (16%), facial make-up products (10%), nail cosmetics (9%), and hair colours (8%).

Belgium [11]

156 patients with allergic cosmetic dermatitis were investigated [11]. This represented 3.0% of the patients patch tested during the period of the investigation. Most reactions were caused by soaps and shampoos (41%), followed by make-up and skin care products (37%), hair dyes and other hair preparations (27%), fragrance products (14%), and shaving preparations (13%).

Comment: It seems highly unlikely that rinse-off products such as soaps and shampoos could be responsible for 41% of all cosmetic allergic reactions.

The Netherlands [5]

49 patients with allergic cosmetic dermatitis were investigated [5]. This represented 0.3% of all patients seen, and 3.5% of the number of patients patch tested during the period of the investigation. The products involved are shown in Table 23.5. Most reactions were caused by skin care products (45%), followed by shaving preparations (10%), nail cosmetics (8%), deodorants/antiperspirants (7%), and eye make-up products (7%).

The Netherlands [12]

119 patients with allergic cosmetic dermatitis were investigated [12]. This represented approximately 0.6% of the number of patients seen, and 5.4% of the number of patients patch tested during the period of the investigation. The products involved are shown in Table 23.5. Most reactions were caused by skin care products (51%), followed by nail cosmetics (12%), fragrance products (8%), hair cosmetics (5%), and deodorants/antiperspirants (5%).

These studies suggest the following:

1. Of dermatological patients patch tested for suspected allergic contact dermatitis, 3–5% are allergic to cosmetic products. More recent information points at a percentage of 10–15 [13].

2. Although the results of the studies vary widely, it appears that skin care products, nail cosmetics, hair cosmetics and fragrance products cause most cases of allergic cosmetic dermatitis.

Risk grading

23.6 The data for the *incidence of side effects* are not directly correlated to the actual risk of a product. Risk grading is only possible if the number of cosmetic units involved has also been counted or estimated in the reports. This is the case in two reports only [3,14]. The results of risk grading are summarized in Table 23.6.

The risk index is defined as the number of cosmetic units that caused one untoward cosmetic experience. Risk grading (high-, medium- and low-risk cosmetics) is based on these calculated risk indices. Some striking discrepancies are shown, for example:

- Eye make-up: high incidence of reports, but only 'medium-risk' cosmetic
- Depilatory: low incidence of reports, but graded as 'high-risk' cosmetic.
- An example of a cosmetic product with a high incidence of untoward experiences and also a 'high-risk' product is a deodorant–antiperspirant.

Table 23.6. Risk index of cosmetic products

Cosmetic product category	Average risk index*	
	500,000 A	1500 B
Hair		
Shampoo	L	L
Hair conditioner	L	L
Hair spray, setting lotion	L	H (700)
Permanent wave	M	L
Hair straightener	H (87,000)	L
Hair colour, bleach	M	H (800)
Hair dressing, growth promotion	L	L
Face, mouth		
Face: moisturising–cleansing cream	M	H (800)
Face: mask	M	–
Face: anti-acne	M	M
Face: skin bleach	H (55,000)	–
Face: make-up	M	M
Eye make-up	M	M
Lipstick	M	M
Toothpaste	L	L
Mouth freshener	L	L
Aftershave	L	L
Other shaving aids	L	L

(continued)

Table 23.6 *(continuation)*

Cosmetic product category	Average risk index* 500,000 A	1500 B
Body, parts of the body		
Hand and body lotion	M	L
Body talc	L	M
Deodorant-antiperspirant	M	H (250)
Feminine hygiene cosmetics	M	M
Soap	L	M
Bath foam, oil	M	H (800)
Perfume, cologne	L	M
Sun cosmetics	M	L
Depilatories	H (26,000)	H (250)
Nail cosmetics	L	M
Foot cosmetics	L	L

A. From US manufacturers' file, 1975 (18-month period: FDA's Voluntary Cosmetic Regulation Program [14]). Risk grading: L(ow) = more than 750,000 units per experience; M(edium) = 100,000–750,000 units per experience; H(igh) = less than 100,000 units per experience.
B. From FDA pilot study (1974: Westat report) among 10,000 US families [3]. Only for the month of September. Risk grading: L(ow) = more than 4,000 units per experience; M(edium) = 1,000–4,000 units per experience; H(igh) = less than 1,000 units per experience.
H ( ) indicates high-risk cosmetics, with the number of cosmetic units to cause one adverse reaction.
*Risk index = number of cosmetic units to cause one adverse reaction.

The role of contact allergy in the spectrum of adverse effects caused by cosmetics and toiletries

23.7 It is generally assumed that irritation is the most common side effect of cosmetic products. The contribution of contact allergic reactions to the spectrum of cosmetic-related adverse events has been investigated in two studies only [1,4]. From the UK study no valid conclusions can be drawn (§ 23.1). A Dutch study suggests that no more than 10% of all reactions is caused by contact allergy [4].

Of 982 clients of beauticians interviewed, 254 (26%) claimed to have experienced an adverse reaction to cosmetic and/or toiletry products in the preceding 5 years. Of the 254, 150 women were patch-tested with the European Standard Series and a 'cosmetic series' of 15 allergens commonly implicated in cosmetic allergy.

In the European standard series, only a few positive reactions were seen to allergens which may be present in cosmetics: fragrance mix ($n = 3$), wool alcohols ($n = 3$), formaldehyde ($n = 2$), balsam Peru ($n = 1$), and rosin ($n = 1$). In the cosmetic series only Kathon CG elicited positive patch test reactions ($n = 3$). Cosmetic allergy was considered to be 'proven' in 3 patients (2%), and 'possible' in 7 (5%).

It was concluded that contact allergy is responsible for a minority (<10%) of all reactions to cosmetics/toiletries. The majority of reactions are due to irritation from personal cleanliness products such as soaps, shampoos, bath foams and from deodorants. Additionally it was found that pre-existing dermatoses such a seborrhoeic dermatitis and acne may be worsened by irritation from cosmetics [4].

23.8 REFERENCES

1. Consumers' Association (1979): *Reactions of the Skin to Cosmetic and Toiletry Products*. Consumers' Association. London.
2. De Groot, A.C., Nater, J.P., van der Lende, R. and Rycken, B. (1987): Adverse effects of cosmetics: A retrospective study in the general population. *Int. J. Cosm. Science, 9*, 255–259.
3. Westat Inc. (1975): *An Investigation of Consumers' Perceptions of Adverse Reactions to Cosmetic Products*. National Technical Information Service, US Department of Commerce, Springfield.
4. De Groot, A.C., Beverdam, E.G.A., Tjong Ayong, C., Coenraads, P.J. and Nater, J.P. (1988): The role of contact allergy in the spectrum of adverse effects caused by cosmetics and toiletries. *Contact Dermatitis, 19*, 195–201.
5. De Groot, A.C. (1987): Contact allergy to cosmetics: causative ingredients. *Contact Dermatitis, 17*, 26–34.
6. Schorr, W.F. (1974): Cosmetic allergy: Diagnosis, incidence, and management. *Cutis, 14*, 844–850.
7. Skog, E. (1980): Incidence of cosmetic dermatitis. *Contact Dermatitis, 6*, 449–451.
8. Romaguera, C., Camarasa, J.M.G., Alomar, A. and Grimalt, F. (1983): Patch tests with allergens related to cosmetics. *Contact Dermatitis, 9*, 167–168.
9. Ngangu, Z., Samsoen, M. and Foussereau, J. (1983): Einige Aspekte zur Kosmetika-Allergie in Strassburg. *Dermatosen, 31*, 126–129.
10. Adams, R.M. and Maibach, H.I. (1985): A five-year study of cosmetic reactions. *J. Am. Acad. Derm., 13*, 1062–1069.
11. Broeckx, W., Blondeel, A., Dooms-Goossens, A. and Achten, G. (1987): Cosmetic intolerance. *Contact Dermatitis, 16*, 189–194.
12. De Groot, A.C., Bruynzeel, D.P., Bos, J.D. et al. (1988): The allergens in cosmetics. *Arch. Dermatol., 124*, 1525–1529.
13. De Groot, A.C. (1990): Labelling cosmetics with their ingredients. *Br. Med. J., 300* , 1636–1638.
14. *Tabulation of Cosmetic Product Experience Report*, submitted to the Food and Drug Administration under Voluntary Cosmetic Regulatory Program (Jan. 1974–June 1975). Food and Drug Administration, Division of Cosmetic Technicology. Washington, DC, USA.

24. Contact allergy to cosmetics

CLINICAL PICTURE OF ALLERGIC COSMETIC DERMATITIS

24.1 The clinical picture of allergic cosmetic dermatitis depends on the type of products used (and consequently, the sites of application) and the degree of the patient's sensitivity. Usually, cosmetics and their ingredients are weak allergens, and the dermatitis resulting from cosmetic allergy is mild: erythema, mild edema, desquamation and papules. Weeping vesicular dermatitis rarely occurs, although some products, especially the permanent hair dyes, may cause fierce reactions. Allergic reactions to the permanent hair dyes usually are most prominent on the face and ears rather than on the scalp.

Contact allergic dermatitis from cosmetic products can sometimes be easily recognized. Examples include reactions to deodorant, eye-shadow, perfume and lipstick. In more than half of all cases, however, the diagnosis of cosmetic allergy is suspected neither by the patient nor by the doctor [1,2]. The typical patient suffering from allergic cosmetic dermatitis is a woman aged 20–45 with mild erythema, edema and scaling of the eyelids. The face itself is also frequently involved and often the dermatitis is limited to the face and/or eyelids. Other predilection sites for cosmetic dermatitis are the neck, the arms and the hands. However, all parts of the body may be involved. Most often, the cosmetics have been applied to previously healthy skin (especially products used on the face), nails or hair. However, allergic cosmetic dermatitis may also be caused by products used on previously damaged skin, notably irritant contact dermatitis (hands) and atopic dermatitis (hands, arms and legs) [1].

THE PRODUCTS CAUSING COSMETIC ALLERGY

These are discussed in Chapter 23.

THE ALLERGENS

STUDIES INVESTIGATING THE ALLERGENS IN COSMETICS

24.2 Although there are many publications on contact allergy to cosmetics and toiletries, only 2 studies [1,2] have systematically investigated the allergens in such products. This may be explained by a general lack of information on their ingredients and by the fact that many cosmetic ingredients are not easily obtained. Data on the constituents of the individual marketed cosmetic products are readily available only in the United States where, since 1978, regulations have required that all ingredients, other than components of flavours and fragrances be declared on cosmetic products labels. According to EC regulations, cosmetic companies are required to provide information on the ingredients of their products to the proper authorities (under provision of secrecy), for purposes of medical treatment. Indeed, most companies are quite cooperative, and dermatologists pursuing the matter usually succeed in obtaining the information necessary for ingredient patch testing. Nevertheless, much time and energy often has to be spent, and this has generally discouraged dermatologists from such investigations. In addition, the identification of the causative allergen(s) usually has little practical value for the patient, as without product ingredient labelling he/she would still be unable to choose products not containing the offending substances [3]. Fortunately, full cosmetic ingredient labelling will be implemented in the EC in 1997, which will boost scientific investigation of cosmetic allergens [4].

USA [2]

During 64 months (1977–1983) the members of the North American Contact Dermatitis Group (NACDG) studied 713 patients with cosmetic dermatitis [2]. Cosmetic allergy was observed in 578 (81%). To identify the causative ingredients, 273 patients (38%) were patch tested with the suspected cosmetics and some of their ingredients; 130 patients (18%) were tested with all ingredients. This resulted in identification of 87 ingredients or classes of ingredients that had caused allergic cosmetic dermatitis (Table 24.1). Fragrance and fragrance ingredients were responsible for the greatest number of reactions (n = 161). In most cases (n = 67) the individual fragrance component could not be determined, but when it could, the most frequent causes were cinnamic alcohol (n = 17), hydroxycitronellal (n = 11), musk ambrette (n = 11), isoeugenol (n = 10) and geraniol (n = 8). Preservatives were the second most frequent causes of reactions (n = 149), followed by *p*-phenylenediamine (n = 41), lanolin and derivatives (n = 29), and glyceryl thioglycolate and propylene glycol (25 each). The preservative ingredients causing the greatest number of reactions were quaternium-15 (n = 65), imidazolidinyl urea (n = 21), parabens (unspecified as to type, n = 19), 2-bromo-2-nitropropane-1,3-diol (n = 16) and formaldehyde (n = 16).

Table 24.1. Causative ingredients in 578 patients with cosmetic allergy [2]

Ingredient	No. of reactions	Ingredient	No. of reactions
Acrylate, unspecified	1	Jasmine, synthetic	2
Allantoin	2	Lanolin	15
α-Amylcinnamic aldehyde	2	Lanolin alcohol	12
Beeswax	1	Lanolin oil	2
Benzalkonium chloride	2	Methacrylate monomer (unspecified)	1
Benzocaine*	2	Microcrystalline wax	1
Benzoin	2	Mineral oil	1

(continued)

Table 24.1 *(continuation)*

Ingredient	No. of reactions	Ingredient	No. of reactions
Benzophenone (unspecified)	1	Musk ambrette	11
Benzophenone-4	2	Neomycin*	1
Benzophenone-8	1	Nitrocellulose	1
Benzyl alcohol	3	2-Nitro-*p*-phenylenediamine	1
Benzyl benzoate	1	Oak moss	3
Benzyl salicylate	1	Octyl dimethyl PABA	5
BHA	3	Oleamide DEA	1
Bismuth oxychloride	1	Oleyl alcohol	1
2-Bromo-2-nitropropane-1,3-diol	16	Oxyquinoline	1
Butyl acetate	1	PABA	3
Captan	2	Paraben (unspecified)	19
Cetearyl alcohol	1	PEG-4 dilaurate	1
Cetyl alcohol	1	Pentyl dimethyl PABA	2
Cherry pit oil	1	Peru balsam	3
Chloroxylenol	1	*p*-Phenylenediamine	41
Cinnamal	6	Potassium sorbate	2
Cinnamic alcohol	17	Propylene glycol	25
Clove oil	1	Propyl gallate	1
Coal tar	1	Quaternium-15	65
Costus oil	1	Resorcinol	3
Coumarin	4	Sandalwood oil	3
Dibutyl phthalate	1	Shellac	1
Diethylene glycol dimethacrylate	1	Sodium bisulfite	1
Disodium mono-oleamido sulfosuccinate	1	Sorbic acid	6
Ethyl methacrylate	5	Stearamidoethyl diethylamine	3
Eugenol	4	Stearic acid	1
Formaldehyde	16	TEA-stearate	1
Fragrance (unspecified)	67	Tetrachlorsalicylanilide*	1
Geraniol	8	Tetrahydrofurfuryl methacrylate	1
Glyceryl PABA	5	Thimerosal	1
Glyceryl thioglycolate	25	Thioglycolate (unspecified)	1
Hydrolyzed animal protein	1	Tocopherol	2
Hydroxycitronellal	11	Toluenesulfonamide/formaldehyde resin	23
Imidazolidinyl urea	21	Tribomsalan*	1
Isoeugenol	10	Triclosan	1
Jasmine, absolute	3	Triethanolamine	3
		UV-absorber (unspecified)	1

*Prohibited in cosmetics in EC.

The Netherlands [1]

Between March 1, 1986 and July 31, 1987, the members of the Dutch Contact Dermatitis Group investigated the allergens in 119 patients with proven cosmetic-related allergic contact dermatitis. 102 patients (86%) were woman, 17 (14%) men. Their ages ranged from 12 to 78 years, with an average of 36 years. Eighty-one patients (68%) were tested with all ingredients of the suspected cosmetic products, 38 (32%) with 1 or more allergens known to be present in cosmetics used.

The results of patch testing were as follows: in the European standard series, most reactions were observed to the fragrance mix (n = 31; 26%). Next was nickel sulfate (n = 17; 14%), followed by Balsam Peru (n = 12; 10%), formaldehyde (n = 10; 8%), wool alcohols (n = 6; 5%), quaternium-15 (n = 5; 4%) and colophony (rosin) (n = 5; 4%). Ingredient patch testing revealed a total of 53 cosmetic allergens (Table 24.2). The most frequent contact allergen was methylchloroisothiazolinone/methylisothiazolinone (Kathon CG), reacting in 33 patients (28%). Second was toluenesulfonamide/formaldehyde resin, causing cosmetic allergy in 15 patients (13%), followed by oleamidopropyl dimethylamine (13 patients, 11%). 15 reactions (13%) were caused by "fragrance, unspecified". 4 patients reacted to eugenol and hydroxycitronellal; 3 reacted to diazolidinyl urea, quaternium-15 and cocamidopropyl betaine. Reactions to the following allergens were observed in 2 patients each: imidazolidinyl urea, propylparaben, cinnamic alcohol, citronellol, geraniol, isoeugenol, cocamide DEA, isopropyl-dibenzoylmethane, 4-methylbenzylidene-camphor and myristyl alcohol. To the other 34 allergens only 1 positive patch test reaction was observed.

The classes of cosmetic allergens are shown in Table 24.2. Due to the large number of patients reacting to Kathon CG, preservatives were the most important category implicated with 47 reactions (32%). Fragrances followed with 39 reactions (27%) and emulsifiers (mostly oleamidopropyl dimethylamine) with 21 reactions (14%).

Table 24.2. Causative (classes of) ingredients (n = 147) in 119 patients with cosmetic allergy

			No. pat.
Preservatives			47 (32%)
Methylchloroisothiazolinone/ methylisothiazolinone (Kathhon CG)	33	Benzoxonium chloride	1
Diazolidinyl urea	3	2-Bromo-2-nitropropane-1,3-diol	1
Quaternium-15	3	Chloroacetamide	1
Imidazolidinyl urea	2	Formaldehyde	1
Propylparaben	2		
Fragrances			39 (27%)
UNSPECIFIED	15		

(continued)

Table 24.2 *(continuation)*

				No. pat.
SPECIFIED	24			
Eugenol	4	Coumarin	1	
Hydroxycitronellal	4	Hexylcinnamic aldehyde	1	
Cinnamic alcohol	2	Linalool	1	
Citronellol	2	Linalyl acetate	1	
Geraniol	2	Lyral	1	
Isoeugenol	2	γ-Methylionone	1	
α-Amylcinnamic aldehyde	1	Pelargol	1	
Emulsifiers				21 (14%)
Oleamidopropyl dimethylamine	13			
Cocamide DEA	2			
Cocamidopropyl betaine	3			
Lauramide DEA	1			
PEG-32 stearate	1			
Stearic acid	1			
Toluenesulfonamide/formaldehyde resin				15 (10%)
Lanolin (derivatives)				4 (3%)
Acetylated lanolin	1			
Eucerit	1			
Lanolin	1			
Lanolin oil	1			
Miscellaneous				21 (14%)
Isopropyl-dibenzoylmethane	2	Laurylpyridinium chloride	1	
4-Methylbenzylidene-camphor	2	Mineral oil	1	
Myristyl alcohol	2	Octyl gallate	1	
Arnica extract	1	Propolis	1	
Avocado oil	1	PVP/hexadecene copolymer	1	
t-Butyl hydroquinone	1	Rosin (Colophony)	1	
Butyl methoxydibenzoylmethane	1	Selenium sulfide	1	
Calendula extract	1	Sodium PCA	1	
Cyclomethicone	1	Zinc pyrithione	1	

24.3 THE ALLERGENS RESPONSIBLE FOR COSMETIC ALLERGY [8]

Fragrances

Fragrances are the most frequent cause of cosmetic allergy [1,2], both from products primarily used for their perfume (perfumes, colognes, eaux de toilettes, aftershaves, deodorants) and from other scented cosmetics. Patients may react on patch testing to the product and to the fragrance mix in the European standard series and/or to the 'indicator allergens' for fragrance sensitivity: balsam of Peru and rosin (colophony). The fragrance mix contains eight very commonly used fragrance materials (each 1%): eugenol, isoeugenol, oak moss absolute, geraniol, cinnamic aldehyde, amylcinnamaldehyde, hydroxycitronellal and cinnamic alcohol, emulsified with sorbitan sesquioleate. This fragrance-mix possibly detects 70–80% of cases of fragrance sensitivity [5]. A perfume may contain 10–300 fragrance compounds. The exact allergen is usually not sought after, but when it is, most reactions have proved to be caused by the components of the fragrance mix. However, changes in the popularity of ingredients used for new fragrances require a periodic reappraisal of the composition of the fragrance mix.

Patients allergic to fragrances may use fragrance-free cosmetics. In individuals sensitive to perfumes a fragrance may sometimes be applied to clothing or hair without eliciting an allergic response. However, they should be avoided altogether in fragrance-sensitive individuals who have active eczema. It may be difficult for an individual with hand eczema to totally avoid fragrance contact, and it may be necessary to consider connubial contact with fragrances.

Musk ambrette, used as a fragrance fixer, has been an important cause of photocontact allergy [6]. Its incorporation into new products has been discouraged and its presence in old formulations has been reduced or removed. It is an occult allergen for those already sensitized, with numerous sources of contact remaining in perfumed or flavoured noncosmetic products.

Preservatives

Preservatives are added to water-containing cosmetics to inhibit the growth of nonpathogenic and pathogenic microorganisms, which may cause degradation of the product or endanger the health of the consumer. The most commonly used preservatives, their spectra of antimicrobial activity and their use concentrations are listed in Table 24.3.

Frequently, mixtures of several preservatives are used; such mixtures are frequently traded as ready-to-use ingredients for the cosmetic industry. Emulsions are often preserved with a "system" consisting of a water-soluble and a lipophilic antimicrobial compound, but aqueous products can also contain a number of chemicals in order to attain the required antimicrobial spectrum.

Table 24.3. Commonly used preservatives [7]

Name	Action spectrum	Use concentration
Methylisothiazolinone + methylchloroisothiazolinone (Kathon CG, Euxyl K100)	Broad spectrum: bacteria, yeasts, fungi	3–15 ppm
Formaldehyde	Broad spectrum: fungicide and bactericide	0.05–0.2%
Quaternium-15 (Dowicil 200)	Broad spectrum: bacteria, moulds, yeasts	0.02–0.3%
Imidazolidinyl urea (Germall 115)	Broad spectrum, especially in combination with parabens	0.05–0.5%
Diazolidinyl urea (Germall II)	Broad spectrum, especially active against gram-negative bacteria, often combined with parabens or other antifungal preservatives	0.03–0.3%
2-Bromo-2-nitropropane-1,3-diol (Bronopol)	Broad spectrum: most effective against bacteria	0.01–0.1%
DMDM hydantoin (Glydant)	Broad spectrum, less active against yeasts	0.15–0.4%
Parabens	Primarily fungi and gram-positive bacteria, little activity against gram-negative bacteria	use at maximum solubility (0.3%)

Isothiazolinones [9,83,84]

A mixture of methylisothiazolinone and methylchloroisothiazolinone (MI/MCI) was introduced as a cosmetic preservative around 1980 [9]. The commercial products of the biocide mixture which are used for cosmetic preservation are known as Kathon CG (CG stands for cosmetic grade) and Euxyl K100. Kathon CG contains 1.5% active ingredients in an inert carrier and Euxyl K100 also contains benzyl alcohol. Variations in the mixtures are used in biocides for industrial purposes.

In a Dutch study investigating the allergenic ingredients in cosmetics [1] MI/MCI was noted to be the most frequent cause of cosmetic allergy in the cohort evaluated. Contact allergy to MI/MCI was observed to occur frequently in various European countries in patients suspected of contact dermatitis routinely tested with this preservative system. High prevalence rates have been reported [9–11] from Finland (2.9%), Germany (5.7% and 3.4%), the Netherlands (5.0%), Italy (8.4%), Sweden (4.2%), and Switzerland (3.5%). Lower rates (approximately 1%) have been recorded in the United Kingdom, Denmark and Belgium. Of positive reactions to MI/MCI, 70–80% have been considered relevant to patients' complaints. Most cases have been caused by leave-on cosmetics, especially skin care products. With few exceptions, the preservative is safe when used in rinse-off products at low concentrations (<5 ppm), but examples have been observed of

MI/MCI sensitivity induced by shampoos, causing allergic contact dermatitis of the hands in hairdressers.

Because the concentration of MI/MCI in cosmetics is usually below 15 ppm, the products themselves often do not induce positive patch test responses in patients allergic to MI/MCI. However, the mixture of MI/MCI at a concentration of 100 ppm in water (which will detect most but not all cases of sensitization [85]) is included in the European standard series. Cosmetics in which Kathon CG was the sensitizer include: moisturising creams [86,89,90], shampoos [86–88], eye make-up remover [86,87], cleansing milk [87], hand cream [87], deodorant [88], sunscreen cream [89,91], hair conditioner [91], mascara [91], facial make-up [91] and eye gel [92].

Formaldehyde

Formaldehyde is a frequent sensitizer and ubiquitous allergen, with numerous noncosmetic sources of contact. Routine testing in patients with suspected allergic contact dermatitis yields prevalence rates of sensitization of 3% or more [12]. Because of this, the cosmetic industry uses small but effective concentrations, with the amount of free formaldehyde not exceeding 0.2% [13], and restricting its use almost exclusively to rinse-off products. Until recently, most shampoos contained formaldehyde. This practice rarely gave rise to cases of allergic cosmetic dermatitis [14]. In recent years, it has largely been replaced by other preservatives (such as MI/MCI), because formaldehyde (when inhaled as gas) is suspected of being a possible human carcinogen [15]. It is still used for plant sanitation and preservation of raw materials, and traces will often be present in the finished cosmetic product. Some biocides are formaldehyde donors. Many patients allergic to formaldehyde were found to have contact dermatitis from cosmetics containing formaldehyde donors [94].

Formaldehyde Donors

Formaldehyde donors are preservatives which, in the presence of water, release formaldehyde. Therefore, cosmetics preserved with such chemicals will contain free formaldehyde, the amount depending on the preservative used, its concentration, the amount of water present in the product and the pH and composition of the product. The antimicrobial effects of formaldehyde donors are said to be intrinsic properties of the parent molecules and not related to formaldehyde release. Formaldehyde-donors used in cosmetics and toiletries include quaternium-15, imidazolidinyl urea, diazolidinyl urea and DMDM hydantoin. In anionic shampoos the amount of formaldehyde released by such donors increases in the order: imidazolidinyl urea < dimethylol dimethyl (DMDM) hydantoin < diazolidinyl urea < quaternium-15 [16]. 2-Bromo-2-nitropropane-1,3-diol (Bronopol®) is sometimes also listed as a formaldehyde donor, but it releases formaldehyde only by decomposition at extreme pH, an error where its application is considered. Whereas the use of formaldehyde as a preservative has drastically decreased in recent years, the increased popularity of the formaldehyde donors in the cosmetic industry suggests that an increase in the prevalence of sensitivity to them can be expected [17].

Quaternium-15 (Dowicil 200). Patients sensitized to formaldehyde may frequently experience cosmetic dermatitis from using leave-on preparations containing quaternium-15. The threshold for eliciting allergic contact dermatitis for most individuals is approximately 30 ppm formaldehyde [18]. At a concentration of 0.1%, quaternium-15 releases about 100 ppm of free formaldehyde. In some European countries such as Belgium [19] and The Netherlands [10], allergy to quaternium-15 is infrequent. In the United Kingdom, however, routine testing has yielded a prevalence rate of sensitization of 2.6% (3.3% in women, 1.4% in men) [20]. Also in the United Kingdom, 6.9% of female patients with facial dermatitis were allergic to quaternium-15 [21]. In the USA, a prevalence rate of 6.3% was found [93]. Cosmetics in which quaternium-15 was the sensitizer include [93,94]: moisturisers, hair preparations, (eye) make-up, deodorant, baby products and face masks. Quaternium-15 is included in the European standard series.

Imidazolidinyl Urea (Germall 115). Imidazolidinyl urea releases only small amounts of formaldehyde, and consequently poses little threat to formaldehyde-sensitive subjects. Contact allergy to imidazolidinyl urea occurs occasionally [19,20]. In 1175 patients tested with the preservative 2% aq. in Belgium, only eight (0.7%) positive reactions were observed, of which one was to formaldehyde [19]. In the United States, where imidazolidinyl urea is part of the routine series, 1.5% of patients patch tested react to the preservative [17]. Cross-reactions to and from the structurally related diazolidinyl urea may be observed [19,22]. Cosmetics in which imidazolidinyl urea was the sensitizer include [94]: skin care products, shampoo, deodorant, face masks and mascaras.

Diazolidinyl Urea (Germall II). Diazolidinyl urea, the newest and most active member of the imidazolidinyl urea group, has only been used since 1982. Several case reports of cosmetic allergy from diazolidinyl urea have been published [22,23]. In a Dutch study of 2142 patients with eczema patch tested with diazolidinyl urea 2% aq, 12 (0.6%) reacted. In 5 of these 12, the patients were also allergic to formaldehyde and formaldehyde donors [24]. The members of the North American Contact Dermatitis Group tested 647 patients with diazolidinyl urea 1% in water, and obtained 12 (1.9%) positive reactions [17]. Patients may become sensitized to diazolidinyl urea without reacting to formaldehyde, but individuals allergic to formaldehyde may experience cosmetic dermatitis from using leave-on preparations preserved with diazolidinyl urea [18]. Cross-reactions to and from imidazolidinyl urea occur [18,20]. Diazolidinyl urea appears to be a stronger sensitizer than imidazolidinyl urea [25].

DMDM Hydantoin (Dimethylol Dimethyl Hydantoin, Glydant). No cases of cosmetic allergy from DMDM hydantoin have been reported. However, routine testing with DMDM hydantoin 3% aq. in 501 patients resulted in four positive reactions; all four were also allergic to formaldehyde [29]. Subsequent testing in patients allergic to formaldehyde resulted in positive reactions to DMDM hydantoin down to concentrations of 0.3% [30]. Also, repeated open application to the skin of a cream containing 0.25% w/w DMDM hydantoin elicited a positive response in some patients. Consequently, patients sensitized to formaldehyde may experience cosmetic dermatitis from using leave-on products preserved with DMDM hydantoin.

Parabens

The paraben esters (methyl, ethyl, propyl, butyl and benzyl esters of *p*-hydroxybenzoic acid) are the most widely used preservatives in cosmetic products. Because the parabens are active primarily against fungi and gram-positive bacteria, but not against gram-negative bacteria such as *Pseudomonas,* they are usually combined with other preservatives such as imidazolidinyl urea. With many dermatologists, the parabens have a bad reputation as notorious sensitizers. However, most cases of paraben sensitivity are caused by topical drugs applied to leg ulcers or used on eczematous skin [31]. Routine testing in the European standard series yields low prevalence rates of sensitization [32]. At the usual concentration of 0.1–0.3% in cosmetics, parabens rarely cause adverse reactions. Parabens are not included in the North American standard series of contact allergens as the allergen causes problems only uncommonly. Sensitized individuals may be able to tolerate products containing parabens, a phenomenon which has been called the "paraben paradox". Tolerance is related to concentration, duration and site of application, and skin status.

2-Bromo-2-nitropropane-1,3-Diol (Bronopol). Bronopol is not a frequent cause of contact allergy in Europe [1,19,20,26]. In the United States, however, bronopol was found to be such a common cause of cosmetic allergy from Eucerin cream [27,28] that the manufacturer decided to replace it. Another concern is that its interaction with amines and amides can result in the formation of nitrosamines of nitrosamides, suspected carcinogens. Cosmetics in which bronopol was the allergen include [94]: liquid soap and moisturizers.

Methyldibromoglutaronitrile. Methyldibromoglutaronitrile (1,2-dibromo-2,4-dicyanobutane, Tektamer®) is present, together with phenoxyethanol, in the preservative system Euxyl K400®. It is an important contact allergen in moist toilet paper in the Netherlands [95], and may become more important as cosmetic allergen in the near future. Cosmetics in which methyldibromoglutaronitrile was the sensitizer include skin care products [95,96], shampoo [97] and massage products [97].

Lanolin and derivatives

Lanolin and lanolin derivatives are used extensively in cosmetic products as emollients and emulsifiers. Lanolin has a bad reputation among some dermatologists, as routine testing with wool alcohols in the European standard series reveals many cases of lanolin sensitivity in some centres [12]. However, the majority of individuals have been sensitized by using topical pharmaceutical preparations containing lanolin, especially for treating varicose ulcers and stasis dermatitis (a similar situation to that of parabens) [33]. The presence of lanolin or its derivatives in cosmetics may cause cosmetic dermatitis in lanolin-sensitive individuals, but the risk of sensitization by using such products is small [33]. Purification and chemical modification may enhance its safety [33,34].

Toluenesulfonamide/formaldehyde resin

Toluenesulfonamide/formaldehyde resin (Santolite resin) is the usual resin in nail varnishes (lacquers) and nail hardeners. It is used in preference to the less allergenic polyester resins because it is resistant to chipping. It is a common cause of cosmetic allergy [1,2,35]. The diagnosis of nail lacquer dermatitis should particularly be suspected in patients presenting with a patchy dermatitis on the neck or eyelids, but the pattern of the eczema may be indistinguishable from that of seborrhoeic eczema. Other possible sites of nail lacquer dermatitis include the upper chest, the external auditory meatus, the vulva and the anus.

Sculptured nails based on methyl methacrylate can cause a nail varnish dermatitis and a nail dystrophy in sensitized individuals [36]. Nail adhesives based on *p-tert*-butylphenol formaldehyde resin have caused similar dystrophy [37].

p-Phenylenediamine and related dyes

p-Phenylenediamine and related hair dyes are important sensitizers. Safer permanent dyes with a lower risk of contact allergy, but with the same technical qualities, are not available. Many cases of sensitization were reported in the 1930s and sensitization was considered so great a hazard that its use in hair dyes was prohibited in several countries. Currently, its incorporation in cosmetic products is allowed in the European Community to a maximum concentration of 6% (as free base).

In recent years, the incidence of dermatitis due to hair dyes containing *p*-phenylenediamine (or derivatives) appears to have decreased [38]. This is attributed to the provision of cautionary notices on the products, awareness of the risk, patch testing the product, improvements in the technical quality of the cosmetic product and improvements in the technique of application of these dyes. Nevertheless, *p*-phenylenediamine and related dyes remain an important cause of cosmetic allergy [98] and are now being seen relatively more frequently in Asian men who dye their hair and beards. These oxidation dyes are also an occupational hazard for hairdressers and beauticians [39]. The chemistry of and adverse reactions to oxidation colouring agents have been reviewed [40]. Semipermanent and temporary dyes rarely cause allergic cosmetic dermatitis. Hair colours that have caused cosmetic allergy are listed in Table 26.6.

Glyceryl thioglycolate

Glyceryl thioglycolate, a waving agent used in acid permanent waving products, occasionally sensitizes consumers [41], but it is usually an occupational hazard for the hairdresser [39,42].

UV filters

Ultraviolet light filters (UV filters) are used in sunscreens to protect the consumer from harmful UV irradiation from the sun. They are also incorporated in some cosmetics to inhibit UV photodegradation of the product and thereby increase its shelf life. UV filters have been identified in increasing frequency as allergens and photoallergens but reactions to them remain uncommon. (Photo)allergic reactions can easily be overlooked, as the resulting dermatitis may be interpreted by the patient/consumer as failure of the product to protect against sunburn or as worsening of the (photo)dermatosis for which the sunscreen was used. Most reactions are currently caused by dibenzoylmethanes, a new class of broad-spectrum UV absorbers, with their main absorption properties in the UVA region (315–400 nm). Several series of patients with (photo)contact allergy to isopropyldibenzoylmethane have been reported [43–45], and its use is now waning.

Cross-reactions to other dibenzoylmethanes such as methoxydibenzoylmethane have been observed [45]. Other UV filters that have caused (photo)contact allergy by their presence in cosmetics are listed in Tables 6.5 and 30.13.

Propolis [74]

Propolis is a lipophilic, yellow-brown to dark brown or sometimes dark greenish material. It is hard and wax-like when cool, but softens and turns resinous and sticky when warm; hence the name bee-glue. Bees use it to seal hive walls and strengthen the borders of the combs as well as the hive entrance. The bee product propolis is used in dental medicine as topical anaesthetic and is present in many toothpastes, mouth-wash preparations for the treatment of gingivitis, cheilitis and stomatitis. It has also found its way into pharmaceutical and cosmetic products such as face creams, ointments, lotions and solutions [74].

Since the first description of contact dermatitis in a bee-keeper in 1915, numerous cases have been observed and published. While formerly remaining chiefly an occupational skin disease in bee-keepers, propolis allergy today is a disease of individuals who use 'bio-cosmetics' [74]. The main allergen in propolis is 'LB-1', which consists of 3-methyl-2-butenyl caffeate (54%), 3-methyl-3-butenyl caffeate (28%), 2-methyl-2-butenyl caffeate (4%), phenyl ethyl caffeate (8%), caffeic acid (1%) and benzyl caffeate (1%) [75]. Poplar bud constituents are probably responsible for propolis allergy [76]. In Prague, 605 consecutive patients were patch tested with a 10% alcoholic solution and 25 (4.2%) reacted. Thirteen of them also had a positive patch test to balsam of Peru. Most of the patients had used propolis as a folk remedy for the treatment of various dermatoses [78]. Cosmetics in which propolis was the sensitizer include face cream [77, 79], face lotion [77], lipstick [75,81] and toothpaste [80,82].

Antioxidants

Antioxidants are added to cosmetics to prevent the deterioration of unsaturated fatty acids and are an occasional cause of cosmetic allergy [1,2], though the actual prevalence may be underestimated [46]. Antioxidants that have caused cosmetic allergy include [10]: BHA (butylated hydroxyanisole) [46], BHT (butylated hydroxytoluene) [46], *t*-butyl hydroquinone [46], 2,5-di-*t*-butyl hydroquinone, nordihydroguiaretic acid, propyl gallate [47] and tocopherol.

Other allergens

Emulsifiers are infrequent causes of cosmetic allergy. Oleamidopropyl dimethylamine, present in a particular baby lotion containing 0.3% of the emulsifier [48], was responsible for allergic contact reactions in many patients in The Netherlands. Other ingredients of cosmetics which are occasional causes of cosmetic allergy include: cetyl alcohol [49], rosin (colophony) [50,51], phenyl salicylate [52], propylene glycol [1] and colours [55]. A comprehensive literature survey on cosmetic allergy is provided in [10] and Chapters 26 to 29.

INGREDIENTS WHICH USED TO BE IMPORTANT COSMETIC ALLERGENS

D & C Red No. 31 (CI 15800:1)

Since the latter half of the 1950s, many cosmetic dermatitis patients with accompanying bizarre pigmentation have been observed in Japan [56]. The descriptive term pigmented cosmetic dermatitis has been proposed for this disease [57]. Most of these patients were found to be allergic to colour-containing cosmetic products such as rouge, lipsticks and face powders [58]. Many of them proved to be hypersensitive to certain coal tar dyes used in such products, especially D & C Red no. 31 (Brilliant lake Red R) and other 1-phenylazo-2-naphthol derivatives [58]. Brilliant lake Red R was considered to be the most important causative agent of pigmented cosmetic dermatitis in Japan [59]. The commercial dye was found to contain many impurities [60], of which 1-phenylazo-2-naphthol (CI 12055, Solvent Yellow 14, Sudan I) was probably the major allergenic ingredient [61]. The role of fragrances and photocontact allergy proved to be far less important [58] than previously suspected [57]. After 1976, cosmetic products containing D & C Red no. 31 rapidly disappeared from the Japanese market, and the incidence of pigmented cosmetic dermatitis soon decreased.

D & C Red no. 21 (Eosin)

Eosin (CI 45380:2, Solvent Red 43, D & C Red no. 21, tetrabromofluorescein) in lipstick used to be the most common cause of cosmetic allergy in the 'fifties [62]. Calnan and Sarkany saw 110 cases within a period of 5 years; this represented approximately half the number of patients with contact dermatitis due to cosmetics [62]. The allergen is not D & C Red no. 21 itself, but an impurity [63–65]; all patients allergic to the colour have reacted more weakly to patch tests with D & C Red no. 21 purified by crystallisation than to the original impure dye [63–65]. The exact chemical identity of the allergen has not been established. The incidence of D & C Red no. 21 sensitivity fell rapidly after 1960 [66] because: (i) paler shades of lipstick, not requiring the routine addition of D & C Red no. 21, became more fashionable; and (ii) much purer (and consequently less allergenic) D & C Red no. 21 became available. Nowadays, lipstick is a relatively infrequent cause of cosmetic allergy, although a large number of its ingredients have been described as sensitisers (Table 27.16).

Halogenated salicylanilides

In the 1960s, the halogenated salicylanilides and related antibacterial and antifungal compounds caused almost an epidemic of photoallergic reactions. Tetrachlorosalicylanilide (TCSA) was responsible between 1960 and 1961 for an estimated 10,000 cases in England [67] before it was removed from general use. Subsequently, a number of related phenolic compounds were incorporated into soaps and other vehicles to combat infection, reduce body odour, act as preservatives and destroy fungi. Photocontact reactions were induced by many of these agents, including bithionol, the brominated salicylanilides, hexachlorophene, dichlorophene, triclocarban, (trichlorocarbanilide), 2,2′-thiobis (4-phenol) (Fenticlor), Multifungin® (5-bromo-4′-chlorosalicylanilide), Jadit (a mixture of buclosamide and salicylic acid [68,69]) and chloro-2-phenylphenol [70].

There has been a rapid decline in the induction of photocontact dermatitis by the halogenated salicylanilides and related compounds since 1968 [71]; this probably as a result of the removal of the more potent of these photosensitizers from general use. Often patients (also) had a 'plain' contact allergy in addition to photoallergy [72].

Zirconium

In 1956–58, American dermatologists were confronted with a unique and highly distinctive clinical entity. The dermatosis was invariably found in the axillae, and was characterised by a chronic papular eruption. Pruritus and acute inflammation were occasionally present. Most patients were women, who were in the habit of shaving their axillae. All used deodorants containing zirconium salts, notably sodium zirconium lactate. The eruption was often chronic, persisting for months or years. No therapy was effective, and in most cases there has been gradual spontaneous involution. Histologically, a granulomatous reaction was observed in the dermis. Six such cases were presented by Shelley and Hurley [73], who also reviewed 64 cases reported previously. It was demonstrated that the 'zirconium deodorant granulomas' were allergic in nature. Patch tests were always negative, but the hypersensitivity was demonstrated by intradermal testing.

ACKNOWLEDGEMENT

Several parts of this chapter have been adapted from de Groot, A.C. and White, I.R. (1992): Cosmetics and skin care products. In: R.J.G. Rycroft et al. (Eds.), *Textbook of Contact Dermatitis*. Chapter 14.1, pp. 158–473. Springer Verlag, Heidelberg; with kind permission of this publisher and Dr. Ian R. White.

24.4 REFERENCES

1. De Groot, A.C., Bruynzeel, D.P., Bos, J.D., van der Meeren, H.L.M., van Joost, T., Jagtman, B.A. and Weyland, J.W. (1988): The allergens in cosmetics. *Arch. Dermatol., 124,* 1525–1529.
2. Adams, R.M. and Maibach, H.I. (1985): A five-year study of cosmetic reactions. *J. Am. Acad. Dermatol., 13,* 1062–1069.
3. De Groot, A.C. (1990): Labelling cosmetics with their ingredients. *Br. Med. J., 300,* 1636–1638.
4. De Groot, A.C. and White, I.R. (1991): Cosmetic ingredient labelling in the European Community. *Contact Dermatitis, 25,* 273–275.
5. Larsen, W,G. and Maibach, H.I. (1982): Fragrance contact allergy. *Semin. Dermatol., 1,* 85–90.
6. Wojnarowska, F. and Calnan, C.D. (1986): Contact and photocontact allergy to musk ambrette. *Br. J. Dermatol., 114,* 667–675.
7. Decker, R.L. Jr. and Wenninger, J.A. (1987): Frequency of preservative use in cosmetic formulas as disclosed to FDA-1987. *Cosmet. Toilet., 102,* 21–40.
8. De Groot, A.C. and White, I.R. (1992): Cosmetics. In: R.J.G. Rycroft et al. (Editors), *Textbook of Contact Dermatitis*, pp. 459–475. Springer Verlag, Heidelberg.
9. De Groot, A.C. and Herxheimer, A. (1989): Isothiazolinone preservative: cause of a continuing epidemic of cosmetic dermatitis. *Lancet, i,* 314–316.
10. De Groot, A.C. (1988): Adverse reactions to cosmetics. Thesis, State University of Groningen.
11. Frosch, P.J. and Schulze-Dirks, A. (1987): Kontaktallergie auf Kathon CG. *Hautarzt, 38,* 422–425.
12. Enders, F., Przybilla, B., Ring, J., Burg, G. and Braun-Falco, O. (1988): Epicutantestung mit einer Standardreihe. *Hautarzt, 39,* 779–786.

13. Cosmetic Ingredient Review (1984): Final report on the safety assessment of formaldehyde. *J. Am. Coll. Toxicol., 3,* 157–184.
14. Bruynzeel, D.P., van Ketel, W.G. and de Haan, P. (1984): Formaldehyde contact sensitivity and the use of shampoos. *Contact Dermatitis, 10,* 179.
15. Council on Scientific Affairs (1989): Formaldehyde. *JAMA, 261,* 1183–1187.
16. Rosen, M. and McFarland, A.G. (1984): Free formaldehyde in anionic shampoos. *J. Soc. Cosmet. Chem., 35,* 157–169.
17. Storrs, F.J., Rosenthal, L.E., Adams, R.M., Clendenning, W., Emmett, E.A., Fisher, A.A., Larsen, W.G., Maibach, H.I., Rietschel, R.L., Schorr, W.F. and Taylor, J.S. (1989): Prevalence and relevance of allergic reactions in patients patch tested in North America - 1984 to 1985. *J. Am. Acad. Dermatol., 20,* 1038–1045.
18. Jordan, W.P., Sherman, W.T. and King, S.E. (1979): Threshold response in formaldehyde-sensitive subjects. *J. Am. Acad. Dermatol., 1,* 44–48.
19. Dooms-Goossens, A., de Boulle, K., Dooms, M. and DeGreef, H. (1986): Imidazolidinyl urea dermatitis. *Contact Dermatitis, 14,* 322–324.
20. Ford, G.P. and Beck, M.H. (1986): Reactions to quaternium-15, bronopol and Germall 115 in a standard series. *Contact Dermatitis, 14,* 271–274.
21. White, I.R. (1986): Prevalence of sensitivity to Dowicil 200 (quaternium-15). Data presented at the 8th International Symposium on Contact Dermatitis, Cambridge, 20–22 March 1986.
22. De Groot, A.C., Bruynzeel, D.P., Jagtman, B.A. and Weyland, J.W. (1988): Contact allergy to diazolidinyl urea (Germall II). *Contact Dermatitis, 18,* 202–205.
23. Kantor, G.R., Taylor, J.S., Ratz, J.L. and Evey, P.L. (1985): Acute allergic contact dermatitis from diazolidinyl urea (Germall II) in a hair gel. *J. Am. Acad. Dermatol., 13,* 116–119.
24. Perret, C.M. and Happle, R. (1989): Contact sensitivity to diazolidinyl urea (Germall II). In: Frosch, P.J., Dooms-Goossens, A., Lachapelle, J.M., Rycroft, R.J.G. and Scheper, R.J. (Eds.), *Current Topics in Contact Dermatitis.* pp. 92–94. Springer, Berlin, Heidelberg, New York,
25. Jordan, W.P. (1984): Human studies that determine the sensitizing potential of haptens. Experimental allergic contact dermatitis. *Dermatol. Clin., 2,* 533–538.
26. Frosch, P.J., White, I.R., Rycroft, R.J.G., Lahti, A., Burrows, D., Camarasa, J.G., Ducombs, G. and Wilkinson, J.D. (1990): Contact allergy to Bronopol. *Contact Dermatitis, 22,* 24–26.
27. Storrs, F. and Bell, D.E. (1983): Allergic contact dermatitis to 2-bromo-2-nitropropane-1,3-diol in a hydrophilic ointment. *J. Am. Acad. Dermatol., 8,* 157–164.
28. Peters, M.S., Connolly, S.M. and Schroeter, A.L. (1983): Bronopol allergic contact dermatitis. *Contact Dermatitis, 9,* 397–401.
29. De Groot, A.C., Bos, J.D., Jagtman, B.A., Bruynzeel, D.P., van Joost, T. and Weyland, J.W. (1986): Contact allergy to preservatives (II). *Contact Dermatitis, 15,* 218–222.
30. De Groot, A.C., van Joost, T., Bos, J.D., van der Meeren, H.L.M. and Weyland, J.W. (1988): Patch test reactivity to DMDM hydantoin. Relationship to formaldehyde. *Contact Dermatitis, 18,* 197–201.
31. Wilkinson, J.D., Hambly, E.M. and Wilkinson, D.S. (1980): Comparison of patch test results in two adjacent areas of England. II. Medicaments. *Acta. Derm. Venereol (Stockh.), 60,* 245–249.
32. Menné, T. and Hjorth, N. (1988): Routine testing with paraben esters. *Contact Dermatitis, 19,* 189–191.
33. Kligman, A.M. (1983): Lanolin allergy: crisis or comedy. *Contact Dermatitis, 9,* 99–107.
34. Edman, B. and Möller, H. (1989): Testing a purified lanolin preparation by a randomized procedure. *Contact Dermatitis, 20,* 287–290.
35. De Wit, F.S., De Groot, A.C., Weyland, J.W. and Bos, J.D. (1988): An outbreak of contact dermatitis from toluenesulfonamide formaldehyde resin in a nail hardener. *Contact Dermatitis, 18,* 280–283.
36. Fisher, A.A. (1980): Cross-reactions between methyl methacrylate monomer and acrylic monomers presently used in acrylic nail preparations. *Contact Dermatitis, 2,* 345.
37. Burrows, D. and Rycroft, R.J.G. (1981): Contact dermatitis from PTBP resin and tricresyl ethyl phthalate in a plastic nail adhesive. *Contact Dermatitis, 7,* 336.
38. Cronin, E. (1980): Contact Dermatitis. Churchill Livingstone, Edinburgh, p. 121.
39. Guerra, L., Tosti, A., Bardazzi, F., et al. (1992): Contact dermatitis in hairdressers: the Italian experience. *Contact Dermatitis, 26,* 101–107.
40. Zviak, C. (ed) (1986): The science of hair care. Dekker, New York.
41. Tosti, A., Melino, M. and Bardazzi, F. (1988): Contact dermatitis due to glyceryl monothioglycolate. *Contact Dermatitis, 19,* 71–72.

42. Storrs, F. (1984): Permanent wave contact dermatitis. Contact allergy to glyceryl monothioglycolate. *J. Am. Acad. Dermatol., 11,* 74–85.
43. English, J.S.C., White, I.R. and Cronin, E. (1987): Sensitivity to sunscreens. *Contact Dermatitis, 17,* 159–162.
44. De Groot, A.C., van der Walle, H.B., Jagtman, B.A. and Weyland, J.W. (1987): Contact allergy to 4-isopropyldibenzoylmethane and 3-(4′-methylbenzylidene)-camphor in the sunscreen Eusolex 8021. *Contact Dermatitis, 16,* 249–254.
45. Schauder, S. and Ippen, H. (1988): Photoallergisches und allergisches Kontaktekzem durch Dibenzoylmethan-Verbindungen und andere Lichtschutzfilter. *Hautarzt, 39,* 435–440.
46. White, I.R., Lovell, C.R. and Cronin, E. (1984): Antioxidants in cosmetics. *Contact Dermatitis, 11,* 265–267.
47. Wilson, A.G.McT., White, I.R. and Kirby, J.D.T. (1989): Allergic contact dermatitis from propyl gallate in a lip balm. *Contact Dermatitis, 20,* 145–146.
48. De Groot, A.C. (1989): Oleamidopropyl dimethylamine. *Dermatosen, 37,* 101–105.
49. Hausen, B.M. and Kulenkamp, D. (1985): Kontaktallergie auf Fludroxycortid und Cetylalkohol. *Dermatosen, 33,* 27–28.
50. Fisher, A.A. (1988): Allergic contact dermatitis due to rosin (colophony) in eyeshadow and mascara. *Cutis, 42,* 507–508.
51. Hausen, B.M. and Mohnert, J. (1989): Contact allergy due to colophony. *Contact Dermatitis, 20,* 295–301.
52. Calnan, C.D., Cronin, E. and Rycroft, R.J.G. (1981): Allergy to phenyl salicylate. *Contact Dermatitis, 7,* 208–211.
53. Schuler, T.M. and Frosch, P.J. (1988): Kontaktallergie auf propolis (Bienen-Kittharz). *Hautarzt, 39,* 139–142.
54. Hausen. B.M., Wollenweber, E., Senff, H. and Post, B. (1987): Propolis allergy (I). Origin, properties, usage and literature review. *Contact Dermatitis, 17,* 163–170.
55. English, J.S.C. and White, I.R. (1985): Dermatitis from D & C Red no. 36. *Contact Dermatitis, 13,* 335.
56. Nakayama, H., Harada, R. and Toda, M. (1976): Pigmented contact dermatitis. *Int. J. Dermatol., 15,* 673–675.
57. Nakayama, H., Hanaoka, H. and Oshiro, A. (1974): Allergen controlled system. *Tokyo: Kanehara Shuppan.*
58. Sugai, T., Takahashi, Y. and Takagi, T. (1977): Pigmented cosmetic dermatitis and coal tar dyes. *Contact Dermatitis, 3,* 249–256.
59. Mid-Japan Contact Dermatitis Research Group. (1978): Incidence of allergic reactions to coal tar dyes in patients with cosmetic dermatitis. *J. Dermatol. (Tokyo), 5,* 291–295.
60. Kozuka, T., Tashiro, M., Sano, S. et al. (1979): Brilliant lake Red R as a cause of pigmented contact dermatitis. *Contact Dermatitis, 5,* 297–304.
61. Kozuka, T., Tashiro, M., Sano, S. et al. (1980): Pigmented contact dermatitis from azo dyes. I. Cross-sensitivity in humans. *Contact Dermatitis, 6,* 330–336.
62. Calnan, C.D. and Sarkany, I. (1957): Studies in contact dermatitis. II. Lipstick cheilitis. *Trans. St. John's Hosp. Derm. Soc., 39,* 28–36.
63. Hecht, R., Schwarzschild, L. and Sulzberger, M.B. (1939): Sensitization to simple chemicals. V. Comparison between reactions to commercial and to purified dyes. *NY State J. Med., 39,* 2170–2173.
64. Sulzberger, M.B. and Hecht, R. (1941): Acquired specific hypersensitivity to simple chemicals. VI. Further studies on the purification of dyes in relation to allergic reaction. *J. Allergy, 12,* 129–137.
65. Calnan, C.D. (1959): Allergic sensitivity to eosin. *Acta Allergologica, 13,* 493–499.
66. Cronin, E. (1980): Contact dermatitis, Edinburgh: Churchill Livingstone, 142–143.
67. Wilkinson, D.S. (1961): Photodermatitis due to tetrachlorosalicylanilide. *Br. J. Derm., 73,* 213–219.
68. Herman, P.S. and Sams, W.M. Jr. (1972): Soap photodermatitis. Springfield, Illinois: Thomas.
69. Epstein, J.H. (1972): Photoallergy: A review. *Arch. Derm., 106,* 741–748.
70. Adams, R.M. (1972): Photoallergic contact dermatitis to chloro-2-phenylphenol. *Arch. Derm., 106,* 711–714.
71. Smith, S.Z. and Epstein, J.H. (1977): Photocontact dermatitis to halogenated salicylanilides and related compounds. *Arch. Derm., 113,* 1372–1374.
72. Calnan, C.D., Harman, R.R.M. and Wells, G.C. (1961): Photodermatitis from soaps. *Brit. Med. J., 2,* 1266–1269.
73. Shelley, W.B. and Hurley, H.J. (1958): The allergic origin of zirconium deodorant granulomas. *Br. J. Dermatol., 70,* 75–101.

74. Hausen, B.M., Wollenweber, E., Senff, H. and Post, B. (1987): Propolis allergy. (I). Origin, properties, usage and literature review. *Contact Dermatitis, 17,* 163–170.
75. Hausen, B.M. and Wollenweber, E. (1988): Propolis allergy. (III). Sensitization studies with minor constituents. *Contact Dermatitis, 19,* 296–303.
76. Ginanneschi, M., Acciai, M.C., Bracci, S. and Sertoli, A. (1991): Studies on propolis components. *Am. J. Contact Dermatitis, 2,* 60–64.
77. Hausen, B.M., Wollenweber, E., Senff, H. and Post, B. (1987): Propolis allergy (II). *Contact Dermatitis, 17,* 171–177.
78. Machác-Ková, J. (1988): The incidence of allergy to propolis in 605 consecutive patients patch tested in Prague. *Contact Dermatitis, 18,* 210–212.
79. Pecegueiro, M and Bordalo, O. (1991): Dermite de contacto por propolis em cosméticos. Boletim Informativo. *Group Português de Estudo Das Dermites de Contacto, no.5,* 63–64.
80. Monti, M., Berti, E., Carminati, G. and Cusini, M. (1983): Occupational and cosmetic dermatitis from propolis. *Contact Dermatitis, 9,* 163.
81. Tosti, A., Caponeri, M., Bardazzi, F., Melino, M. and Veronesi, S. (1985): Propolis contact dermatitis. *Contact Dermatitis, 12,* 227–228.
82. Young, E. (1987): Sensitivity to propolis. *Contact Dermatitis, 16,* 49–50.
83. De Groot, A.C. and Weyland, J.W. (1988): Kathon CG: A review. *J. Am. Acad. Dermatol., 18,* 350–358.
84. De Groot, A.C. (1990): Methylisothiazolinone/methylchloroisothiazolinone (Kathon CG) allergy: an updated review. *Am. J. Contact Dermatitis, 1,* 151–156.
85. Färm, G. and Wahlberg, J.E. (1991): Isothiazolinones (MCI/MI): 200 ppm versus 100 ppm in the standard series. *Contact Dermatitis, 25,* 104–107.
86. Ledieu, G., Martin, P. and Thomas, P. (1991): L'Allergie de contact au Kathon® CG. *Ann. Dermatol. Venereol, 118,* 181–189.
87. Foussereau, J. (1990): An epidemiological study of contact allergy to 5-chloro-3-methyl isothiazolinone/3-methyl isothiazolinone in Strasbourg. *Contact Dermatitis, 22,* 68–70.
88. Cronin, E., Hannuksela, M., Lachapelle, J.M., Maibach, H.I., Malten, K. and Meneghini, C.L. (1988): Frequency of sensitization to the preservative Kathon® CG. *Contact Dermatitis, 18,* 274–279.
89. Foussereau, J., Brändle, I. and Boujnah-Khouadja, A. (1984): Allergisches Kontaktekzem durch Isothiazolin-3-on-Derivate. *Dermatosen, 32,* 208–211.
90. Hannuksela, M. (1986): Rapid increase in contact allergy to Kathon® CG in Finland. *Contact Dermatitis, 15,* 211–214.
91. De Groot, A.C. (1988): *Adverse Reactions to Cosmetics*, pp. 111–112. Thesis, University of Groningen.
92. Cronin, E. (1987): Allergy to cosmetics. *Acta. Derm. Venereol, Suppl. 134,* 77–82.
93. Parker, L.U. and Taylor, J.S. (1991): A 5-year study of contact allergy to quaternium-15. *Am. J. Contact Dermatitis, 2,* 231–234.
94. Flyvholm, M.A. and Menné, T. (1992): Allergic contact dermatitis from formaldehyde. *Contact Dermatitis, 27,* 27–36.
95. De Groot, A.C., Bruynzeel, D.P., Coenraads, P.J. et al. (1991): Frequency of allergic reactions to methyldibromoglutaronitrile (1,2-dibromo-2,4-dicyanobutane) in the Netherlands. *Contact Dermatitis, 25,* 270–271.
96. Torres, V. and Soares, A.P. (1992): Contact allergy to dibromodicyanobutane in a cosmetic cream. *Contact Dermatitis, 27,* 114.
97. Fuchs, Th., Enders, F., Przybilla, B. et al. (1991): Contact allergy to Euxyl K400. *Dermatosen, 39,* 151–153.
98. Guerra, L., Bardazzi, F. and Tosti, A. (1992): Contact dermatitis in hairdressers' clients. *Contact Dermatitis, 26,* 108–111.

25. Patch testing with cosmetic preparations

25.1 Ideally, when a cosmetic is suspected of having caused a contact allergic reaction, all ingredients should be tested separately, in a suitable patch testing vehicle and at an adequate concentration [1]. Unfortunately, this procedure is rarely performed, as such an analysis to determine the actual cause of sensitivity poses several practical difficulties, all of which make the investigation very laborious:

1. Unlike in the United States, the cosmetic industry in many countries is not committed to declare the ingredients on cosmetic products labels. Most companies require an individual request to be written for each product before providing ingredient information for their products (if at all!).
2. Patients often use several cosmetic preparations, and it is frequently impossible to decide which one of these has caused the adverse reaction.
3. Cosmetics are often composed of numerous ingredients.
4. Many of the cosmetic ingredients have no published documentation as to proper non-irritating patch test concentrations. Serial dilutions and control tests must then be performed [1].

25.2 For the above reasons, the cosmetic as such is usually used for patch testing. However, there are several pitfalls to this procedure:

1. False-positive reactions may be noted, as many cosmetics act as weak irritants when tested under occlusion; such reactions are sometimes hard to distinguish from weak allergic reactions. Irritant reactions are frequently seen with testing of cosmetics that contain volatile chemicals (which may be irritants), such as hair lacquers, liquid mascaras, and nail lacquers. It is advisable to allow such cosmetics to dry on the skin before they are covered with patch testers. In addition, all detergent-containing cosmetics (soap, shampoo, bath and shower foam) have to be diluted to 1–2% to avoid false-positive (irritant) reactions, which, even then, they still frequently induce.
2. False-negative reactions frequently occur because the concentration of the sensitizer in the cosmetic may be too low to elicit a positive patch test reaction. This is seen especially in cases of contact allergy to preservatives and fragrance materials. Additionally, when detergent-containing products are diluted (which is necessary to avoid false-positive reactions), the actual allergen is also diluted, often down to a concentration below the threshold for elicitation of a positive patch test reaction (false-negative reaction).
3. Patch testing under occlusion with undiluted cosmetics may (rarely) carry the risk of sensitizing the patient, as has been noted with hair dyes.

25.3 When patch testing with a cosmetic yields a weak positive reaction, the patch test should be repeated; weak irritant reactions are less likely to be reproducible than allergic ones. Control tests should also be performed. Sometimes a Repeated Open Application Test (ROAT) may be helpful: the cosmetic is applied 2–3 times daily to the same area of one forearm for 7 days and, subsequently, the reaction is recorded. Whereas a positive open test indicates the patch test reaction to be allergic in nature, a negative result does not exclude the possibility of a cosmetic allergy.

The patient should then be instructed to use the cosmetic as she/he would normally have done, and reappear for clinical examination. Nevertheless, confirmation of contact allergy by patch testing with the ingredients of the cosmetic separately is always advisable, if not mandatory. A guideline to the testing of cosmetics is provided in § 25.4 (adapted from de Groot and White [2]). Concomitant testing of a 'cosmetic series' containing well known cosmetic sensitizers may often identify the sensitizer in the implicated product. A suggested cosmetic screening series is shown in Table 25.2.

25.4 **Table 25.1. Recommended test concentrations for cosmetic products. Most cosmetics not mentioned in this table can be tested undiluted**

Cosmetic product	Typical ingredients	Test concentration and vehicle
bleach	ammonium persulfate	1% pet
depilatory	thioglycolate	1% pet
foaming bath product		1% water
foaming cleanser		1% water
hair dyes		2% water
mascara		pure (allow to dry)
nail cuticle remover		individual ingredients
nail glue		individual ingredients
nail polish		pure (allow to dry)
nail polish remover		individual ingredients
permanent wave solution	glyceryl thioglycolate	1% pet
shampoo		1% water
shaving lather or cream		1% water
skin lightener	hydroquinone	1% pet
soap or detergent		1% water
straightener		individual ingredients
toothpaste		2% water

25.5 Many ingredients of cosmetic preparations are also used in non-cosmetic topical preparations. Only those compounds that have caused side effects *by their presence in cosmetic products* will be listed in this part of the book. An exception is made for plant products used for cosmetics; the side effects mentioned usually do not relate to the use of these compounds in cosmetics (with the exception of fragrances). For ingredients of cosmetics that have caused adverse reactions *in non-cosmetic topical preparations only*, the reader is referred to Chapter 5.

Table 25.2. Suggested allergens for a 'cosmetic screening series'

Allergen	Function	Test conc. & vehicle
Amerchol L 101 (mineral oil and lanolin alcohol)	emulsifier	50% pet
benzophenone-3 (oxybenzone)	sunscreen	2% pet
benzophenone-10 (mexenone)	sunscreen	2% pet
BHA (butylated hydroxyanisole)	antioxidant	2% pet
2-bromo-2-nitropropane-1,3-diol (bronopol)	preservative	0.5% pet
cetearyl alcohol	emulsifier	30% pet
chloroacetamide	preservative	0.2% pet
cocamidopropyl betaine	surfactant	1% aqua
diazolidinyl urea	preservative	2% pet
fragrance-mix (ICDRG)	fragrance	8×1% pet
glyceryl thioglycolate	permanent waving agent	1% pet
hydrogenated lanolin	emulsifier	pure
imidazolidinyl urea	preservative	2% pet
4-isopropyldibenzoylmethane	sunscreen	2% pet
methyl(chloro)isothiazolinone (Kathon CG)	preservative	100 ppm in water
methyldibromoglutaronitrile	preservative	0.05% pet
musk ambrette	fragrance	5% pet
octyl dimethyl PABA	sunscreen	2% pet
PABA	sunscreen	2% pet
parabens	preservatives	5×3% pet
propolis	natural ingredient	10% pet
propyl gallate	antioxidant	1% pet
propylene glycol	humectant	2% pet
toluenesulfonamide/formaldehyde resin	nail lacquer resin	10% pet

25.6 REFERENCES

1. De Groot, A.C. (1993): *Patch Testing. Test Concentrations and Vehicles for 2800 Allergens, 2nd edition.* Elsevier Science Publishers, Amsterdam.
2. De Groot, A.C. and White, I.R. (1992): Cosmetics. In: *Textbook of Contact Dermatitis*, Chapter 14.1, pp. 459–475. Editors: R.J.G. Rycroft et al. Springer Verlag, Heidelberg.

26. Hair cosmetics

SHAMPOO AND ANTI-DANDRUFF SHAMPOO

26.1 A shampoo cleans the hair by removing dirt, excessive fat and scaling by means of surfactants. It should not clean too much and should leave sufficient natural sebum on the hair. The shampoo-washed hair must be manageable (in wet as well as in dry condition), easily set in style and not dull in appearance. When a shampoo accidentally comes into contact with the eye, the product should not sting.

A shampoo has a very short contact time with the skin of the scalp and is generally diluted several times with water; it is washed off thoroughly after use. Because of this, no serious side effects are to be expected [82]. In general, most complaints relate to itching or stinging of the eyes after accidental contact with the shampoo.

A typical **shampoo** formula is:

Ingredients		Example
50–70%	water	water
7–15%	anionic surfactant (principal)	TEA-lauryl sulfate
3–5%	foam builder	lauramide MEA
0.5–1%	thickener	sodium chloride
ca. 1%	additive for pearlescent appearance	PEG-8 distearate
ca. 2%	conditioner	polyquaternium-10
ca. 0.2%	preservatives	formaldehyde
ca. 0.005%	colour	Acid Yellow 23
ca. 0.5%	perfume	perfume

Shampoos are aqueous products which are generally preserved with water soluble preservatives. Commonly used are formaldehyde donors (DMDM Hydantoin, imidazolidinyl urea), methyldibromoglutaronitrile and isothiazolinones (Kathon CG). More apolar preservatives like the parabens are also used, however.

Anti-dandruff shampoos are shampoos to which 1–2% active ingredients have been added. The following anti-dandruff agents are mentioned in the literature:
- captan
- coal tar
- climbazole
- ketoconazol (drug)
- piroctone olamine
- pyrithione disulfide Mg-sulfate (prohibited in the EC)
- salicylic acid
- selenium sulfide (sold as drug)
- sodium pyrithione (prohibited in EC)
- sulfur (colloidal)
- undecylamide DEA/MEA
- undecylenic acid
- zinc pyrithione

Quaternary ammonium compounds (e.g. benzalkonium chloride) are sometimes used as anti-dandruff agents, but their efficacy is rather doubtful.

Shampoos have to be diluted to 1–2% aqueous for a closed patch test of 5% aqueous for an open test to avoid irritation. However, even then irritant reactions occur frequently (false-positive reactions). In addition, in those patients actually sensitized, false-negative reactions also occur, as the causative allergen is diluted to a low concentration which cannot elicit a positive patch test reaction. Therefore, in cases of suspected allergy, the properly diluted ingredients of the incriminated product should always be tested separately.

Side effects of shampoo ingredients are listed in § 26.2 and 26.3.

26.2 Contact allergy to ingredients of shampoos

Ingredient	Use	Patch test conc. & vehicle (§ 5.2)	Cross-reactions (§ 5.5)	Comment	Ref.
captan	anti-dandruff agent	0.1% pet		*Photoallergy* (§ 6.5)	19
carbon tetrachloride	solvent for fat	10% o.o.		No controls tested	46
cetrimonium bromide (cetrimide)	conditioner	0.01% aqua			81
cinnamic alcohol	fragrance	2% pet			
chloromercaptodicar-boximide (captan)				*See under* Captan	
cocamide DEA	nonionic surfactant	0.5% pet	lauramide DEA		80 123
cocoamidopropyl betaine	detergent	1% aqua		occupational allergy: Ref. [124]	79 83
coco-betaine	amphoteric detergent	2% aqua	cocamidopropyl betaine (Tegobetain®)		61

(continued)

§ **26.2** *(continuation)*

Ingredient	Use	Patch test conc. & vehicle (§ 5.2)	Cross-reactions (§ 5.5)	Comment	Ref.
formaldehyde	preservative	1% aqua			1 6 49
lauramide DEA	nonionic surfactant	1% pet/aqua	cocamide DEA		80
linalool	fragrance	30% pet			123
miranols (imidazole derivatives)	amphoteric surfactants	1% aqua		Testing with miranols in 3% conc. may sensitize. Miranols are amphoteric surfactants to which anionic detergents have sometimes been added	56
perfume(?)		1% o.o.			44
potassium cocohydrolyzed animal protein	detergent	5% and 30% aqua	TEA coco-hydrolyzed animal protein. Potassium undecylenoyl hydrolyzed animal protein. TEA oleyl-polypeptide	The patient primarily became sensitized to TEA-oleylpolypeptide, and later cross-reacted to potassium coco-hydrolyzed animal protein in shampoo	78
selenium sulfide	anti-dandruff agent	2% pet.		Contact allergy not proven in [18]	18 123
sodium laureth sulfate (sodium laurylether sulfate)	in dish-washing liquids and possibly also in shampoos (amphoteric surfactant)	1% aqua		Contained allergic reactions caused by an impurity, i.e. sultones	12 53 61
sodium pyrithione (Sodium omadine®)	anti-dandruff agent	0.3% aqua		For occupational allergy in a metallurgical worker, *see* [76]	75
TEA PEG-3 cocamide sulfate	amphoteric detergent	1% aqua		Concomitant (?) reaction to cocamidopropyl betaine	83
zinc pyrithione	anti-dandruff agent	1% pet	possibly piperazine, etylene diamine and hydroxyzine		38 59 77

26.3 Other adverse reactions to ingredients of shampoos

Ingredient	Use	Side effect	Comment	Ref.
alcohol in a beer-containing shampoo	fragrance enhancer	antabuse effect in a patient taking disulfiram for alcoholism		74
cetrimonium bromide	hair conditioner	matting of the hair (bird's nest hair), irritant dermatitis	Irreversible matting may be caused by a viscous fluid (probably a deposit from shampoos) or bending of the hairs through 180° [84]	16
cinnamon oil	fragrance	contact urticaria, *see* § 7.5		45
medicated shampoos		wash the colour out of dyed hair		52
PVP (polyvinyl pyrrolidone)	hair sprays	pneumonitis		126
selenium sulfide	anti-dandruff agent	irritant dermatitis, reversible hair loss and oiliness of the scalp, systemic toxicity		
shampoo ingredient, not specified	shampoo	contact urticaria		74
sorbic acid	preservative	contact urticaria		45
surfactant in shampoo		irritant dermatitis in subjects employed in shampoo manufacture; also in hairdressers		3 51
zinc pyrithione	anti-dandruff agent	postinflammatory hyper- and hypopigmentation; photosensitization and actinic reticuloid; peripheral neuritis (?)		38 59 85
?	hair spray	nail damage	Weak evidence for causal relationship	125

CONDITIONING SHAMPOO AND HAIR CONDITIONER (AFTER-SHAMPOO RINSE)

26.4 Shampooed hair (in particular when slightly damaged by repeated colouring, bleaching of waving) is often in a bad condition. It such (wet) hair is treated with an after-shampoo rinse, significant improvement may be obtained: better lustre and feel, good combability and ease of styling. It has been assumed that the presence of many negatively charged sites on the hair surface is the cause of the bad condition. The active after-shampoo ingredients are large positively charged (cationic) molecules that neutralize the anionic sites.

In several shampoos conditioning agents are formulated; in these cases the use of an after-shampoo rinse is not necessary. The classical conditioning shampoo is based on the addition of a cationic conditioner and has to be formulated carefully, because incompatibility of the anionic principal surfactant and the cationic conditioner easily results in inactivation of the conditioning properties. This formulation problem has been alleviated by the introduction of silicone derivatives as the conditioning agent. Silicones carry no charge and are compatible with anionic detergents. A typical example is dimethicone copolyol.

Shortly after their introduction it has been suggested that these silicone based '2-in-1' shampoos gave rise to increased loss of hair, but there is no evidence that this is the case.

The most important hair conditioning agents are:
- quaternary ammonium compounds (see § 30.15.3)
- amphoteric surfactants (see § 30.15.3)
- amine oxides
- hydrolyzed animal protein
- silicone derivatives (dimethicone copolyol, amodimethicone, etc.)

A typical formula of an **after-shampoo rinse** is:

Ingredients		Example
ca. 93%	water	water
2–5%	hair conditioning agent	stearalkonium chloride, lauramine oxide
ca. 2%	lipid	cetyl alcohol, glyceryl stearate
ca. 0.5%	thickener	carbomer
ca. 0.2%	perfume	perfume
ca. 0.05%	colour	FD&C Blue No. 1

A typical formula of a **'2-in-1' shampoo** is:

Ingredients		Example
60–80%	water	water
10–30%	anionic detergent	ammonium laureth sulfate
3–5%	foam builder	cocamide MEA
3–5%	conditioner	amodimethicone
3–5%	opacifying agent	glycol distearate
0.5–1%	thickener	hydroxyethyl cellulose
0.2%	preservative	diazolidinyl urea
<0.5%	perfume	perfume
<0.5%	colour	FD&C Blue No. 1

HAIR COLOURS

26.5 There are 5 types of hair colours, each with a specific composition and action mechanism. Therefore, when an adverse reaction from a hair colour is suspected, it is important to find out which type of product is used by the patient.

1. Hair restorers are hair dressings which gradually (after several days) darken grey hair to a brownish-black colour. The active ingredient is (ca 1%) lead acetate and colloidal sulfur or sodium thiosulfate, which forms black lead sulfide on the hair surface. For toxicological and/or regulatory reasons lead acetate has been replaced by bismuth citrate in some countries, but unfortunately this gives less satisfactory results.

A typical **hair restorer** formula is:

Ingredients		Example
0–10%	water	water
ca. 10%	polyol	glycerin
70–80%	lipid	petrolatum, lanolin
0–1%	surfactant	ceteth-20
ca. 2%	active ingredients	lead acetate, sulfur (colloidal)
ca. 0.5 %	perfume	perfume

2. Vegetable hair dyes: in particular henna, the powdered leaves of *Lawsonia alba*. The active ingredient is lawsone (2-hydroxy-1,4-naphthoquinone), which colours the hair in approximately one hour. It can be applied as an aqueous (hot water) paste of the dried leaves, but the long reaction time is not very convenient. The colour obtained is reddish. Other vegetable materials which can be used are indigo leaves, chamomile flowers, and powdered walnuts. Synthetic Lawson®, which is commercially available, or other naphthoquinones may be added to enhance the colouring power. Henna extracts mixed with ordinary shampoo bases are also available.

3. Temporary dyes (washable after one shampooing) are particularly applied in *hair colour setting lotions*.

4. Semi-permanent dyes (which will withstand 4–5 shampooings) are formulated in shampoo bases. Direct colours used are of small molecular size, which facilitates the penetration of the dye into the hair cortex. Some of these dye ingredients are also used in the *permanent* type.

A typical formula of a **semi-permanent hair colour shampoo** is:

Ingredients		Example
70%	water	water
ca. 10%	principle surfactant	sodium laureth sulfate
ca. 1%	thickener	carbomer-914
ca. 0.2%	preservatives	2-bromo-2-nitropropane-1,3-diol
1–3%	semi-permanent hair colours	HC Blue 2, HC Red 3, 2-nitro-*p*-phenylenediamine

Examples of hair colours which are used as **semi-permanent hair colours** are (see also § 30.11):
- Aminonitrophenols (several isomers)
- Disperse Blue 1 and 3
- Disperse Violet 1 and 4
- HC Blue 2-4-5
- HC Orange 1
- HC Red 1-3
- HC Yellow 2-3-4-5
- Nitrophenylene diamines (several isomers)

5. Oxidation hair colours or **permanent hair colours**. This is the most important type; it is easily applied and the colours will withstand more than 10 shampooings, because the colour is formed within the hair cortex. Oxidation hair colours are easily recognized. The two separate parts should be mixed just before use. One part is a mixture of the colour intermediates and the other is a hydrogen peroxide solution or a peroxide powder in a shampoo or a viscous lotion base. The mixture should be immediately applied to the hair after mixing. Two different reactions occur in the mixture: the hydrogen peroxide bleaches the original hair melanin (the bleached hair permits better colouring), the other reaction is a complex (new) colour formation (for a part within the hair cortex by the hydrogen peroxide and the colour intermediates). After 15 minutes, when sufficient new colour has formed, the product is washed off.

A typical formula is:

Colour shampoo of intermediates (Part I)

Ingredients		Example
ca. 70%	water	water
ca. 10%	surfactant	TEA lauryl sulfate
ca. 1%	thickener	carbomer-914
0.5–4%	hair colour (intermediates)	toluene-2,5-diamine, *m*-aminophenol, resorcinol
ca. 1%	antioxidant: stabilizer	erythorbic acid, sodium sulfite
ca. 1%	ammonia	ammonia

Hydrogen peroxide lotion (Part II)

Ingredients		Example
ca. 85%	water	water
ca. 5%	lipid	cetyl alcohol
ca. 2%	surfactant: nonionic	ceteth-20
3–5%	hydrogen peroxide	hydrogen peroxide
ca. 1–2%	stabilizer and pH adjusting agent	EDTA, phenacetine, potassium phosphate

Colour formation results from a complicated reaction, in which oxidation of the primary intermediates by hydrogen peroxide produces highly reactive benzoquinone mono- or di-imines, which rapidly react with other compounds present, known as couplers. Depending on the choice of intermediates and the reaction conditions, a wide variety of shades can be obtained.

Examples of colour intermediates (see § 30.11) are:

Primary intermediates	Couplers
diamines	resorcinol, chlororesorcinol, 2-methylresorcinol
p-phenylenediamine	naphthol, 1,5- and 1,7-dihydroxynaphthalene
2,5-diaminotoluene	*m*-aminophenol, 4-methyl-5-aminophenol,
2-chloro-*p*-phenylenediamine	*o*-aminophenol
N-phenyl-*p*-phenylenediamine	*m*-phenylene diamine
N,N-bis(2-hydroxyethyl)-*p*-phenylene diamine	1,5-dihydroxynaphtalene
	1,7-dihydroxynaphtalene
aminophenols	4-methyl-5-(2-hydroxyethyl) aminophenol
p-aminophenol	
N-methyl-*p*-aminophenol	

The allergenicity of hair dyed with *p*-phenylenediamine

Some investigations indicate that *p*-phenylenediamine-sensitive individuals can come into intimate contact with hairs or furs coloured with this dye, without risking an allergic contact dermatitis. Once the *p*-phenylenediamine is oxidized, which happens very rapidly in the hair, the resultant *p*-benzoquinone-diimine that is formed is not allergenic [20].

This statement however is only valid when the hair has been correctly dyed. Unreacted not fully oxidized dye (because of inadequate mixing or rinsing after dyeing) may result in residues of unreacted *p*-phenylenediamine remaining in the hair [24,57] which are then capable of inducing contact-allergic reactions in sensitized individuals.

Tabulation of side effects to hair colour ingredients

Side effects of ingredients of hair colours are tabulated in § 26.6 (contact allergy) and § 26.7 (other side effects).

26.6 Contact allergy to ingredients of hair colours

Ingredient	Patch test conc. & vehicle (§ 5.2)	Cross-reactions (§ 5.5)	Comment	Ref.
m-aminophenol	2% pet.	related compounds		4
p-aminophenol	2% pet.	related compounds	Ortho- and paraaminophenol patch-testing may sensitize	4 47
Basic blue 99 (CI 56059)	1% pet		Aminoketone colour	108
henna (dried leaves of *Lawsonia alba*, containing 2-hydroxy-1,4-naphthoquinone = lawsone)	prick test with 10 mg henna powder in 100 ml aqua, ether and ethanol		Immediate-type reaction: sneezing, facial swelling, urticaria, asthma [68]. One patient reacted to lawsone (test concentration not specified [113]). In an old publication, a patient was reported to have died from a contact allergic reaction to henna hair dye [121]	13 68 113
N-(β-hydroxyethyl)-2-nitro-4-hydroxy-aminobenzene	1% pet	possibly to other aminobenzenes		109
1-hydroxy-3-nitro-4-aminobenzene	0.2% pet	possibly to other aminobenzenes		109
1-hydroxyethylamino-3-nitro-4-aminobenzene	1% pet	possibly to other aminobenzenes		109
lead acetate	1% aqua		The reported case may have been due to patch-test sensitization	64
2-nitro-*p*-phenylenediamine	1% pet.			41
p-phenylenediamine	1% pet.			14 29 42 57
N-phenyl-*p*-phenylenediamine (*p*-aminodiphenylamine)	0.25% pet.	4-isopropylaminodiphenylamine and other related compounds, diphenylamine [60]		4 48
pyrocatechol	2% pet.	hydroquinone		110
quinaphtalone (in DC Yellow 12)	0.1% pet			111
resorcinol	2% pet.			4 12
toluene-2,4-diamine	1% pet	related compounds		4
toluene-2,5-diamine	1% pet.	related compounds		4 14 35

See for cross-sensitivity between para-dyes and certain antihistamines MacKie and MacKie [34].

26.7 Other side effects of ingredients of hair colours

Ingredient	Side effect	Ref.
4-amino-2-nitrophenol	mutagenic (?)	28
copper in cosmetic plant extracts	green hair	
4-methoxy-*m*-phenylenediamine	mutagenic (?), carcinogenic (?)	28
4-nitro-*o*-phenylenediamine	mutagenic (?), carcinogenic (?)	28
2-nitro-*p*-phenylenediamine	mutagenic (?), carcinogenic (?)	28
m-phenylenediamine	mutagenic (?), carcinogenic (?)	28
p-phenylenediamine	systemic absorption with darkening of the urine	36,37
	vertigo, anaemia, gastritis, exfoliative dermatitis and death	73
	chromosomal damage (?)	32
	mutagenic (?)	28
	aplastic anaemia (?)	55
	immediate-type hypersensitivity with edema and difficulty in breathing	9
toluene-2,4-diamine	mutagenic (?), carcinogenic (?)	28
toluene-2,5-diamine	mutagenic (?)	28

Teratogenicity due to hair dyes has not been documented [114]. Embryotoxicity has been suggested in older publications [122], but remains unconfirmed.

The mutagenicity and animal carcinogenicity data available for hair dyes and their ingredients suggest that they may have the potential to constitute a human health risk. However, epidemiological and human monitoring studies, with few exceptions [116,120], have not detected any such risk in the exposed human populations [115,117–119]. The issue has not been settled at the time of writing [115].

Percutaneous penetration of hair dyes under usage conditions has been reported [72]: diaminoanisole (0.015%), *p*-phenylenediamine (0.14%) and HC Blue 1 (0.09%).

PERMANENT WAVE

26.8 Permanent waving of hair is performed nowadays without the application of heat (cold wave). For a cold wave a dual solution is needed, the components of which are used separately and successively:

1. an alkaline thioglycolate solution of pH 8–10 (*waving fluid*);
2. an acid hydrogen peroxide solution (*fixation* or *neutralization fluid*).

The hair is pretreated with an alkaline shampoo to make the hair surface more permeable to the waving fluid. The hair is then set in curls and wetted with the waving fluid. The alkaline reaction swells the hair to almost 150% of its original size, which promotes the action of the thioglycolate. Even the strong S–S bridges of the keratin filaments are broken. This treatment lasts for 10–20 minutes.

The thioglycolate solution is subsequently removed thoroughly with the aid of a towel while the hair is still in curls. The second fluid is then applied to the hair. The acid reaction stops the action of residual thioglycolate, and the hydrogen peroxide restores the S–S bridges. As this happens in the curly state of the hair, the curl becomes permanent. The fixation takes about 15 minutes.

A typical formula for a **waving fluid** is:

Ingredients		Example
ca. 90%	water	Water
5–11%	thioglycolic acid	thioglycolic acid
ca. 1%	cloudifier	styrene/acrylates copolymer, laureth-20, carbomer-941
ca. 0.05%	colour	FD&C Blue No. 1
ca. 0.1%	perfume	perfume
	ammonia sufficient for a pH of 8.5	ammonia

The thioglycolate solution can also be applied as an aerosol foam. The following is a typical formula for an **aerosol waving fluid**:

Ingredients		Example
ca. 80%	water	water
ca. 5%	propellant	butane, isobutane
ca. 10%	MEA-thioglycolate	MEA-thioglycolate
ca. 5%	lipid	dibutyl phthalate
ca. 1%	surfactant	laureth-20
ca. 0.1%	perfume	perfume

Permanent waves based on thioglycolic acid are quite alkaline and consequently irritating. In an attempt to provide alternatives which lack the irritating properties of the classical cold waves, products based on glyceryl thioglycolate, the glyceryl ester of thioglycolic acid, are currently marketed. Glyceryl thioglycolate is generally packaged separately (as a solution in anhydrous glycerin) in order to prevent hydrolysis, and has to be mixed with a second solution containing additional ingredients to prepare the waving solution. These permanent waves are known as '**acid waves**', though the pH after the mixing of the solutions may be slightly alkaline. Usually, however, the pH will be between 6.5 and 7.

A typical formula of an **acid perm wave** is:

Ingredients			Example
1	12%	waving agent	glyceryl thioglycolate
	8%	solvent	glycerin
II	80%	water	water
	0.5–1%	surfactant	coceth-8
	0.1–0.4%	fragrance	fragrance

Solutions I and II are mixed before use.

A typical formula for the **fixation fluid** is:

Ingredients		Example
ca. 95%	water	water
ca. 4%	hydrogen peroxide	hydrogen peroxide
0.1%	stabilizer for hydrogen peroxide	phenacetine
ca. 0.5%	citric acid	citric acid
ca. 1%	cloudifier	styrene/acrylates copolymer, laureth-20, Carbomer-941

Irritation from the alkaline thioglycolate solutions occurs frequently in hairdressers [5]. Glyceryl thioglycolate has become a major contact allergen in those occupationally exposed. With proper application techniques, sensitization of the customer is infrequent (§ 26.14).

In case of a suspected allergic reaction, other cosmetic materials such as setting materials, colouring agents, perfumes etc. should also be investigated as a possible cause.

Side effects of ingredients of permanent wave cosmetics are tabulated in § 26.14 (contact allergy) and § 26.15 (other side effects).

HAIR SPRAY, HAIR SETTING LOTION AND STYLING FOAM

26.9 Styled hair can be kept in place by applying a film polymer around the hair filament. A few flushes of an aerosol hair spray is a very convenient and popular way to perform this operation. Until recently, chlorofluorocarbons were the first choice propellants, but the alleged breakdown of the ozone layer from chlorofluorocarbons has resulted in a change of the choice of propellants. The first alternatives were simple hydrocarbons like propane and isobutane, but due to regulatory pressure, hydrocarbons as the sole propellants are being partly substituted more and more by dimethylether. Similar considerations, and its possible mutagenicity, have made the once popular solvent methylene chloride (dichloromethane) lose much of its former significance, although it is still being used in Europe.

A typical aerosol **hair spray** formula is:

Ingredients		Example
1–5%	film polymer	PVM/VA copolymer
ca. 0.1–0.5%	polymer neutralizer	aminomethyl propanol
30–40%	solvent	alcohol, water
35–60%	propellant	dimethyl ether/isobutane/propane

One should be aware that the volatile propellants evaporate almost immediately; consequently, the concentration in which the ingredients reach the skin is much higher than indicated above.

Styling foams are a variation on the hair spray, in which the addition of a foam builder (for example cocamide DEA) produces a mousse rather than a spray. The mousse is spread through the (wet or dry) hair and left to dry.

Increased environmental consciousness of consumers has led to an increased popularity of **pump sprays**, which until recently could not compete with aerosol sprays. The basic formulation principle is the same as for aerosol sprays, but no propellants are used. Instead, the spray is dispensed by a small manually powered pump. **Setting lotions** are similar to pump sprays, but lack the pump system.

All these hair styling products may have additional ingredients to provide for hair conditioning (quaternary ammonium compounds, silicone derivatives, panthenol, etc.), colouring of the hair (temporary hair dyes) or UV protection (benzophenones, etc.).

A fashionable alternative to hair spray is the **styling gel**. It consists basically of (much) water, a thickener and a film polymer. Sometimes these gels contain titanated mica for glitter effects.

A typical formula for a **styling gel** is:

Ingredients		Example
4–5%	film former	PVP/VA copolymer
1%	viscosity increasing agent	carbomer-940
1–30%	alcohol	alcohol
0.1–1.0%	preservative colour	DMDM hydantoin
0.1–0.5%	fragrance	fragrance
ad 100%	water	water

Side effects

For side effects of ingredients of hair-spray and hair-setting lotions see § 26.14 and § 26.15.

HAIR BLEACH

26.10 There are two types of hair bleaches: one is based on the action of hydrogen peroxide or a 'per-salt', and the second is based on zinc formaldehyde sulfoxylate; the latter is used mainly to bleach artificially coloured hair.

The type based on hydrogen peroxide is most frequently used. The simplest product is an acidic solution of hydrogen peroxide in a pump spray, which is popular among blondes to lighten their hair to a 'summer blond' shade.

Stronger home bleaches, suitable for lightening darker shades of hair, add 'boosters' and often contain multiple separated packages per unit, to assure stability of the hydrogen peroxide. The various components are mixed just before use, and this will result in an viscous paste which is easily applied to the hair. After 10–40 minutes, depending on the desired degree of bleaching, the paste is rinsed off thoroughly to avoid traces of the peroxide being left on the hair, which can cause brittleness.

A typical 3-parts **home bleach** is as follows (1 + 2 + 3 to be mixed just before use):

Ingredients		Example
Cream with hydrogen peroxide (Part I):		
ca. 60%	water	water
ca. 5%	lipid	glyceryl stearate
ca. 2%	emulsifier	PEG-100 stearate
ca. 0.5%	stabilizer	phenacetine
ca. 0.1%	stabilizer	EDTA
ca. 1%	acid agent	phosphoric acid
5–8%	bleaching agent	hydrogen peroxide
'Oily' liquid (so-called 'bleach base') (Part II):		
ca. 80%	water	water
ca. 1%	foam builder	oleamide DEA
ca. 2%	emulsifier	nonoxynol-10
5–10%	emulsifier	ammonium oleate
ca. 1%	alkaline agent	ammonia
ca. 0.01%	colour	colour
Powder containing a 'booster' to increase bleaching power (Part III):		
ca. 20%	sodium persulfate	
ca. 75%	magnesium carbonate	
ca. 5%	sodium lauryl sulfate	

Frequent bleaching with hydrogen peroxide will cause increased brittleness of the hair.

The second type of hair bleach, used to bleach artificially coloured hair, contains 5–7% zinc formaldehydesulfoxylate (Rongalit®) which is a condensation product of two bleaching agents: formaldehyde and sodium sulfite.

Tabulation of side effects

Side effects of ingredients of hair bleaches are tabulated in § 26.14 (contact allergy) and § 26.15 (other side effects).

HAIR DRESSING

26.11 The 'classic' hair care consists of a daily application of a hair dressing, which is mainly an oil as such, or an emulsion of an oil with water.

A typical formula for a **hair dressing** (non-aqueous type) is:

Ingredients		Example
ca. 99%	lipid	petrolatum, lanolin oil
ca. 0.05%	antioxidant	BHT
ca. 1%	perfume	perfume
ca. 0.01%	colour	chlorophyllin–copper complex (CI 75810)

A typical formula for a **hair dressing emulsion** is:

Ingredients		Example
ca. 20%	water	water
ca. 80%	lipid	mineral oil, beeswax
ca. 2%	surfactant	sodium borate (reacts with beeswax to a soap emulsifier)
ca. 0.5%	perfume	perfume

Anti-dandruff hair dressings are formulated by addition of approx. 0.1% of an antidandruff agent (e.g. zinc pyrithione). Colouring hair dressings have been mentioned under *hair restorers* (§ 26.5).

Tabulation of side effects

Side effects of ingredients of hair dressings are tabulated in § 26.14 and § 26.15.

HAIR STRAIGHTENER (HAIR RELAXER)

26.12 Straightening curly hair is performed in 3 consecutive steps: (1) the hair is wetted with the straightening fluid for approximately 15 minutes; (2) the hair is subsequently straightened by intermittent combing with a special comb for approximately 15–20 minutes; followed by (3) rinsing off with plenty of water, and neutralizing with neutralizing liquid for 3–5 minutes. Usually, a dual solution is used:

1. The straightening fluid, based on one of the three following agents: sodium (potassium) hydroxide, sodium bisulfite or ammonium thioglycolate.
2. The neutralizing fluid, using special neutralizers for each type:
   for sodium hydroxide: a non-alkaline shampoo is sufficient;
   for sodium bisulfite: sodium bicarbonate;
   for ammonium thioglycolate: hydrogen peroxide.

N.B. The thioglycolate solution is basically similar to the permanent wave fluid and neutralizer.

A typical formula for the **sodium hydroxide hair straightener** is:

Ingredients		Example
ca. 65%	water	water
ca. 2%	sodium hydroxide	sodium hydroxide
25–30%	lipid	cetyl alcohol, mineral oil, petrolatum
ca. 4%	surfactant	sodium lauryl sulfate

A typical formula for a **sulfite hair straightener** is:

Ingredients		Example
70–80%	water	water
ca. 8–9%	sodium bisulfite	sodium bisulfite
ca. 25%	gelling agent	poloxamer 407

A typical formula for a **thioglycolate hair relaxer** is:

Ingredients		Example
5–10%	active ingredient	thioglycolic acid
qs	pH adjuster	ammonia
50–80%	water	water
10–20%	lipid	cetearyl alcohol, decyl oleate
2–5%	emulsifier	oleth-10, cocamide DEA
0.1–0.5%	fragrance	fragrance

Tabulation of side effects

Side effects of hair straighteners are tabulated in § 26.14 and § 26.15.

HAIR GROWTH PROMOTION

26.13 In spite of the lack of any scientific proof for remedies to cure baldness, to promote hair growth or to prevent hair loss, these products are still on the market. Many of the active ingredients are rubefacients. which promote blood circulation near the hair follicles.

The following 'active' ingredients are mentioned in an OTC-proposed monograph (*Fed. Reg., Vol. 45, No. 218*, November 7, 1980):

allantoin	lanolin
amino acids	olive oil
ammonium lauryl sulfate	polyethylene glycol (PEG)
ascorbic acid	polysorbate 80
benzethonium chloride	propylene glycol
benzoic acid	proteins
dichlorophene	tar
estradiol	tetracaine hydrochloride
eucalyptus oil	vitamins
hormones	wheat germ oil
isopropyl alcohol	

Other 'active' ingredients mentioned in the literature are:

aloe	methyl salicylate
androgenic hormones	methyl nicotinate
benzyl nicotinate	nicotinamide
cantharidine	nicotinic acid
capsicum oleoresin	panthenol
cinchona extract	pilocarpine
diazoxide	quinine
diethylstilbestrol (DES)	resorcinol
estrogenic hormones	salicylic acid
4-(5-methoxyheptyl)-hexahydro-2(1H)-pentalenone	

In 1989, the Food and Drug Administration of the USA issued a final rule establishing "that any over-the-counter (OTC) hair grower or hair loss prevention drug product for external use is not generally recognized as safe and effective *and is misbranded.*" Consequently, any such product is subject to regulatory action [90].

Recently, however, it was found that minoxidil, an oral hypertensive drug, caused hypertrichosis in many patients. The effectiveness of topical minoxidil (branded in 1988 as Regaine® or Rogaine®) in the treatment of alopecia androgenetica (male pattern baldness) has subsequently been investigated in many trials. It was established that topical minoxidil indeed stimulates the growth of new hair, although this rarely results in cosmetically satisfactory results. Continued application does, however, prevent the hair from further falling out [91,92]. The side effects of topical minoxidil are discussed elsewhere in this book (e.g. § 16.45).

A typical formula for a **hair tonic** is:

Ingredients		Example
ca. 70%	water	water
ca. 20%	solvent	isopropanol, alcohol, propylene glycol
ca. 1–2%	active ingredients	cantharidine, quinine tincture, panthenol
0–0.02%	colour	CI 19140
ca. 0.1%	perfume	perfume

Side effects

Side effects of hair cosmetics (shampoos and colours excluded) are tabulated in § 26.14 (contact allergy) and § 26.15 (other side effects).

26.14 Contact allergy to ingredients of hair preparations (shampoos and colours excluded)

Ingredient	Cosmetic	Patch test conc. & vehicle (§ 5.2)	Cross-reactions (§ 5.5)	Comment	Ref.
ammonium persulfate (bleaching agent)	hair bleach	2.5% pet.		For occupational contact allergy, *see* [105]. For rashes amongst workers employed in the manufacture of persulfates, *see* [62]	21 58
ammonium thioglycolate (hair waving agent)	permanent wave	2.5% pet.		Has also caused irritant dermatitis. Occupational contact dermatitis in hairdressers, *see* [104]	17 50
benzoin (resin)	hair lacquer	10% pet. or alc.		Also contact allergy to benzoin in rose water	66
BHA (butylated hydroxyanisole) (antioxidant)	hair cream	2% pet.			98
compound tincture of benzoin (fragrance)	permanent wave	10% pet. or alc.			25
cyclohexanone-formaldehyde resin (resin)	hair lacquer spray	1% acet. and pet.			89
D&C Yellow No. 11 (Solvent Yellow 33; CI 47000) (colour)	hair cream	0.1% pet.			93
diazolidinyl urea (preservative)	hair gel	1% pet. or aqua	imidazolidinyl urea		88
dye	coloured hair setting lotion	0.1% pet.		Dye possibly a 'polyamino anthraquinone'	40
eugenol (fragrance)	hair cream	2% pet.	isoeugenol		123
fenticlor (antidandruff agent)	hair cream	1% pet.		Caused *photosensitivity* in the reported case	2

(continued)

§ **26.14** *(continuation)*

Ingredient	Cosmetic	Patch test conc. & vehicle (§ 5.2)	Cross-reactions (§ 5.5)	Comment	Ref.
glutaral (glutaraldehyde) (preservative)	hair conditioner	1% pet.			97
glyceryl thioglycolate (waving agent)	acid permanent waves	2.5% pet.	diglyceryl dithioglycolate ammonium thioglycolate	Glyceryl thioglycolate is a frequent cause of occupational allergic contact dermatitis in hairdressers, but clients may also be sensitized. Glyceryl thioglycolate-related allergen is retained in hair for up to 3 months after the permanent, which explains the long-lasting dermatitis that occurs in sensitized clients [99]. For the chemistry of waving, *see* [103].	99 100 101 102
hexamidine isethionate	hair lotion	0.15% aqua		The patient had been sensitized by an antiseptic product containing hexamidine isethionate	86
hinokitiol (β-thujaplicin) (hair growth stimulant)	hair liquid	0.1% alc.		Mainly used in Japan	63
Ineral®* (formaldehyde cyanoguanide and polyvinyl pyrrolidon solution) (hair film polymer)	hair strengthener	10% aqua pet.		Has caused irritant dermatitis	7 30 31 33
laurylpyridinium chloride (conditioner)	hair conditioner	0.1% aqua		The test concentration used is slightly irritant. Connubial dermatitis	87
maleic anhydride				*See under* Rosin	
methylisothiazolinone and methylchloroisothiazolinone (preservative)	hair conditioner	100 ppm aqua		Active ingredients in Kathon CG® and Euxyl K100®	123
panthenyl ethyl ether (hair conditioning agent)	hair lotion	30% pet.			96

(continued)

§ **26.14** *(continuation)*

Ingredient	Cosmetic	Patch test conc. & vehicle (§ 5.2)	Cross-reactions (§ 5.5)	Comment	Ref.
petrolatum (highly refined) (hair dressing)	hair tonic	7% in alc. 30%		No controls tested. The patient did *not* react to crude liquid petrolatum. Contact allergy not proven.	39
procaine hydrochloride (local anaesthetic, hair growth promoter)	hair lotion	1% pet.		Prohibited in cosmetics in the EC	9
pyridoxine dioctanoate (antiseborrhoeic drug)	hair liquid	1% pet.	pyridoxine hydrochloride		63
resorcinol (hair dye, hair growth promoter)	hair tonic	2% pet.	hexylresorcinol	Contact allergy not proven	54
rosin (colophony) (resin) and maleic anhydride	hair lacquer	rosin: 20% pet. maleic anhydride: ?		Possibly the many cases reported were *irritant* dermatitis	69 70
sodium bisulfite (antioxidant, waving agent)	cold permanent wave	2% pet.		Connubial dermatitis. The test concentration may be irritant. When improperly applied, irritant dermatitis may be frequent. Immediate-type allergy with asthma, urticaria and syncope reported.	106
Sulfated castor oil (hair dressing)	hair conditioner spray	pure?		Repeated insult patch tests were positive in 10% of normal volunteers.	65
thioglycerin (depilatory)	depilating cream	10% aqua			23
dimercaprol (1,2-dithio-glycerol, BAL) (chelating agent)	permanent wave	10% aqua		Has also caused irritant dermatitis	8 17
tioxolone	'hair product'	1% pet.			11
zinc pyrithione (antidandruff)	medicated hair cream	1% pet.			38

*The product 'Ineral' has been reformulated: the active ingredient in current use is dihydroxymethyl-1,3-thione-2-imidazolidine (DHMTI). This product polymerizes spontaneously in acid medium when applied to the hair or nails.

26.15 Other side effects of hair preparations (shampoos and colours excluded)

Ingredient	Cosmetic	Side effect	Ref.
aerosol propellants (fluoroalkane gases)	hair spray	cardiac arrhythmias 'sudden sniffing death'	43
ammonium persulfate	hair bleach	immediate-type hypersensitivity: – contact urticaria – headache and drowsiness – respiratory symptoms	10 21
ammonium thioglycolate	permanent wave	respiratory symptoms due to immediate-type allergy	26
estrogens	hair tonic cream	systemic side effects *See* § 16.61	
ethanol	hair spray	bronchoconstriction *See also under* Perfume	71
ethylenediamine	hair spray	respiratory symptoms due to immediate-type allergy	26
fixation fluid for permanent wave		contact urticaria: causative ingredient not specified. *See* §7.6	
hair bleach		contact urticaria; causative ingredient not specified. *See* § 7.6. *See also under* Ammonium persulfate	
hair spray		contact urticaria: causative ingredient not specified. *See* § 7.6	
hexamethylene tetramine	hair spray	respiratory symptoms due to immediate-type allergy	26
Ineral® (*see* § 26.14)	hair strengthener	irritant dermatitis (reversible), nail dystrophy with onycholysis	7 31 33
Lycopod powder (degreasing agent)	powder for the treatment of greasy hair	Rhinitis and asthma in the partners. Nasal provocation tests were positive	95
monoethanolamine	hair setting lotion	respiratory symptoms due to immediate-type allergy	26
perfume (?)	hair spray	alteration of pulmonary function in persons with preexisting disease such as asthma [67] and healthy individuals [71]	67 71
permanent wave fluid		contact urticaria: causative ingredient not specified. *See* § 7.6	
phenolic derivatives	hair tonic	pigmentation of palms, temples and hair margins	22
polyvinyl pyrrolidone (PVP)	hair setting preparation	thesaurosis in the lung. The relationship has been disputed [107]	27
thioglycolate solution	permanent wave	nickel release from nickel-plated clips due to the alkalinicity of the solution	15

26.16 REFERENCES

1. Ancona-Alayon, A., Jiminez-Castilla, J.L. and Gomez-Alvarez, E.M. (1976): Dermatitis from epoxy resin and formaldehyde in shampoo packers, *Contact Dermatitis, 2,* 356.
2. Beer, W.E. (1970): Sensitivity to fentichlor. *Contact Dermatitis Newsl. 8,* 188.
3. Black, M.M. and Russell, B.F. (1973): Shampoo dermatitis in apprentice hairdressers. *J. Soc. Occ. Med., 23*, 120.
4. Borelli, S. (1958): Die Verträgliehkeit gebräuchlicher Haarfärbungspräparate, Farbstoffgrundsubstanzen und verwandter chemischer Verbindungen. *Hautarzt, 9*, 19.
5. Borelli, S. and Manok, M. (1961): Ergebnisse von Untersuchungen bei Berufsanfängern im Friseurgewerbe. *Berufsdermatosen, 9,* 271.
6. Bork, K., Heise, D. and Rosinus, A. (1979): Formaldehyd in Haarshampoos. *Beruf u. Umwelt., 27*, 10.
7. Bourgeois-Spinasse, J. and Grupper. M.Ch. (1971): Insuffisance des tests prophétiques, nouvelles méthodes d'investigation allergique. *Bull. Soc. Fr. Derm. Syph., 78*, 571.
8. Burckhardt, W. (1953): Coiffeurekzem verursacht durch ein neues Kaltdauerwellenwasser. *Dermatologica (Basel), 107*, 253.
9. Calnan, C.D. (1967): Hair dye reaction. *Contact Dermatitis Newsl., 1,* 16.
10. Calnan, C. D. and Shuster, S. (1963): Reactions to ammonium persulphate. *Arch. Dermatol., 88,* 812.
11. Camarasa, J.G. (1981): Contact dermatitis to thioxolone. *Contact Dermatitis, 7*, 213.
12. Conner, D.S., Ritz, H.L., Ampulsti, R.S., Kowollik, H.G., Lim, P., Thomas, D.W. and Parkhurst, R. (1975): Identification of sultones as the sensitizers in alkylethoxysulfate. *Fette, Seifen, Anstrichm., 72*, 25.
13. Nigram, P.K. and Saxena, A.K. (1988): Allergic contact dermatitis from henna. *Contact Dematitis, 18,* 55–56.
14. Cronin, E. (1980): Cosmetics. In: *Contact Dermatitis.* pp. 93–170. Churchill Livingstone, Edinburgh.
15. Dahlquist, I., Fregert, S. and Grauberger, B. (1979): Release of nickel from plated utensils in permanent wave liquids. *Contact Dermatitis, 5,* 52.
16. Dawber, R.P.R. and Calnan, C.D. (1976): Bird's nest hair. Matting of scalp hair due to shampooing. *J. Clin. Exp. Derm., 1,* 155.
17. Downing, J.G. (1951): Dangers involved in dyes, cosmetics and permanent wave solutions applied to hair and scalp. *Arch. Dermatol., 63*, 561.
18. Eisenberg, B.C. (1955): Contact dermatitis from selenium sulfide shampoo. *Arch. Dermatol., 72*, 71.
19. Epstein, S. (1968): Photoallergic contact dermatitis; report of a case due to Dangard. *Cutis (N.Y.), 4*, 856.
20. Fisher, A.A. (1975): Is hair dyed with PPD allergenic? *Contact Dermatitis, 1,* 266.
21. Fisher, A.A. and Dooms-Goossens, A. (1976): Persulphate hair bleach reactions. *Arch. Dermatol., 112,* 1407.
22. Forman, L. (1975): Pigmentation of the palms and scalp probably due to proprietary hair tonics containing various phenols and phenolic derivatives. *Br. J. Dermatol., 93*, 718.
23. Foussereau, J. and Benezra, Cl. (1970): *Les Eczémas Allergiques Professionels*, p. 385. Masson et Cie, Paris.
24. Foussereau, J., Reuter, G. and Petitjean, J. (1980): Is hair dyed with PPD-like dyes allergenic? *Contact Dermatitis, 6*, 143.
25. Garnier, G. (1955): Dermatitis bullosa due to wave set containing tincture of benzoin. *Bull. Soc. Fr. Derm. Syph., 57*, 397.
26. Gelfand, H.H. (1963): Respiratory allergy due to chemical compounds encountered in the rubber, lacquer, shellac and beauty culture industries. *J. Allergy, 34*, 374.
27. Gowdy, J.M. and Wagstoff, M. J. (1972): Pulmonary infiltration due to aerosol thesaurosis. *Arch. Environm. Hlth., 25*, 1-10.
28. Hanlon, J. (1978): Tint of suspicion. *New Scientist, May 11,* 352.
29. Hindson, C. (1975): o-Nitro-paraphenylenediamine in hair dye — an unusual dental hazard. *Contact Dermatitis, 1,* 333.
30. Hjorth, N. (1973): Occupational dermatitis from Ineral (new formula). *Contact Dermatitis Newsl., 3*, 385.
31. Hjorth, N. and Niordson, A.M. (1972): Occupational dermatitis with onycholysis in hairdressers. *Contact Dermatitis Newsl., 11*, 254.
32. Kirkland, D.J., Lawler, S.D. and Venitt, S. (1978): Chromosomal damage and hair dyes. *Lancet, 2*, 124.
33. Lepine, M.J. and Fachot, M.L. (1971): Dermatite allergique des mains des coiffeurs par un nouveau produit capillaire: I'Ineral. *Bull. Derm. Syph., 78,* 150.

34. MacKie. B.S. and MacKie. L.E. (1964): Cross-sensitisation in dermatitis due to hair dyes. *Aust. J. Derm., 7,* 189.
35. Magnusson, B. (1974): The allergenicity of paraphenylenediamine versus that of paratoluenediamine. *Contact Dermatitis Newsl., 15,* 432.
36. Maibach, H.I., Leaffer, M.A. and Skinner, W.A. (1975): Percutaneous penetration following use of hair dyes. *Arch. Dermatol., 111,* 1444.
37. Marshall, S. and Palmer, W.S. (1973): Dark urine after hair colouring. *J. Am. Med. Assoc., 226,* 1010.
38. Goh, C.L. and Lim, K.B. (1984): Allergic contact dermatitis to zinc pyrithione. *Contact Dermatitis, 11,* 120.
39. Niles, H.D. (1941): Dermatitis of hands caused by liquid petrolatum in a proprietary hair tonic. *Arch. Derm. Syph., 43,* 689.
40. Osmundsen, P.E. (1975): Contact dermatitis from a hair dye. *Contact Dermatitis, 1,* 186.
41. Pasricha, J.S., Gupta, R. and Panjwani, S. (1980): Contact dermatitis to Henna (Lawsonia). *Contact Dermatitis, 6,* 288.
42. Rajka, G. and Blohm, S.G. (1970): The allergenicity of paraphenylenediamine. *Acta Derm.-Venereol. (Stockh.), 50,* 51.
43. Reinhardt, C.F., Azar, A., Maxfield, E., Smith, P.E. and Mullin, L.S. (1971): Cardiac arrhythmias and aerosol sniffing. *Arch. Environm. Hlth.,* 22, 265.
44. Ridley, C.M. (1978): Perfume in shampoo dermatitis. *Contact Dermatitis, 4,* 170.
45. Rietschel, R.L. (1978): Contact urticaria from synthetic cassia oil and sorbic acid limited to the face. *Contact Dermatitis, 4,* 347.
46. Romaguera, C. and Grimalt, F. (1980): Sensitization to benzoyl peroxide, retinoic acid and carbontetrachloride. *Contact Dermatitis, 6,* 442.
47. Rudzki, E., Napriorkowska, T. and Grzywa, Z. (1980): Active sensitization to ortho- and paraaminophenol with negative patch test to meta-aminophenol. *Contact Dermatitis, 6,* 501.
48. Schønning, L. and Hjorth, N. (1969): Cross sensitisation between hair dyes and rubber chemicals. *Berufsdermatosen, 17,* 100.
49. Bruynzeel, D.P., van Ketel, W.G. and de Haan, P. (1984): Formaldehyde in shampoos and toiletries. *Contact Dermatitis Newsl., 10,* 179–180.
50. Schulz, K.H. (1961): Durch Thioglykolsäurederivate ausgelöste Kontaktekzeme im Friseurberuf. *Berufsdermatosen, 9,* 244.
51. Sheffrin, S. (1974): Shampoo dermatitis. *J. Soc. Occ. Med., 24,* 31.
52. Spoor, H.J. (1977): Shampoos and hair dyes. *Cutis, 20,* 189.
53. Sylvest, B., Hjorth, N. and Magnusson, B. (1975): Laurylether sulphate dermatitis in Denmark. *Contact Dermatitis, 1,* 359.
54. Templeton, H.J. (1940): Cheilitis and dermatitis from resorcinol and a derivative. *Arch. Derm. Syph., 42,* 138.
55. Toghill, P.J. and Wilcox, R.G. (1976): Aplastic anaemia and hair dye. *Br. Med. J., 4,* 502.
56. Verbov, J.L. (1969): Contact dermatitis from Miranols. *Trans. St. John's Hosp. Derm. Soc. (Lond.), 55,* 192.
57. Warin, A.P. (1976): Contact dermatitis to partner's hair dye. *Clin. Exp. Derm. 1,* 283.
58. Widström, L. (1977): Allergic reactions to ammonium persulphate in hair bleach. *Contact Dermatitis, 3,* 343.
59. Yates, V.M. and Finn, O.A. (1980): Contactallergic sensitivity to zinc pyrithione followed by the photosensitivity dermatitis and actinic reticuloid. *Contact Dermatitis, 6,* 349.
60. Calnan, C.D. (1978): Diphenylamine. *Contact Dermatitis, 4,* 301.
61. Van Haute, N. and Dooms-Goossens, A. (1983): Shampoo dermatitis due to cocobetaine and sodium lauryl ether sulphate. *Contact Dermatitis, 9,* 169.
62. White, I.R., Catchpole. H.E. and Rycroft, R.J.G. (1982): Rashes amongst persulphate workers. *Contact Dermatitis, 8,* 168.
63. Fujita, M. and Aoki, T. (1983): Allergic contact dermatitis to pyridoxine ester and hinokitiol. *Contact Dermatitis, 9,* 61.
64. Edwards, E.K. Jr. and Edwards, E.K. (1982): Allergic contact dermatitis to lead acetate in a hair dye. *Cutis, 30,* 629.
65. Fisher, L.B. and Berman, B. (1982): Contact allergy to sulfonated castor oil. *Contact Dermatitis, 8,* 339.
66. Garnier, M.G. (1950): Dermite bulleuse par un fixateur d'ondulations. *Bull. Soc. Fr. Derm. Syph., 57,* 397.

67. Schleuter. D.P., Soto, R.J., Baretta, E.D. et al. (1979): Airway response to hair spray in normal subjects and subjects with hyperreactive airways. *Chest, 75*, 544.
68. Starr, J.C., Yunginger, J. and Brahser, G.W. (1982): Immediate type I asthmatic response to henna following occupational exposure in hairdressers. *Ann. Allergy, 48*, 98.
69. Schwartz. L. (1943): An outbreak of dermatitis from hair lacquer. *Publ. Hlth Rep.*, 58, 1623.
70. Ginsburg, L. and Ellis, F.A. (1944): Hair lacquer pad dermatitis. *Arch. Derm. Syph.*, 49, 198.
71. Zuskin, E., Bouhuys, A. and Beck, G. (1978): Hair sprays and lung function (Letter). *Lancet, 2*, 1203.
72. Maibach, H.I. and Wolfram, L.J. (1981): Percutaneous penetration of hair dyes. *J. Soc. Cosmet. Chem., 32*, 223.
73. D'Arcy, P.F. (1982): Fatalities with the use of a henna dye. *Pharm. Int., 3*, 217.
74. Stoll, D. and King, L.E. Jr. (1980): Disulfiram-alcohol skin reaction to beer-containing shampoo (Letter). *J. Am. Med. Assoc., 244*, 2045.
75. de Boer, E.M., van Ketel, W.G. and Bruynzeel, D.P. (1989): Dermatoses in metal workers. Allergic contact dermatitis. *Contact Dermatitis, 20,* 280–286.
76. Tosti, A., Piraccini, B. and Brasile, G.P. (1990): Occupational contact dermatitis due to sodium pyrithione. *Contact Dermatitis, 22,* 118–119.
77. Brandrup, F. and Menné, T. (1985): Zinc pyrithione (Zinc Omadine®) allergy. *Contact Dermatitis, 12,* 50.
78. Dooms-Goossens, A., Debusschere, K., Dupré, K. and Degreef, H. (1988): Can eardrops induce a shampoo dermatitis? A case study. *Contact Dermatitis, 19,* 143–144.
79. Vilaplana, J., Grimalt, F. and Romaguera, C. Contact dermatitis by cocamidopropyl betaine. Data presented at the 9th International Symposium on Contact Dermatitis, 17–19 May 1990, Stockholm, Sweden: p. 102.
80. De Groot, A.C., de Wit, F.S., Bos, J.D. and Weyland, J.W. (1987): Contact allergy to cocamide DEA and lauramide DEA in shampoos. *Contact Dermatitis, 16,* 117–118.
81. Sharvill, D. (1965): Reaction to chlorhexidine and cetrimide. *Lancet, i,* 771.
82. Benke, G.M. and Larsen, W.G. (1984): Safety evaluation of perfumed shampoos: dose/response relationships for product use testing by presensitized subjects. *J. Toxicol-Cut & Ocular Toxicol., 3,* 65–72.
83. Andersen, K.E., Roed-Petersen, J. and Kamp, P. (1984): Contact allergy related to TEA-PEG-3 cocamide sulfate and cocamide propyl betaine in a shampoo. *Contact Dermatitis, 11,* 192–194.
84. Wilson, C.L., Ferguson, D.J.P. and Dawber, R.P.R. (1990): Matting of scalp hair during shampooing — a new look. *Clin. exp. Dermatol., 15,* 139–142.
85. Beck, J.E. (1978): Zinc pyrithione and peripheral neuritis. *Lancet, i,* 444.
86. Dooms-Goossens, A., van Daele, M., Bedert, R. and Marien, K. (1989): Hexamidine isethionate: a sensitizer in topical pharmaceutical products and cosmetics. *Contact Dermatitis, 21,* 270.
87. Bruynzeel, D.P., De Groot, A.C. and Weyland, J.W. (1987): Contact dermatitis to lauryl pyridinium chloride and benzoxonium chloride. *Contact Dermatitis, 17,* 41–42.
88. Kantor, G.R., Taylor, J.S., Ratz, J.L. and Evey, P.L. (1985): Acute allergic contact dermatitis from diazolidinyl urea (Germall II) in a hair gel. *J. Am. Acad. Dermatol., 13,* 116–119.
89. Heine, A. and Laubstein, B. (1990): Contact dermatitis from cyclohexanone-formaldehyde resin (L_2 resin) in a hair lacquer spray. *Contact Dermatitis, 22,* 108.
90. Food and Drug Administration (1989): Hair grower and hair loss prevention drug products for over-the-counter human use. Final rule. *Federal Register, 54,* 28772–28777.
91. Katz, H.I. (1989): Topical minoxidil: a review of efficacy and safety. *Cutis, 43,* 94–98.
92. De Groot, A.C., Nater, J.P. and Herxheimer, A. (1987): Minoxidil: hope for the bald? *Lancet, i,* 1019–1021.
93. Monk, B. (1987): Allergic contact dermatitis to D & C Yellow 11 in a hair cream. *Contact Dermatitis, 17,* 57–58.
94. Dooms-Goossens, A., Swinnen, E., Vandermaesen, J., Mariën, K. and Dooms, M. (1987): Connubial dermatitis from a hair lotion. *Contact Dermatitis, 16,* 41–42.
95. Pradalier, A., Dry, J. and Valla, D. (1984): Hypersensibilité à la poudre de lycopode. *Rev. fr. Allergol., 24,* 85–86.
96. van Ketel, W.G. (1984): Hair lotion dermatitis with sensitization to d-panthenyl ethyl ether. *Contact Dermatitis, 10,* 48.
97. Jaworsky, C., Taylor, J.S., Evey, P. and Handel, D. (1987): Allergic contact dermatitis to glutaraldehyde in a hair conditioner. *Cleveland Clin. J. Med., 54,* 443–444.
98. White, I.R., Lovell, C.R. and Cronin, E. (1984): Antioxidants in cosmetics. *Contact Dermatitis, 11,* 265–267.

99. Morrison, L.H. and Storrs, F.J. (1988): Persistence of an allergen in hair after glyceryl monothioglycolate-containing permanent wave solutions. *J. Am. Acad. Dermatol., 19,* 52–59.
100. Tosti, A., Melino, M. and Bardazzi, F. (1988): Contact dermatitis due to glyceryl monothioglycolate. *Contact Dermatitis, 19,* 71–72.
101. Fisher, A.A. (1989): Management of hairdressers sensitized to hair dyes or permanent wave solutions. *Cutis, 43,* 316–318.
102. Storrs, F.J. (1984): Permanent wave contact dermatitis. Contact allergy to glyceryl monothioglycolate. *J. Am. Acad. Dermatol., 11,* 74–85.
103. Wickett, R.R. (1987): Permanent waving and straightening of hair. *Cutis, 39,* 496–497.
104. Yamasaki, R., Dekio, S. and Jidoi, J. (1984): Allergic contact dermatitis to ammonium thioglycolate. *Contact Dermatitis, 11,* 255.
105. Kellett, J.K. and Beck, M.H. (1985): Ammonium persulphate sensitivity in hairdressers. *Contact Dermatitis, 13,* 26–28.
106. Fisher, A.A. (1989): Dermatitis due to sulfites in home permanent preparations. Part II. *Cutis, 44,* 108–109.
107. Brunner, M.J., Giovacchini, R.P., Wyatt, J.P., Dunlap, F.E. and Calandra, J.C. (1963): Pulmonary disease and hair-spray polymers: a disputed relationship. *JAMA, 184,* 95–101.
108. De Groot, A.C. and Weyland, J.W. (1990): Cosmetic allergy from the amino ketone colour Basic Blue 99 (CI 56059). *Contact Dermatitis, 23,* 56–57.
109. Perno, P. and Lisi, P. (1990): Psoriasis-like contact dermatitis from a hair nitro dye. *Contact Dermatitis, 23,* 123–124.
110. Andersen, K.E. and Carlsen, L. (1988): Pyrocatechol contact allergy from a permanent cream dye for eyelashes and eyebrows. *Contact Dermatitis, 18,* 306–307.
111. Komamura, H., Kozuka, T., Ishii, M., Yoshikawa, K. and Iyoda, M. (1989): Allergic contact sensitivity to quinophthalone. *Contact Dermatitis, 20,* 177–181.
112. Vilaplana, J., Romaguera, C. and Grimalt, F. (1991): Contact dermatitis from resorcinol in a hair dye. *Contact Dermatitis, 24,* 151–152.
113. Gupta, B.N., Mathur, A.K., Agarwal, C. and Singh, A. (1986): Contact sensitivity to henna. *Contact Dermatitis, 15,* 303–304.
114. Koren, G. and Bologa, M. (1989): Teratogenic risk of hair care products. *JAMA, 262,* 2925.
115. Kirkland, D.J. (1983): The mutagenicity and carcinogenicity of hair dyes. *Int. J. Cosm. Sci., 5,* 51–71.
116. Nasca, P.C., Lawrence, L.E., Greenwald, P. et al. (1980): Relationship of hair dye use, benign breast disease and breast cancer. *J. Nat. Cancer Inst., 64,* 23–28.
117. Cordle, F. and Thompson, G.E. (1981): An epidemiologic assessment of hair dye use. *Regulatory Toxicol. Pharmacol., 1,* 388–400.
118. Clemmesen, J. (1981): Epidemiological studies into the possible carcinogenicity of hair dyes. *Mutat. Res., 87,* 65–79.
119. Spengler, J. and Bracher, M. (1990): Toxicological tests and health risk assessment of oxidative hair dye mixtures. *Cosm. Toiletries, 105,* 67–76.
120. Skov, T., Andersen, A., Malker, H., Pukkala, E., Weiner, J. and Lynge, E. (1990): Risk for cancer of the urinary bladder among hairdressers in the Nordic countries. *Am. J. Industr. Med., 17,* 217–223.
121. Gougerot, H. and Sclafer, H. (1945): Mort par tenture du coiffeur. *Bull. Acad. Med., 129,* 664–665.
122. Notter, A. and Perrot, L. (1963): Néphrite subaiguë toxique avec mort feotale au 6e mois de la gestation après shampooing colorant à la diamine. *Ann. Méd. Leg., 43,* 245–248.
123. De Groot, A.C. (1988): Adverse reactions to cosmetics, p.112. Thesis, University of Groningen.
124. Taniguchi, S., Katoh, J., Hisa, T., Tabata, M. and Hamada, T. (1992): Shampoo dermatitis due to cocamidopropyl betaine. *Contact Dermatitis, 26,* 139.
125. Daniel, C.R. III. and Scher, R.K. (1991): Nail damage secondary to a hair spray. *Cutis, 47,* 165–166.
126. Stringer, G.C., Hunter, S.W. and Bonnabeau, R.L. (1977): Hypersensitivity pneumonitis following prolonged inhalation of hair spray. *JAMA, 238,* 888–889.
127. Tosti, A., Mattioli, D. and Misciali, C. (1991): Green hair caused by copper present in cosmetic plant extracts. *Dermatologica, 182,* 204–205.

27. Face cosmetics

FACE CREAM (MOISTURIZING CREAM)

27.1 For facial care creams, lotions and milks are used, which are sold under various names: cold cream, emollient cream, day cream, night cream, moisturizing cream, vanishing cream, etc. They all have the same basic emulsion formulation, and they will therefore all be considcred here as moisturizing cream/milk.

A typical basic formula for a **moisturizing cream/milk/lotion** is as follows:

Ingredients		Example
20–90%	water	water
1–5%	polyol	sorbitol
10–80%	lipid	stearic acid, cetearyl alcohol, squalane
2–5%	surfactant	polysorbate 40, TEA-oleate
0–5%	special moisturizer	polyamino sugar condensate
ca. 0.3%	preservative	methyl and propylparaben, DMDM hydantoin
ca. 0.2%	perfume	perfume

As many possibilities exist for the choice of the functional ingredients, endless variations can be made (see § 21.3).

For all these emulsions the water/lipid ratio determines the result. Ratios of 7–9 make fluid products (milks/lotions). Most oil-in-water creams have ratios of 1–2: they are the most popular types. The 'oily' water-in-oil creams have ratios of 0.5–1.

For many (often expensive) moisturizing creams a large variety of 'skin conditioning' ingredients is available, often referred to in advertising as 'active ingredients'. These active ingredients can be divided (rather arbitrarily) into emollients, humectants, occlusive skin conditioning agents, and a category of miscellaneous compounds.

Emollients are mostly lipids, which can help to maintain a soft and smooth appearance of the skin. Many lipids may be used as emollients, and it is not always clear whether such lipids are supposed to function as the 'active ingredient' or merely as the cream base.

Skin conditioning agents — emollients

avocado oil
fatty alcohols (cetyl alcohol, cetearyl alcohol)
fatty acid glycerides (caprylic/capric triglyceride)
esters of fatty acids and fatty alcohols (cetyl myristate)
isopropyl lanolate
lanolin, lanolin oil, lanolin alcohol
mineral oil
mink oil
octyldodecanol
PEG-8 ceteth-2
propylene glycol dioctanoate
soy sterol
squalene
wheat germ glycerides

Occlusive agents are also mostly lipids. They function by retarding the evaporation of water from the skin surface, so increasing the water content of the skin. Many emollients exert the same properties, so the distinction is not sharp.

Skin conditioning agents — occlusive

acetylated lanolin
aluminum lanolate
avocado oil
caprylic/capric triglyceride
dimethicone
hydrogenated castor oil
jojoba oil
mink oil
paraffin
petrolatum
shea butter
shark liver oil
shellac wax
synthetic wax
tristearin

Humectants are ingredients intended to increase the water content of the top layers of the skin. They are generally hygroscopic agents, chemically characterized by a small molecular size and the possession of polar functional groups. Typical examples are:

Skin conditioning agents – humectants

acetamide MEA
amino acids (histidine, serine, alanine, etc.)
disaccharides (lactose)
glycerin
honey
maltitol
mannitol
methylgluceth
polyamino sugar condensate
sodium lactate
sodium PCA
sorbitol
TEA lactate
urea

A large group of miscellaneous special additives remains. In some respects they have similar functions to the previous groups, but among them are also vitamins, peptides, rubefacients, skin protecting agents, etc. In addition, this group contains many proteins and protein derivatives from natural sources which, advertisers would have the consumer believe, have the ability to 'repair' skin or proteins, e.g. collagen amino acids and elastin. Some of the miscellaneous ingredients are listed below.

Miscellaneous skin conditioning agents:

Ingredient	function	Ingredient	Function
adenosine phosphate		hydrolyzed human placental protein	
adenosine triphosphate		hydrolyzed silk	
allantoin (and derivatives)	skin protectant	keratin	protein
aloe	moisturizer	methionine	
animal collagen amino acids	protein hydrolysate	menthol	topical analgesic
animal elastin amino acids	protein hydrolysate	milk	
animal keratin amino acids	protein hydrolysate	niacin	vitamin
ascorbic acid	vitamin	potassium DNA	
botanicals	*see* § 30.16	pregnenolone acetate	hormone
camphor	topical analgesic	pyridoxine (and derivatives)	vitamin
casein	protein	resorcinol acetate	keratolytic agent
desamido animal collagen	modified protein	retinol and its acetate and palmitate esters	vitamin
dried buttermilk		salicylic acid	keratolytic agent
dried egg yolk		silk	protein
estrogenic hormones	hormone	sodium riboflavin phosphate	vitamin
ethisteron	hormone	soluble animal collagen	protein
ethyl urocanate	moisturizer	sulfur	anti-acne
folic acid	biological additive	thiamine HCl and nitrate	vitamin
methyl nicotinate	rubefacient	threonine	essential amino acid
human placental protein	protein	tocopheryl acetate and other esters	vitamin
hyaluronic acid	moisturizer	tyrosine	melanin precursor
hydrolyzed animal elastin	protein hydrolysate	urocanic acid	moisturizer
hydrolyzed animal keratin	protein hydrolysate	whey protein	protein
hydrolyzed animal protein	protein hydrolysate		

Liposomes

A more recent development in skin care is the use of liposomes. Liposomes have, for more than a decade, been a promising research subject in the pharmaceutical sciences, because it is believed that they might be used for drug targeting. The merit of their introduction in cosmetics is debated, opinions varying between 'a mere marketing trick' and 'a revolution in cosmetic science'.

Liposomes are spherical bilayered vesicles, varying in size between 25 and 5000 nm and composed of suitable amphophilic molecules, which combine to form a membrane. These molecules are mainly phospholipids, consisting of a phosphatidyl moiety (two fatty acids ester bridged to glycerolphosphate) coupled to a hydrophilic group. Suitable hydrophilic groups are, for example, choline, ethanolamine or glycerol. When the dispersion medium (and the core) is water, the molecules arrange in such a way that the outer layers of the membrane are formed by the hydrophilic heads of the molecules, while the lipophilic tails of the molecules form a lipophilic double layer between the two hydrophilic layers. Niosomes are essentially similar, but the building materials are nonionic surfactants like polyoxyethylene alkylethers or polyethylene alkyesters.

Liposomes can be *loaded* with 'active' ingredients. Water soluble substances (for example humectants) can be captured in the aqueous interior of the liposome, while lipophilic substances (like tocopheryl palmitate) load in the amphophilic membrane itself. Loaded this way, liposomes are supposed to be useful as carriers of 'active' cosmetic ingredients, enabling the targeting of these ingredients into the deeper layers of the stratum corneum and the dermis. Such a mechanism is doubtful, however, because their size makes it improbable that liposomes could penetrate through the intercellular spaces of the epidermis; the distance between the laminar structures of the lipid layers in the intercellular spaces spans about 5–10 nm, smaller than the smallest liposomes. Although after application of liposome preparations to the skin, liposome-like structures have been found several layers deep in the stratum corneum, the actual migration is probably in dispersed form, the liposome-like structure forming again in situ. Nevertheless, a number of investigations report better results from the application of topical drugs in liposome creams than from normal creams, either in terms of local concentration or of healing rates. Examples are studies of the application in liposome creams of econazole [107], hydrocortisone [108] and triamcinolone [109]; noteworthy is also a report that suggests increased sensitization potential of propyl gallate when attached to liposomes [105].

Meanwhile, it remains to be decided whether or not the effects of liposomes are primarily dependent on the physico-chemical properties of the material, rather than on their superstructure.

More and more cosmetics for the face contain sunscreens, both for the protection of the product and the skin of the user. Preservation is often by means of parabens, but almost all other preservatives may occur.

Tabulation of side effects

Side effects of ingredients of moisturizing creams are tabulated in § 27.3.

CLEANSING LOTION

27.2 Cleansing milks/lotions are used to aid cleansing the face with a tissue in order to remove excessive fat, make-up residues and dirt. The cleansing agents in these products are always oils and surfactants. The formulas of cleansing lotion and moisturizing cream bases are the same.

The following is a typical formula for cleansing milk (emulsion type):

Ingredients		Example
60–80%	water	water
ca. 2%	polyol	propylene glycol
20–30%	lipid	mineral oil, isopropyl myristate
2–8%	surfactants	sodium lauryl sulfate
ca. 0.3%	preservative	2-bromo-2-nitropropane-1,3-diol
ca. 0.2%	perfume	perfume

Almond meal and pumice may also be incorporated as extra cleansing aids.

The concentration of surfactants in cleansing products may be high. Cleansing milk should not be patch-tested undiluted. A 5–10-fold dilution with water is necessary to avoid irritant reactions.

Perioral dermatitis has been linked to the regular and abundant use of moisturizing creams [84]. The report remained unconfirmed, however.

Tabulation of side effects

Side effects of ingredients of cleansing lotions are tabulated in § 27.3.

27.3 Contact allergy to moisturizing and cleansing preparation

Ingredient	Use	Patch test conc. & vehicle (§ 5.2)	Cross-reaction (§ 5.5)	Comment	Ref.
α-amylcinnamic aldehyde in skin care product	fragrance	2% pet.			97
beeswax in cold cream	vehicle constituent	30% pet.			20
bornelone in a facial cream	sunscreen	5% pet.			95
2-bromo-2-nitropropane-1,3-diol (bronopol) in skin care product	preservative	0.5% pet.			97
castor oil in make-up remover	lipid	pure			64
chloroacetamide in 'anti-wrinkle' serum	preservative	0.2% pet.			91
chloroacetamide in facial spray astringent	preservative	0.2% pet.			90
chloroacetamide in skin care product	preservative	0.2% pet.			97
citronellol in skin care product	fragrance	1–2% pet.			97

(continued)

§ **27.3** *(continuation*

Ingredient	Use	Patch test conc. & vehicle (§ 5.2)	Cross-reaction (§ 5.5)	Comment	Ref.
cocamidopropyl betaine in skin care product	surfactant	1% aqua			97
cocamidopropyl betaine in eye make-up remover	surfactant	1% aqua			80
cyclomethicone in skin care product	emollient	pure			97
DEA-dihydroxypalmityl phosphate and isopropyl hydroxypalmityl ether in lotion	surfactant	2.5% aqua			86
drometrizole in skin care product	sunscreen	1% pet.; 5% pet. [49]			20
Eucerit® (lanolin alcohol) in skin care product	emollient	30% pet.			97
Eusolex® 8021 in moisturizing cream	sunscreen	2% pet.		Eusolex® 8021 is a mixture of 4-methyl-benzylidene camphor and isopropyl dibenzoyl-methane. The actual allergen was not determined	43
formaldehyde released from imidazolidinyl urea in facial cream	preservative	1% aqua			87
hexylcinnamic aldehyde in skin care product	fragrance	2% pet.			97
hydroxycitronellal in skin care product	fragrance	2% pet.			97
imidazolidinyl urea in skin care product	preservative	2% pet.			97
lanolin in facial cream	lipid	pure			16
methylisothiazolinone and methyl-chloroisothiazolinone in skin care product	preservative	100 ppm aqua		Active ingredients of Kathon CG® and Euxyl® K100	97
methyldibromo glutaronitrile (1,2-dibromo-2,4-dicyanobutane) in anti-wrinkle lotion	preservative	0.05% pet.		Main active ingredient of Euxyl® K400	78

(continued)

§ **27.3** *(continuation*

Ingredient	Use	Patch test conc. & vehicle (§ 5.2)	Cross-reaction (§ 5.5)	Comment	Ref.
methylheptine carbonate in facial cream	fragrance	0.5% pet.			30
γ-methylionone in skin care product	fragrance	10% pet.			97
myristyl alcohol in skin care product	lipid	5% pet.			97
myristyl alcohol in moisturizing cream	lipid	5% pet.			83
parabens in facial cream	preservatives	each 3% pet.			39
PEG-32 stearate in skin care product	emulsifier	20% pet.			97
pelargol in skin care product	fragrance	5% pet.			97
perfume in facial tissue				The patient reacted to cinnamic alcohol and cinnamic aldehyde	60
o-phenylphenol in foundation cream	preservative	1% pet.			20
propyl gallate in cosmetic cream	antioxidant	2% pet.			76 105
propyl gallate in skin care product	antioxidant	1% pet.			100
PVP/hexadecene copolymer in skin care product	dispersant, film former	5% pet.			97
quaternium-15 in skin care product	preservative	1% pet.		Formaldehyde donor	97
sodium PCA in skin care product	humectant	2% aqua			97
solvent red 3 (CI 12010) in soothing oil	colour	1% pet.			94
stearic acid in facial moisturizer	emollient, emulsifier	5% pet.	sodium stearate		82
TEA-coco-hydrolyzed animal protein in facial skin cleanser	mild surfactant	5 and 50% aqua.			24
tocopheryl acetate (vitamin E) in facial cream	skin conditioning agent, antioxidant	10% pet.			79 89

FACIAL MAKE-UP

27.4 There are make-up products for the entire facial area and the neck, and products for the cheeks only (rouge); the basic formula for both products is the same. The functional part is always a colour pigment mixture of the following composition:

20–80%	talc as the powder base	
ca. 10%	kaolin or rice starch for adsorption of fat	
ca. 5%	zinc stearate for improving skin adherence	
ca. 2%	magnesium carbonate as carrier for perfume	
0–10%	titanium dioxide to increase covering power	
10–70%	coloured pigments to obtain the desired tint, e.g.	
	– yellow, brown, reddish	iron oxides (CI 77491)
	– red:	D&C Red No. 31 (CI 15800), calcium lake carmine (CI 75470)
		many other red pigments (see § 30.10)
	– pearlescent pigments:	titanated mica, bismuth oxychloride coated mica, silk powder

Facial make-up products are available in various forms: as a loose powder, compact powder, cream make-up, and fluid make-up. The following typical formulas will illustrate the various products.

Face powder (loose)

ca. 99%	colour pigment mixture	see § 27.4
ca. 1%	(fused) silica	to improve 'free flow'

Compact face powder or compact rouge

95%	colour pigment mixture	see § 27.4
ca. 5%	lipid, as binder	acetylated lanolin
0–0.3%	preservative	methylparaben

Cream make-up or cream rouge

30–60%	colour pigment mixture	see § 27.4
40–60%	cream base composed of water, polyol, lipid, surfactant-emulsifier, preservative and perfume	see § 27.1

Fluid make-up or fluid rouge

ca. 30%	colour pigment mixture	see § 27.4
ca. 70%	water	
ca. 5%	suspending agent for the pigments	magnesium aluminum silicate, quaternium-18 hectorite
ca. 0.3%	preservative	quaternium-15

Tabulation of side effects

Side effects of ingredients of facial make-up cosmetics are tabulated in § 27.6.

FACE MASK

27.5 Masks have been designed to provide intensive care (cleaning and moisturizing) for the face, within a relatively short period of time. Masks are muddy pastes or viscous liquids that will easily adhere to the skin of the face after being applied. There are several types, which may be characterized by the following typical formulas.

Face mask formulations

Mask (paste ready for use)

Ingredients		Example
10–40%	water	water
30–80%	powder base	kaolin, magnesium aluminum silicate
ca. 3%	binder	hydroxyethylcellulose
0–5%	abrasive	almond meal
0–30%	active ingredients	methyl nicotinate, allantoin, honey
ca. 0.5%	preservative	methylparaben, DMDM hydantoin

Mask powder (to be mixed with an aqueous fluid. e.g. water, milk, cucumber juice, yoghurt, just before use; preservatives are unnecessary)

Ingredients		Example
30–80%	powder base	bentonite, yeast
ca. 3%	binder	magnesium aluminum silicate
0–5%	abrasive	rice bran, wheat bran
0–50%	active ingredients	arnica flowers, wheat flour, oat flour, zinc peroxide

Peeling masks (this is a viscous liquid that will dry to a colourless film, which can be peeled off after use)

Ingredients		Example
50–60%	water	water
10–20%	alcohol	alcohol
10–15%	polyvinyl alcohol	polyvinyl alcohol
ca. 1%	lipid	lanolin oil
ca. 1%	surfactant	buteth-45
ca. 1%	perfume	perfume

27.6 Contact allergy to ingredients of facial make-up products

Ingredient	Use	Patch test conc. & vehicle (§ 5.2)	Cross-reactions (§ 5.5)	Comment	Ref.
benzoin in 'party make-up'	fragrance	10% alc.			29
BHA (butylated hydroxy-anisole) in cream blusher	antioxidant	2% pet.			77
citronellol	fragrance	2% pet.			97
D&C Red No. 17 (CI 26100, Sudan III) in blush-on	colour	1% pet.			3
D&C Red No. 31 (Brilliant Lake Red R, CI 15800:1) in blusher	colour	1% pet.	related dyes (see § 4.3)		31 32
D&C Red No. 36 (CI 12085) in face powder	colour	1% pet.			3
D&C Red No. 36 (CI 12085) in blusher	colour	1% pet.			92
D&C Yellow No. 11 (CI 47000) in blush-on	colour	0.1% pet.	D&C Yellow No. 10 (0.1% pet.) [55]	Patch testing with the dye 1% may sensitize [51]. D&C Yellow 11 proved to be a sensitizer in human [53,54] and animal [52] experiments	7 34 51 55
D&C Yellow No. 11 (CI 47000) in colour stick	colour	0.1% pet.		Concomitant sensitization to D&C Red No. 17	62
dichlorophene in liquid make-up base	preservative	1% pet.			25

(continued)

§ **27.6** *(continuation)*

Ingredient	Use	Patch test conc. & vehicle (§ 5.2)	Cross-reactions (§ 5.5)	Comment	Ref.
diisopropanolamine in blush-on	pH-adjuster	1% aqua			20
geraniol	fragrance	2% pet.			97
hydroxycitronellal in cream make-up	fragrance	2% pet.			9
methylisothiazolinone and methylchloroisothiazolinone	preservative	100 ppm aqua		Active ingredients of Kathon CG® and Euxyl® K100	97
musk moskene	fragrance	2% pet.		Pigmented contact dermatitis	102
potassium sorbate in face powder	preservative	5% pet.	sorbic acid		59
rosin in blush-on	binder, film former	20% pet.			28

Other side effects

Irritant dermatitis due to face painting with tempera pigments in a commercial dishwashing liquid was described by Mathias [36].

AFTERSHAVE

27.7 An aftershave is primarily intended to be a perfume for men. Sometimes ingredients are added for the purpose of astringency and counterirritancy.

Aftershaves are of two types: lotions and emulsions. The emulsion type aftershave is formulated basically the same as the moisturizing milks described in § 27.1

A typical formula for **aftershave lotion** is:

Ingredients		Example
25–60%	water	water
40–60%	alcohol	alcohol
2–5%	polyol	glycerin
ca. 0.5%	perfume compound mixture	perfume
0.01%	colour	Acid Yellow 23 (CI 19140)
0–1%	special additives	panthenol, allantoin, benzethonium chloride

Side effects from aftershave cosmetics are mainly caused by the perfume compound mixture. A typical fragrance ingredient is *musk*. The following synthetic musks may be ingredients of aftershaves:

- 5-acetyl-1,1,2,3,3,6-hexamethylindan (Phantolide®)
- 4-acetyl-6-tert-butyl-1,1-dimethylindan (Celestolide®)
- acetylethyltetramethyltetralin (AETT, Versalide®) (neurotoxic, use abandoned in 1977)
- ambrettolide
- ethylene brassylate
- hexahydrohexamethylcyclopentabenzopyran (Galaxolide®)
- musk ambrette
- musk ketone
- musk tibetene
- musk xylol

Tabulation of side effects

Side effects of ingredients of aftershaves are tabulated in § 27.8. See also the chapter on contact allergy to fragrance materials (§ 5.10–5.15).

27.8 Contact allergy to ingredients of aftershave products

Ingredient	Use	Patch test conc. & vehicle (§ 5.2)	Cross-reactions (§ 5.5)	Comment	Ref.
atranorin in aftershave lotion	fragrance	0.5% pet.	fumarprotocetraric acid	Present in oak moss perfumes	22
benzyl alcohol in aftershave lotion	fragrance	5% pet.			27
cinnamic alcohol in aftershave lotion	fragrance	2% pet.			41
eugenol	fragrance	2% pet.			97
fumarprotocetraric acid in aftershave lotion	fragrance	0.1% acet.	atranorin	Present in oak moss perfumes	22
geraniol in shaving foam	fragrance	2% pet.			97
hydroxycitronellal in aftershave lotion	fragrance	2% pet.	linalool ? [44]		41 44
lanolin oil	emollient	30% pet.			97
linalool in aftershave lotion	fragrance	30% pet.	hydroxycitronellal (?)	Caused facial psoriasis in the reported case	44
methylheptine carbonate in aftershave	fragrance	0.5% pet.			41
musk ambrette in aftershave lotion	fragrance				
triethanolamine in shaving foam	pH adjuster	2.5% pet.			98
triethanolamine in shaving cream	pH adjuster	5% pet.			50

OTHER SHAVING AIDS

27.9 Shaving aids include shaving foams (aerosol) and beard softeners (paste, cream).

A typical formula for an **aerosol shaving foam** is:

Ingredients		Example
ca. 10%	propellant	butane, isobutane, propane
ca. 90%	concentrate:	
	ca. 90% water	water
	ca. 5% foam surfactant	TEA-cocoate, lauramide DEA
	ca. 3% polyol	propylene glycol
	ca. 0.2% perfume	perfume

A typical formula for a **cream beard softener** is:

Ingredients		Example
ca. 80%	water	water
ca. 15%	lipid	stearic acid
ca. 1%	polyol	polypropylene glycol
ca. 1%	surfactant: emulsifier	potassium stearate
ca. 0.2%	preservative	methylparaben, propylparaben, DMDM hydantoin
ca. 0.1%	perfume	perfume

Some beard softeners are designed to exert a depilatory effect. The following typical formula for this type of cosmetic is a powder, that is mixed with water to a paste, just before use:

Powder beard softener (depilating)

Ingredients		Example
ca. 80%	powder base	kaolin, calcium carbonate
ca. 5%	binder	dextrin
3–5%	depilating agent	strontium thioglycolate, barium sulfide
ca. 1%	surfactant	nonoxynol-10
ca. 0.5%	perfume	perfume

EYE MAKE-UP

27.10 Eye make-up products include eye shadow, eye liner, mascara and eyebrow pencil. Typical formulas are:

Eye shadow: compact powder

(This cosmetic has the same basic structure as compact face powder)

40–60%	talc as powder base
ca. 7%	zinc stearate for skin adherence
ca. 1%	magnesium carbonate as perfume carrier
ca. 5%	lipid binder: e.g. decyl oleate, isopropyl lanolate
ca. 5%	titanium dioxide to improve covering power
10–30%	coloured pigments (see § 30.10)
	– green: chromium hydroxide green, chrome oxide greens (CI 77289, 77288)
	– blue: ultramarine or ferric ferrocyanide (CI 77007-77510)
	– red: carmine, Pigment Red 57:2; Barium lake (CI 15850:2)
	– brown-black: iron oxides (CI 77489, CI 77491, CI 77492, CI 77499), carbon black (CI 77266)
	– yellow: Acid Yellow 104 Aluminum lake (CI 15985:1)
	– orange: Acid Yellow 23 Aluminum lake (CI 19140)
	– pearl pigments: titanated or bismuthoxychloride-coated micas

Eye shadow: stick

This has the same formula as eye shadow compact powder, but with a considerably higher content of the lipid binder: 60–80%. Examples for the lipid binder are: *mineral oil, petrolatum, paraffin wax, beeswax.*

To prevent rancidity of these lipids approximately 0.05% antioxidants are added, for example: BHA (butylated hydroxyanisole) (see § 30.5 for an extensive list).

Eye liner fluid:

ca. 25% polymer as an emulsion (e.g. styrene/butadiene emulsion)

ca. 10% pigments (see § 27.4)

ca. 3% suspending agent (e.g.: magnesium aluminum silicate)

ca. 1% surfactant

ca. 0.5% preservative

Mascara: paste or a block

(Mascara blocks mix easily with water to form a paste.)

Ingredients		Example
ca. 70%	water (absent in solid block)	water
5–10%	pigments (see § 27.4)	iron oxides, chrome oxide greens
ca. 5%	surfactants	TEA-oleate
ca. 3%	suspending agents	magnesium aluminum silicate
ca. 20%	lipids	lanolin, carnauba wax, oleic acid
0–5%	rayon fibres	rayon
0.05–0.3%	preservative	thiomersal

Mascara ('waterproof'): These cosmetics should be removed at night, otherwise the eyelashes may be pulled out.

Ingredients		Example
ca. 65%	hydrocarbon solvent	petroleum distillate
ca. 2%	solvent thickener	aluminum stearate
ca. 20%	lipids	beeswax, hydroabietyl alcohol, lanolin
ca. 10%	pigments	carbon black
ca. 0.05%	antioxidants	BHA

Although many patients ascribe their eye complaints to the use of mascara or other eye make-up products, true contact allergic reactions seem to be infrequent. Most cases of complaints are of an irritant character.

Patch tests with mascara 'as is' may frequently cause false positive irritant reactions and should therefore be interpreted with care. Testing of the ingredients in the suitable concentrations and vehicles is advisable. On the other hand, in cases of relevant eye cosmetic dermatitis, patch testing with eye cosmetics often gives false negative reactions. It has been suggested that the mascara rubbed on to the patch-tester be mixed with a drop of dimethyl sulfoxide 50% before patch-testing [41]. Control tests with eye cosmetics are necessary, usage and open tests may be helpful.

Tabulation of side effects

Side effects of ingredients of eye cosmetics are tabulated in § 27.11.

27.11 Contact allergy to ingredients of eye cosmetics

Ingredient	Use	Patch test conc. & vehicle (§5.2)	Cross-reactions (§ 5.5)	Comment	Ref.
BHA (butylated hydroxyan-isole) in eyeshadow	antioxidant	2% pet.			77
t-butyl hydroquinone in eyeshadow	antioxidant	1% pet.			77
chloroacetamide in eye cream	preservative	0.2% pet.			4 81
D&C Red No. 17 (CI 26100) in eye cream	colour	1% pet.			8
D&C Yellow No. 11 (CI 47000 in eye cream	colour	0.1% pet.	D&C Yellow No. 10 (0.1% pet.) [55]		11 51 55
dihydroabietyl alcohol (abitol) in mascara	binder	10% pet.	cross-reaction to rosin (colophony) and abietic acid possible		23
diisopropanolamine in eyeshadow	pH adjuster	1% aqua		25% of controls reacted to the undiluted ingredient	19
di-*t*-butylhydroquinone in eyeshadow	antioxidant	1% pet.			6
imidazolidinyl urea (Germall® 115) in liquid eyeliner	preservative	1% pet./aqua			25 26
isoeugenol in 'eye cosmetics'	fragrance	2% pet.			63
lanolin alcohol (wool alcohols) in 'eye cosmetics'	emollient; vehicle constituent	30% pet.		The patient also reacted to isoeugenol in the cosmetics	63
lanolin in eyeshadow	emollient, lipid	pure			38
methylisothiazolinone and methylchloroisothiazoli-none in mascara	preservative	100 ppm aqua		Active ingredients of Kathon CG® and Euxyl® K100	97
mineral oil in eyeshadow	emollient, pigment binder	pure			97
nickel in eyeshadow	contaminant	5% pet.			42
perfume in eye cream		0.1% ?		Contact allergy to e.g. angelica root oil (as is) and alcohol C-8 (as is)	33
perfume in mascara		1% pet.			8
rosin (colophony) in mascara	binder, film former	20% pet.			94
rosin in eyeshadow	binder, film former	20% pet.			94
thiomersal in eyeshadow	preservative	0.1% pet.			103

Allergic granuloma from cosmetic eyebrow tattoos due to chromium has been reported [96].

Other side effects of eye cosmetics

Stinging and burning, which are noted directly or soon after the application of the eye cosmetics, are the most common side effects. Subjective irritation may be induced by the evaporation of volatile ingredients, e.g. mineral spirits, isoparaffins and cyclomethicone or by non-volatile chemicals such as propylene glycol, soap emulsifiers, surfactants and other silicones. Irritant dermatitis (objective irritation) also occurs. Conjunctivitis may be elicited by physical and chemical irritants as well as by allergens. Physical irritants include mascara that may be washed into the conjunctival sac by the lacrimal fluid or the inadvertent entry of lash extenders and flakes of eyeshadow. Solvents, surfactants, and soap emulsifiers are among the chemical irritants involved [67]. Chronic conjunctivitis and blepharitis due to contaminated eyeliner and mascara have been reported [56,66,70]. Some cases of corneal ulceration due to contamination with Pseudomonas aeruginosa have been documented [57]. Conjunctival pigmentation may occur when eyeliner or mascara is applied to the mucosal aspect of the lid instead of the exterior or of the excessive use of mascara washed into the conjunctival sac by lacrimal fluid [68]. Many eyeshadows are radio-opaque, and may mimic orbital calcification on X-ray examination [69].

ANTI-ACNE PRODUCTS

27.12 Although it would clearly be advisable to regard and regulate anti-acne products as drugs (as is the case in the USA), many of them are sold in Europe as cosmetic preparations. They are available as creams, clear lotions, and as gels.

Anti-acne products may contain the following active ingredients:

- allantoin
- benzalkonium chloride
- benzoyl peroxide (prohibited in cosmetics in the EC)
- resorcinol
- resorcinol acetate
- salicylic acid
- sulfur (colloidal)
- tioxolone (hydroxy-oxo-benzoxathiole)
- tocopheryl acetate
- tretinoin (vitamin A acid) (prohibited in cosmetics in the EC)
- triclosan
- Vibenoid® (an aromatic retinoid-amide)

Typical formulas for the various types of products are:

I. Cream

Ingredients		Example
40–70%	water	water
ca. 2%	polyol	propylene glycol
30–50%	lipid	cetearyl alcohol, caprylic/capric triglyceride
2–5%	surfactant	polysorbate 40, sorbitan stearate
0–5%	anti-acne agent	benzoyl peroxide
0.3%	preservative	methylparaben
0.1%	perfume	perfume

II. Clear lotion

Ingredients		Example
50–80%	water	water
20–50%	alcohol	alcohol, isopropanol
ca. 2%	polyol	glycerin
1–2%	surfactant	cocamidopropyl betaine
ca. 0.5%	organic acid	citric acid
ca. 1%	anti-acne agent	salicylic acid, triclosan

III. Clear gel

Ingredients		Example
ca. 70%	water	water
ca. 10%	alcohol	alcohol
ca. 20%	block polymer	poloxamer 407
ca. 1%	anti-acne agent	resorcinol, triclosan

Adverse reactions to the various active ingredients (*from other sources*) are mentioned elsewhere in this book.

CAMOUFLAGE AND GREASEPAINT ('SCHMINK')

27.13 These cosmetics are make-up products with a high content of coloured pigments in order to obtain a high covering power. Basically they have similar formulations, typical formulas being:

Camouflage cream

Ingredients		Example
ca. 20%	water	water
ca. 25%	lipid	stearic acid, acetylated lanolin
ca. 2%	surfactant	TEA lauryl sulfate
40–50%	colour pigments	titanium dioxide, iron oxides
ca. 0.2%	preservative	methylparaben, propylparaben, imidazolidinyl urea
0–0.1%	perfume	perfume

Greasepaint stick (black)

Ingredients		Example
ca. 40%	lipid	ozokerite, mineral oil, petrolatum
ca. 1%	surfactant	sorbitan stearate
ca. 60%	colour pigments	carbon black
ca. 0.1%	antioxidant	BHT

Theatre compact powder

See facial make-up: compact face powder (§ 27.4).

TOOTHPASTE AND MOUTHWASH

27.14 These products and their side effects are discussed in Chapter 13.

LIPSTICK AND LIP BALM

27.15 These products intended for the care and the make-up of the lips, are mainly lipid mixtures of suitable composition; they are sufficiently rigid, and can therefore be easily applied to lips. Indelible lipsticks contain xanthene dyes (acid form; CI numbers start with 45...) which are dissolved in special solvents (castor oil, oleyl alcohol, hexylene glycol, diisopropyladipate). Such solutions are pale-red coloured, but streak bright red on the skin or lip, leaving an indelible colour.

Typical formulas are:

Lipstick

Ingredients		Example
ca. 60%	lipid–wax mixture	carnauba wax, beeswax
ca. 30%	lipid solvent	castor oil, oleyl alcohol
5–8%	colour and pigments	titanium dioxide, Solvent Red 43 (CI 45380:2), Pigment Red No. 4 (CI 12085), D&C Red No. 6 Barium lake (CI 15830:2)
ca. 0.05%	antioxidant	*p*-hydroxyanisole
ca. 0.1%	perfume	perfume

Lip balm

Ingredients		Example
ca. 95%	lipid–wax mixture	lanolin oil, beeswax, jojoba oil
1–2%	UV absorber	benzophenone-2
0.5%	perfume	perfume
0.05%	antioxidant	octyl gallate, BHA

Cheilitis caused by an allergic reaction to one of the ingredients of lipstick has nowadays become infrequent, mainly because of the use of better purified xanthene dyes, e.g. D&C Red No. 21 (eosin). Lipstick may be patch-tested 'as is'.

27.16 Contact allergy to lipstick ingredients

Ingredient	Use	Patch test conc. & vehicle (§5.2)	Cross-reactions (§5.5)	Comment	Ref.
acetylated lanolin	lipid; vehicle constituent	30% pet.			97
azulene	skin conditioner	1% pet.			17
Basic Violet No. 10 (CI 45170; Rhodamine B; *formerly*: D&C Red No. 19)	colour	1% pet.		Discontinued in the USA; prohibited in EC	17
benzoin	resin of natural origin	10% alc.			47
benzophenone-3 (oxybenzone)	sunscreen	2% pet.			104
BHA (butylated hydroxyanisole)	antioxidant	2% pet.			77

(continued)

§ **27.16** *(continuation)*

Ingredient	Use	Patch test conc. & vehicle (§5.2)	Cross-reactions (§5.5)	Comment	Ref.
BHT (butylated hydroxytoluene)	antioxidant	2% pet.			77
bromofluorescein derivatives	colour	?			2
t-butyl hydroquinone	antioxidant	1% pet.			12 77
butyl methoxydibenzoyl-methane	sunscreen	2% pet.	isopropyl dibenzoylmethane		75
carmine in lip salve	colour	pure			37
castor oil in lipstick/cream	lipid; vehicle constituent	pure		The offending chemical possibly was ricinoleic acid (30% pet. and pure). The test concentration is slightly irritant [58]	46 58 65
cinnamic aldehyde	fragrance	1% pet.		Cinnamal in toothpaste aggravated the cheilitis	71
cinnamic alcohol	fragrance	2% pet.			97
D&C Red No. 17 (CL 26100; Sudan III)	colour	1% pet.	possibly other azo-dyes		8
D&C Red No. 22 (CI 45380; eosin)	colour	50% pet.	possibly other bromofluorescein derivatives	Contact allergy very rare nowadays; actual allergen unknown	2 14
D&C Red No. 31 (CI 15800:1, calcium salt; Brilliant Lake Red R)	colour	1% pet.	other azo-dyes		17
D&C Red No. 36 (CI 12085)	colour	1% pet.			3
D&C Yellow No. 11 (CI 47000)	colour	0.1% pet.	D&C Yellow No. 10	Patch testing with the dye may sensitize	7 51
ester gum?	thickener?	0.1% pet.		Actual allergen not identified	72
geraniol	fragrance	2% pet.			13
glyceryl isostearate	emollient	35% pet.	isostearyl alcohol		73
isopropyl dibenzoylmethane	sunscreen	1% pet.		Concomitant reaction to 4-methylbenzylidene camphor in the sunscreen Eusolex® 8021	99 106

(continued)

§ **27.16** *(continuation)*

Ingredient	Use	Patch test conc. & vehicle (§5.2)	Cross-reactions (§5.5)	Comment	Ref.
isostearyl alcohol	emollient	0.25% pet.	glyceryl isostearate		73
lanolin	emollient; vehicle constituent	pure			38
lanolin alcohol (wool wax alcohols)	vehicle constituent	30% pet.			63
4-methylbenzylidene-camphor	sunscreen	2% pet.			99
methylheptine carbonate	fragrance	0.5% pet.			1
microcrystalline wax	emollient	pure		Exact composition and actual allergen not identified	48
p-nitrobenzene-azo-beta-naphthol (para-Red Dark)	colour	?	possibly other azo-dyes		40
octyl gallate	antioxidant	0.25% pet.			97
oleyl alcohol	surfactant; emollient	30% pet.			15
PEG-5 lanolate (Lanpol 5)	surfactant; emulsifier	5% pet.			74
pentyl dimethyl PABA (amyl dimethyl PABA, Padimate A®)	sunscreen	1% pet.		Prohibited in the EC	10
perfume		*see* § 5.8			17
phenyl salicylate (salol)	sunscreen	1% pet.	other aryl salicylates [45]		13 45
Pigment Orange 5 (CI 12075; *formerly*: D&C Orange No. 17)	colour	1% pet.	possibly other azo-dyes	Discontinued in the USA; prohibited in the EC	3
propyl gallate	antioxidant	1% pet.			21
rosin (colophony) in lipstick sealant	binder; film former	30% pet.			74
shellac (in lipstick sealant)	binder; film former	pure			74
sodium salt of m-xylene-azo-beta-naphthol-3,6-disulfonic acid	colour		possibly other azo-dyes		40
1-sulfo-beta-naphthalene-azo-beta-naphthol	colour		possibly other azo-dyes		40

27.17 REFERENCES

1. Baer, H.L. (1935): Lipstick dermatitis. *Arch. Dermatol., 32*, 726–734.
2. Calnan, C.D. (1959): Allergic sensitivity to eosin. *Acta Allerg., 13*, 493–499.
3. Calnan, C D. (1967): Reactions to artificial colouring materials. *J. Soc. Cosmet. Chem., 18*, 215–223.
4. Calnan, C.D. (1971): Chloroacetamide dermatitis from a cosmetic. *Contact Dermatitis Newsl. 9*, 215.
5. Fisher, A.A., (1988): Allergic contact dermatitis due to rosin (colophony) in eyeshadow and mascara. *Cutis, 42*, 507–508.
6. Calnan, C.D. (1973): Ditertiary butylhydroquinone in eye-shadow. *Contact Dermatitis Newsl., 14*, 402.
7. Calnan, C.D. (1976): Quinazoline yellow SS in cosmetics. *Contact Dermatitis, 2*, 160.
8. Calnan, C.D. (1976): Dermatocosmetic relations. *J. Soc. Cosmet. Chem., 77*, 491.
9. Calnan, C.D. (1979): Perfume dermatitis from the cosmetic ingredients oakmoss and hydroxycitronellal. *Contact Dermatitis, 5*, 194.
10. Calnan, C.D. (1980): Amyldimethylamino benzoic acid causing lipstick dermatitis. *Contact Dermatitis, 6*, 233.
11. Calnan, C.D. (1981): Quinazoline yellow dermatitis (D and C Yellow 11) in an eye cream. *Contact Dermatitis, 7*, 271.
12. van Joost, Th., Liem, D.H. and Stolz, E. (1984): Allergic contact dermatitis to monotertiary-butylhydroquinone in lipgloss. *Contact Dermatitis, 10*, 189–190.
13. Calnan, C.D., Cronin, E. and Rycroft, R.J.G. (1981): Allergy to phenyl salicylate. *Contact Dermatitis, 7*, 208.
14. Calnan, C.D. and Sarkany, I. (1957): Studies in contact dermatitis: II. Lipstick cheilitis. *Trans. St. John's Hosp. Derm. Soc. (Lond.), 39*, 28–36.
15. Calnan, C.D. and Sarkany, I. (1960): Studies in contact dermatitis: XII. Sensitivity to oleyl alcohol. *Trans. St. John's Hosp. Derm. Soc. (Lond.), 44*, 47.
16. Cronin, E. (1966): Lanolin dermatitis. *Br. J. Derm., 78*, 167.
17. Cronin, E. (1967): Contact dermatitis from cosmetics. *J. Soc. Cosmet. Chem., 18*, 681.
18. Cronin, E. (1972): Clinical prediction of patch test results. *Trans. St. Johns Hosp. Derm. Soc. (Lond.), 58*, 153.
19. Cronin, E. (1973): Di-isopropanolamine in an eye-shadow. *Contact Dermatitis Newsl., 13*, 364.
20. Cronin, E. (1980): Cosmetics. In: *Contact Dermatitis*, pp. 93–170. Churchill Livingstone, Edinburgh.
21. Wilson, A.G.M., White, I.R. and Kirby, J.D.T. (1989): Allergic contact dermatitis from propyl gallate in a lip balm. *Contact Dermatitis, 20*, 145–146.
22. Dahlquist, I. and Fregert, S. (1980): Contact allergy to atranorin in lichens and perfumes. *Contact Dermatitis, 6*, 111.
23. Dooms-Goossens, A., Degreef, H. and Luytens, E. (1979): Dihydroabietylalcohol (Abitol), a sensitizer in mascara. *Contact Dermatitis, 5*, 350.
24. Emmett, E.A. and Wright, R.C. (1976): Allergic contact dermatitis from TEA-coco hydrolyzed protein. *Arch. Dermatol., 112*, 1008.
25. Epstein, E. (1966): Dichlorophene allergy. *Ann. Allergy, 24*, 437–439.
26. Fisher, A.A. (1975): Allergic contact dermatitis from Germall 115, a new cosmetic preservative. *Contact Dermatitis, 1*, 126.
27. Fisher, A.A. (1975): Allergic paraben and benzyl alcohol hypersensitivity — relationship of the 'delayed' and immediate varieties. *Contact Dermatitis, 1*, 281.
28. Foussereau, J. (1975): A case of allergy to colophony in a facial cosmetic. *Contact Dermatitis, 1*, 259.
29. Hoffmann, T.E. and Adams, R.M. (1978): Contact dermatitis to benzoin in greasepaint makeup. *Contact Dermatitis, 4*, 379.
30. Hoffman, M.J. and Peters, J. (1935): Dermatitis due to facial cream, caused by methyl heptine carbonate. *J. Am. Med. Assoc., 104*, 1072.
31. Kozuka, T., Tashiro, M., Sano, S., Fujimoto, K., Nakamura, Y., Hashimoto, S. and Nakaminami, G. (1979): Brilliant Lake Red as a cause of pigmented contact dermatitis. *Contact Dermatitis, 5*, 297.
32. Kozuka, T., Tashiro, M., Sano, S., Fujimoto, K., Nakamura, Y., Hashimoto, S. and Nakaminami, G. (1980): Pigmented contact dermatitis from azo dyes. I. Cross-sensitivity in humans. *Contact Dermatitis, 6*, 330.
33. Larsen, W.G. (1975): Cosmetic dermatitis due to a perfume. *Contact Dermatitis, 1*, 142.
34. Larsen, W.G. (1975): Cosmetic dermatitis due to a dye (D and C yellow no. 11). *Contact Dermatitis, 1*, 61.
35. Mandy, S.H. (1974): Contact dermatitis to substituted imidazolidinyl-urea — a common preservative in

cosmetics. *Arch. Dermatol., 110*, 463.

36. Mathias, C.G.T. (1980): Contact dermatitis in children due to face paints. *Cutis, 26*, 584.
37. Sarkany, I., Meara, R.H. and Everall, J. (1961): Cheilitis due to carmine in lip salve. *Trans. St. John's Hosp. Derm. Soc. (Lond.), 46*, 39.
38. Schorr, W. F. (1973): Lip gloss and gloss-type cosmetics. *Contact Dermatitis Newsl. 14*, 408.
39. Simpson, J.R. (1978): Dermatitis due to parabens in cosmetic creams. *Contact Dermatitis, 4*, 311.
40. Sulzberger, M.B., Goodman, J., Byrne, L.A. and Mallozzi, E.D. (1938): Acquired specific hypersensitivity to simple chemicals. II. Cheilitis, with special reference to sensitivity to lipsticks. *Arch. Derm. Syph., 37*, 597–615.
41. Van Ketel, W.G. (1979): Patch testing with eye cosmetics. *Contact Dermatitis, 5*, 402.
42. Goh, C.L., Ng, S.K. and Kwok, S.F. (1989): Allergic contact dermatitis from nickel in eyeshadow. *Contact Dermatitis, 20*, 380–381.
43. Woods, B. (1981): Dermatitis from Eusolex 8021 sunscreen agent in a cosmetic. *Contact Dermatitis, 7*, 108.
44. De Groot, A.C. and Liem, D.H. (1983): Facial psoriasis caused by contact allergy to linalool and hydroxycitronellal in an after-shave. *Contact Dermatitis, 9*, 230.
45. Marchand, B., Barbier, P., Ducombs, G. et al. (1982): Allergic contact dermatitis to various salols (phenyl salicylates). *Arch. Derm. Res., 272*, 61.
46. Sai, S. (1983): Lipstick dermatitis caused by castor oil. *Contact Dermatitis, 9*, 75.
47. Hjorth, N. (1987): Skin reactions to balsams and perfumes. *Clin. Exp. Dermatol., 7*, 1–9.
48. De Darko, E. and Osmundsen, P.E. (1984): Allergic contact dermatitis to Lipcare® lipstick. *Contact Dermatitis, 11*, 46.
49. De Groot. A.C. and Liem, D.H. (1983): Contact allergy to Tinuvin® P. *Contact Dermatitis, 9*, 324.
50. Curtis, G. and Netherton, E.W. (1940): Cutaneous hypersensitivity to triethanolamine. *Arch. Derm. Syph., 41*, 729.
51. Björkner, B. and Magnusson, B. (1981): Patch test sensitization to D & C Yellow no. 11 and simultaneous reaction to Quinoline Yellow. *Contact Dermatitis, 7*, 1.
52. Lamson, S.A., Kong, B.M. and De Salva, S.J. (1982): D & C Yellow Nos. 10 and 11: delayed contact hypersensitivity in the guinea pig. *Contact Dermatitis, 8*, 200.
53. Rapaport, M.J. (1980): Allergy to D & C Yellow No. 11. *Contact Dermatitis, 6*, 364.
54. Weaver, J.E. (1983): Dose response relationships in delayed hypersensitivity to quinoline dyes. *Contact Dermatitis, 9*, 309.
55. Björkner, B. and Niklasson, B. (1983): Contact allergic reaction to D & C Yellow No. 11 and Quinoline Yellow. *Contact Dermatitis, 9*, 263.
56. Ahearn, D.G. and Wilson, L.A. (1976): Microflora of the outer eye and eye area cosmetics. *Devel. Indus. Microbiol., 17*, 23.
57. Wilson, L.A. and Ahearn, D.G. (1977): Pseudomonas-induced corneal ulcers associated with contaminated eye mascaras. *Am. J. Ophthal., 84*, 112.
58. Andersen, K.E. and Nielsen, R. (1984): Lipstick dermatitis related to castor oil. *Contact Dermatitis, 11*, 253–254.
59. Fisher, A.A. (1980): Cutaneous reactions to sorbic acid and potassium sorbate. *Cutis, 25*, 350, 352, 423.
60. Guin. J.D. (1981): Contact dermatitis to perfume in paper products. *J. Am. Acad. Dermatol., 4*, 733.
61. Rapaport, M.J. (1980): Sensitization to Abitol. *Contact Dermatitis, 6*, 137.
62. Calnan, C.D. (1973): Allergy to D and C Red 17 and D and C Yellow 11. *Contact Dermatitis Newls., 14*, 405.
63. Schorr, W.F. (1973): Lip gloss and gloss type cosmetics. *Contact Dermatitis Newsl., 14*, 408.
64. Brandle, I., Boujnah-Khouadja, A. and Foussereau, J. (1983): Allergy to castor oil. *Contact Dermatitis, 9*, 424.
65. Sai, S. (1983): Lipstick dermatitis caused by ricinoleic acid. *Contact Dermatitis, 9*, 524.
66. Thomas E.T. and Barton, S.N. (1978): The role of eye cosmetic contaminants in the pathogenesis of eye infection: an epidemiologic investigation. *Alabama J. Med. Sci., 15*, 246–251.
67. Pascher, F. (1982): Adverse reactions to eye area cosmetics and their management. *J. Soc. Cosm. Chem., 33*, 249–258.
68. Platia, E.V., Michaels, R.G. and Green, W.R. (1978): Eye cosmetic-induced conjunctival pigmentation. *Ann. Ophthalmol., 10*, 501–504.
69. Forman, W.H., McDowell, R.V., Shivers, J.A. and Steele, J.R. (1977): Cosmetic eye shadow mimicking orbital calcification. *JAMA*, 2695.

70. Reid, F.R. and Wood T.O. (1979): *Pseudomonas* corneal ulcer. The causative role of contaminated eye cosmetics. *Arch. Ophthalmol., 97*, 1640–1641.
71. Maibach, H.I. (1986): Cheilitis: occult allergy to cinnamic aldehyde. *Contact Dermatitis, 15*, 106–107.
72. Hayakawa, R., Matsunaga, K., Arima, Y. and Ohtsu, Y. (1990): Allergic contact dermatitis due to ester gum in a lipstick. *Ninth Int. Symp. on Contact Dermatitis, 17–19 May 1990, Stockholm, Sweden. Book of Abstracts*, p. 85.
73. Hayakawa, R., Matsunaga, K., Suzuki, M., Arima, Y. and Ohkido, Y. (1987): Lipstick dermatitis due to C_{18} aliphatic compounds. *Contact Dermatitis, 16*, 215–219.
74. Rademaker, M., Kirby, J.D. and White, I.R. (1986): Contact cheilitis to Shellac, Lanpol 5 and colophony. *Contact Dermatitis, 15*, 307–308.
75. De Groot, A.C. and Weyland, J.W. (1987): Contact allergy to butyl methoxydibenzoylmethane. *Contact Dermatitis 16*, 278.
76. Bardazzi, F., Misciali, C., Borrello, P. and Capobianco, C. (1988): Contact dermatitis due to antioxidants. *Contact Dermatitis, 19*, 385–386.
77. White, I.R., Lovell, C.R. and Cronin, E. (1984): Antioxidants in cosmetics. *Contact Dermatitis, 11*, 265–267.
78. Senff, H., Exner, M., Görtz, J. and Goos, M. (1989): Allergic contact dermatitis from Euxyl K400. *Contact Dermatitis, 20*, 381–382.
79. De Groot, A.C., Berretty, P.J.M., van Ginkel, C.J.W., den Hengst, C.W., van Ulsen, J. and Weyland, J.W. (1991): Allergic contact dermatitis from tocopheryl acetate in cosmetic creams. *Contact Dermatitis, 25*, 302–304.
80. Ross, J.S. and White, I.R. (1991): Eyelid dermatitis due to cocamidopropyl betaine in an eye make-up remover. *Contact Dermatitis, 25*, 64.
81. Dooms-Goossens, A., Bedert, R., Degreef, H. and Vandaele, M. (1990): Airborne allergic contact dermatitis from kitasamycin and midecamycin. *Contact Dermatitis, 23*, 118–119.
82. De Groot, A.C., van der Meeren, H.L.M. and Weyland, J.W. (1988): Cosmetic allergy from stearic acid and glyceryl stearate. *Contact Dermatitis, 19*, 77–78.
83. De Groot, A.C., Bruynzeel, D.P., van Joost, Th. and Weyland, J.W. (1988): Cosmetic allergy from myristyl alcohol. *Contact Dermatitis, 19*, 76–77.
84. Fritsch, P., Pichler, E. and Linser, I. (1989): Periorale dermatitis. *Hautarzt, 40*, 475–479.
85. Sun, C.C. (1987): Allergic contact dermatitis of the face from contact with nickel and ammoniated mercury in spectacle frames and skin lightening creams. *Contact Dermatitis, 17*, 306–309.
86. Dooms-Goossens, A., Debusschere, K., Gladys, K. and DeGreef, H. (1988): Contact allergy to an emulsifier in a cosmetic lotion. *Contact Dermatitis, 18*, 249–250.
87. De Groot, A.C. and Weyland, J.W. (1987): Hidden contact allergy to formaldehyde in imidazolidinyl urea. *Contact Dermatitis, 17*, 124–125.
88. Spier, H.W. and Sirt, I. (1953): Lorbeer als Träger eines wenig beacheten kontaktekzematogenen Allergens. *Derm. Wschrift., 128*, 805–810.
89. Fisher, A.A. (1987): Cosmetic warning: this product may be detrimental to your purse. *Cutis, 39*, 23–24.
90. Koch, S.E., Mathias, T. and Maibach, H.I. (1985): Chloracetamide: an unusual cause of cosmetic dermatitis. *Arch. Dermatol., 121*, 172–173.
91. De Groot, A.C. and Weyland, J.W. (1986): Contact allergy to chloroacetamide in an "anti-wrinkle serum". *Contact Dermatitis, 15*, 97–98.
92. Englich, J.S.C. and White, I.R. (1985): Dermatitis from D & C Red no. 36. *Contact Dermatitis, 13*, 335.
93. Whittington, C.V. (1985): Elicitation of contact lens allergy to thimerosal by eye cream. *Contact Dermatitis, 13*, 186–187.
94. Gollhausen, R., Przybilla, B. and Ring, J. (1986): Contact allergy to CI. Solvent Red 3. *Contact Dermatitis, 14*, 123–124.
95. De Groot, A.C., Bos, J.D. and Liem, D.H. (1984): Contact allergy to bornelone. *Contact Dermatitis, 10*, 45–46.
96. Eun, H.C. and Kim, K.H. (1989): Allergic granuloma from cosmetic eyebrow tattooing. *Contact Dermatitis, 21*, 276–278.
97. De Groot, A.C. (1988): Adverse reactions to cosmetics, p. 111–112. Thesis, University of Groningen.
98. Curtis, G. and Netherton, E.W. (1940): Cutaneous hypersensitivity to triethanolamine. *Arch. Dermatol., 41*, 729–731.
99. De Groot, A.C., van der Walle, H.B., Jagtman, B.A. and Weyland, J.W. (1987): Contact allergy to 4-isopropyldibenzoylmethane and 3-(4′-methylbenzylidene) camphor in the sunscreen Eusolex 8021.

Contact Dermatitis, 16, 249–254.
100. Marston, S. (1992): Propyl gallate on liposomes. *Contact Dermatitis, 27,* 74–76.
101. Peter, C. and Hoting, E. (1992): Contact allergy to cocamidopropyl betaine (CAPB). *Contact Dermatitis, 26,* 282–283.
102. Hayahawa, R., Hirose, O. and Arima, Y. (1991): Pigmented contact dermatitis due to musk moskene. *J. Dermatol., 18,* 420–421.
103. Podmore, P. and Storrs, F.J. (1989): Contact lens intolerance: allergic conjunctivitis? *Contact Dermatitis, 20,* 98–103.
104. Aguirre, A., Izu, R., Gardeazabal, J. et al. (1992): Allergic contact cheilitis from a lipstick containing oxybenzone. *Contact Dermatitis, 27,* 267–268.
105. Marston, S. (1992): Propylgallate on liposomes. *Contact Dermatitis, 27,* 74–76.
106. Alomar, A. and Cerda, M.T. (1989): Contact allergy to Eusolex® 8021. *Contact Dermatitis,* 74–75.
107. Raab, R. (1988): Liposomen — eine neue Form dermatologischer Wirkstofftrager. *Arzliche Kosmetologie, 18,* 213–224.
108. Wohlrab, W. and Lasch, J. (1989): Penetration kinetics of liposomal hydrocortisone in human skin. *Dermatologica, 174,* 18.
109. Mezei, M. (1988): Liposomes in the topical application of drugs. In: G.G. Gregoridis (Editor), *Liposomes as Drug Carriers*, pp. 663–667. Wiley, New York.

28. Nail cosmetics

28.1 The nail-line of cosmetics consists of: lacquer, lacquer remover, hardener, elongator, cuticle softener and cream. Lacquers are the most popular nail cosmetics. Typical formulas are:

Nail lacquer

Ingredients		Example
ca. 15%	film polymer	nitrocellulose
ca. 7%	polymer resin	toluenesulfonamide/formaldehyde resin* (Santolite MHP or MS®)
ca. 7%	lipid plasticizer	dibutyl phthalate, camphor, castor oil
ca. 70%	solvent mixture	toluene, butyl acetate, *n*-butyl alcohol, ethyl acetate
0.1%	colour pigments mixture	titanium dioxide, Pigment Red 57:2 Barium Lake (CI 15850:2)
ca. 1%	suspending agent	quaternium-18 hectorite

*Toluenesulfonamide/formaldehyde resins are indispensable in nail lacquer technology; they have outstanding properties. Sensitization, however, is not infrequent. There is always a small amount of free formaldehyde present, at least in the preparations available in Holland. The Enschede laboratory found levels of 0.15% free formaldehyde in 22 commercial nail lacquers of different brands, and only in 2 samples was the concentration lower than 0.01%. The presence of toluenesulfonamide-formaldehyde resins was confirmed by infrared spectroscopy.

Nail lacquer remover

Ingredients		Example
ca. 98%	solvent mixture	butyl acetate, ethyl acetate, ethoxyethanol (Cellosolve®), acetone
ca. 2%	lipid	castor oil, lanolin oil

Nail hardener (formaldehyde type)

Ingredients		Example
ca. 80%	water	water
ca. 5%	hardening agent	formaldehyde*
ca. 1%	organic acid	lactic acid

*Limited to 5% in the EEC Cosmetic Directive (1976).

Nail elongator (other names: nail extender, liquid nails, artificial nail set)

There are two types: one using plastic nails to be glued with a special glue (e.g. ethylcyanoacryl-type glue), the other type is a dual product of the following typical formulas:

Elongator I (powder)

Ingredients		Example
ca. 97%	acryl-type polymer (powder)	polymethylmethacrylate
ca. 3%	polymerization initiator	benzoylperoxide

Elongator II (liquid)

Ingredients		Example
ca. 99%	acryl-type monomer	methylmethacrylate (monomer)
ca. 1%	stabilizer	hydroquinone, *p*-dimethylaminochlorobenzene

Powder I and liquid II are mixed before use and applied as an extension of the nail. It hardens after ca. 15 minutes.

Cuticle removers or **softeners** are dilute solutions of alkali. A typical formula is:

Ingredients		Example
ca. 90%	water	water
1–5%	softening agent	potassium hydroxide
5–1%	thickener	sorbitol, magnesium aluminum silicate
0.1%	perfume	perfume

Nail cream is an ordinary water-in-oil moisturizing cream, with low water (ca. 30%) and a high lipid content (typical lipids: lanolin, propolis, jojoba oil, carrot oil). It is applied to combat brittleness and splitting of the nails.

A typical formula is:

Ingredients		Example
ca. 30%	water	water
ca. 65%	lipids	beeswax, lanolin wax, jojoba oil, turtle oil
ca. 2%	emulsifier	sodium lauryl sulfate
ca. 0.2%	preservative	2-bromo-2-nitropropane-1,3-diol

Dermatitis from nail cosmetics may be localized on:
- the eyelids
- the lower part of the face (in the majority of patients)
- the neck and upper chest
- the skin around the nails (less frequent)
- the external auditory meatus (rare)
- the skin behind the ears (rare)
- the pinnae (rare)
- the lips and the corners of the eyes (rare)
- perineum and groins (rare);

It can also be generalized (rare).

Nail varnish may be tested 'as is' but should be allowed to dry before patch testing. The majority of contact allergic reactions to nail cosmetics are due to the resins.

Tabulation of side effects

Side effects of ingredients of nail cosmetics are tabulated in § 28.2 (contact allergy) and § 28.3 (other side effects). For a survey of adverse reactions, see also Refs. [20,23]. For adverse reactions to acrylate sculptured nails and glues, see Refs. [26].

28.2 Contact allergy to ingredients of nail cosmetics

Ingredient	Use	Patch test conc. & vehicle (§ 5.2)	Cross-reaction (§ 5.5)	Ref.
aryl-sulfonamide resin (toluenesulfonamide/ formaldehyde resin)	polymer resin	10% pet.	sulfanilamide formaldehyde. Contact allergy to toluene sulfonamide/ formaldehyde resin in nail hardeners: see Ref. [24]	3 8

(continued)

§ **28.2** *(continuation)*

Ingredient	Use	Patch test conc. & vehicle (§ 5.2)	Cross-reaction (§ 5.5)	Ref.
drometrizole	UV-absorber in nail varnish	5% pet.		18
formaldehyde	nail hardener	1% aqua		5
glyceryl phthalate resin	polymer resin	10% pet.		3
guanine	pearlescent pigment	pure		15
methacrylic acid esters	monomers		Cross-reactions between methyl methacrylate monomers and acrylic monomers are possible. Sensitization results in onychia and paronychia. Dystrophic nail changes may persist for several months and permanent loss of fingernails, sometimes with prolonged paraesthesia, has been observed [19,26]. Permanent paraesthesia from sculptured nails of an irritant phenomenon has been reported [27]. For irritant and allergic reactions to acrylates and methacrylates *see also* [4]	10 7 9
– methyl methacrylate	monomer	1% pet.		
– ethyl methacrylate	monomer	1% pet.		
– butyl methacrylate	monomer	1% pet.		
– isobutyl methacrylate	monomer	2% pet.		
– tetrahydrofurfuryl methacrylate	monomer	1% pet.		
– methacrylic acid	monomer	1% pet.		
– diethylene glycol dimethacrylate	monomer	1% pet.		
– trimethylol propane trimethacrylate	monomer	0.1% pet. or acet.		
nitrocellulose	film polymer	10% aqua		21
polyester nail varnish	resin	?	The resin consisted of trimellitic anhydride, adipic acid, neopentyl glycol and cyclohexane dimethanol 70% in butyl acetate	25
p-tertiary butylphenol resin	resin in plastic nail adhesive	1% pet.		16 17
tricresyl ethyl phthalate	plasticizer in artificial nail	5% pet.		17

28.3 Other side effects of ingredients of nail cosmetics

Ingredient	Use	Side effects	Comment	Ref.
acrylates	artificial nails	onycholysis	Contact allergy not excluded	22
formaldehyde	nail hardener	paronychia, subungual hyperkeratosis, subungual haemorrhages, leukonychia, onycholysis, lip haemorrhages in nail biters	These effects may be allergic or non-allergic in nature	6 11 14
nail varnish	contact urticaria	causative ingredient not specified	*See* § 7.6	
phenol formaldehyde resin	polymer resin	subungual haemorrhage, red-brown discoloration of the nail plate, onycholysis, subungual hyperkeratosis	These effects may both be allergic or non-allergic in nature	13 16
toluenesulfonamide/ formaldehyde resin	polymer resin	onycholysis	The validity of this report was questioned by Brauer [1]	12
Transparent Yellow Lake (CI 16901)		orange discoloration of the nail		2

28.4 REFERENCES

1. Brauer, E.W. (1980): Letter to the Editor. *Cutis, 26*, 588.
2. Calnan, C.D. (1967): Reactions to artificial colouring materials. *J. Soc. Cosmet. Chem., 18*, 215.
3. Calnan, C.D. and Sarkany, I. (1958): Studies in contact dermatitis, III. Nail varnish. *Trans. St. John's Hosp. Derm. Soc. (Lond.), 40*, 1.
4. Cavelier, C., Jelen, G., Hervé-Bazin, B. and Foussereau, J. (1981): Irritation et allergie aux acrylates et methacrylates. *Ann. Derm. Vénéréol. (Paris), 108*, 549.
5. Epstein, E. and Maibach, H.I. (1966): Formaldehyde allergy. *Arch. Dermatol., 94*, 186.
6. Fisher. A.A. (1979): Current contact news. *Cutis, 23*, 743, 746, 753, 847, 852, 855, 863, 871.
7. Fisher, A.A. (1980): Cross reactions between methyl methacrylate monomer and acrylic monomers presently used in acrylic nail preparations. *Contact Dermatitis, 6*, 345.
8. Keil, H. and van Dijck, L.S. (1944): Dermatitis due to nail polish. *Arch. Dermatol., 50*, 39.
9. Maibach, H.I. et al. (1978): Butyl methacrylate monomer and ethyl methacrylate monomer-frequency of reaction. *Contact Dermatitis, 4*, 60.
10. Marks Jr., J.F., Bishop, M.E. and Willis, W.P. (1979): Allergic contact dermatitis to sculptured nails. *Arch. Dermatol., 115*, 100.
11. Mitchell, J.C. (1981): Non-inflammatory onycholysis from formaldehyde-containing nail hardener. *Contact Dermatitis, 7*, 173.
12. Paltzick, R.L. and Enscoe, I. (1980): Onycholysis secondary to toluene sulfonamide formaldehyde resin used in nail hardener mimicking onychomycosis. *Cutis, 75*, 647.
13. Rein, C.R. and Rogin, J.R. (1950): Allergic eczematous reaction of the nail bed due to 'undercoats'. *Arch. Dermatol., 61*, 971.
14. Rice, E.G. (1968): Allergic rcactions to nail hardeners. *Cutis, 4*, 971.
15. Stritzler, C. (1958): Dermatitis of the face caused by guanine in pearly nail lacquer. *Arch. Dermatol., 78*, 252.
16. Rycroft, R.J.G., Wilkinson, J.D., Holmes, R. and Hay, R.J. (1980): Contact sensitization to p-tertiary butylphenol (PTBP) resin in plastic nail adhesive. *Clin. Exp. Dermatol., 5*, 441.

17. Burrows, D. and Rycroft, R.J.G. (1981): Contact dermatitis from PTBP resin and tricresyl ethyl phthalate in a plastic nail adhesive. *Contact Dermatitis, 7*, 336.
18. De Groot, A.C. and Liem, D.H. (1983): Contact allergy to Tinuvin®. *Contact Dermatitis, 9*, 324.
19. Fisher, A.A. (1980): Permanent loss of fingernails from sensitization and reaction to acrylic in a preparation designed to make artificial nails. *J. Derm. Surg. Oncol., 6*, 70.
20. Scher, R.K. (1982): Cosmetics and ancillary preparations for the care of nails. *J. Am. Acad. Dermatol., 6*, 523.
21. Dobes, W.L. and Nippert, P.H. (1944): Contact eczema due to nail polish. *Arch. Derm. Syph., 49*, 183.
22. Goodwin, P. (1976): Onycholysis due to acrylic nail applications. *Clin. Exp. Dermatol., 1*, 191.
23. Baran, R. (1982): Pathology induced by the application of cosmetics to the nail. In: *Principles of Cosmetics for the Dermatologist, Chapter 24*, pp. 181–184. Editors.: Ph. Frost and S.N. Horwitz. C.V. Mosby Company, St. Louis, U.S.A.
24. De Wit, F.S., de Groot, A.C., Weyland, J.W. and Bos J.D. (1988): An outbreak of contact dermatitis from toluenesulfonamide formaldehyde resin in a nail hardener. *Contact Dermatitis, 18*, 280–283.
25. Shaw, S. (1989): A case of contact dermatitis from hypoallergenic nail varnish. *Contact Dermatitis, 20*, 385.
26. Fisher, A.A. and Baran, R.L. (1991): Adverse reactions to acrylate sculptured nails with particular reference to prolonged paresthesia. *Am. J. Contact Dermatitis, 2*, 38–42.
27. Baran, R.L. and Schibli, H. (1990): Permanent paresthesia to sculptured nails. A distressing problem. *Dermatologic Clinics, 8*, 139–141.
28. Shelley, E.D. and Shelley, W.B. (1988): Nail dystrophy and periungual dermatitis due to cyanoacrylate glue sensitivity. *J. Am. Acad. Dermatol., 19*, 574–575.

29. Cosmetics for the body and parts of the body

BATH AND SHOWER COSMETICS

29.1 These cosmetics, which consist mainly of foam and fragrance, have the following typical formulas:

Foam bath (bubble bath), foam shower: basically a shampoo formulation (see § 26.1) but with the emphasis on the foam building surfactants.

Ingredients		Example
70–80%	water	water
10–20%	surfactant: foam builder	sodium laureth sulfate, lauramide DEA
0–1%	thickener	sodium chloride
ca. 1%	perfume	perfume
ca. 0.2%	preservative	2-bromo-2-nitropropane-1,3-diol, methylparaben
ca. 0.02%	colour	D&C Green No. 5 (CI 61570)

Bath oil (floating type): when this bath oil is poured into the bath, oil floats on the water surface and will partly stay on the body after bathing.

Ingredients		Example
ca. 95%	lipid	oleyl alcohol, mineral oil
ca. 0.5%	surfactant	polyethylene glycol, glyceryl cocoate
ca. 0.5%	perfume	perfume
ca. 0.05%	antioxidant	BHA

Bath oil (dispersible type): when poured into the bath, a milky dispersion instantly appears.

Ingredients		Example
ca. 80%	lipid	decyl oleate, mineral oil
5–10%	surfactant	sulfated castor oil, PEG-150 dioleate
1–5%	perfume	perfume
ca. 0.05%	antioxidant	BHA

Bath cream: bath cream has the same properties as dispersible bath oil, but it gives more foam.

Ingredients		Example
60–70%	water	water
ca. 5%	lipid	isopropyl myristate
ca. 5%	surfactant: pearlescent additive	PEG-8 distearate
20–30%	surfactant	TEA lauryl sulfate
ca. 0.3%	preservative	imidazolidinyl urea, methylparaben
ca. 1%	perfume	perfume
ca. 0.05%	antioxidant	BHA, BHT

Bath salt: bath salts are added to baths to imitate natural mineral water, but most formulas contain only one or more of the following salts: disodium phosphate, magnesium sulfate, sea salt, sodium bicarbonate, sodium carbonate, sodium chloride, sodium iodide, sodium sesquicarbonate, sodium thiosulfate.

Ingredients		Example
ca. 99%	salts (see list above)	sodium chloride, potassium iodide, sodium bicarbonate
ca. 0.5%	perfume	perfume
ca. 0.01%	colour	Basic Violet No. 14 (CI 42510)

Effervescent bath tablet: these are added to baths for a steady release of carbon dioxide or oxygen gas.

Ingredients		Example
10–25%	salts for CO_2 gas release	citric acid, sodium sesquicarbonate
	or: salts for O_2 gas release	sodium perborate, manganese sulfate
ca. 20%	filler additives	sodium chloride, kaolin, talc
ca. 0.5%	perfume	perfume
ca. 0.01%	colour	Basic Violet 14 (CI 42510)

HAND AND BODY LOTION

29.2 These products are popular as 'all-purpose' lotions and creams, but they are especially and very widely used for treating mild 'housewives eczema'. The composition is basically similar to ordinary moisturizing and cleansing milks:

Hand and body lotion/cream

Ingredients		Example
60–80%	water	water
ca. 5%	polyol	sorbitol
20–30%	lipid	mineral oil, glyceryl stearate, cetyl alcohol
2–5%	surfactant: emulsifier	TEA lauryl sulfate, trioleth-8-phosphate
ca. 7 ppm–0.3%	preservative	methylisothiazolinone and methylchloroisothiazolinone
ca. 0.02%	colour	Acid Red No. 27 (CI 16185)
ca. 0.2%	perfume	perfume

Fragrance materials and their side effects are discussed in Chapter 5. The side effects of bath, shower and body cosmetics are tabulated in § 29.3.

29.3 Contact allergy to ingredients of bath and shower and hand and body cosmetics

Ingredient	Cosmetic	Patch test conc. & vehicle (§ 5.2)	Cross-reactions (§ 5.5)	Comment	Ref.
benzoin (resin)	hand cream	10% alc.			72
benzoxonium chloride (preservative)	ointment	0.05% aqua	benzalkonium chloride domiphen bromide		109

(continued)

§ **29.3** *(continuation)*

Ingredient	Cosmetic	Patch test conc. & vehicle (§ 5.2)	Cross-reactions (§ 5.5)	Comment	Ref.
BHA (butylated hydroxyanisole) (antioxidant)	hand cream	2% pet.			113
2-bromo-2-nitro-propane-1,3-diol (preservative)	moisturizing lotion	0.5% pet.			153
cinnamic alcohol (fragrance)	moist toilet paper	2% pet.			109
chloroacetamide (preservative)	hand lotion	0.2% pet.			64
chloroxylenol (preservative)	body lotion	1% pet.			8
cocamide DEA (foam builder)	hand gels	0.5% pet.		Also in handwashing liquids and shampoos	37
cocamide DEA	bath foam	0.5% aqua or pet.			112
decyl oleate (emollient)	body lotion	1% pet.			156
diazolidinyl urea (preservative)	day and night cream, body lotion	2% pet.			154
glyceryl stearate (emollient)	body lotion	20% pet.			111
Labilin®	lotions, towels and powder	2% aqua		Labilin® is casein hydrolyzed with papain, and 2.5% methylparaben. Report later revoked [157]	115
lauramine oxide (ammonyx LO®) (foam builder)	dish washing detergents, shampoos, foam bath, surgical scrubs	3.7% aqua			35
methyldibromo glutaro-nitrile (1,2-dibromo-2,4-dicyanobutane) (preservative)	antiwrinkle lotion and moist toilet paper	0.05% pet.			105 106
myristyl alcohol (emollient)	moisturizing cream	5% pet.			110

(continued)

§ **29.3** *(continuation)*

Ingredient	Cosmetic	Patch test conc. & vehicle (§ 5.2)	Cross-reactions (§ 5.5)	Comment	Ref.
nordihydroguaiaretic acid (antioxidant)	cream	2% pet.		Case quoted by Fisher [113]	113
octyldodecanol (emollient)	moisturizing lotion	30% pet. 13.5% aqua			69
oleamidopropyl dimethylamine (emulsifier)	baby body lotion	0.1–0.3% aqua	ricinoleamidopropyl dimethylamine lactate stearamidopropyl dimethylamine lactate behenamidopropyl dimethylamine isostearamidopropyl dimethylamine tallowamidopropyl dimethylamine lauramidopropyl dimethylamine myristamidopropyl dimethylamine cocamidopropyl dimethylamine minkamidopropyl dimethylamine palmitamidopropyl dimethylamine		103 104
o-phenylphenol (preservative)	'medicated cream'	1% pet.			68
phenyl salicylate (sunscreen)	moisturizing cream	1% pet.			102
propylene glycol (solvent)	body cream and lotion	2% pet.			117
propyl gallate (antioxidant)	moisturizing cream and (baby) body lotion	1% pet.	octyl gallate dodecyl gallate		100 101
quaternium-15 (preservative)	hand and body lotion	1% pet.		Formaldehyde donor	116
stearamidoethyl dimethylamine phosphate (emulsifier)	skin lotion	0.4% aqua			114

(continued)

§ **29.3** *(continuation)*

Ingredient	Cosmetic	Patch test conc. & vehicle (§ 5.2)	Cross-reactions (§ 5.5)	Comment	Ref.
tocopheryl acetate (vitamin E) (antioxidant, natural ingredient)	cream	10% pet.	tocophenyl nicotinate		107
triethanolamine (pH adjuster)	hand lotion moisturizing cream	2.5% pet.			54 119
trilaureth-4 phosphate (emulsifier)	hand and body lotion	0.5–1% pet.			116

Allergic contact urticaria due to a wheat bran bath has been reported in an atopic child, whose eczema improved on a gluten-free diet [86]. A baby with a strong history of cow's milk allergy developed anaphylaxis following application of a casein-containing ointment to an inflamed diaper area. RAST testing showed a significant elevation in IgE antibodies to milk and milk proteins [118]. Excessive use of bubble baths may lead to urinary tract irritation, especially in children [123]. Vitamin E in baths can produce a follicular eruption [89].

BODY TALC

29.4 Body talc is widely used in the Americas. It is mainly a fragrance product. The formula is very simple, as can be seen from the following example:

Body talc

Ingredients		Example
90–98%	talc	talc
0.5%	silica (fused) to improve free flow	silica (fused)
ca. 2%	carrier for perfume	magnesium carbonate
ca. 0.5%	perfume	perfume

Another type of body talc has additional properties: relief of itching, deodorizing, antiseptic, absorption of perspiration. A typical example is:

Dusting powder

Ingredients		Example
80–90%	talc	talc
0.5%	silica (fused) to improve free flow	silica (fused)
ca. 10%	active ingredients	salicylic acid, boric acid, zinc oxide, lanolin, menthol
ca. 2%	perfume carrier	magnesium carbonate
ca. 0.5%	perfume	perfume

SOAP

29.5 The classic toilet soap bar, which is still very popular, is almost entirely the sodium salt of fatty acids (either a single salt or a natural mixture).

A typical formula for **toilet soap bars** is:

Ingredients		Example
85–95%	sodium salt of fatty acids	sodium cocoate, sodium tallowate
ca. 0.5%	perfume	perfume
ca. 0.1%	antioxidant and chelating agent	*o*-tolylbiguanide, EDTA
ca. 0.01%	colour	titanium dioxide

Various ingredients may be added to obtain special soap types:

Ingredients		Soap type
lipids:	lanolin paraffin	super-fatty soap
polyols:	sucrose glycerin	transparent soap
antimicrobials:	triclocarban dichlorophene triclosan sulfur (colloidal)	deodorant soap

Syndet soap bars consist entirely or partially of synthetic detergents ('syndets'). The development of these products was largely due to some undesirable properties of soaps such as the alkalinicity, leading to skin irritation, and incompatibility with hard water, leading to precipitation of calcium fatty acid salts.

The use of syndet soap bars has increased considerably, especially for medical use, where frequent hand washing is inevitable. In many countries the term 'soap' is protected and may be used only for the classic type of soap.

A typical formula of **syndet soap bars** is:

Ingredients		Example
50–95%	synthetic surfactant	dioctyl sodium sulfosuccinate, sodium lauryl sulfate, cocamidopropyl betaine
0–50%	soap: sodium salt of fatty acids	sodium cocoate
5–20%	additives to aid technologic performance	kaolin, sorbitol, paraffin, sodium silicate, cellulose gum
1–5%	pH adjusting agent (to a pH of ca. 5.5)	lactic acid, citric acid
ca 0.1%	antioxidant and chelating agent	*o*-tolylbiguanide, edetic acid
ca 0.5%	perfume	perfume

Side effects of soaps on the skin include:
1. irritant contact dermatitis;
2. allergic contact dermatitis (to ingredients of soaps);
3. a combination of irritant and allergic reactions.

Irritant side effects

Soaps exert a weak toxic effect on the skin, thus slightly damaging it; prolonged or repeated contact will lead to irritant dermatitis. This reaction may be provoked by prolonged contact with a soap solution on practically every skin, although there is a great variety in individual susceptibility; atopic individuals are particularly susceptible.

The eruption often starts under a ring, and is associated with wet work (kitchen personnel, hairdressers, housewives, bartenders): it is diagnosed as 'housewives eczema' or 'soap dermatitis'. Excessive use of soap on the vulva may be an important cause of dysuria [121].

Allergic side effects

Soaps themselves are not sensitizing, but sometimes chemicals are added that may cause allergic reactions; these include perfumes [75,120], lanolin, rosin [74], sodium ricinoleic monoethanolamido sulfosuccinate derivative (?) in hand cleanser [48], chloroxylenol [23,25], D&C Yellow No. 11 [122], stearic acid [152], tocopherol (vitamin E) [156], formaldehyde [158], undecylenamide DEA [159], and mercury [70]. *Apricot soap* has been reported to cause pruritus ani et vulvae due to contact allergy [61]. *Monosulfiram soap* has caused allergic contact dermatitis in a patient sensitive to tetramethylthiuram disulfide [16]. Patients sensitized to DC Yellow 11 in maximization tests exhibited an allergic contact dermatitis from the use of soap containing this dye [76, 77]. Halogenated salicylanilides have caused epidemics of photoallergic reactions (§ 6.5). Photodermatitis from chlorophenylphenol in soap has been reported in two patients [97]. Contact allergy to chromium in a toilet soap caused 'pigmented cosmetic dermatitis' [99].

FLUID SOAP AND HAND CLEANER

29.6 Fluid soaps (particularly in use to clean the hands) have gained in popularity, because when supplied with special dispensing bottles, they are more hygienic in use than soap bars. Liquid soaps found their way into the medical profession because they can be formulated to a pH in accordance with the skin (ca. 5.5); it has been wrongly assumed that this would cause less irritation of the skin, even when used frequently. Because of the hygienic advantages fluid soaps are popular for use in public buildings and are penetrating into the family home. One should be aware that the term *'liquid soap'* is protected in many countries and restricted to pure 'salts of fatty acids'. Therefore, product names like *hand cleaner, hand washing lotion*, etc. are in use. The typical formulas for these products are basically similar to those for shampoos, but special attention is given to the pH of the product (5.5) and surfactants of low skin-irritancy are selected. Examples of such mild acting surfactants are:

Protein-fatty acid condensates (Lamepon®, Maypon®, different types)
- potassium coco hydrolyzed animal protein (Lamepon POTR®)
- sodium soya hydrolyzed animal protein (Maypon K®)
- TEA coco hydrolyzed animal protein (Lamepon STR®)
- TEA oleoyl hydrolyzed animal protein (Lamepon POTR®)

Amino acid-fatty acid condensates
- sodium cocoyl glutamate (Amisoft CS11®)
- sodium cocoyl sarcosinate (Sarkosine KA®)
- sodium hydrogenated tallow glutamate (Amisoft HS11®)
- sodium lauroyl glutamate (Amisoft LS11®)
- sodium lauroyl sarcosinate (Sarkosyl NL30®, Medialan LD®, Maprosil 30®)
- sodium myristoyl sarcosinate (Hamposyl M30®)
- TEA cocoyl glutamate (Amisoft CT12®)

Phosphate esters
- lecithin
- trilaneth-4 phosphate (Hostaphat KW340N®)
- trioleth-8 phosphate (Hostaphat KO380®)
- trioleyl phosphate (Hostaphat KO300®)

Amphoteric surfactants (see § 30.15.5)
- sodium cocoamphoacetate (Miranol CMconc®)
- disodium cocoamphodiacetate (Miranol C2Mconc®)
- disodium cocoamphodiacetate and sodium lauryl sulfate and hexylene glycol (Miranol 2MC® modified)
- cocamidopropyl betaine (Tegobetain L7®)
- coco-betaine (Emcol CC37-18®, Dehyton AB30®, Standapol AB45®)

A typical formula for a **handwashing lotion (handcleaner)** is:

Ingredients		Example
60–80%	water	water
ca. 15%	surfactant (principal)	disodium cocoamphodiacetate, disodiummonoundecylenamido MEA-sulfosuccinate
ca. 1%	surfactant: foam builder	lauramide MEA
ca. 1%	thickener	carbomer-934
ca. 2%	lipid: super-fatty agent	lanolin oil
ca. 1%	organic acid: pH-adjusting agent	citric acid
10 pp.–ca. 0.3%	preservative	methylisothiazolinone and methylchloroisothiazolinone
ca. 0.01%	colour	Acid Yellow No. 23 (CI 19140)
ca. 0.3%	perfume	perfume

DEPILATORY PREPARATIONS

29.7 Hair can be removed by mechanical pulling with the aid of an *epilating wax*. The wax has a melting point near 45°C and is poured on the skin in melted condition. When the wax has solidified, the hair may be pulled off with the wax. Removing hair by mechanical epilation has no permanent effect.

A typical formula for **epilating wax** is:

Ingredients		Example
ca. 70%	rosin	rosin
ca. 30%	lipids: waxes and oils	beeswax, linseed oil
ca. 0.2%	perfume	perfume

The most popular method of removing hair is depilating with a paste [124]. The active ingredients are alkali (pH 12.5) and one or more of the following depilating agents: calcium or strontium thioglycolate, barium or calcium sulfide, or sodium stannite. These products are applied as a paste to the skin for 5–10 minutes. Thus the hair is weakened and can be removed, together with the paste, with a spatula. Residual alkali should be rinsed off immediately with water in order to prevent irritation. 'After-depilating' creams, containing lactic acid or citric acid as active ingredients are used to assure the neutralization of alkali. Hair removal by this method is not permanent.

A typical formula for a **depilating cream/paste** is:

Ingredients		Example
60–70%	water	water
ca. 5%	thickener: inorganic	magnesium aluminum silicate
20–30%	lipid	cetyl alcohol, mineral oil
2–5%	surfactant: emulsifier	sodium lauryl sulfate
ca. 2%	alkaline agent to adjust pH to 12.5	calcium hydroxide
3–5%	depilating agent	sodium stannite, calcium thioglycolate
ca. 0.5%	perfume	perfume

Other mercapto-type depilating agents are: *thiolactic acid* and *thioglycerin*.

Permanent removal of hair is claimed by means of enzymatic (protease: papain for keratinase) inactivation of the hair follicle. Pre-removal by epilating the hair is necessary in order to allow contact of the enzyme with the hair papilla. To prevent inactivation of the proteinase enzyme, the product is sold as a powder (containing the enzyme) and a liquid, which are mixed before use. The mixture is applied with a brush and should contact the hair follicle. If the pre-removal of the hair is not complete the procedure will fail.

A typical formula for an **enzymatic depilator** is:

I. Powder

Ingredients		Example
ca. 90%	inert powder	kaolin
ca. 2%	surfactant: nonionic	polysorbate 80
ca. 1%	thickener	pectin
ca. 3%	proteinase	keratinase

II. Liquid

Ingredients		Example
ca. 99%	water	water
ca. 1%	buffering salt for optimum pH	dipotassium phosphate

SKIN BLEACHING AGENTS

29.8 Skin bleaching agents are applied to the skin of the face and other parts of the body for depigmentation of hyperpigmented lesions, usually for a relatively long period of time. Some of these products are also known as 'summer freckles cream': the active ingredients in both preparations are the same. Most skin bleaching creams also contain a sunscreen (UV-B absorber) in order to prevent repigmentation of the treated skin. The compounds used in skin bleaching creams are listed in Table 29.9. The most commonly used skin bleaching agent is hydroquinone [126]. In products manufactured in third world countries, monobenzone (hydroquinone benzylether) and hydroquinone methylether are employed; such products can also be found in ethnic shops in the western world. Ethers of hydroquinone are prohibited in cosmetics in the EC.

A typical formula of a **skin bleaching cream** is:

Ingredients		Example
40–70%	water	water
ca 5%	polyol	sorbitol
30–50%	lipid	olive oil, lanolin, decyl oleate
2–5%	surfactant	TEA-coco hydrolyzed animal protein
1–5%	skin bleaching agent	hydroquinone
ca. 2%	UV-B absorber	octyl dimethyl PABA
0.3%	preservative	methylparaben, dehydroacetic acid
0.2%	perfume	perfume

29.9 Skin bleaching agents

ammoniated mercury*	niacinamide
ascorbic acid	niacin
ascorbyl palmitate	sodium bisulfite
ascorbyl-3-phosphate	sodium hydrosulfite
hydrogen peroxide	sodium hypochlorite (may be tested in 0.5% aqua [38])
hydroquinone	sodium metabisulfite
monobenzone*	zinc formaldehyde sulfoxylate (Rongalite®)
monomethyl ether of hydroquinone*	zinc peroxide

*Prohibited in the EC.

Side effects of ingredients of skin bleaching agents are tabulated in § 29.10 (contact allergy) and § 29.11 (other side effects).

29.10 Contact allergy to ingredients of skin bleaching agents

Ingredient	Patch test conc. & vehicle	Cross-reactions	Comment	Ref.
ammoniated mercury	1% pet.		Formerly used for the treatment of psoriasis	36 125
fragrance, unspecified	10% pet.			152
hydroquinone	1% pet.			3 52 62
monobenzone (monobenzyl ether of hydroquinone)	1% pet.	*p*-hydroxybenzoic acid ester, bisphenol-A, diethylstilbestrol (?)	Patch test sites have become depigmented	6 17 51

29.11 Other adverse reactions to ingredients of skin bleaching agents (see also § 10)

Ingredient	Adverse reactions	Comment	Ref.
ammoniated mercury	nephrotic syndrome	Systemic absorption has been studied by Barr et al. [5]	4
	chronic mercury poisoning (for symptoms and signs of mercury poisoning, *see* § 16.43)	Topical use of ammoniated mercury containing drugs has caused pigmentation of the skin (§ 10.1)	60

(continued)

§ **29.11** *(continuation)*

Ingredient	Adverse reactions	Comment	Ref.
hydroquinone	irritant dermatitis	Especially with higher concentrations (4–5%)	3 52
	ochronosis		19 82 83
	brown discoloration of the nails		84
	post-inflammatory hyperpigmentation		6
	pigmented colloid milium		19 83
	leukoderma		78
monobenzone (monobenzylether of hydroquinone)	irritant dermatitis		51
	leukoderma		79
monomethyl ether of hydroquinone	leukoderma		80

DEODORANT-ANTIPERSPIRANT

29.12 The use of deodorant-antiperspirants has considerably increased during the last thirty years [134]. In particular the underarm-deo is very popular. Feminine hygiene deodorants ('intimate sprays') were popular some years ago, but they have lost their popularity nowadays, because serious side effects have occurred from their use.

Deodorant-antiperspirant products are available as *aerosols* (or *pump-sprays*), as viscous liquids (*lotion, roller*) and as *solid sticks*. They often contain one or more of the following active ingredients:

A: **antiperspirant agents**
- alcloxa (aluminum chlorohydroxy allantoinate)
- aldioxa (aluminum dihydroxy allantoinate)
- aluminum chloride
- aluminum chlorohydrate
- aluminum chlorohydrex
- aluminum zirconium chlorohydrates
- aluminum sulfate
- methenamine (hexamine)
- sodium aluminum chlorohydroxylactates

B: **anticholinergic agents**
- propantheline bromide
- scopolamine bromide

N.B. Anticholinergic agents are very rarely used in market products, and are prohibited in cosmetics in the EC.

C: **antimicrobials**
- chlorhexidine digluconate
- dichlorophene
- triclocarban
- triclosan

D: **odour eliminators**
- citronellyl senecionate (Sinodor®)
- zinc ricinoleate

E: **perfume**; to mask minor residues of malodour

The following typical formulas will illustrate most types of market products:

Aerosol antiperspirant

Ingredients		Example
ca. 90%	propellant	propane, isobutane, dimethyl ether
ca. 10%	concentrate:	
	– ca. 30% antiperspirant	aluminum chlorohydrate
	– ca. 60% carrier liquid	isopropyl myristate
	– ca. 3% anticaking agent	quaternium-18 hectorite
	– ca. 1% perfume	perfume

Aerosol deodorant

Ingredients		Example
ca. 80%	propellant	butane, isobutane, propane
ca. 20%	concentrate:	
	– organic solvent	alcohol
	– carrier fluid	propylene glycol
	– antimicrobial	triclosan
	– perfume	perfume

Intimate spray

Ingredients		Example
ca. 95%	propellants	chlorofluorocarbon 11 and 12*
ca. 5%	concentrate:	
	– ca. 95% lipid carrier	isopropyl myristate; wheat germ triglycerydes
	– 1–3% antimicrobial	triclosan
	– 1–2% perfume	perfume

*Due to their alleged effect on the oxone layer, chlorofluorocarbons have become less popular recently and are being replaced with 'ozone-friendly' propellants or pump-sprays.

Deo pump-spray

Ingredients		Example
5–30%	water	water
10–30%	alcohol	alcohol
5–15%	lipid	decyl oleate
ca. 5%	surfactant	sodium lauryl sulfate
1–3%	antimicrobial	triclosan
1–2%	perfume	perfume

Deo roller or lotion/cream

Ingredients		Example
60–80%	water	water
ca. 5%	polyol	propylene glycol
5–15%	lipid	stearic acid, mineral oil, beeswax
2–5%	surfactant (non-ionic)	polysorbate-40, sorbitan oleate
ca. 10%	antiperspirant	alcloxa
1–3%	antimicrobial	triclosan
ca. 0.5%	perfume	perfume

Deo stick

Ingredients		Example
ca. 10%	ethanol	alcohol
ca. 60%	polyol	propylene glycol
ca. 5%	lipid	stearic acid
ca. 8%	soap surfactant	sodium stearate
ca. 0.5%	antimicrobial	triclosan
ca. 10%	antiperspirant	aldioxa
ca. 1.5%	perfume	perfume

Tabulation of side effects

The side effects of deodorants, antiperspirants and ferminine hygiene cosmetics are tabulated in § 29.13.

29.13 Contact allergy to ingredients of deodorants, antiperspirants and feminine hygiene cosmetics

Ingredient	Use	Patch test conc. & vehicle (§5.2)	Cross-reactions (§5.5)	Comment	Ref.
aluminum salt	antiperspirant	aluminum powder: pure; aluminum chloride 2% aqua		Axillary granulomas from aluminum deodorants, *see* [128]	127
atranorin	fragrance	1% pet.	fumarprotocetraric acid	Present in oak moss perfumes	15
benzethonium chloride*	antimicrobial	0.05% aqua	benzalkonium chloride		20
cetalkonium chloride	antimicrobial	0.05% aqua			49
chlorhexidine*	antimicrobial	0.5% aqua and pet.			20
chlorofluorocarbon 11 (freon 11)	propellant	pure	ethyl chloride (?)	Inhaled chlorofluorocarbons may be hallucinogenic [137]	55
chlorofluorocarbon 12 (freon 12)	propellant	pure	ethyl chloride (?)	Inhaled chlorofluorocarbons may be hallucinogenic [137]	55 136
chlorphenesin	antifungal	1% pet.			133
cocamidopropyl betaine	emulsifier	1% aqua			160
dibutyl phthalate	vehicle	5% pet.	*not* to dimethyl and diethyl phthalate		50 95
evernic acid	fragrance	0.1% acet.		Present in oak moss perfumes	15
fenticlor	antimicrobial	1% pet.			9
formaldehyde	antiperspirant	1% aqua		In the 1950s very important contact allergen in antiperspirants in Scandinavia	13

(continued)

§ **29.13** *(continued)*

Ingredient	Use	Patch test conc. & vehicle (§5.2)	Cross-reactions (§5.5)	Comment	Ref.
fumarprotocetraric acid	fragrance	0.1% acet.	atranorin	Present in oak moss perfumes	15
glutaral (glutaraldehyde)	antimicrobial	1% aqua (not stable)	*not* to formaldehyde		31
glyceryl stearate	vehicle constituent	30% pet.			46
hexachlorophene	antimicrobial	1% pet.	dichlorophene		129
hydroxycitronellal	fragrance	2% pet.			152
isoeugenol	fragrance	2% pet.			152
isopropyl myristate*	vehicle constituent	5% pet.			20
isostearyl alcohol	vehicle constituent	5% alc.		The patients were sensitized by a Draize test with a pump-spray deodorant	93
lilial	fragrance	1% pet.			63
linalyl acetate	fragrance	3% pet.			152
lyral	fragrance	2% pet.			152
paraben	preservative	3% pet.		The patient had previously been sensitized to parabens in a corticosteroid cream	87
perfumes		*see* § 5.8			58 135
propantheline bromide	anticholinergic agent	5% pet.			24 71
propylene glycol	vehicle constituent	2% pet.			2 117
propyl gallate	antioxidant	1% pet.			132
tocopherol	antioxidant	10% pet.			1 34
triclocarban	antimicrobial	1% pet.			2
triclosan	antimicrobial	2% pet.			57 94

(continued)

§ **29.13** *(continued)*

Ingredient	Use	Patch test conc. & vehicle (§5.2)	Cross-reactions (§5.5)	Comment	Ref.
usnic acid	antimicrobial	0.1% pet.		Present in lichens, air-borne contact dermatitis	130
zinc ricinoleate	antiperspirant	comm. prep. pure	hydrogenated castor oil; sulfated castor oil; glyceryl ricinoleate; PEG-400 ricinoleate; sodium sulforicinate		132
zirconium compounds	antiperspirants	patch testing on normal skin is negative; 2–4% veh. (?) on skin, denuded of epidermis; also intra-dermal testing with sodium zirconium lactate 1/1000 and 1/10,000 aqueous		Has caused granulomatous skin reactions	18 47

*In feminine hygiene cosmetics.

BODY MAKE-UP

29.14 Body make-up is chiefly used at parties and during carnival time. It is applied over large surfaces of the skin (arms, legs, trunk) and therefore preferably formulated as fluids, such as fluid make-up.

A typical formula for **body paint** is:

Ingredients		Example
ca 75%	water	water
ca. 15%	colour pigment mixture (*see* facial make-up)	titanium dioxide, iron oxides
ca. 2%	suspending agent	magnesium aluminum silicate
ca. 1%	surfactant	dioctyl sodium sulfosuccinate
ca. 0.3%	preservative	quaternium-15
ca. 0.1%	perfume	perfume

SUN AND SOLARIA COSMETICS

29.15 Sun cosmetics are designated primarily to protect the human skin (white skin in particular) against harmful effects of sunlight, notably sunburn, premature ageing of the skin, and the induction of premalignant and malignant skin lesions.

Until recently, attention had mainly been focused on protection against shortwave ultraviolet rays (UVB region: 290–320 nm), but in view of recent knowledge of skin photobiology, an increasing tendency is noticeable to extend the protection to the UVA region (320–400 nm) also. Pigmentary changes as seen in PUVA-treated patients have also been observed from cosmetic tanning-bed use: 'sunbed lentigines' [161].

The active protecting ingredients of sun cosmetics are the so-called 'sunscreens'. Sunscreens fall into two major classes [151]:

1. *Chemical absorbers*: UV-absorbing compounds of organic synthetic nature. Such sunscreens are invisible, and therefore cosmetically elegant. A list of currently used sunscreens is provided in § 30.13. Usually these chemical absorbers are efficient only in the UVB region. The benzophenones, however, may provide protection against UV waves up to 360 nm. Special UVA absorbers are the dibenzoylmethanes (isopropyl dibenzoylmethane and butyl methoxydibenzoylmethane) [142,143]. Anthranilates absorb UVA up to 350 nm.

2. *Reflectors*: These include the white pigments titanium dioxide and zinc oxide, which are effective reflectors and scatterers of both ultraviolet (UVB/UVA) and visible radiation.

Although sunscreens containing reflectors are opaque, they may still have a reasonable cosmetic acceptability, provided care is taken to incorporate in the formulation colouring agents which can be varied to suit the individual user. Other, less frequently used reflectors are red veterinary petrolatum, talc and iron oxide.

Sunscreens are also used to protect patients suffering from photosensitive dermatoses (§ 29.18). The use of appropriate absorbers or reflectors is an intrinsic part of the management of these affections. The absorption spectra of some sunscreens are listed in § 29.17. It should be stressed that adverse effects to sunscreens, which are used to protect photosensitive individuals, occur frequently in these patients, and photo (patch) tests should be performed in cases of worsening or therapy resistance of the photosensitive dermatoses [163].

The protection given by a sunscreen preparation is measured by the Sun Protection Factor (SPF). The SPF is defined as the quotient of the minimal dose of UV-radiation causing erythema in the protected skin and the minimal dose causing erythema in the unprotected skin. It should be noted that since erythema is caused by UV-B radiation, the SPF only measures protection against UV-B. The actual measurement of the SPF is complicated, and several countries (Germany, USA and Australia) prescribe methods for its reproducible measurement. Since these norms differ considerably, the SPF values measured are not fully comparable.

Recommendations for the SPF for photoprotection in 'normal' individuals are given in § 29.16.

29.16 Skin types and SPF recommendation of sunscreen products

Skin type	Sensitivity to UV radiation	Skin complexion	Susceptibility to suntan and sunburn*	Recommended SPF value of sunscreens
I	very sensitive	very fair	burns easily; never tans	15 or greater
II	very sensitive	fair	burns easily; only a slight tan	15
III	sensitive	light	burns moderately; a moderate tan	10–15
IV	moderately sensitive	medium	burns minimally; tans well	6–10
V	minimally sensitive	dark	rarely burns; tans instantly	4–6
VI	very insensitive	very dark	never burns; deeply pigmented	4 or less

*Approximately one hour of midday summer sun without a prior tan or sunscreen protection.

29.17 Absorption spectra of some sunscreen [90,142]

Chemical (class)	Absorption spectrum (nm)	Maximum absorption (nm)
PABA (derivatives)	250–320	288
Salicylates		
homosalate (homomenthyl salicylate)	295–315	306
octyl salicylate (2-ethylhexyl salicylate)	280–320	300
menthyl salicylate	270–330	
Anthranilates	322–350	340
Cinnamates		
octyl methoxycinnamate (2-ethylhexyl-*p*-methoxy-cinnamate)	290–320	307–310
cinoxate (2-ethoxyethyl-*p*-methoxy-cinnamate)	280–320	310
DEA methoxycinnamate	280–310	285–290
Benzophenones		
oxybenzone	270–350	287–290
Camphor derivatives	280–320	
methylbenzylidene camphor	280–315	300
4-methylbenzylidene camphor	280–315	300
Dibenzoylmethanes	320–380	360
isopropyl dibenzoylmethane	320–370	345
butyl methoxydibenzoylmethane	320–390	360
dimethoxydibenzoylmethane	320–390	360
Miscellaneous		
phenylbenzimidazole sulfonic acid	290–320	302
dibenzalazine	up to 330 nm	
digalloyl trioleate	270–320	300

Sun protective factor (SPF) values of various sunscreen classes are given below [98]. It should be appreciated that these values were obtained by indoor testing; the percentage of chemical, bases used, and other factors can influence these values. The SPF values on proprietary products may be misleading [149]. It should also be appreciated that the SPF gives an indication only of the UV-B, not of the UV-A protection. The best protection against UV-A is provided by a combination of dibenzoylmethanes and physical agents [14].

SPF values of sunscreening agents:

PABA	4– 8
PABA esters	6–10
Benzophenones	4– 6
Cinnamates	4– 6
Salicylates	2– 6
Anthranilates	2– 6
PABA esters-benzophenones	10–15

29.18 Action spectra of various normal and abnormal responses of human skin to solar radiation [22,88]

Condition	Range of effectiveness wavelength (nm)	Maximum reaction (nm)
I *Normal individuals*		
Sunburn reaction (solar)	290–320	305–307
Sunburn reaction (artificial light source)	250–320	250–
Immediate pigment darkening (IPD) or tanning reaction	320–700	340–380
Delayed tanning (melanogenesis)	290–480	290–320
II *Photosensitivity*		
A. Phototoxic reaction		
Oral or internal (drugs)	300–400	320–380
Topical or external (drugs)	300–400	320–380
Phytophotodermatitis (plants)	320–400	320–360
Phototoxicity in chemically induced porphyria or hematoporphyrins	380–600	380–420
B. Photoallergic reaction		
Drug photoallergy (delayed hypersensitivity, topical, or systemic)	290–450	320–380
Certain solar urticarias (immediate hypersensitivity)	290–380	290–320 320–400
C. Persistent photosensitivity (persistent light reactions or actinic reticuloid)	290–400	290–320
III *Degenerative and neoplastic*		
Chronic actinic elastosis	290–400	290–320
Actinic keratosis	290–320	290–315
Basal cell epithelioma	290–320	290–315

(continued)

§ **29.18** *(continued)*

	Condition	Range of effectiveness wavelength (nm)	Maximum reaction (nm)
	Squamous cell carcinoma	290–320	290–315
	Malignant melanoma (?)	290–320	290–315
IV	*Genetic and metabolic*		
	Xeroderma pigmentosum	290–320	290–320
	Albinism	290–400	290–320
	Ephelides (freckles)	290–400	290–320
	Erythropoietic porphyria	390–600	390–420
	Erythropoietic protoporphyria	390–600	390–420
	Porphyria cutanea tarda	390–600	390–420
	Variegate porphyria	390–600	390–420
	Vitiligo (macules)	290–320	290–315
	Hartnup syndrome	290–320	
	Cockayne's syndrome	290–320	
	Darier–White disease	290–320	
	Bloom's syndrome	290–320	
	Rothmund–Thomson syndrome	290–320	
	Hailey–Hailey disease	290–320	
V	*Nutritional*		
	Kwashiorkor	290–400	
	Pellagra	290–400	
VI	*Infections (viral)*		
	Lymphogranuloma venereum	290–320	
	Herpes simplex	290–320	
VII	*Miscellaneous* (light and abnormal skin or diseases)		
	Hydroa aestivale	290–400 infrared	290–320
	Hydroa vacciniforme	290–400 infrared	290–320
	Polymorphous photodermatoses, including variants such as papular, plaques, papulovesicular and eczematous eruptions	290–400	290–320
	Disseminated superficial actinic porokeratosis	290–320	290–320
	Discoid lupus erythematosus	290–320	290–320
	Systemic lupus erythematosus	290–230	
	Dermatomyositis	290–320	
	Photosensitive eczema	290–320	

Sometimes ingredients are added to sun cosmetics for secondary (cosmetic) effects: artificial tanning, suntan promotion, skin healing, skin moisturizing, insect repelling, local anaesthesia. These effects may be obtained by the following compounds:

dihydroxyacetone	artificial tanner
walnut extract (Juglans regia)	artificial tanner
juglon (5-hydroxy-1,4-naphthoquinone)	artificial tanner
5-methoxypsoralen	suntan promoter
allantoin	skin healing agent
diethyl toluamide	insect repellent
benzocaine	local anaesthetic
lidocaine	local anaesthetic
skin conditioning agents (*see* § 27.1)	

In some sunscreens oil of bergamot or 5-methoxypsoralen (bergapten) is incorporated. The manufacturers claim that the formulations can stimulate a quick tanning response and subsequently the acquired tan can provide the possible advantages against the harmful effects of sunlight in the form of enhanced photoprotection resulting from the increased melanin pigment. However, the photoreactive 5-MOP is not only cytotoxic and phototoxic to melanocytes, but can also be highly mutagenic and carcinogenic to the epidermal melanocytes and keratinocytes. Therefore it is felt that the widespread use of these sunscreens may provoke unwanted effects similar to those seen in oral photochemotherapy (Chapter 18), notably the risk of cutaneous carcinoma to the normal human population. According to some investigations, their application should therefore be discouraged [88,92], but the issue is controversial [91,150,162].

Sun cosmetics are available in various forms: milks/creams (most popular), oils, gels, lotions and aerosol foams. Typical formulas are:

Sun milk/cream

Ingredients		Example
40–75%	water	water
ca. 5%	polyol	propylene glycol
15–30%	lipid	lanolin, decyl oleate
ca. 2%	surfactant/emulsifier	TEA lauryl sulfate
1–8%	UV absorber	isopropyl dibenzoylmethane, 4-methylbenzylidene camphor
0–2%	reflectors	titanium dioxide
0–5%	secondary active agents	allantoin
ca. 0.2%	preservative	parabens, phenoxyethanol
ca. 0.1%	perfume	perfume

Sun oil

Ingredients		Example
ca. 90%	lipid	peanut oil, isopropyl myristate
1–8%	UV absorber	homosalate, benzophenone-1
ca. 0.05%	antioxidant	tocopheryl acetate
ca. 1%	perfume	perfume

Sun gel

Ingredients		Example
50–60%	water	water
ca. 5%	polyol	sorbitol
ca. 2%	thickener: gelling agent	carbomer 914, TEA
10–30%	organic solvent	alcohol
1–8%	UV absorber	allantoin PABA, benzophenone-9
ca. 0.05%	perfume	perfume
ca. 0.2%	preservative	DMDM hydantoin, methylparaben

Sun lotion

Ingredients		Example
60–95%	water	water
10–40%	alcohol	alcohol
10–20%	polyol	glycerin
5–10%	lipid	glyceryl stearate, oleic acid
ca. 2%	surfactant: emulsifier	sodium lauryl sulfate
1–8%	UV absorber	octyl dimethyl PABA
ca. 0.2%	preservative	2-bromo-2-nitropropane-1,3-diol
ca. 0.1%	perfume	perfume

Sun aerosol foam

Ingredients		Example
ca. 10%	propellant	isobutane, propane, dimethylether
ca. 90%	concentrate:	
	– ca. 70% water	water
	– ca. 5% polyol	propylene glycol
	– ca. 20% lipid	acetylated lanolin, stearic acid
	– ca. 2% surfactant: emulsifier	TEA lauryl sulfate, polysorbate 40
1–5%	UV absorber	phenylbenzimidazole sulfonic acid, guanine
ca. 1%	other active agents	polyamino sugar condensate, sodium lactate, dihydroxyacetone
ca. 0.2%	preservative	quaternium-15, *o*-phenylphenol
ca. 0.1%	perfume	perfume

After-sun milk/cream

Ingredients		Example
40–70%	water	water
ca. 5%	polyol	sorbitol
10–30%	lipid	lanolin oil, wheat germ glycerides
2–5%	surfactant: emulsifier	sodium lauryl sulfate
ca. 2%	moisturizer	collagen
ca. 2%	skin healing agent	allantoin
0–0.5%	local anaesthetics	benzocaine
0.2%	preservative	methylparaben, propylparaben
0.1%	perfume	perfume

Solaria oils are used to prevent drying of the skin from solaria treatments: they contain a UV absorber, and rarely a tanning promoter.

Solaria oil

Ingredients		Example
ca. 98%	lipid	isopropyl palmitate, caprylic/capric triglyceride
ca. 2%	UV absorber	4-methylbenzylidene camphor
0–75 ppm	UVA tanning promoter	5-methoxypsoralen
ca. 0.05%	antioxidant	BHA

Side effects of topical sunscreens include [163]:
1. irritant dermatitis [40]
2. phototoxic dermatitis (though this seems rather paradoxical); see Chapter 6
3. photoallergic dermatitis; see Chapter 6
4. allergic contact dermatitis. Sunscreens that have caused contact allergy are listed in § 29.19.

Cases have been caused both by products intended to protect against the sun ('sunscreen preparations') and by a variety of cosmetic products (creams, lotions, lipsticks). The literature on adverse reactions to sunscreen has been reviewed [163].

29.19 Contact allergy to topical sunscreens (review, see Ref. [163])

Sunscreen	Patch test conc. & vehicle (§5.2)	Cross-reactions (§5.5)	Comment	Ref.
amyl dimethyl PABA			*See* pentyl dimethyl PABA	
benzophenone-4 (sulisobenzone)	2% pet.			41 80
benzophenone-8 (dioxybenzone)	2% pet.	oxybenzone		39 81
benzophenone-10 (mexenone)	2% pet.			144
benzotriazole derivatives	1% pet.			30
benzyl salicylate	1% pet.			32
butyl methoxydibenzoyl-methane	2% pet.	isopropyl dibenzoylmethane		142 144 145
cinoxate (2-ethoxyethyl-*p*-methoxycinnamate)	1% pet.	balsam Peru, benzyl cinnamate, methyl cinnamate, cinnamyl alcohol, cinnamal, *p*-methoxyisoamyl cinnamate [163]		12 140 144
digalloyl trioleate	3.5% pet.			43
drometrizole	5% pet.		UV-absorber in nail varnish in the reported case	73
glyceryl PABA	1–5% pet.	benzocaine, other para-compounds and PABA-derivatives [163]	The actual allergen may be either benzocaine or an unknown impurity [11]	11 28 44 140
glyceryl-3-(glyceroxy)-anthranilate	5% pet.		UVA filter in Contralume Cream®	56

(continued)

§ **29.19** *(continued)*

Sunscreen	Patch test conc. & vehicle (§5.2)	Cross-reactions (§5.5)	Comment	Ref.
homosalate (homomenthyl salicylate)	2% pet.		Has caused a follicular eruption	42
isopropyl dibenzoylmethane	2% pet.	butyl methoxydi-benzoylmethane	Together with 4-methylbenzylidene camphor the sunscreen Eusolex 8021®	59 142 143
menthyl salicylate	2% pet.		Patch test sensitization may occur	21
4-methylbenzylidene camphor (Eusolex 6300®)	2% pet.		Together with isopropyl dibenzoylmethane the sunscreen Eusolex 8021®	59 142 143
mexenone			*See* benzophenone-10	
octyl dimethyl PABA	2% pet.	benzocaine, PABA and derivatives [163]		140 144 148
oxybenzone (benzophenone-3)	2% pet.	dioxybenzone	Some cases reported as photoallergy were probably 'plain' contact [146]	39 53
PABA (*p*-aminobenzoic acid)	2–5% pet.	paraphenylene diamine, procaine, sulfonamides, azo-dyes and other para-compounds, PABA derivatives	Stains light-coloured fabrics	29 140 147
pentyl dimethyl PABA (amyl dimethyl PABA)	2% pet.	PABA (derivatives), benzocaine	Has caused burning after sun exposure	7 10 33 140 144
phenylbenzimidazole sulfonic acid	1% aqua	possibly to 2-phenyl-5-methylbenzoxazol (witisol) [143]		3 14
phenyl salicylate	2% pet.			27
sulisobenzone			*See* benzophenone-4	41 80
witisol (2-phenyl-5-methyl-benzoxazol)	1% pet.	possibly to phenyl-benzimidazole sulfonic acid [143]		85 143

Contact allergic reactions to commercial sunscreens are not always caused by the UV-absorber, other ingredients which have caused contact allergy include TEA stearate [65], *t*-butyl alcohol [66], avocado oil [138], methylparaben [65], phenyldimethicone [139], Solvent Red 1 (CI 12150) and 3 (CI 12010) [140], dexpanthenol [141], quaternium-15 [147] and methylisothiazolinone and methylchloroisothiazolinone [152].

SPORT AND MASSAGE OILS

29.20 Sport and massage oils and liniments (emulsions) are mainly smooth lipid mixtures, to which rubefacients and counterirritants are added. Typical formulas are:

Sport massage oil

Ingredients		Example
ca. 80–90%	lipid	mineral oil, isopropyl myristate
0.5–5%	rubefacient-counterirritant	glycol salicylate, methyl nicotinate
0.05%	perfume	perfume

Massage liniment

Ingredients		Example
ca. 40–50%	water	water
ca. 30%	lipid	caprylic/capric triglyceride, decyl oleate
ca. 2%	surfactant	sodium lauryl sulfate
0.5–5%	rubefacient-counterirritant	ammonia, capsicum oleoresin, camphor
0.05%	perfume	pine oil

Sport massage aerosol

Ingredients		Example
ca. 60%	propellants	isobutane, propane, dimethyl ether
ca. 40%	concentrate:	
	– ca. 60% solvent	isopropyl alcohol
	– ca. 35% lipid carrier	isopropyl myristate
	– ca. 5% rubefacient-counterirritant	methyl nicotinate, methyl salicylate, arnica extract
	– ca. 0.05% perfume	camphor oil, pine needle oil

The following counterirritants and rubefacients are frequently used in sport massage products:

ammonia
arnica extract
camphor oil
capsicum oleoresin
cajuput oil
glycol salicylate
methyl nicotinate
methyl salicylate
pine oil
rosemary extract
turpentine

Side effects

Contact allergy to chloroacetamide in a body massage cream has been reported [67].

FOOT COSMETICS

29.21 Foot care products have one or more of the following properties: refreshing, anti-pruritic, callus-softening, deodorizing and antiperspirant, cleansing, moisture absorbing, antiseptic or antifungal. Various types of products are available: powders, tablets, creams, lotions, aerosols.

Typical foot cosmetics formulas are:

Foot powder

Ingredients		Example
80–90%	powder base	talc, kaolin, rice starch, boric acid
0–10%	functional ingredients	thymol, camphor, menthol, triclosan
ca. 0.1%	perfume	pine needle oil

Foot cream

Ingredients		Example
40–60%	water	water
ca. 5%	polyol	glycerin
20–40%	lipid	glyceryl stearate, cetyl alcohol
ca. 2%	surfactant	TEA lauryl sulfate, polysorbate 20
0–10%	functional ingredients	zinc oxide, zinc undecylenate, menthol, alcloxa
ca. 0.2%	preservative	methylparaben, propylparaben
ca. 0.1%	perfume	camphor oil

Foot aerosol

Ingredients		Example
ca. 40%	propellant	isobutane, propane
ca. 60%	concentrate:	
	– ca. 1% functional ingredient	dichlorophene, triclosan, aluminum chlorohydrate
	– ca. 5% lipid carrier	isopropyl myristate
	– 0-10% polyol	propylene glycol
	– ca. 80% solvent	alcohol
	– ca. 2% surfactant	laureth-4
	– ca. 0.1% perfume	perfume

Foot tablet (for foot bath)

Ingredients		Example
ca. 20%	CO_2-generating ingredients	sodium bicarbonate, citric acid
ca. 10%	oxygen-generating salts	sodium perborate
10–50%	salts	magnesium sulfate, sodium chloride
ca. 0.5%	colour	DC Yellow 8 (CI 45350)
ca. 1%	perfume	pine needle oil
ca. 2%	surfactant	laureth-4

29.22 Examples of other typical functional ingredients for foot cosmetics are:

alcloxa	(antiperspirant)	menthol	(refreshing agent, antipruritic)
aldioxa	(antiperspirant)	methenamine (hexamine)	(antimicrobial)
allantoin	(skin-healing agent)	methyl salicylate	(herbal fragrance)
aluminum chloride	(antiperspirant)	paraben: methyl-ethyl-propyl-butyl	(antimicrobial)
aluminum chlorohydrate	(antiperspirant)	phenol	(antipruritic, antimicrobial)
aluminum hydroxide	(antiperspirant)	pine oil	(herbal fragrance)
balsam Peru	(balsamic fragrance, antimicrobial)	salicylic acid	(callus-softening agent)
benzalkonium chloride	(antimicrobial)	sodium borate (borax)	(callus-softening agent)
benzocaine*	(antipruritic)	sodium perborate	(oxygen-releasing agent)
boric acid	(antimicrobial)	sodium persulfate	(oxygen-releasing agent)
camphor	(antipruritic, soothing)	sodium phosphate	(callus-softening agent)
captan*	(antifungal)	sorbic acid	(antifungal)
chlorhexidine digluconate	(antimicrobial)	rice and potato starch	(moisture absorber)
chlorphenesin	(antifungal)	sulfur (colloidal)	(antifungal)
climbazole	(antifungal)	thymol	(antipruritic, herbal fragrance)
dehydroacetic acid DHA	(antifungal)	triclosan	(antimicrobial)
dichlorophene	(antimicrobial)	undecylenamide DEA	(antifungal)
disodium undecylenamido-MEA-sulfosuccinate	(antifungal)	undecylenamide MEA	(antifungal)
hexachlorophene*	(antimicrobial)	undecylenic acid	(antifungal)
kaolin	(moisture absorbent)	zinc oxide	(skin healing, antiphlogistic agent)
lidocaine*	(antipruritic)	zinc undecylenate	(antifungal)

*Not allowed in the EC.

Contact allergy to triclosan (Irgasan DP 300®) in foot powder has been reported [94].

BARRIER CREAM

29.23 Barrier creams are used to protect the skin against corrosive agents during working conditions. Although mechanical protection of the hands by gloves is more effective, application of barrier creams is more convenient. Such creams should be easy to apply, and easily washed off at the end of the work. As the cream stays in contact with the skin for a long time, the ingredients should be carefully selected on minimal irritation in producing and developing effective barrier creams. Extensive testing is necessary to achieve optimal protection and performance.

Four main types of barrier creams with typical formulas are:

Cream barrier against dust

Ingredients		Example
ca. 65%	water	water
ca. 10%	polyol	glycerin
ca. 20%	active barrier ingredient: solid lipid and zinc stearate	stearic acid zinc stearate
ca. 2%	surfactant: emulsifier	sodium stearate
ca. 0.3%	preservative	methylparaben, propylparaben, quaternium-15
ca. 0.05%	perfume	perfume

Cream barrier against organic solvents

Ingredients		Example
ca. 50%	water	water
ca. 2%	polyol	glycerin
ca. 30%	active barrier ingredient: soap surfactant, starch	potassium stearate, sodium lauroyl glutamate, rice starch
ca. 0.3%	preservative	methylparaben, propylparaben, phenoxyethanol
ca. 0.05%	perfume	perfume

Cream barrier against aqueous solvents

Ingredients		Example
ca. 65%	water	water
ca. 2%	polyol	glycerin
ca. 25%	active barrier ingredient: semisolid lipid, silicones	petrolatum, beeswax cyclomethicone
ca. 2%	surfactant	sodium lauryl sulfate, cocamidopropyl betaine
ca. 0.3%	preservative	2-bromo-2-nitropropane-1,3-diol
ca. 0.05%	perfume	perfume

Ointment (anhydrous type) barrier against aqueous solvents

Ingredients		Example
ca. 99%	active barrier ingredient:	petrolatum, squalene, beeswax
	semisolid lipid, zinc stearate	zinc stearate
ca. 0.05%	antioxidant	ascorbyl palmitate
ca. 0.05%	perfume	perfume

Barrier creams are advocated as a practical means to prevent the occurrence of (irritant as well as allergic) industrial dermatoses. The invisible protecting glove effect, produced when the cream is applied properly, should prevent the penetration of noxious substances, and facilitate the washing process. The requirements of barrier creams were discussed in detail by Schneider et al. [45]. The usefulness of these creams is still in doubt. The layer formed on the skin by the cream is very thin, and the quantity of protective material is generally insufficient, as compared with the amount of deleterious substance against which it should protect the skin. Besides, part of the applied protective substance gets lost by friction and perspiration. Furthermore, the oily layer might even facilitate the penetration of substances into the epidermis! Thus, the protection offered by barrier creams seems to be small. On the other hand, organic solvents may damage the natural skin barrier by the extraction of epidermal lipids, thus promoting penetration of toxic and allergenic substances. In such circumstances lipid-containing barrier creams might provide a substitute for the lost natural lipids, reestablishing the skin barrier function.

The interest in barrier creams increased with the introduction of silicone oils after the Second World War. However, from the results of a comparative study Herrmann [26] concluded that barrier creams containing silicone oil did not have advantages over those without these oils.

Patch tests with barrier creams under occlusion may cause false positive irritant reactions. This is due to the surfactant fraction. Patch tests with separate ingredients are to be preferred.

Side effects

Contact allergy to parabens in a barrier cream [96] and to quaternium-15 [155] has been reported.

29.24 REFERENCES

1. Aeling, J.L., Panagotacos, P.J. and Andreozzi, R.J. (1973): Allergic contact dermatitis to vitamin E in aerosol deodorant. *Arch. Dermatol., 108*, 579.
2. Agren-Jonsson, S. and Magnusson, B. (1976): Sensitization to propantheline bromide, trichlorocarbanilide and propylene glycol in an antiperspirant. *Contact Dermatitis, 2*, 79.
3. Arndt, K.A. and Fitzpatrick, T.B. (1965): Topical use of hydroquinone as a depigmenting agent. *J. Am. Med. Assoc., 194*, 965.
4. Barr, R.D., Rees, P.H., Cordy, P.E., Kungu, A.. Woodger, B.A. and Cameron, H.M. (1972): Nephrotic syndrome in adult Africans in Nairobi. *Br. Med. J., 2*, 131.

5. Barr, R.D., Woodger, B.A. and Rees, P.H. (1973): Levels of mercury in urine correlated with the use of skin lightening creams. *Am. J. Clin. Pathol., 59*, 36.
6. Bentley-Phillips, B. and Bayler, M.A.H. (1975): Cutaneous reactions to topical application of hydroquinone. S. Afr. Med. J., 49, 1391.
7. Blank, H. (1971): Immediate cutaneous reactions to sunscreens. *Arch. Dermatol., 103*, 461.
8. Calnan, C.D. (1962): Contact dermatitis from drugs. *Proc. Roy. Soc. Med., 55*, 39.
9. Calnan, C.D. (1975): Dihydroxydichlorodiphenylmonosulphide in a deodorant. *Contact Dermatitis, 1*, 127.
10. Calnan, C.D. (1980): Amyldimethylaminobenzoic acid causing lipstick dermatitis. *Contact Dermatitis, 6*, 233.
11. Bruze, M., Gruvberger, B. and Thune, P. (1988): Contact and photocontact allergy to glyceryl para-aminobenzoate. *Photodermatol., 5*, 162–165.
12. Cronin, E. (1980): Photosensitisers. In: *Contact Dermatitis*, pp. 102 and 454. Churchill Livingstone, Edinburgh.
13. Marcussen, P.V. (1962): Dermatitis caused by formaldehyde resins in textiles. *Dermatologica, 125*, 101–111.
14. Roelandts, R. (1991): Which components in broad spectrum sunscreens are most necessary for adequate UVA protection ? *J. Am. Acad, Dermatol., 25*, 999–1004.
15. Dahlquist, I. and Fregert, S. (1980): Contact allergy to atranorin in lichens and perfumes. *Contact Dermatitis*, 6, 111.
16. Dick, D.C. and Adams, R.H. (1979): Allergic contact dermatitis from monosulfiram (Tetmosol) soap. *Contact Dermatitis, 5*, 199.
17. Dorsey, C.S. (1960): Dermatitic and pigmentary reactions to monobenzyl ether of hydroquinone. *Arch. Dermatol., 81*, 245.
18. Epstein, W.L. and Allen, J.R. (1964): Granulomatous hypersensitivity after use of zirconium-containing poison oak lotions. *J. Am. Med. Assoc., 190*, 940.
19. Findlay, G.H., Morrison, J.G.L. and Simson I.W. (1975): Exogenous ochronosis and colloid milium from hydroquinone bleaching creams. *Br. J. Dermatol., 93*, 613.
20. Fisher, A.A. (1973): Allergic reactions to feminine hygiene sprays. *Arch. Dermatol., 108*, 801.
21. Fisher, A.A. (1973): The role of patch testing in allergic contact dermatitis. In: *Contact Dermatitis, 2nd Edition*, p. 33. Lea and Febiger. Philadelphia.
22. Fitzpatrick. T.B., Pathak, M.A. and Parrish, J.A. (1974): Protection of human skin against sunburn. In: *Sunlight and Man, Normal and Abnormal Photobiologic Responses*, p. 753. University of Tokyo Press. Tokyo.
23. Libow, L.F., Ruszowski, A.M. and DeLeo, V.A. (1989): Allergic contact dermatitis from para-chloro-meta-xylenol in Lurosep soap. *Contact Dermatitis, 20*, 67–68.
24. Hannuksela, M. (1975): Allergy to propantheline in an antiperspirant. *Contact Dermatitis, 1*, 244.
25. Ranchoff, R.E., Steck, W.D., Taylor, J.S. and Evey, P. (1986): Electrocardiograph electrode and hand dermatitis from parachlorometaxylenol. *J. Am. Acad. Dermatol., 15*, 348–350.
26. Herrmann, W.A. (1957): Barrier creams (1). *Acta Derm.-Venereol. (Stockh.) 37,* 276.
27. Hindson, C. (1980): Phenylsalicylate (Salol) in a lip salve. *Contact Dermatitis, 6*, 216.
28. Hjorth. N., Wilkinson, D., Magnusson, B., Bandmann, H.J. and Maibach, H.I. (1978): Glyceryl-p-aminobenzoate patch testing in benzocaine-sensitive subjects. *Contact Dermatitis, 4*, 4.
29. Horio, T. and Higuchi, T. (1978): Photocontact dermatitis from p-aminobenzoic acid. *Dermatologica (Basel), 156*, 124.
30. Joo, I. and Simon, N. (1974): Die Benzotriazolderivate als UV-Absorber. *Arch. Derm. Forsch., 249*, 13–19.
31. Jordan, W.P., Dahl, M.V. and Albert, H.L. (1972): Contact dermatitis from glutaraldehyde. *Arch. Dermatol., 105*, 94.
32. Kahn, G. (1971): Intensified contact sensitization to benzylsalicylate. *Arch. Dermatol., 103*, 497.
33. Kaidbey, K.H. and Kligman, A.M. (1978): Phototoxicity to a sunscreen ingredient. *Arch. Dermatol., 114*, 547.
34. Minkin, W., Cohen. H.J. and Frank, S.B. (1973): Contact dermatitis from deodorants. *Arch. Dermatol., 107*, 775.
35. Muston, H.L., Boss, J.M. and Summerlym R. (1977): Dermatitis from Ammonyx LO, a constituent of a surgical scrub. *Contact Dermatitis, 3*, 347.
36. North American Contact Dermatitis Group (1973): Epidemiology of contact dermatitis in North America: 1972. *Arch. Dermatol., 108*, 537.

37. Nurse. D.S. (1980): Sensitivity to coconut diethanolamide. *Contact Dermatitis, 6*, 502.
38. Osmundsen, P.E. (1980): Contact dermatitis due to sodium hypochlorite. *Contact Dermatitis, 4*, 177.
39. Pariser, R.J. (1977): Contact dermatitis to dioxybenzone. *Contact Dermatitis, 3*, 172.
40. Parrish, J.A., Pathak, M.A. and Fitzpatrick, T.B. (1975): Facial irritation due to sunscreen products. *Arch. Dermatol., 111*, 525.
41. Ramsay, D.C., Cohen, H.J. and Baer, R.L. (1972): Allergie reaction to benzophenone. *Arch. Dermatol., 105*, 906.
42. Rietschel, R.L. and Lewis, C.W. (1978): Contact dermatitis to homomenthylsalicylate. *Arch. Dermatol., 114*, 442.
43. Sams. W.R. (1956): Contact photodermatitis. *Arch. Derm. Syph., 73*, 142.
44. Satulsky, E.M. (1950): Photosensitization induced by monoglycerol para-aminobenzoate. *Arch. Derm. Syph., 62*, 711.
45. Schneider, W., Tronnier, H. and Wagner, H. (1962): Protektiver Hautschutz. In: *Dermatologie und Venereolagie*, Bd 1/2 1070. Editors: H.A. Gottron and W.J. Schönfeld. G. Thieme Verlag, Stuttgart.
46. Schwartzberg. S. (1961): Allergic eczematous contact dermatitis caused by sensitisation by glycerol monostearate. *Ann. Allergy, 19*, 402.
47. Shelley, W.B. and Hurley, H.J. (1958): The allergic origin of zirconium deodorants granulomas in man. *Br. J. Dermatol., 70*, 75–101.
48. Reynold, N.J. and Peachey, R.D.G. (1990): Allergic contact dermatitis from a sulfosuccinate derivative in a hand cleanser. *Contact Dermatitis, 22*, 59–60.
49. Shmunes, E. and Levy, E.J. (1972): Quaternary ammonium compound contact dermatitis from a deodorant. *Arch. Dermatol., 105*, 91.
50. Sneddon, I.B. (1972): Dermatitis from dibutylphtalate in an aerosol antiperspirant and deodorant. *Contact Dermatitis Newsl., 12*, 308.
51. Spencer, M.C. (1962): Leukoderma following monobenzyl ether of hydroquinone bleaching. *Arch. Dermatol., 86*, 615.
52. Spencer, M.C. (1965): Topical use of hydroquinone for depigmentation. *J. Am. Med. Assoc., 194*, 962.
53. Thompson, G.. Maibach, H.I. and Epstein, J. (1977): Allergic contact dermatitis from sunscreen preparations complicating photodermatitis. *Arch. Dermatol., 113*, 1252.
54. Thyresson, N., Lodin, A. and Nilzen, A. (1956): Eczema of the hands due to triethanolamine in cosmetic hand lotions for housewives. *Acta Derm.-Venereol. (Stockh.), 36*, 355.
55. Van Ketel, W.G. (1976): Allergic contact dermatitis from propellants in deodorant sprays in combination with allergy to ethylchloride. *Contact Dermatitis, 2,* 115.
56. Van Ketel. W.G. (1977): Allergic contact dermatitis from an aminobenzoic acid compound used in sunscreens. *Contact Dermatitis, 3*, 283.
57. Wahlberg, J.E. (1976): Routine patch testing with Irgasan DP 300. *Contact Dermatitis, 2*, 292.
58. Wishart, J.M. (1974): Generalized exfoliative dermatitis due to contact with an antiperspirant. *Br. J. Clin. Pract., 28*, 264.
59. de Groot, A.C., van der Walle, H.B., Jagtman, B.A. and Weyland, J.W. (1987): Contact allergy to 4-isopropyldibenzoylmethane and 3-(4′-methylbenzylidene) camphor in the sunscreen Eusolex 8021. *Contact Dermatitis, 16*, 249–254.
60. Wüstner, H., Orfanos, C.E., Steinbach, K., Käferstein, H. and Herpers, H. (1975): Nagelverfärbung und Haarausfall. *Dtsch. Med. Wschr., 100*, 1694.
61. Yaffee, H.S. (1978): Apricot allergy. *Schoch Letter, 28*, July. Item 46.
62. Romaguera, C. and Grimalt, F. (1983): Dermatitis from PABA and hydroquinone. *Contact Dermatitis, 9*, 226.
63. Larsen, W.G. (1983): Allergic contact dermatitis to the fragrance material lilial. *Contact Dermatitis, 9*, 158.
64. Suhonen, R. (1983): Chloracetamide — a hidden contact allergen. *Contact Dermatitis, 9*, 161.
65. Edwards, E.K. Jr. and Edwards, E.K. (1983): Allergic reaction to triethanolamine stearate in a sunscreen. *Cutis, 31*, 195.
66. Edwards, E.K. Jr. and Edwards, E.K. (1982): Allergic reaction to tertiary butyl alcohol in a sunscreen. *Cutis, 29*, 476.
67. Dooms-Goossens. A., Degreef, H., VanHee, J. et al. (1981): Chlorocresol and chloracetamide: Allergens in medications, glues and cosmetics. *Contact Dermatitis, 7*, 51.
68. Adams, R.M. (1981): Allergic contact dermatitis due to o-phenylphenol. *Contact Dermatitis, 7*, 332.

69. Tucker. W.F.G. (1983): Contact dermatitis to Eutanol G. *Contact Dermatitis, 9*, 88.
70. Alomar, A., Camarasa, J.G. and Barnadas, M. (1983): Addison's disease and contact dermatitis from mercury in a soap. *Contact Dermatitis, 9*, 76.
71. Przybilla, B., Schwab, U., Hölze, E. and Ring, J. (1983): Kontaktsensibilisierung durch ein Antiperspirant mit dem Wirkstoff Propanthelinbromid. *Hautarzt, 34*, 459–462.
72. Mann, R.J. (1982): Benzoin sensitivity. *Contact Dermatitis, 8*, 263.
73. De Groot, A.C. and Liem, D.H. (1983): Contact allergy to Tinuvin® P. *Contact Dermatitis, 9*, 324.
74. Cooke, M.A. and Kurwa, A.R. (1975): Colophony sensitivity. *Contact Dermatitis, 2*, 192.
75. Rothenborg, H.W. and Hjorth, N. (1968): Allergy to perfumes from toilet soaps and detergents in patients with dermatitis. *Arch. Dermatol., 97*, 417.
76. Jordan, W.P. Jr. (1981): Contact dermatitis from D & C Yellow 11 dye in a toilet bar soap. *J. Am. Acad. Dermatol., 4*, 613.
77. Weaver, J.E. (1983): Dose response relationships in delayed hypersensitivity to quinoline dyes. *Contact Dermatitis, 9*, 309.
78. Fisher, A.A. (1982): Can bleaching creams containing 2% hydroquinone produce leukoderma? *J. Am. Acad. Dermatol., 7*, 134.
79. Grojean, M.F., Thivolet, J. and Perrot. H. (1982): Leucomélanodermies accidentelles provoquées par les topiques depigmentants. *Ann. Derm. Venereol. (Paris), 109*, 641.
80. Colomb. D. (1982): Dépigmentation en confettis après application de Leucodinine B[R] sur un chloasma (Letter). *Ann. Derm. Venereol. (Paris), 109*, 899.
81. Eiermann, H.J., Larsen, W., Maibach, H.I. and Taylor, J.S. (1982): Prospective study of cosmetic reactions: 1977–1980. *J. Am. Acad. Dermatol., 6*, 909.
82. Cullison, D., Abele, D.C. and O'Quinn, J.L. (1983): Localized exogenous ochronosis. Report of a case and review of the literature. *J. Am. Acad. Dermatol., 8*, 882.
83. Findlay, G.H. (1982): Ochronosis following skin bleaching with hydroquinone. *J. Am. Acad. Dermatol., 6*, 1092.
84. Mann. R.J. and Harman, R.R.M. (1983): Nail staining due to hydroquinone. *J. Am. Acad. Dermatol., 6*, 1092.
85. Mørk, N.J. and Austad, J. (1984): Contact dermatitis from witisol, a sunscreen agent. *Contact Dermatitis, 10*, 122–123.
86. Langeland, T. and Nyrud, M. (1982): Contact urticaria to wheat bran bath: A case report. *Acta Derm.-Venereol. (Stockh.), 62*, 82.
87. Fisher, A.A. (1982): Cortaid cream dermatitis and the 'paraben paradox'. (Letter). *J. Am. Acad. Dermatol., 6*, 116.
88. Pathak, M.A. (1982): Sunscreens: Topical and systemic approaches for protection of human skin against harmful effects of solar radiation. *J. Am. Acad. Dermatol., 7*, 285.
89. Fisher, A.A. (1982): Contact dermatitis from topical medicaments. *Semin. Derm., 1*, 49.
90. Roelandts, R., Van Hee, J., Bonamie, A. et al. (1983): A survey of ultraviolet absorbers in commercially available sun products. *Int. J. Dermatol., 22*, 247.
91. Levine, N., Don, S., Owens, C. et al. (1989): The effects of bergapten and sunlight on cutaneous pigmentation. *Arch. Dermatol., 125*, 1225–1230.
92. Morison, W.L. (1989): To tan or not to tan. A burning question. *Arch. Dermatol., 125*, 1258–1260.
93. Aust, L.B. and Maibach. H.I. (1980): Incidence of human skin sensitization to isostearyl alcohol in two separate groups of panelists. *Contact Dermatitis, 6*, 269.
94. Roed-Petersen, J., Auken, G. and Hjorth, N. (1975): Contact sensitivity to Irgasan DP 300. *Contact Dermatitis, 1*, 293.
95. Calnan, C.D. (1975): Dibutyl phthalate. *Contact Dermatitis, 1* 388.
96. Husain, S.L. (1975): Sensitivity to parabens in Codella barrier cream. *Contact Dermatitis, 1*, 395.
97. Adams, R.M. (1972): Photodermatitis from chlorophenylphenol. *Contact Dermatitis Newsl., 11*, 276.
98. Rapaport, M.J. (1983): Sunscreening agents and sun protective factors. *Int. J. Dermatol., 22*, 293.
99. Mathias, C.G.T. (1982): Pigmented cosmetic dermatitis from contact allergy to a toilet soap containing chromium. *Contact Dermatitis, 8*, 29.
100. Bois, G., Nicklasson, B. and Svensson, A. (1987): Allergic contact dermatitis to propyl gallate. *Contact Dermatitis, 17*, 294–298.
101. Heine, A. (1988): Contact dermatitis from propyl gallate. *Contact Dermatitis, 18*, 313–314.
102. Fimiani, M., Casin, L. and Bocci, S. (1990): Contact dermatitis from phenyl salicylate in a galenic cream. *Contact Dermatitis, 22*, 239.

103. De Groot, A.C. and Liem, D.H. (1984): Contact allergy to oleamidopropyl dimethylamine. *Contact Dermatitis, 11*, 298–301.
104. De Groot, A.C., Jagtman, B.A., van der Meeren, H.L.M et al. (1988): Cross-reaction pattern of the cationic emulsifier oleamidopropyl dimethylamine. *Contact Dermatitis, 19*, 284–289.
105. Senff, H., Exner, M., Görtz, J. and Goos, M. (1989): Allergic contact dermatitis from Euxyl K 400. *Contact Dermatitis, 20*, 381–382.
106. De Groot, A.C. and Weyland, J.W. (1991): Contact allergy to methyldibromoglutaronitrile in the cosmetics preservative Euxyl K 400. *Am. J. Contact Dermatitis, 2*, 31–32.
107. De Groot, A.C., Berretty, P.J.M., van Ginkel, C.J.W., den Hengst, C.W., van Ulsen, J. and Weyland, J.W. (1991): Allergic contact dermatitis from tocopheryl acetate in cosmetic creams. *Contact Dermatitis, 25*, 302–304.
108. De Groot, A.C., Baar, J.J.M., Terpstra, H. and Weyland, J.W. (1991): Contact allergy to moist toilet paper. *Contact Dermatitis, 24*, 135–136.
109. De Groot, A.C., Conemans, J. and Liem, D.H. (1984): Contact allergy to benzoxonium chloride (Bradophen®). *Contact Dermatitis, 11*, 324–325.
110. De Groot, A.C., Bruynzeel, D.P., van Joost, Th. and Weyland, J.V. (1988): Cosmetic allergy from myristyl alcohol. *Contact Dermatitis, 19* , 76–77.
111. De Groot, A.C., van der Meeren, H.L.M. and Weyland, J.W. (1988): Cosmetic allergy from stearic acid and glyceryl stearate. *Contact Dermatitis, 19*, 77–78.
112. De Groot, A.C., van der Meeren, H.L.M., de Wit, F.S., Bos, J.D. and Weyland, J.W. (1988): Contact allergie voor cocamide DEA. *Bull. Contact Dermatosen, 2*, 42–45.
113. Fisher, A.A. (1976): Reactions to antioxidants in cosmetics and foods. *Cutis, 17*, 21–28.
114. Taylor, J.S., Jordan, W.P. and Maibach, H.I. (1984): Allergic contact dermatitis from stearamidoethyl diethylamine phosphate: a cosmetic emulsifier. *Contact Dermatitis, 10*, 74–76.
115. Ippen, H. (1985): Labilin® — a little-known contact allergen. *Contact Dermatitis, 13*, 200–201.
116. Neill, S.M. and du Vivier, A. (1984): Contact dermatitis to trilaureth phosphate. *Contact Dermatitis, 11*, 130–131.
117. Fisher, A.A. (1978): Propylene glycol dermatitis. *Cutis, 21*, 166–78.
118. Jarmoc, L.M. and Primack, W.A. (1987): Anaphylaxis to cutaneous exposure to milk protein in a diaper rash ointment. *Clinical Pediatrics, 26*, 154–155.
119. Srinivas, C.R., Padhee, A. and George, N.D. (1990): Triethanolamine-induced allergic contact dermatitis over a tuberculoid leprosy lesion. *Int. J. Leprosy, 58*, 382–384.
120. Burry, J.N. (1986): Environmental dermatitis. Contact dermatitis from perfumes in soap. *Med. J. Austral., 145*, 160–161.
121. Ravnskov, U. (1984): Soap is the major cause of dysuria. *Lancet, ii*, 1027–1028.
122. Fisher, A.A. (1984): Allergic reactions to D&C Yellow No. 11 dye. *Cutis, 34*, 344–348.
123. Jass, H.E. (1986): Bubble bath warning. *Cosmetics and Toiletries, 101*, 13.
124. Natow, A.J. (1986): Chemical removal of hair. *Cutis, 38*, 91–92.
125. Sun, C.-C. (1987): Allergic contact dermatitis of the face from contact with nickel and ammoniated mercury in spectacle frames and skin-lightening creams. *Contact Dermatitis, 17*, 306–309.
126. Engasser, P.G. and Maibach, H.I. (1981): Cosmetics and dermatology: bleaching creams. *J. Am. Acad. Dermatol., 5*, 143–147.
127. Fisher, A.A. (1984): Reactions to aluminum and its salts. *Cutis, 33*, 154–159.
128. Williams, S. and Freemont, A.J. (1984): Aerosol antiperspirants and axillary granulomata. *Br. Med. J., 288*, 1651–1652.
129. Epstein, E. (1966): Dichlorophene allergy. *Ann. Allergy, 24*, 437–439.
130. Heine, A. and Tarnick, M. (1987): Allergisches Kontaktekzem durch Usninsäure in Deodorant sprays. *Derm. Mschr., 173*, 221–225.
131. Kraus, A.L., Stotts, J., Altringer, A. and Allgood G.S. (990): Allergic contact dermatitis from propyl gallate: dose response comparison using various application methods. *Contact Dermatitis, 22*, 132–136.
132. Dooms-Goossens, A., Dupré, K., Borghuis, A., Swinnen, C., Dooms, M. and Degreef, H. (1987): Zinc ricinoleate: sensitizer in deodorants. *Contact Dermatitis, 16*, 292–294.
133. Goh, C.L. (1987): Dermatitis from chlorphenesin in a deodorant. *Contact Dermatitis, 16*, 287.
134. Emery, I.K. (1987): Antiperspirants and deodorants. *Cutis, 39*, 531–532.
135. Rogers, S., Cooke, S. (1989): Allergic contact dermatitis due to stick deodorant. *Contact Dermatitis, 21*, 112–113.

136. Valdivieso, R., Pola, J., Zapata, C. et al. (1987): Contact allergic dermatitis caused by Freon 12 in deodorants. *Contact Dermatitis, 17*, 243–245.
137. Clayton, J.W. (1967): Fluorocarbon toxicity. Past, present, future. *J. Soc. Cosm. Chemists, 18*, 33–38.
138. De Groot, A.C., van der Meeren, H.L.M. and Weyland, J.W. (1987): Contact allergy to avocado oil in a sunscreen. *Contact Dermatitis, 16,* 108–109.
139. Edwards, E.K. Jr. and Edwards, E.K. (1984): Allergic reaction to phenyldimethicone in a suncreen. *Arch. Dermatol., 120,* 575.
140. Thune, P. (1984): Contact and photocontact allergy to suncreens. *Photodermatol., 1,* 5–9.
141. Jeanmougin, M., Manciet, J.R., Moulin, J.P., Blanc, F., Pons, A. and Civatte, J. (1988): Contact allergy to dexpanthenol in sunscreens. *Contact Dermatitis, 18,* 240.
142. Schauder, S. and Ippen, H. (1986): Photoallergic and allergic contact dermatitis from dibenzoylmethanes. *Photodermatology, 3,* 140–147.
143. Schauder, S. and Ippen, H. (1988): Photoallergisches und allergisches Kontaktekzem durch Dibenzoylmethan Verbindungen und andere Lichtschutzfilter. *Hautarzt, 39,* 435–440.
144. English, J.S.C., White, I.R. and Cronin, E. (1987): Sensitivity to sunscreens. *Contact Dermatitis, 17,* 159–162.
145. De Groot, A.C. and Weyland, J.W. (1987): Contact allergy to the UV-absorber butyl methoxydibenzoyl methane. *Contact Dermatitis, 16,* 278.
146. Knobler, E., Almeida, L., Ruzkowski, A.M., Held, J., Harber. L. and deLeo, V. (1989): Photoallergy to benzophenone. *Arch. Dermatol., 125,* 801–804.
147. Freeman, S. and Frederiksen, P. (1990): Sunscreen allergy. *Am. J. Contact Dermatitis, 1,* 240–243.
148. Kleinhans, D. (1988): Kontaktallergie gegen UV-Filtersubstanzen in Lichtschutzpräparaten. *Derm. u. Kosmet., 29,* 28–34.
149. Garmyn, M.A., Murphy, G.M., Gibbs, N.K. and Hawk, J.L.M. (1986): Are the protection factors assigned to proprietary sunscreen products misleading ? *Photodermatol., 3,* 104–106.
150. Young, A.R. (1990): To tan or not to tan. Morison, W.L. (Reply). *Arch. Dermatol., 126,* 681–682.
151. Pathak, M.A. (1986): Sunscreens, topical and systemic approaches for the prevention of acute and chronic sun-induced skin reactions. *Dermatologic Clinics, 4,* 321–334.
152. De Groot, A.C. (1988): Adverse reactions to cosmetics, p. 111-112. Thesis, University of Groningen.
153. Storrs, F.J. and Bell, D. (1983): Allergic contact dermatitis to 2-bromo-2-nitropropane-1,3-diol in a hydrophilic ointment. *J. Am. Acad. Dermatol., 8,* 157–170.
154. De Groot, A.C., Bruynzeel, D.P., Jagtman, B.A. and Weyland, J.W. (1988): Contact allergy to diazolidinyl urea (Germall II®). *Contact Dermatitis, 18,* 202-205.
155. Parker, L.U. and Taylor, J.S. (1991): A 5-year study of contact allergy to quaternium-15. *Am. J. Contact Dermatitis, 2,* 231–234.
156. Garcia-Bravo, B. and Mozo, P. (1992): Generalized contact dermatitis from Vitamin E. *Contact Dermatitis, 26,* 280.
157. Grob, W. and Ippen, H. (1990): Labilin. *Contact Dermatitis, 23,* 62–63.
158. Flyvholm, M.A. and Menné, T. (1992): Allergic contact dermatitis from formaldehyde. *Contact Dermatitis, 27,* 27–36.
159. Christersson, S. and Wrangsjö, K. (1992): Contact allergy to undecylenamide diethanolamide in a liquid soap. *Contact Dermatitis, 27,* 191–192.
160. Peter, C. and Hoting, E. (1992): Contact allergy to cocamidopropyl betaine (CAPB). *Contact Dermatitis, 26,* 282–283.
161. Kadunce, D.P., Piepkorn, M.W. and Zone, J.J. (1990): Persistent melanocytic lesions associated with cosmetic tanning bed use: "Sunbed lentigines". *J. Am. Acad. Dermatol., 23,* 1029–1031.
162. Young, A.R., Potten, C.S. and Chadwick, C.A. et al. (1991): Photoprotection and 5-MOP photochemoprotection from UVR induced DNA damage in humans, the role of skin type. *J. Invest. Dermatol., 97,* 942–948.
163. Dromgoole, S.H. and Maibach, H.I. (1990): Sunscreening agent intolerance: contact and photocontact sensitization and contact urticaria. *J. Am. Acad. Dermatol., 22,* 1068–1078.

30. Tabulation of ingredients of cosmetics

30.1 In this chapter, tabulations are given of the following groups of ingredients of cosmetics:

- Antimicrobials and antioxidants (§ 30.5)
- Fragrance materials (§ 30.7)
- Colours (§ 30.9–11)
- Sunscreens (§ 30.13)
- Lipids and surfactants (§ 30.15)
- Botanical ingredients (§ 30.16)
- Miscellaneous cosmetic ingredients (§ 30.17)

The patch test concentrations and vehicles given in the following tables have usually been taken from: De Groot, A.C. Patch testing: test concentrations and vehicles for 2800 allergens, 2nd Edition. Amsterdam, Elsevier, 1994. The sign "†" following a patch test concentration and vehicle indicates that the authors have patch-tested one or more patients with this compound in this concentration and vehicle without observing irritant reaction(s). Reference numbers given under "Patch test concentration and vehicle and reference" and "Comment" refer to the following publications:

30.2 REFERENCES

1. Lahti, A. and Hannuksela, M. (1980): Immediate contact allergy to birch leaves and sap. *Contact Dermatitis, 6,* 464–465.
2. Nater, J.P. and de Groot, A.C. (1985): Plant products in cosmetics. In: *Unwanted Effects of Cosmetics and Drugs in Dermatology, 2nd Edition.* Chapter 26, pp. 377–388. Elsevier, Amsterdam.
3. Roed-Petersen, J. (1975): Allergic contact hypersensitivity to ivy (Hedera helix). *Contact Dermatitis, 1,* 57–59.
4. Foussereau, J., Muller, J. and Benezra, C. (1975): Contact allergy to Frullania and Laurus nobilis, cross-sensitization and chemical structure of the allergen. *Contact Dermatitis, 1,* 223–237.
5. van Ketel, W.G. (1982): Allergy to Matricaria chamomilla. *Contact Dermatitis, 8,* 143-144.
6. CIR 1981. Final Reports. *Cosmetic Ingredient Review.* 1110 Vermont Ave. N.W., Suite 8, Washington DC 2008.
7. Fisher, A.A. (1975): Patch testing with perfume ingredients. *Contact Dermatitis, 1,* 166.
8. Rapaport, M.J. (1980): Patch testing of color additives. *Contact Dermatitis, 6,* 231.
9. Kozuka, T., Tashiro, M., Sano, S. et al. (1980): Pigmented cosmetic dermatitis from azo dyes. I. Cross-sensitivity in humans. *Contact Dermatitis, 6,* 330.
10. Sertoli, A., Fabbri, P., Campoli, P. and Panconesi, E. (1978): Allergic contact dermatitis to Salvia officinalis, Inula viscosa and Conyza Bonariensis. *Contact Dermatitis, 4,* 314–316.

11. Eiermann, H.J. (1980): Regulatory issues concerning AETT and 6-MC. *Contact Dermatitis, 6,* 120.
12. Thune, P.O. and Solberg, Y.J. (1980): Photosensitivity and allergy to aromatic lichen acids, Compositae oleoresins and other plant substances. *Contact Dermatitis, 6,* 81–84.
13. Rudzki, E. (1977): Contact urticaria from silk. *Contact Dermatitis, 3,* 53.
14. Rudzki, E. and Grzywa, Z. (1977): Contact urticaria from egg. *Contact Dermatitis, 3,* 103.
15. Thune, P. (1984): Contact and photocontact allergy to sunscreens. *Photodermatol., 1,* 5–9.
16. Bilsland, D. and Strong, A. (1990): Allergic contact dermatitis from the essential oil of French marigold (Tagetes patula) in an aromatherapist. *Contact Dermatitis, 23,* 55–56.
17. Fregert, S. (1981): *Manual of Contact Dermatitis. 2nd Edition.* Munksgaard, Copenhagen.
18. Bruynzeel, D.P. and Niklasson, B. (1992): The patch test dilution of oleamidopropyl dimethylamine. *Contact Dermatitis, 23,* 190–191.
19. Adams, R.M. and Maibach, H.I. (1985): A five-year study of cosmetic reactions. *J. Am. Acad. Dermatol., 13,* 1062–1069.
20. Mitchell, J.C., Adams, R.M. and Glendenning, W.E. et al. (1982): Results of standard patch tests with substances abandoned. *Contact Dermatitis, 8,* 336.
21. Roed-Petersen, J. (1980): Allergic contact dermatitis from butyl acetate. *Contact Dermatitis, 6,* 55.
22. Larsen, W.G. (1975): Cosmetic dermatitis due to a perfume. *Contact Dermatitis, 1,* 142.
23. Rudzki, E., Grzywa, Z. and Bruo, W.S. (1976): Sensitivity to 35 essential oils. *Contact Dermatitis, 2,* 196.
24. Rudzki, E. and Grzywa, Z. (1976): Sensitizing and irritating properties of star anise oil. *Contact Dermatitis, 2,* 305.
25. Metz, J., Hundertmark, U. and Pevny, I. (1980): Vitamin C allergy of the delayed type. *Contact Dermatitis, 6,* 172–174.
26. Cavelier, C., Foussereau, J. and Tomb, R. (1988): Allergie de contact et colorants. *Cahiers de notes documentaires,* 1–54. (ISSN 0007-9952) (ISBN 2-85599-853-0).
27. Belsito, D.V. (1987): Contact dermatitis to ethyl-cyanoacrylate containing glue. *Contact Dermatitis, 17,* 234–236.

30.3 **Frequency of use** (Freq. use) is defined as frequency of use in 20,000 formulas listed in FDA File, 1992, obtained from A.L. Harper, FDA, Washington DC, USA.

Contact Allergy: If contact allergy has been reported, this is indicated by "+" in the columns headed 'Cont. all.'. Reference to the relevant paragraphs is made in the 'Comment' columns. Consult the index also for additional information on contact allcrgy and other (side) effects.

Nomenclature: with the exception of fragrance compounds (§ 30.7) and colours (§ 30.10) the nomenclature employed in the tables corresponds to the CTFA adopted names as included in the CTFA International Cosmetic Ingredient Dictionary, Ed. IV, (1991).

Ingredients not listed in the Dictionary are denoted by "‡".

Abbreviations:

DEA	diethanolamine
MEA	monoethanolamine
MIPA	monoisopropylamine
PEG	polyethyleneglycol/polyoxyethylene
PEI	polyethyleneimine
PG	propylene glycol
PPG	polypropyleneglycol
TEA	triethanolamine

ANTIMICROBIALS AND ANTIOXIDANTS

30.4 Antimicrobials and antioxidants are tabulated as follows:
- Antioxidants and chelating agents (§ 30.5.1)
- Antimicrobials; acids — esters — alcohols — amides (§ 30.5.2)
- Formaldehyde and donor compounds (§ 30.5.3)
- Mercurials (§ 30.5.4)
- Phenols — halogenated phenols — organohalogen compounds (§ 30.5.5)
- Cationic compounds (§ 30.5.6)
- All other antimicrobials (§ 30.5.7).

Preservatives permitted in the EEC: Agents marked * in the 'Comment' columns of the tables are preservatives listed in Annex VI of EC Council Directive 76/768/EC and subsequent amendments up until the 15th Commission Directive (92/86/EC) of 21.10.1992 (permitted preservatives).

30.5.1 Antioxidants and chelating agents

Name	Synonym®	Advised patch test conc. & veh. (§ 30.1)	Freq. use (§ 30.3)	Cont. all. (§ 30.3)	Comment (§ 30.3 and § 30.4)
ascorbic acid		pure	267	+	Ref. 25
ascorbyl palmitate			290		
BHA (butylated hydroxyanisole)	Tenox BHA	2% pet.	1826	+	*See* § 5.7
BHT (butylated hydroxytoluene)	Ionol, Tenox BHT	2% pet.	1287	+	*See* § 5.7
t-butyl hydroquinone (TBHQ)		1% pet.	3	+	‡ *See* § 27.16
di-*t*-butylhydroquinone (DTBHQ)		1% pet.	15	+	*See* § 27.11
citric acid		1% aqua	2073		
cysteine			16		
cysteine hydrochloride			11		
diamylhydroquinone	Santovar				
dilauryl thiodipropionate			55		
2,6-*ditert*-butyl-4-hydroxymethyl-phenol	Ionox 100				‡
EDTA (ethylenediamine tetraacetate)		1% pet.	724	+	*See* § 5.7
– disodium EDTA			746		
– tetrasodium EDTA			965		
– trisodium EDTA			773		

(continued)

§ 30.5.1 *(continuation)*

Name	Synonym®	Advised patch test conc. & veh. (§ 30.1)	Freq. use (§ 30.3)	Cont. all. (§ 30.3)	Comment (§ 30.3 and § 30.4)
erythorbic acid (= isoascorbic acid)			307		
– sodium erythorbate			17		
ethoxyquin (= 6-ethoxy-1,2-dihydroxy-2,2,4-trimethyl-quinoline)		0.5% aqua or pet.		+	*See* § 5.43
gallates					*See* § 5.7 *under* gallate esters
– butyl gallate		1% pet.†			‡
– cetyl gallate					
– dodecyl gallate		0.1% pet.		+	
– octyl gallate		0.25% pet.	15	+	‡
– propyl gallate		1% pet.	308	+	
HEDTA (hydroxyethyl ethylene diamine triacetic acid)			12		
– trisodium HEDTA			184		
hydroxytetramethylchromane carboxylic acid	Trolox C				‡
monomethyl ether of hydroquinone			5		
monosulfiram		1% pet.		+	‡ *See* § 29.5
mono-tert-butylhydroquinone					‡ *See t*-butyl-hydroquinone
nordihydroguaiaretic acid (NDGA)		2% pet.		+	*See* § 5.7
pentasodium pentetate (= pentasodium diethylenetriamine pentaacetate)			322		
sodium bisulfite		10% aqua	160		
sodium hexametaphosphate		1% aqua †	42		
sodium metabisulfite		5% aqua	77	+	*See* § 5.7
sodium sulfite		2-5% pet.	624	+	*See* § 5.7
stearic hydrazide			10		
tetrasodium etidronate (= tetrasodium hydroxyethane diphosphonate)	Turpinal 4NL		34		

(continued)

§ **30.5.1** *(continuation)*

Name	Synonym®	Advised patch test conc. & veh. (§ 30.1)	Freq. use (§ 30.3)	Cont. all. (§ 30.3)	Comment (§ 30.3 and § 30.4)
tetrasodium pyrophosphate			17		
3,3-thiodipropionic acid (= TDPA)					‡
tocopherol (mixed isomers)		10% pet.	666	+	*See* § 5.7
dl-α-tocopherol		10% pet.	19	+	‡ *See* § 27.3
tocopheryl acetate		10% pet.	386	+	*See* § 27.3
dl-α-tocopheryl acetate		10% pet.	427	+	‡ *See* § 27.3
tocopheryl linoleate		10% pet.	163		
tocopheryl nicotinate		10% pet.	5	+	*See* § 27.3
tocopheryl succinate					
o-tolylbiguanide	Sopanox	2% pet.	10		
trihydroxybutyrophenone (= THBP)					‡
trimethyl-tris(di-tert-butylhydroxy-benzyl) benzene	Sopant				‡
trisodium nitrilotriacetate		0.25% aqua†			

30.5.2 Antimicrobials: acids, esters, alcohols, amides

Name	Synonym®	Advised patch test conc. & veh. (§ 30.1)	Freq. use (§ 30.3)	Cont. all. (§ 30.3)	Comment (*§ 30.3 and § 30.4)
benzoic acid		5% pet.	154	+	**See* § 5.7
benzyl alcohol		5-10% pet.	298	+	**See* 5.7
dehydroacetic acid		0.1% and 1% pet.	202	+	**See* § 5.7
disodium undecylene-amido MEA sulfosuccinate	Steinazid SBU 185		4		*
formic acid		1% aqua	4		*
p-hydroxybenzoic acid		5% pet.			* ‡
isopropyl sorbate		3% pet. †			*
parabens					*See* § 5.7
– benzylparaben		3% pet.	5	+	*

(continued)

§ **30.5.2** *(continuation)*

Name	Synonym®	Advised patch test conc. & veh. (§ 30.1)	Freq. use (§ 30.3)	Cont. all. (§ 30.3)	Comment (*§ 30.3 and § 30.4)
– butylparaben		3% pet.	1329	+	*
– ethylparaben		3% pet.	904	+	*
– methylparaben		3% pet.	7573	+	*
– propylparaben		3% pet.	6234	+	*
– sodium methylparaben			30		*
– sodium propylparaben			3		*
phenoxyethanol (phenoxetol)		1% pet.	685	+	**See* § 5.7
phenoxyisopropanol			5		*
potassium sorbate		5% pet.	136	+	**See* § 5.7
propionic acid					*
salicylic acid		2% pet.	82	+	**See* § 5.37
sodium benzoate		5% pet.	142	+	**See* § 5.7
sodium dehydroacetate		3% aqua †	355		*
sodium salicylate			6		*
sodium formate					*
sorbic acid		2% pet.	283	+	**See* § 5.7
undecylenamide DEA	Steinazid DU 185	1% aqua †			*
undecylenamide MEA	Steinazid U 185		4		*
undecylenic acid		2.5% pet.	8	+	**See* § 5.30
usnic acid		0.1% pet.		+	*See* § 5.7 and § 5.14
usnic acid copper salt					‡

30.5.3 Formaldehyde and donor compounds

Name	Synonym®	Advised patch test conc. & veh. (§ 30.1)	Freq. use (§ 30.3)	Cont. all. (§ 30.3)	Comment (*§ 30.3 and § 30.4)
benzylhemiformal	Preventol D2				*

(continued)

§ **30.5.3** *(continuation)*

Name	Synonym®	Advised patch test conc. & veh. (§ 30.1)	Freq. use (§ 30.3)	Cont. all. (§ 30.3)	Comment (* § 30.3 and § 30.4)
2-bromo-2-nitropropane-1,3-diol	Bronopol	0.5% pet.	307	+	**See* § 5.7
diazolidinyl urea	Germall II	2% aqua or pet.	447	+	**See* § 5.7
DMDM hydantoin (dimethylol dimethylhydantoin)	Glydant	1-3% aqua	771	+	**See* § 5.7
formaldehyde (and paraformaldehyde)		1% aqua	43	+	**See* § 5.7
imidazolidinyl urea	Germall 115	1% pet. or aqua	2118	+	**See* § 5.7
MDM hydantoin (monomethylol dimethylhydantoin)		3% aqua †	13	+	**See* § 5.7 *under* DMDM hydantoin
methenamine (= hexamine)		2% pet.	7	+	**See* § 5.7
methylolchloracetamide		0.2% pet.		+	‡ **See* § 5.7
quaternium-15 (chloroallylhexaminium chloride)	Dowicil 200	1% pet.	885	+	**See* § 5.7 *under* quaternary ammonium compounds
trihydroxyethyl hexahydrotriazine	Grotan BK	1% pet.		+	‡**See* § 5.7 *under* hexahydro-1,3,5-tris(2-hydroxyethyl)-triazine

30.5.4 Mercurials

Name	Synonym®	Advised patch test conc. & veh. (§ 30.1)	Freq. use (§ 30.3)	Cont. all. (§ 30.3)	Comment (* § 30.3 and § 30.4)
phenylmercuric acetate		0.01% aqua	46	+	**See* § 5.7
phenylmercuric benzoate					*
phenylmercuric borate		0.01% aqua		+	**See* § 5.7
phenylmercuric chloride					*‡
phenylmercuric nitrate		0.01% aqua		+	‡**See* § 5.7
thimerosal (thiomersal; sodium ethyl-mercurithiosalicylate)	merthiolate	0.1% pet.	35	+	*See* § 5.7

30.5.5 Phenols, halogenated phenols, organohalogen compounds

Name	Synonym®	Advised patch test conc. & veh. (§ 30.1)	Freq. use (§ 30.3)	Cont. all. (§ 30.3)	Comment (* § 30.3 and §30.4)
bithionol		1% pet.		+	‡*See* § 5.7: prohibited in EC; Annex II, no. 352
bromochlorophene		2% pet.		+	**See* § 5.7
5-bromo-5-nitro-1,3-dioxane	Bronidox	0.5% pet. †	42		*
2-bromo-2-nitropropane-1,3,-diol	Bronopol	0.5% pet.	307	+	**See* §5.7
captan	Vancide 89RE	0.1–0.25% pet.	18	+	*See* [10] *and* § 26.2; prohibited in EC; Annex II, no. 370
chloroacetamide		0.2% pet.	86	+	**See* § 5.7
chlorhexidine diacetate	Arlacide A	0.5% and 1% aqua	9	+	**See* § 5.7
chlorhexidine digluconate	Hibitane	0.5% and 1% aqua	28	+	**See* § 5.7
chlorhexidine dihydrochloride	Arlacide H	0.5% and 1% aqua	6	+	**See* § 5.7
chlorobutanol (= trichlorbutanol)		5% pet.		+	**See* § 5.7
p-chloro-*m*-cresol (= chlorocresol, PCMC)		1% pet.	15	+	**See* § 5.7
chlorophene (= 2-benzyl-4-chlorphenol)	Preventol BP	1% pet.			*
chloroxylenol (*p*-chloro-*m*-xylenol, PCMX)	Emericide 1199	1% pet.	64	+	**See* 5.7
climbazole (= imidazolyl-chlorphenoxydimethylbutanon)					*
cloflucarban (= halocarban)	Irgasan CF3	0.5% pet.			
o-cymene-5-ol	Biosol		11		
dibromohexamidine diisethionate					*‡
dibromopropamidine diisethionate		1-5% pet.		+	*See* § 5.7
dibromsalan		1% pet.			‡ prohibited in EC; Annex II; no.359
dichlorobenzylalcohol (= 2,4-dichlorobenzylalcohol)	Myacide SP	2% pet. †	11		*
3,4-dichlorobenzylalcohol					‡
dichlorophene	G-4	1% pet.	7	+	**See* § 5.7

(continued)

§ **30.5.5** *(continuation)*

Name	Synonym®	Advised patch test conc. & veh. (§ 30.1)	Freq. use (§ 30.3)	Cont. all. (§ 30.3)	Comment (* § 30.3 and §30.4)
dichloro-*m*-xylenol (DCMX)		1% pet.			* *See* § 5.7 *under* *p*-chloro-*m*-xylenol
Euxyl K100®				+	*See* methylchloro-isothiazolinone
Euxyl K400®				+	*See* methyldibromoglutaronitrile
fenticlor		1% pet.		+	‡ *See* § 5.7
glyceryl-*p*-chlorophenyl ether (= chlorphenesin)		1% pet.		+	‡ * *See* § 5.32 *under* chlorphenesin
hexachlorophene	G-11	1% pet.		+	*See* § 5.7: prohibited use in EC; Annex II, no. 371
isopropyl-*m*-cresol		1% pet.		+	* *See* § 5.7 *under* thymol
Kathon CG®				+	‡ *See* methyl-chloroiso-thiazolinone
methylchloroisothiazolinone/methylisothiazolinone	Kathon CG®	100 ppm. aqua	647	+	* *See* § 5.7
methyldibromoglutaronitrile (1,2-dibromo-2,4-dicyanobutane)	Euxyl K400® (mixture with phenoxy-ethanol); Tektamer 38®	0.05% pet.	7	+	* *See* § 5.7
o-phenylphenol		1% pet.	9	+	* *See* § 5.7
– sodium salt			5		*
tetrabrom-*o*-cresol			8		‡
tribromsalan (TBS)		1% pet.			‡ prohibited in EC; Annex II, no. 373
trichlorobutanol					‡* *See* chlorobutanol
triclocarban (TCC)		2% pet.	17	+	* *See* § 5.7
triclosan	Irgasan DP300	2% pet.	370	+	* *See* § 5.7

30.5.6 Cationic compounds

Name	Synonym®	Advised patch test conc. & veh. (§ 30.1)	Freq. use (§ 30.3)	Cont. all. (§ 30.3)	Comment (*§ 30.3 and § 30.4)
benzalkonium chloride	Zephiran	0.01% and 0.1% aqua	100	+	*See § 5.7 *under* quaternary ammonium compounds
benzethonium chloride	Hyamine 1622	0.01% and 0.1% aqua	77	+	*See § 5.7 *under* quaternary ammonium compounds
cetearalkonium bromide					
cetrimonium bromide (= cetrimide)		0.01% and 0.1% aqua	37	+	*See § 5.7 *under* quaternary ammonium compounds
cetrimonium chloride		0.01% and 0.1% aqua	138		*See § 5.7 *under* quaternary ammonium compounds
cetylpyridinium chloride		0.01% and 0.1% aqua	18	+	*See* § 5.7 *under* quaternary ammonium compounds
chlorhexidine					
– diacetate	Arlacide A	0.5% and 1% aqua	9	+	*See § 5.7
– digluconate	Hibitane	0.5% and 1% aqua	28	+	*See § 5.7
– dihydrochloride	Arlacide H	0.5% and 1% aqua	6	+	*See § 5.7
dibromohexamidine isethionate					‡ *See § 30.5.5
dibromopropamidine isethionate					*See* § 30.5.5
dodecylguanidine acetate	Dodine				‡
hexamidine *p*-hydroxybenzoate					*‡
hexamidine isethionate	Hexomedine	0.15% aqua	18	+	*See § 5.7
hexetidine		0.1% pet.		+	*See § 5.30
piroctone olamine	Octopirox				*
polyhexamethylenebiguanide chloride	Arlagard C				*‡
(other) quaternary ammonium compounds		0.1% and 0.01% aqua			‡*See* § 30.15.3
stearalkonium chloride		0.01% and 0.1% aqua	387		*

30.5.7 All other antimicrobials

Name	Synonym®	Advised patch test conc. & veh. (§ 30.1)	Freq. use (§ 30.3)	Cont. all. (§ 30.3)	Comment (* § 30.3 and § 30.4)
chlorquinaldol	Sterosan	3% pet.		+	‡*See* § 5.7
coal tar		5% pet.	6	+	*See* § 5.37
decominol (INN)					*‡
diiodohydroxyquin	Diiodoquin	3% pet.		+	‡*See* § 5.7
dimethoxane (= 6-acetoxy-2,4-dimethyl-*m*-dioxane)		0.1% - 1% pet.	18		‡ Has caused photosensitivity; (§ 6.5) prohibited in EC; Annex II, no. 368
dimethyloxazolidine	Oxadine A				*
ethacridine lactate	Rivanol	1-2% pet.		+	‡*See* § 5.7
7-ethylbicyclooxazolidine					‡*
glutaral (= glutaraldehyde)		0.5-1% aqua (not stable)	115	+	**See* § 5.7
2-hydroxypyridine-*N*-oxide	Oxypyrion				‡
iodine		0.5% aqua open test	3	+	‡*See* § 5.7; prohibited in EC; Annex II, no. 213
iodopropenyl butylcarbamate	Glydant plus				*
iodochlorohydroxyquinoline	Vioform	3% pet.		+	*See* § 5.7 *under* quinoline derivatives
oxyquinoline (= 8-hydroxyquinoline)		3% pet.	5	+	**See* § 5.7 *under* quinoline derivatives
– benzoate (salt)					*
– benzoate (ester) (= benzoxyquine)					*
– sulfate (salt)			13		*
povidone-iodine (PVP-iodine)		10% solution and comm. prep.		+	*See* § 5.7
proflavine dihydrochloride		0.1%-1% pet.		+	*See* § 5.7
pyrithiones					
– aluminum pyrithione camsylate					*
– pyrithione disulfide	in Omadine MDS				*
– sodium pyrithione		0.3% aqua	3	+	prohibited in EC; Annex II, no. 369 *See* § 26.2

(continued)

§ **30.5.7** *(continuation)*

Name	Synonym®	Advised patch test conc. & veh. (§ 30.1)	Freq. use (§ 30.3)	Cont. all. (§ 30.3)	Comment (*§ 30.3 and § 30.4)
– zinc pyrithione	Zinc Omadine	1% pet.	45	+	**See* § 5.7 and § 26.2
selenium sulfide		2% pet.		+(?)	*See* § 26.2
sodium hydroxymethylglycinate (= sodium hydroxymethyl-aminoacetate)	Suttocide				*
sulfur, colloidal		1–5% pet.	46	+	*See* § 5.37 and § 5.7
tyrothricin		20% pet.	8	+	*See* § 5.23; prohibited in EC; Annex II no. 392
undebenzophenone (= ethylene glycophenyl undecyl ether *p*-hydroxybenzoate)					*

FRAGRANCE MATERIALS

30.6 The fragrance materials are tabulated in § 30.7. Sources are:

1. Opdyke, D.L.J.: RIFM Monographs, published in *Food and Cosmetic Toxicology, 1973–April 1981.*
2. Opdyke, D.L.J. and Letizia, C. (1982): RIFM Monographs, published in *Food and Cosmetic Toxicology, 20,* 633–851.
3. Ford, R.A., Api, A.M. and Letizia, C.S. (1992): Monographs on Fragrance raw materials in *Food and Chemical Toxicology, 30, Suppl. 1S–138S.*
4. Ford, R.A. (1988): RIFM Monographs, published in *Food and Chemical Toxicology, 26,* 275–415.
5. *Code of Practice, IFRA.* F. Grundschober, 8 rue Charles-Humbert, CH-1205 Geneva, Switzerland.

The **names of the fragrance ingredients** are given according to the RIFM Monographs nomenclature.

Patch test concentrations and vehicles are non-irritating test concentrations in human maximization tests (see also § 5.2)

Quantitative use: defined as use of fragrances in the USA in thousands of lbs per year, according to the RIFM. Note that these figures are taken from the original monographs and may be inaccurate in some cases.

– = no data from RIFM (in the columns on non-irritating patch test conc.)
N = material of natural origin
HMT = human maximization test.

References to IFRA recommendations on the use of specific fragrance ingredients are listed in the 'comments' column; where these involve the recommendation that an ingredient should not be used in fragrances this is indicated.

A better notion of the exposure to fragrance ingredients by their presence in cosmetics can be obtained from data which estimate the frequency of use by chemical analysis of market products.

The following table summarizes the results of the analyses of 400 fragrances from major commercial cosmetic products marketed around the world [1] and the results of the analyses of 300 cosmetic products sold on the Dutch market [2]. The frequencies of occurrence of the most frequently used fragrance ingredients found are respectively:

Rank order	Fragrances found in 400 products [1]	* (%)	Fragrances found in 300 cosmetic products sold in the Netherlands [2]	* (%)
1	linalool	90	linalool	91
2	phenylethyl alcohol	82	phenylethyl alcohol	79
3	linalyl acetate	78	benzyl acetate	78
4	benzyl acetate	74	limonene	71
5	benzyl salicylate	74	citronellol	71
6	coumarin	68	linalyl acetate	67
7	terpineol	66	γ-methylionone	63
8	hedione	56	terpineol	52
9	hexylcinnamic aldehyde	51	β-pinene	51
10	γ-methylionone	51	geraniol	50
11	terpenyl acetate	50	hydroxycitronellal	49
12	lilial	49	benzyl benzoate	49
13	lyral	46	hexylcinnamic aldehyde	48
14	geraniol	43	lilial	48
15	heliotropin	43	coumarin	44
16	galaxolide	41	benzyl salicylate	43
17	vertofix	41	benzyl alcohol	42
18	musk ketone	38	eugenol	36
19	citronellol	38	α-pinene	35
20	amyl salicylate	32	geranyl acetate	35
21	eugenol	26	α-amylcinnamic aldehyde	35
22	vertenex	25	musk ketone	34
23	isobornyl acetate	23	caryophyllene	33
24	α-amylcinnamic aldehyde	21	lyral	33
25	hydroxycitronellal	21	camphor	31

[1] R.S. Penn, Aroma chemical usage trends in modern perfumery (1989): *Perfumer & Flavorist, 14*, 3–10.
[2] Data J.W. Weyland, personal communication 1992.
*Percentage of products containing the fragrances listed.

30.7 Fragrance materials

Name	Non-irritating patch test conc. (RIFM) (§ 30.6)	Quant. use (§ 30.6)	Patch test conc. & veh. (§ 30.1)	Cont. all. (§ 30.3)	Comment (N: § 30.6)
Abies alba (cone) oil	20% pet.	1	2% pet.	+	N. *See* § 30.2 [23]
Abies alba (needle) oil	20% pet.	1	2% pet.	+	N. *See* § 30.2 [23]
acetaldehyde diethyl acetal	10% pet.	1			
acetaldehyde ethyl *cis*-3-hexenyl acetal	10% pet.				
acetaldehyde ethyl-*trans*-3-hexenylacetal	5% pet.	1			
acetaldehyde ethyl hexyl acetal	5% pet.				
acetaldehyde ethyl isoeugenyl acetal	10% pet.				
acetaldehyde ethyl linalyl acetal	6% pet.				
acetaldehyde ethyl phenylethyl acetal	5% pet.				
acetate C-7	8% pet.	1			
acetate C-8	8% pet.	5			
acetate C-9	2% pet.	5			
acetate C-10	8% pet.	1			
acetate C-11	8% pet.	1			
acetate C-12	20% pet.	1			
acetoin	10% pet.	1			
acetophenone	2% pet.	10			
4-acetoxy-2-ethoxybenzaldehyde	4% pet.				
1-acetoxy-1-ethynyl-2-*sec*-butylcyclohexane	14% pet.				
4-acetoxy-3-pentyl-tetrahydropyran	10% pet.				
acetyl butyrol	4% pet.	1			
acetyl carene	10% pet.				
acetyl cedrene	30% pet.	200			

(continued)

§ **30.7** *(continuation)*

Name	Non-irritating patch test conc. (RIFM) (§ 30.6)	Quant. use (§ 30.6)	Patch test conc. & veh. (§ 30.1)	Cont. all. (§ 30.3)	Comment (N: § 30.6)
acetylethyltetra-methyltetralin (AETT, Versalide®)	4% pet.	100			Discontinued in 1977: neurotoxic (*see* § 30.2 [11]): should not be used in fragrances (IFRA recommendation, November 1977, February 1980); EC Annex II, 362
5-acetyl-1,1,2,3,3,6-hexamethylindan (Phantolide®)	4% pet.	6			Phototoxic; (IFRA, October 1987, November 1987)
acetyl isovaleryl	5% pet.	<0.1			Sensitizer in HMT; Should not be used in fragrances (IFRA recommendation, February 1980, May 1983)
acetyl propionyl	4% pet.	1			
4-acetyl-6-*tert*-butyl-1,1-dimethylindan (Celestolide®)	4% pet.	5			
alantroot oil (= elecampane oil)	4% pet.		do not test	+	N. Sensitizer in HMT (due to alantolactone) *See* § 5.39. Should not be used in fragrances (IFRA recommendation, June 1975
alcohol C-6	1% pet.	1			
alcohol C-7	1% pet.	1			
alcohol C-8	2% pet.	10	pure (?)	+	*See* § 30.2 [22]
alcohol C-9	2% pet.	10	pure (?)	+	*See* § 30.2 [22]
alcohol C-10	3% pet.	20			
alcohol C-11	1% pet.	10			
alcohol C-11, undecylenic	4% pet.	1			
alcohol C-12	4% pet.	20			
alcohol C-14, myristic	12% pet.	1			
aldehyde C-6	1% pet.	1			
aldehyde C-7	4% pet.	1	pure (?)	+	*See* § 30.2 [22]

(continued)

§ 30.7 *(continuation)*

Name	Non-irritating patch test conc. (RIFM) (§ 30.6)	Quant. use (§ 30.6)	Patch test conc. & veh. (§ 30.1)	Cont. all. (§ 30.3)	Comment (N: § 30.6)
aldehyde C-7, dimethyl acetal	8% pet.	1			
aldehyde C-8	0.25% pet.	10			
aldehyde C-9	1% pet.	10	pure (?)	+	*See* § 30.2 [22]
aldehyde C-10	–	25	10% isoprop. palm		
aldehyde C-11, undecylenic	1% pet.	20	10% isoprop. palm		
aldehyde C-11, undecylic	5% pet.	20			
aldehyde C-12, lauric	1% pet.	20	10% isoprop. palm		
aldehyde C-12 MNA (methyl *m*-nonylacet-aldehyde)	4% pet.	35			
aldehyde C-14, myristic	1% pet.	2			
ale oil	20% pet.	1	1% alc./2% pet. [7] 1% pet. [17]		N
allo-ocimenol	8% pet.				
allyl-α-ionone*	10% pet.	2			
allyl butyrate*	4% pet.				Test concentration slightly irritating
allyl caproate*	4% pet.	5			
allyl caprylate*	4% pet.	1			
allyl cinnamate*	0.1% pet.				Test concentration slightly irritating
allyl cyclohexylacetate*	4% pet.	2			
allyl cyclohexylpropionate*	4% pet.	30			
allyl isovalerate*	1% pet.				
allyl phenoxyacetate*	1% pet.	1			
allyl phenylacetate*	1.5% pet.	1			Test concentration irritating. Sensitizer in HMT
allyl trimethylhexanoate	4% pet.	1			

(continued)

*__Note on allyl esters__: during human testing with allyl esters delayed type of irritation 2 or 3 days after exposure occasionally occured, which the investigators considered as sensitization. In every case this reaction has been traced to the presence of at least 0.1% of free allyl alcohol.
IFRA recommends only to use allyl esters when the level of free allyl alcohol in the ester is less than 0.1%.

§ **30.7** *(continuation)*

Name	Non-irritating patch test conc. (RIFM) (§ 30.6)	Quant. use (§ 30.6)	Patch test conc. & veh. (§ 30.1)	Cont. all. (§ 30.3)	Comment (N: § 30.6)
almond oil bitter	4% pet.		almond oil pure	+(?)	N. *See* § 5.39. Derived from *Prunus amygdalus amara* (Rosaceae)
			bitter almond oil 10% o.o.		Crude oil is toxic
almond oil bitter FFPA (= free of prussic acid)	4% pet.	50			N
almond oil sweet	4% pet.	1	1% alc./2% pet.[7], 1% pet. [17]		N
ambergris tincture	30% pet.				N
ambrette seed oil	1% pet.	1	1% alc./2% pet. [7], 1% pet. [17]		N
ambrettolide	1% pet.	1			
amyl benzoate	6% pet.	1			
amyl cinnamate	8% pet.	1	32% pet.	+	*See* § 5.14
amylcinnamic acetate	8% pet.				
α-amylcinnamic alcohol	8% pet.	10	2% pet.	+	*See* § 5.14
α-amylcinnamic aldehyde	6% pet.	800	2% pet.	+	*See* § 5.14
amylcinnamic aldehyde diethyl acetal	10% pet.	3			
α-amylcinnamic aldehyde dimethyl acetal	8% pet.	3			
amylcinnamylidene methylanthranilate	8% pet.	1			
4-*tert*-amylcyclohexanone	8% pet.	10			
amylcyclohexyl acetate (mixed isomers)	12% pet.				
amylcyclopentenone	1% pet.				Weak sensitizer in HMT; (IFRA 1987)
amyl formate	3% pet.	1			
amyl hexanoate	1% pet.				
amyl isoeugenol	8% pet.				
amyl salicylate	10% pet.	600	2% pet.		

(continued)

§ **30.7** *(continuation)*

Name	Non-irritating patch test conc. (RIFM) (§ 30.6)	Quant. use (§ 30.6)	Patch test conc. & veh. (§ 30.1)	Cont. all. (§ 30.3)	Comment (N: § 30.6)
amyl vinylcarbinol	10% pet.				
amyl vinyl carbinyl acetate	10% pet.	5			Sensitizer in HMT; (IFRA, July 1989: 1-Octen-3-yl acetate)
amyris oil acetylated	10% pet.	5	1% alc./2% pet. [7], 1% pet. [17]		N
anethole	2% pet.	16	2-5% pet.	+	*See* § 13.3
angelica root oil	1% pet.	1	2% pet.	+	*See* § 30.2 [23] N. Phototoxic; (IFRA, June 1975, October 1978)
angelica seed oil	1% pet.	1			N. Not phototoxic
anise oil	2% pet.	1	0.25% pet.	+	N. *See* § 13.3 Derived from *Pimpinella anisum* (Umbelliferae)
anise (star anise) oil	4% pet.	1	0.25% pet.	+	N. *See* § 13.3. Testing with star anise oil 1% may cause patch test sensitization and irritant patch test reactions. Lower test concentrations give false-negative results (§ 30.2, [24])
anisic aldehyde	10% pet.	50	5% pet.		
anisol	4% pet.	1	0.01% chloroform		
anisyl alcohol	5% pet.	5			
anisyl *n*-butyrate	8% pet.	1			
anisyl formate	4% pet.	1			
anisylidene acetone	2% pet.	1	2% pet. (fresh)	+	*See* § 5.14. Sensitizer in HMT; should not be used in fragrances (IFRA recommendation, November 1984)
anisyl phenylacetate	12% pet.	1			
anisyl propionate	4% pet.	1			

(continued)

§ **30.7** *(continuation)*

Name	Non-irritating patch test conc. (RIFM) (§ 30.6)	Quant. use (§ 30.6)	Patch test conc. & veh. (§ 30.1)	Cont. all. (§ 30.3)	Comment (N: § 30.6)
armoise oil	12% pet.	5	1% alc./2% pet. [7], 1% pet. [17]		N
artemisia oil (wormwood)	2% pet.	1	1% alc./2% pet. [7], 1% pet. [17]		N
baccartol	4% pet.				
balsam Canada	2% pet.	5	25% pet.		N
balsam Copaiba	8% pet.	40			N
balsam Peru	8% pet.		25% pet.	+	N. *See* § 5.14
balsam Tolu	2% pet.	20	20% pet.	+	N. *See* § 5.14
basil oil sweet	4% pet.	2	1% alc./2% pet. [17], 1% pet. [17]		N
bay oil	10% pet.	10	1% pet. [7]		N. Derived from *Pimenta acris* (Myrtaceae)
beeswax absolute	4% pet.		30% pet.	+	N. *See* § 5.38
benzaldehyde	4% pet.	75	5% pet.	+	*See* § 5.14
benzaldehyde dimethyl acetal	4% pet.	1			
benzaldehyde propylene glycol acetal	4% pet.				
benzal glyceryl acetal	4% pet.	1			
benzhydrol	5% pet.	1			
benzoin resinoid	8% pet.	100	10% pet or alc.	+	N. *See* § 5.38
benzonitrile	2% pet.				
benzophenone	6% pet.	100			*See* § 29.19
benzyl acetate	8% pet.	1000	as is [7]		
benzyl alcohol	10% pet.	250	5% pet.	+	*See* § 5.7 and § 5.14
benzyl benzoate	30% pet.	500	5% pet.	+	*See* § 5.40
benzyl butyrate	4% pet.	5			
benzyl cinnamate	8% pet.	20	5% pet.	+	*See* § 5.14
benzyl formate	10% pet.	2			

(continued)

§ 30.7 *(continuation)*

Name	Non-irritating patch test conc. (RIFM) (§ 30.6)	Quant. use (§ 30.6)	Patch test conc. & veh. (§ 30.1)	Cont. all. (§ 30.3)	Comment (N: § 30.6)
benzylidene acetone	2% pet.		0.5% pet.	+	*See* § 5.14. Sensitizer in HMT; should not be used in fragrances (IFRA recommendation, June 1984)
benzyl isoamyl ether	12% pet.	1			
benzyl isobutyrate	4% pet.	1			
benzyl isoeugenol	5% pet.	1			
benzyl isovalerate	4% pet.	1			
benzyl laurate	30% pet.	1			
benzyl phenylacetate	2% pet.	2			
benzyl propionate	4% pet.	8			
benzyl salicylate	30% pet.	300	1% pet.	+	*See* § 5.14
bergamot oil, expressed	30% pet.	300	5% pet.	+	N. Phototoxic; principal phototoxic compound is 5-MOP. *See* § 5.38, § 30.2 [23] and § 5.14 (IFRA, October 1974, June 1992)
bergamot oil, rectified	30% pet.				N. Free of furo-coumarines and non-volatile residues
birch tar oil	2% pet.	1	1% alc./2% pet. [7], 1% pet. [17]		N
bisabolene	10% pet.	1			
black pepper oil	4% pet.	10			N. Weakly phototoxic
bois de rose, acetylated	12% pet.	30	1% alc./2% pet. [7], 1% pet. [17]		N
bois de rose Brasilian	5% pet.	400	1% alc./2% pet. [7], 1% pet. [17]		N
boldo leaf oil	4% pet.	1			N
L-borneol	8% pet.	2			
L-bornyl acetate	2% pet.	3			
bornyl isovalerate	4% pet.	1			
bromstyrol	4% pet.	1			Strongly irritant

(continued)

§ **30.7** *(continuation)*

Name	Non-irritating patch test conc. (RIFM) (§ 30.6)	Quant. use (§ 30.6)	Patch test conc. & veh. (§ 30.1)	Cont. all. (§ 30.3)	Comment (N: § 30.6)
butyl acetate	4% pet.	8	25% o.o.	+	*See* § 30.2 [19] and § 5.43
n-butyl anthranilate	4% pet.	1			
butyl-*n*-butyrate	4% pet.	2			
butyl butyrolactate	4% pet.	1			
n-butyl cinnamate	4% pet.	1			
butyl cinnamic aldehyde	8% pet.	5			
4-*tert*-butylcyclohexanol	4% pet.	10			
2-*sec*-butylcyclohexanone (freskomenthe)	10% pet.				
p-*tert*-butylcyclohexanone	6% pet.				
2-*tert*-butylcyclohexyl acetate (Verdox®)	4% pet.				
4-*tert*-butylcyclohexyl acetate	4% pet.	300			
p-*tert*-butyldihydrocin-namaldehyde	6% pet.				(IFRA recommendation, April 1991)
6-butyl-2,4-dimethyldihy-dropyrane	10% pet.				
butyl isobutyrate	4% pet.	1			
n-butyl isovalerate	1% pet.	1			
butyl lactate	1% pet.	1			
p-*tert*-butyl-α-methyl-hydrocinnamic aldehyde (Lilial®)	4% pet.	1000	1% pet.	+	*See* § 5.14
butyl oleate	10% pet.	1			
p-*tert*-butylphenol	1% pet.	2			Sensitizer in HMT Causes depigmentation; should not be used in fragrances (IFRA rec-ommendation, June 1975)
3-butyl phthalide	2% pet.				
n-butyl propionate	2% pet.	1			
sec-butyl quinoline	2% pet.	4			

(continued)

§ **30.7** *(continuation)*

Name	Non-irritating patch test conc. (RIFM) (§ 30.6)	Quant. use (§ 30.6)	Patch test conc. & veh. (§ 30.1)	Cont. all. (§ 30.3)	Comment (N: § 30.6)
n-butyl salicylate	2% pet.	1			
2-butyl-4,4,6-trimethyl-1,3-dioxane (herboxane)	20% pet.				
butyl undecylenate	8% pet.	1			
n-butyraldehyde	1% pet.	0.5			
n-butyric acid	1% pet.				
cabreuva oil	6% pet.	1	1% alc./2% pet. [7], 1% pet. [17]		N
cade oil rectified (juniper tar)	2% pet.	1	3% pet.		N (IFRA, July 1990)
cadinene	10% pet.	4	1% pet. [7]		
cajeput oil	4% pet.	1	1% alc./2% pet. [7], 1% pet. [17]		N
calamus oil	4% pet.	2	1% alc./2% pet. [7], 1% pet. [17]		N
camphene	4% pet.	6			
camphor oil brown	4% pet.	1	camphor oil 10% pet.		N
camphor oil yellow	4% pet.	20	camphor oil 10% pet.		N
camphor oil white	20% pet.	15	camphor oil 10% pet.		N
camphor USP	4% pet.		10% pet.	+	N. *See* § 5.41
cananga oil	10% pet.	2	2% pet.	+	N. *See* § 5.14 and § 30.2 [23]
capric acid	1% pet.	1			
caprylic acid	1% pet.				
caraway oil	4% pet.		caraway seed oil 25% c.o.		N. Derived from *Carum carvi* (Umbelliferae)
cardamom oil	4% pet.	2	1% alc./2% pet. [7], 1% pet. [17]		N. Derived from *Elettaria cardomomum* (Zingiberaceae)
δ-carene	10% pet.				Weakly phototoxic

(continued)

§ **30.7** *(continuation)*

Name	Non-irritating patch test conc. (RIFM) (§ 30.6)	Quant. use (§ 30.6)	Patch test conc. & veh. (§ 30.1)	Cont. all. (§ 30.3)	Comment (N: § 30.6)
carrot seed oil	4% pet.	1	1% alc./2% pet. [7], 1% pet. [17]		
carvacrol	4% pet.	2	5% pet.	+	*See* § 5.14
L-carveol	4% pet.	1		,	
D-carvone	2% pet.	3	carvone 2-5% pet.	+	*See* § 13.3. Sensitizer in HMT
L-carvone	1% pet.	2	carvone 2-5% pet.	+	*See* § 13.3. Sensitizer in HMT
carvone oxide	–				Sensitizer in HMT (IFRA, October 1979)
L-carvyl acetate	4% pet.	1			
L-carvyl propionate	4% pet.	1			
caryophyllene	4% pet.	20	5% pet.		
caryophyllene acetate	4% pet.	4			
caryophyllene alcohol	4% pet.	5			
cascarilla oil	4% pet.	1	1% alc./2% pet. [7], 1% pet. [17		N
cassia oil	4% pet.	9	2% pet.	+	N. Sensitizer due to cinnamic aldehyde. *See* § 30.2 [23] Weakly phototoxic; (IFRA, October 1974, October 1980)
castoreum	4% pet.	20	1% alc./2% pet. [7], 1% pet. [17]		N
cedar leaf oil	4% pet.	10			N
cedarwood oil Atlas	8% pet.	25	cedarwood oil 10% o.o. [7]; 10% pet.		N
cedarwood oil Texas	6% pet.	25	cedarwood oil 10% o.o. [7]; 10% pet.		N
cedarwood oil Virginia	8% pet.	100	cedarwood oil 10% o.o. [7]; 10% pet.		N
α-cedrene	5% pet.				
cedr-8-ene epoxide	10% pet.				

(continued)

§ **30.7** *(continuation)*

Name	Non-irritating patch test conc. (RIFM) (§ 30.6)	Quant. use (§ 30.6)	Patch test conc. & veh. (§ 30.1)	Cont. all. (§ 30.3)	Comment (N: § 30.6)
cedrenol	8% pet.	8			
cedrenone	20% pet.	1			
cedrenyl acetate	8% pet.	45			
cedrol	8% pet.	50			
cedrol methyl ether	8% pet.	1			
cedryl acetate	8% pet.	100			
cedryl formate	12% pet.	5			
celery seed oil	4% pet.	2	1% alc./2% pet. [7], 1% pet. [17]		N
cetyl alcohol	12% pet.	1	20% pet.	+	*See* § 5.20
chamomile oil German	4% pet.	1	chamomile as is; chamomile oil 25% o.o.		N. *See also* § 5.39 Derived from *Anthemis nobilis* (Compositae)
chamomile oil Roman	4% pet.	3			
chenopodium oil	4% pet.	1	1% alc./2% pet. [7], 1% pet. [17]		N
1,4-cineole (eucalyptol)	16% pet.		5% pet.	+	*See* index
cinnamic acid	4% pet.	1	1–5% pet. [7]		
cinnamic alcohol	4% pet.	150	2% pet.	+	*See* § 5.14 (IFRA, October 1978, June 1992)
cinnamic aldehyde		100	1% pet.	+	*See* § 5.14. Sensitizer in HMT (IFRA, October 1975, March 1978, February 1980)
cinnamic aldehyde dimethyl acetal	10% pet.				
cinnamic aldehyde methyl anthranilate	12% pet.	1			Sensitizer in HMT; (IFRA, June, 1979, May 1983)
cinnamon bark oil Ceylon	8% pet.	4	2% pet.	+	N. *See* § 5.14 *under* cinnamon oil. Derived from *Cinnamomum cassia* (Lauraceae). Sensitizer due to cinnamic aldehyde. Weakly phototoxic. (IFRA, October 1974, October 1978, October 1980)

(continued)

§ **30.7** *(continuation)*

Name	Non-irritating patch test conc. (RIFM) (§ 30.6)	Quant. use (§ 30.6)	Patch test conc. & veh. (§ 30.1)	Cont. all. (§ 30.3)	Comment (N: § 30.6)
cinnamon leaf oil Ceylon	10% pet.	4	2% pet.	+	N. *See* § 5.14 *under* cinnamon oil
cinnamyl acetate	5% pet.	5			
cinnamyl anthranilate	4% pet.	1			Carcinogenic (?)
cinnamyl benzoate	5% pet.	1	10% pet.	+	*See* § 5.14
cinnamyl butyrate	4% pet.	1			
cinnamyl cinnamate	4% pet.	1	8% pet.	+	*See* § 5.14
cinnamyl formate	4% pet.	1			
cinnamyl isobutyrate	4% pet.	1			
cinnamyl isovalerate	2% pet.	1			
cinnamyl nitrile	4% pet.				
cinnamyl propionate	4% pet.	1			
cinnamyl tigliate	4% pet.	1			
citral		75	2% pet. (fresh)	+	*See* § 5.14. Sensitizer in HMT (IFRA, October 1975, February 1980)
citral dimethyl acetal	4% pet.	50			
citral ethylene glycol acetal	5% pet.				
citral methyl anthranilate	12% pet.	1			
citronella oil	8% pet.	400	2% pet.	+	N. *See* § 5.14
citronellal	4% pet.	4	2–4% pet.	+	*See* § 5.14
citronellic acid	2% pet.	1			
citronellol	6% pet.	150	1–2% pet.	+	*See* § 27.3
citronellyl acetate	4% pet.	20			
citronellyl *n*-butyrate	5% pet.	1			
citronellyl crotonate	8% pet.	1			
citronellyl ethyl ether	4% pet.	1			
citronellyl formate	4% pet.	40			
citronellyl isobutyrate	4% pet.				
citronellyl nitrile	6% pet.	5			

(continued)

§ **30.7** *(continuation)*

Name	Non-irritating patch test conc. (RIFM) (§ 30.6)	Quant. use (§ 30.6)	Patch test conc. & veh. (§ 30.1)	Cont. all. (§ 30.3)	Comment (N: § 30.6)
citronellyl oxyacetaldehyde	8% pet.	4	1% pet.		
citronellyl phenylacetate	4% pet.	1			
citronellyl propionate	4% pet.	2			
civet absolute	4% pet.	3.5			N
civetone	4% pet.	1			
clary sage oil	8% pet.	10	2% pet.	+	N. *See* § 30.2 [23]
clove bud oil	5% pet.	100	clove oil 2% pet.	+	N
clove leaf oil Madagascar	5% pet.	30	clove oil 2% pet.	+	N. *See* § 30.2, [19] *and* [23]. Derived from *Eugenia caryophyllus* (Myrtaceae)
clove stem oil	10% pet.	40	clove oil 2% pet.	+	N
cognac oil green	4% pet.	1	1% alc./2% pet. [7], 1% pet. [17]		N
coniferyl alcohol			2% pet.	+	*See* § 5.14
copaiba oil	8% pet.	33	1% alc./2% pet. [7], 1% pet. [17]		N
coriander oil	6% pet.	10	2% pet.	+	N. *See* § 30.2, [23]
corn mint oil	8% pet.	1	1% alc./2% pet. [7], 1% pet. [17]		N
costus root essential oil, absolute and concrete	4% pet.	1	1% pet.	+	N. *See* § 5.14. Sensitizer in HMT; (IFRA, October 1974, June 1982)
coumarin	8% pet.	250	5% pet.	+	*See* § 5.14
p-cresol	4% pet.	2			
p-cresyl acetate	4% pet.	1			
p-cresyl caprylate	4% pet.	1			
p-cresyl isobutyrate	4% pet.	1			
p-cresyl methyl ether	2% pet.	10			
p-cresyl phenylacetate	4% pet.	2			
cubeb oil	8% pet.	1	1% alc./2% pet. [7], 1% pet. [17]		N

(continued)

§ **30.7** *(continuation)*

Name	Non-irritating patch test conc. (RIFM) (§ 30.6)	Quant. use (§ 30.6)	Patch test conc. & veh. (§ 30.1)	Cont. all. (§ 30.3)	Comment (N: § 30.6)
cuminaldehyde	4% pet.	3	15 % pet.	+	*See* § 5.14
cumin oil	4% pet.	2	1% alc./2% pet. [7], 1% pet. [17]		N. Weakly phototoxic; (IFRA, October 1975, June 1986)
cuminyl alcohol	4% pet.	2			
cyclamen alcohol	20% pet.				Sensitizer in HMT; should not be used as such in fragrances (IFRA recommendation, November 1977, October 1978, February 1980)
cyclamen aldehyde	3% pet.	150			
cyclamen aldehyde diethyl acetal	24% pet.				
cyclamen aldehyde dimethyl acetal	24% pet.	1			
cyclamen aldehyde ethyleneglycol acetal	24% pet.	1			
cyclamen aldehyde methylanthranilate	6% pet.				
cyclamen aldehyde propyleneglycol acetal	24% pet.				
cyclohexanol	4% pet.				
cyclohexyl acetate	4% pet.	1			
cyclohexyl butyrate	4% pet.				
2-cyclohexyl cyclohexanone	20% pet.	35			
cyclohexylethyl acetate	4% pet.				
cyclohexylethyl alcohol	4% pet.				
cyclopentadecanolide	10% pet.	3			
cyclopentadecanone	10% pet.	1			
cyclopentanone	10% pet.	1			
cyclopentenyl propionate musk	20% pet.				
p-cymene	4% pet.	9	1% pet.		

(continued)

§ 30.7 *(continuation)*

Name	Non-irritating patch test conc. (RIFM) (§ 30.6)	Quant. use (§ 30.6)	Patch test conc. & veh. (§ 30.1)	Cont. all. (§ 30.3)	Comment (N: § 30.6)
cypress oil	5% pet.	1	1% alc./2% pet. [7], 1% pet. [17]		N
cyste absolute	4% pet.	1			N
davana oil	4% pet.	1	1% alc./2% pet. [7], 1% pet. [17]		N
2,4-decadienal	5% pet.	1			
decahydro-β-naphthol	2% pet.	4			
decahydro-β-naphthyl acetate	12% pet.	1			
decahydro-β-naphthyl formate	12% pet.	1			
γ-decalactone	10% pet.	1			
δ-decalactone	1% pet.	1			
decanal dimethylacetal	4% pet.	1			
2-decen-1-al	4% pet.				
cis-4-decen-1-al	1% pet.	1			
9-decenyl acetate	12% pet.	1			
decylenic alcohol	2% pet.	20			
decyl methyl ether	4% pet.	1			
decyl vinylether (decave)	12% pet.				
deertongue absolute	5% pet.	1			N
deertongue incolore	5% pet.	1			N
deobase (deodorized kerosine)	12% pet.	150			
diacetyl	2% pet.	1	1% aqua		
diallyl disulfide	1% pet.				Patch tested 5% pet. in 23 garlic sensitive patients produced 18 reactions. No reactions were observed with 0.5% pet.

(continued)

§ **30.7** *(continuation)*

Name	Non-irritating patch test conc. (RIFM) (§ 30.6)	Quant. use (§ 30.6)	Patch test conc. & veh. (§ 30.1)	Cont. all. (§ 30.3)	Comment (N: § 30.6)
diallyl sulfide	0.5% pet.				Patch tested 5% pet. in 23 garlic sensitive patients produced no reactions
dibenzyl	8% pet.				
dibenzyl ether	4% pet.	1	2% euc. anh.		
dibutyl sulfide	8% pet.	1			
diethylene glycol monoethyl ether	20% pet.	5			
diethylene glycol monomethyl ether	20% pet.	5			
diethyl ketone	4% pet.				
diethyl maleate	4% pet.	1			Sensitizer in HMT; should not be used in fragrances (IFRA recommendation, June 1975)
diethyl malonate	4% pet.	1			
diethyl sebacate	4% pet.	1	20% alc.	+	*See* § 5.20 and § 5.14
diethyl succinate	4% pet.	1			
dihexyl fumarate	4% pet.	1			
dihydroanethole	10% pet.	1			
dihydrocarveol	4% pet.	1			
dihydrocarvone	20% pet.	1			
dihydrocoumarin	20% pet.	10	5% pet.	+	*See* § 5.14. Sensitizer in HMT; should not be used in fragrances (IFRA, recommendation, October 1974)
dihydroeugenol	8% pet.	2			
6,7-dihydrogeraniol	10% DEP	0			Sensitizer in HMT and human repeated insult patch test; should not be used in fragrances (IFRA recommendation, April 1989)
dihydro-α-ionone	12% pet.	1			

(continued)

§ **30.7** *(continuation)*

Name	Non-irritating patch test conc. (RIFM) (§ 30.6)	Quant. use (§ 30.6)	Patch test conc. & veh. (§ 30.1)	Cont. all. (§ 30.3)	Comment (N: § 30.6)
dihydro-isojasmone	4% pet.	1			
dihydrojasmone	4% pet.	1			
dihydromethyl-α-ionone	4% pet.	2			
dihydromyrcenol	4% pet.	1			
dihydrosafrole	12% pet.	2			
dihydro-α-terpineol	10% pet.	1			
dihydroterpinyl acetate	12% pet.	10			
2,4-dihydroxy-3-methyl-benzaldehyde	4% pet.				Sensitizer in HMT; should not be used in fragrances (IFRA recommendation, October 1980)
dill seed oil, Indian	4% pet.	1	1% alc./2% pet. [7], 1% pet. [17]		N
dill weed oil	4% pet.	1	1% alc./2% pet. [7], 1% pet. [17]		N
dimethyl anthranilate	10% pet.	1			Phototoxic
2,4-dimethylbenzyl acetate	3% pet.				
dimethylbenzyl carbinol	8% pet.	2			
dimethylbenzyl carbinyl acetate	4% pet.	50			
dimethylbenzyl carbinyl butyrate	10% pet.	1			
dimethylbenzyl carbinyl propionate	10% pet.	1			
4,6-dimethyl-8-*tert*-butyl-coumarin	8% pet.				Photoallergic; should not be used in fragrances (IFRA recommendation, February 1979, June 1981)
dimethyl carbonate	4% pet.	1			
dimethyl citraconate	12% pet.				Sensitizer in HMT; should not be used in fragrances (IFRA recommendation, October 1976)

(continued)

§ **30.7** *(continuation)*

Name	Non-irritating patch test conc. (RIFM) (§ 30.6)	Quant. use (§ 30.6)	Patch test conc. & veh. (§ 30.1)	Cont. all. (§ 30.3)	Comment (N: § 30.6)
7,11 dimethyl-4,6,10-dodecatrien-3-one (pseudo methylionone)	8% pet.				Sensitizer in HMT; should not be used in fragrances (IFRA recommendation, February 1979, October 1979, April 1989)
α,α-dimethyl-*p*-ethyl-phenylpropanal	3% pet.				
dimethylheptenal	4% pet.	3			
2,6-dimethyl-2-heptanol	10% pet.				*Syn*: freesiol, lolitol
dimethylheptenol	10% pet.	1			
dimethylhydroquinone	4% pet.	2			
dimethylionone	4% pet.				
dimethyl malonate	8% pet.	1			
3,7-dimethyl-7-methoxy-octan-2-ol	10% pet.				*Syn*: osirol
3,7-dimethyl-2,6-nonadienenitrile	6% pet.				*Syn*: lemonile
3,6-dimethyl-3-octanol	20% pet.	200			
3,7-dimethyl-1-octanol	8% pet.	10	2% pet. [7]		
3,6-dimethyloctan-3-yl acetate	20% pet.	30			
3,7-dimethyloctanyl acetate	8% pet.	3			
3,7-dimethyloctanyl butyrate	10% pet.	1			
2,6-dimethyl-2,4,6-octatriene	1% pet.				
dimethylphenylcarbinol	4% pet.	1			
dimethylphenylethyl carbinol	4% pet.	7			
dimethylphenylethyl carbinyl acetate	4% pet.	1			
dimethyl succinate	4% pet.	2			

(continued)

§ **30.7** *(continuation)*

Name	Non-irritating patch test conc. (RIFM) (§ 30.6)	Quant. use (§ 30.6)	Patch test conc. & veh. (§ 30.1)	Cont. all. (§ 30.3)	Comment (N: § 30.6)
dimethyl sulfide	1% pet.	1			
6,10-dimethyl-3,5,9-undecatriene-2-one (pseudoionone)	8% pet.				Pseudoionone. Sensitizer in HMT; should not be used in fragrances as such; acceptable as impurity in ionones (IFRA recommendation, February 1979, July 1987, April 1989)
dimyrcetol	4% pet.	3			
dimethyltetrahydrobenz-aldehyde (mixed isomers)	4% pet.				
dipentene (D,L-limonene)	20% pet.	1	2% pet.		
diphenylamine	1% pet.	1			
diphenylmethane	8% pet.	4			
diphenyl oxide	4% pet.	100			
dipropylene glycol	20% pet.	50			
γ-dodecalactone	12% pet.				
δ-dodecalactone	12% pet.	1			
eau de brouts absolute	4% pet.	1	1% alc./2% pet. [7], 1% pet. [17]		N
elemi oil	4% pet.	1	1% alc./2% pet. [7], 1% pet. [17]		N
estragon oil	4% pet.	2	1% alc./2% pet. [7], 1% pet. [17]		N
p-ethoxybenzaldehyde	4% pet.	1			
7-ethoxy-3,7-dimethyl-octanal	4% pet.				
ethyl acetate	10% pet.	2	10% pet.		
ethyl acetoacetate	8% pet.	8			
ethyl acetoacetate ethylene glycolketal	20% pet.				

(continued)

§ **30.7** *(continuation)*

Name	Non-irritating patch test conc. (RIFM) (§ 30.6)	Quant. use (§ 30.6)	Patch test conc. & veh. (§ 30.1)	Cont. all. (§ 30.3)	Comment (N: § 30.6)
ethyl acrylate	4% pet.	1			Sensitizer in HMT; should not be used in fragrances (IFRA recommendation, November 1974)
ethyl amyl ketone	2% pet.	2			
ethyl anisate	4% pet.	1			
ethyl anthranilate	4% pet.	1			
ethyl benzene	10% pet.				
ethyl benzoate	8% pet.	5			
ethyl butyl ketone	4% pet.	1			
ethyl butyrate	5% pet.	51			
ethyl caprate	2% pet.	1			
ethyl caproate	4% pet.	3			
ethyl caprylate	2% pet.	1			
ethyl cellulose	12% DEP	1			
ethyl cinnamate	4% pet.	1			
ethyl citral	4% pet.	1			
ethyl crotonate	4% pet.	1			
ethyl *trans*-2,*cis*-4-decadienoate	3% pet				
ethylene brassylate	30% pet.	2000			
ethylene dodecanedioate (Arova 16®: Musk 144®)	20% pet.				
ethyl formate	4% pet.	3			
ethyl heptoate	4% pet.	1			
2-ethylhexanal	2% pet.				
2-ethylhexanol	4% pet.	25			
2-ethyl hexyl acetate	4% pet.	10			
ethyl hexyl palmitate	4% pet.	1			
ethyl hexyl salicylate	4% pet.	1			

(continued)

§ 30.7 *(continuation)*

Name	Non-irritating patch test conc. (RIFM) (§ 30.6)	Quant. use (§ 30.6)	Patch test conc. & veh. (§ 30.1)	Cont. all. (§ 30.3)	Comment (N: § 30.6)
ethyl isobutyrate	8% pet.	1			
ethyl isovalerate	2% pet.	1			
ethyl lactate	8% pet.	10			
ethyl laevulinate	4% pet.	<1			
ethyl laurate	12% pet.	1			
ethyl linalool	30% pet.	2			
ethyl linalyl acetate	4% pet.	<1			
ethyl maltol	10% pet.				
ethyl 2-methoxybenzyl ether	4% pet.				
ethyl methylphenyl-glycidate	1% pet.	5			
ethyl myristate	12% pet.	1			
ethyl octine carbonate	2% pet.				
ethyl oleate	8% pet.	<1			
ethyl pelargonate	12% pet.	1			
ethyl phenylacetate	8% pet.	2			
ethyl phenylglycidate	4% pet.	2			
ethyl propionate	2% pet.	16			
ethyl salicylate	12% pet.	5			
ethyl stearate	12% pet.	1			
ethyl tiglate	5% pet.				
ehtyl undecylenate	8% pet.	<1			
ethyl vanillin	2% pet.	28	10% pet.		
eucalyptol	16% pet.	5	5% o.o	+	*See also* 1,4-cineole
eucalyptus oil	10% pet.	32	2% pet.	+	N. *See* § 30.2, [23]. Derived from *Eucalyptus* sp. (Myrtaceaes)
eucalyptus citriodora oil	10% pet.		1% alc./2% pet. [7], 1% pet. [17]		N

(continued)

§ **30.7** *(continuation)*

Name	Non-irritating patch test conc. (RIFM) (§ 30.6)	Quant. use (§ 30.6)	Patch test conc. & veh. (§ 30.1)	Cont. all. (§ 30.3)	Comment (N: § 30.6)
eucalyptus citriodora oil, acetylated (Citrodyle®)	10% pet.		1% alc./2% pet. [7], 1% pet. [17]		
eugenol	8% pet.	100	2% pet.	+	*See* § 5.14
eugenyl acetate	20% pet.	5			
eugenyl formate	12% pet.	<1			
eugenyl phenylacetate	12% pet.	1			
farnesol	not yet published		4% pet.	+	*See* § 5.14. Sensitizer, if not sufficiently pure. (IFRA, October 1979, February 1980)
fenchone	4% pet.	1			
fenchyl acetate	5% pet.	1			
fenchyl alcohol	4% pet.	1			
fennel oil	4% pet.	4	1% alc./2% pet. [7], 1% pet. [17]		N
fennel oil bitter	4% pet.	1	1% alc./2% pet. [7], 1% pet. [17]		N
fenugreek absolute	2% pet.	1			N
fig leaf absolute	5% pet.	<1			N. Sensitizer; extremely phototoxic; should not be used in fragrances (IFRA recommendation, October 1980, May 1983)
fir balsam Oregon	8% pet.	1			N
fir needle oil Canadian	10% pet.	35	1% alc./2% pet. [7], 1% pet. [17]		N
fir needle oil Siberian	2-5% pet.	35	1% alc./2% pet. [7], 1% pet. [17]		N
flouve oil	4% pet.	1	1% alc./2% pet. [7], 1% pet. [17]		N
foin absolute	4% pet.	1			N
formaldehyde cyclododecyl ethylacetal (Boisambrene Forte®)	2% pet.				

(continued)

§ 30.7 *(continuation)*

Name	Non-irritating patch test conc. (RIFM) (§ 30.6)	Quant. use (§ 30.6)	Patch test conc. & veh. (§ 30.1)	Cont. all. (§ 30.3)	Comment (N: § 30.6)
formaldehyde cyclododecyl methylacetal (Boisambrene®)	2% pet.				
2-formyl-6,6-dimethyl-bicyclo [3.1.1] hept-2-ene (Myrtenal®)	1% pet.				
1-formyl-1-methyl-4(4-methylpentyl)-3-cyclo-hexene (Vernaldehyde®)	4% pet.				
furfural	2% pet.	1			
galbanum oil	4% pet.	15	10% alc. 1-2% pet. [7, 17]		N
galbanum resin (ferula resin)	8% pet.				N
genet absolute	12% pet.	1			N
geranial	1% pet.		1-5% pet.	+	*See* § 5.14. Sensitizer in HMT
geranic acid	4% pet.	1			
geraniol	6% pet.	800	2% pet.	+	*See* § 5.14. Sensitizer in HMT
geranium oil Algerian	10% pet.	100	2% pet.		N
geranium oil Bourbon	10% pet.	100	2% pet.	+	N. *See* § 5.14 *and* § 30.2, [23]
geranium oil Moroccan	10% pet.	100	2% pet.		N
geranyl acetate	4% pet.	100			
geranyl acetoacetate	4% pet.				
geranyl acetone	10% pet.	1			
geranyl benzoate	2% pet.	2			
geranyl butyrate	4% pet.	2			
geranyl caproate	6% pet.				
geranyl crotonate	10% pet.	1			
geranyl ethyl ether	4% pet.	<1			
geranyl formate	2% pet.	10			

(continued)

§ **30.7** *(continuation)*

Name	Non-irritating patch test conc. (RIFM) (§ 30.6)	Quant. use (§ 30.6)	Patch test conc. & veh. (§ 30.1)	Cont. all. (§ 30.3)	Comment (N: § 30.6)
geranyl isobutyrate	10% pet.	1			
geranyl isovalerate	2% pet.	6			
geranyl linalool	1% pet.				
geranyl nitrile	12% pet.				
geranyl oxyacetaldehyde	4% pet.	1			
geranyl phenylacetate	4% pet.	5			
geranyl propionate	4% pet.	5			
geranyl tiglate	6% pet.	1			
ginger oil	4% pet.	2	1% pet. [7]		N. Weakly phototoxic Derived from *Zingiber officinale* (Zingiberaceae)
grapefruit oil, expressed	10% pet.	18	1% alc./2% pet. [7], 1% pet. [17]		N. May contain bergapten (IFRA, June 1992). Derived from *Citrus paradisi* (Rutaceae)
grisalva	1% pet.				N
guaiacol	2% pet.	<1	guaiacol 2-5% pet.		N
guaiac wood acetate	8% pet.	30	guaiacol 2-5% pet.		
guaiac wood oil	8% pet.	50	guaiacol 2-5% pet.	+	N. *See* § 30.2, [23]
guaiene	2% pet.				
gurjun balsam	12% pet.	1			N
gurjun oil	8% pet.	1	1% alc./2% pet. [7], 1% pet. [17]		N
helichrysum oil	4% pet.	1	1% alc./2% pet. [7], 1% pet. [17]		N
heliotropin (piperonal)	6% pet.	150	2-5% pet.	+	*See* § 30.2, [22]
γ-heptalactone	4% pet.	<4			Weak sensitizer in HMT
trans-2-heptenal	4% pet.				Sensitizer in HMT; should not be used in fragrances (IFRA recommendation, February 1985, April 1989)

(continued)

§ 30.7 *(continuation)*

Name	Non-irritating patch test conc. (RIFM) (§ 30.6)	Quant. use (§ 30.6)	Patch test conc. & veh. (§ 30.1)	Cont. all. (§ 30.3)	Comment (N: § 30.6)
heptyl butyrate	1% pet.				
2-*n*-heptyl cyclopentanone	10% pet.	1			
heptyl formate	12% pet.	1			
heptylidene methyl anthranilate	12% pet.	<1			
2-heptyltetrahydrofuran	6% pet.				
hexadecanolide	4% pet.	1			
2,4-hexadienyl isobutyrate	4% pet.				
hexahydrocoumarin	–				Sensitizer in HMT; should not be used in fragrances (IFRA recommendation, February 1980)
trans,trans-2,4-hexadienal	1% pet.				Weak sensitizer in HMT
1,3,4,6,7,8-hexahydro-4,6,6,7,8,8-hexamethyl-cyclopenta-γ-2-benzopyran (Galaxolide®)	15% pet.	50	25% pet.	+	*See* § 5.14 *under* galaxolide
γ-hexalactone	12% pet.	1			
δ-hexalactone	4% pet.	<1			Weak sensitizer in HMT
hexanoic acid	1% pet.				
trans-2-hexenal	0.2% pet.				Sensitizer in HMT (IFRA, April 1989, June 1992)
cis-3-hexenal	2% pet.				
hexen-2-al	4% pet.	1			
trans-3-hexenal	2% pet. (tested as 4% in pet. of a 50% solution in triacitin)				
trans-2-hexenal diethylacetal	8% pet. 4% pet.				Sensitizer in HMT; should not be used in fragrances (IFRA recommendation, February 1985, April 1989)

(continued)

§ **30.7** *(continuation)*

Name	Non-irritating patch test conc. (RIFM) (§ 30.6)	Quant. use (§ 30.6)	Patch test conc. & veh. (§ 30.1)	Cont. all. (§ 30.3)	Comment (N: § 30.6)
trans-2-hexenal dimethylacetal	8% pet.				Sensitizer in HMT; should not be used in fragrances (IFRA recommendation, February 1985, April 1989)
cis-3-hexenol	4% pet.	20			
trans-2-hexenol	4% pet.	3			
2-hexenyl acetate	10% pet.	1			
cis-3-hexenyl acetate	10% pet.	2			
cis-3-hexenyl anthranilate	10% pet.	<1			
cis-3-hexenyl benzoate	10% pet.	1			
hexenyl cyclopentanone	10% pet.				
5-(*cis*-3-hexenyl)dihydro-5-methyl-2(3H)-furanone)	2% pet.				
cis-3-hexenyl formate	10% pet.	1			
cis-3-hexenyl hexanoate	2% pet.				
cis-3-hexenyl isobutyrate	10% pet.	1			
cis-3-hexenyl oxyacetaldehyde	4% pet.	1			
cis-3-hexenyl phenyl acetate	10% pet.	1			
cis-3-hexenyl propionate	10% pet.	1			
trans-2-hexenyl propionate	10% pet.	1			
cis-3-hexenyl salicylate	3% pet.		3% pet.	+	*See* § 5.14
cis-3-hexenyl tiglate	12% pet.	1			
cis-3-hexenyl valerate	2% pet.				
hexoxyacetaldehyde dimethylacetal	10% pet.	1			
hexyl acetate	4% pet.	1			
hexyl benzoate	3% pet.	5			

(continued)

§ **30.7** *(continuation)*

Name	Non-irritating patch test conc. (RIFM) (§ 30.6)	Quant. use (§ 30.6)	Patch test conc. & veh. (§ 30.1)	Cont. all. (§ 30.3)	Comment (N: § 30.6)
hexyl butyrate	12% pet.	1			
hexyl caproate	1% pet.	1			
hexyl caprylate	4% pet.				
hexylcinnamic aldehyde	12% pet.	300	2% pet.	+	§ 5.14
hexyl crotonate	10% pet.	<1			
2-hexyl cyclopentanone	10% pet.				Test concentration slightly irritating
2-hexyl-2-decenal	10% pet.	<1			
hexyl ethyl acetoacetate	4% pet.	1			
hexyl formate	4% pet.				
hexyl isobutyrate	4% pet.	5			
hexyl isovalerate	4% pet.				
hexyl 2-methylbutyrate	10% pet.	<1			
hexyl neopentanoate	4% pet.	<1			
hexyl propionate	12% pet.				
hexyl salicylate	3% pet.				
hexyl tiglate	12% pet.	1			
hibawood oil	12% pet.	1	1% alc./2% pet. [7], 1% pet. [17]		N
ho leaf oil	10% pet.	50	1% alc./2% pet. [7], 1% pet. [17]		N
honeysuckle absolute	3% pet.				N
hyacinth absolute	8% pet.	1			N
hydratropic acetate	12% pet.	1			
hydratropic alcohol	6% pet.	1			
hydratropic aldehyde	2% pet.	25			
hydratropic aldehyde dimethyl acetal	4% pet.	1			

(continued)

§ **30.7** *(continuation)*

Name	Non-irritating patch test conc. (RIFM) (§ 30.6)	Quant. use (§ 30.6)	Patch test conc. & veh. (§ 30.1)	Cont. all. (§ 30.3)	Comment (N: § 30.6)
hydroabietyl alcohol (Abitol®)	10% pet.	9	10% pet.	+	Sensitizer in HMT; should not be used in fragrances (IFRA recommendation, October 1974, May 1976) *See* § 27.11
hydroxycitronellal	5% pet.	500	1% pet.	+	*See* § 5.14; (IFRA, March 1987)
hydroxycitronellal dimethylacetal	10% pet.	4			
hydroxycitronellal methylanthranilate	6% pet.	20			
hydroxycitronellol	10% pet.	1			
3- and 4-(4-hydroxy-4-methylpentyl)-3-cyclo-hexene-1-carboxaldehyde (Lyral®)	10% pet.				
4-(*p*-hydroxyphenyl)-2-butanone	12% pet.	1			
hyssop oil	4% pet.	1	1% alc./2% pet. [7], 1% pet. [17]		N
immortelle absolute	2% pet.	1			N
indole	1% pet.	4			
α-ionol	8% pet.				
β-ionol	8% pet.				
ionone	8% pet.	200	2% pet.	+	*See* § 5.14
α-ionyl acetate	8% pet.				
α-irone	10% pet.	1			
isoamyl alcohol	8% pet.	1			
isoamyl butyrate	3% pet.	2			
isoamyl caproate	2% pet.	1			
isoamyl caprylate	2% pet.	1			
isoamyl formate	3% pet.	1			
isoamyl geranate	8% pet.	1			

(continued)

§ 30.7 *(continuation)*

Name	Non-irritating patch test conc. (RIFM) (§ 30.6)	Quant. use (§ 30.6)	Patch test conc. & veh. (§ 30.1)	Cont. all. (§ 30.3)	Comment (N: § 30.6)
isoamyl isovalerate	2% pet.	1			
isoamyl phenylacetate	2% pet.	1			
isoamyl propionate	4% pet.	1			
isoborneol	10% pet.	10			
isobornyl acetate	10% pet.	200			
isobornyl formate	2% pet.	1			
isobornyl methyl ether	10% pet.				
isobornyl propionate	10% pet.	2			
isobutyl acetate	2% pet.	5			
isobutyl benzoate	2% pet.	2			
isobutyl butyrate	12% pet.	1			
isobutyl caproate	20% pet.	1			
isobutyl cinnamate	8% pet.	1			
isobutyl furylpropionate	2% pet.	1			
isobutyl heptylate	2% pet.	1			
isobutyl isovalerate	1% pet.	<1			
isobutyl linalool	20% pet.	1			
isobutyl phenylacetate	4% pet.	1			
isobutyl quinoline	2% pet.	2			
isobutyl salicylate	10% pet.	3			
isocamphyl cyclohexanol (mixed isomers)	20% pet.	25			
isocyclocitral	4% pet.	1			
isoeugenol	8% pet.	40	2% pet.	+	*See* § 5.14; (IFRA, May 1980, June 1982)
isoeugenyl acetate	10% pet.	1			
isohexenyl cyclohexenyl carboxaldehyde	3% pet.	12			
isojasmone	8% pet.	2			
isomenthone	8% pet.	3			

(continued)

§ **30.7** *(continuation)*

Name	Non-irritating patch test conc. (RIFM) (§ 30.6)	Quant. use (§ 30.6)	Patch test conc. & veh. (§ 30.1)	Cont. all. (§ 30.3)	Comment (N: § 30.6)
2-isopropenyl-5-methyl-4-hexen-1-ol	5% pet.				
p-isopropylbenzyl acetate	12% pet.				
isopropyl cinnamate	6% pet.				
p-isopropylcyclohexanol	5% pet.	1			
6-isopropyl-2-decahydro-naphthalenol	4% pet. 10% pet. 2% DMP				Sensitizer in HMT
6-isopropyl-2-decalol	–				Sensitizer in HMT; should not be used in fragrances (IFRA recommendation, June 1979, April 1989)
2-isopropyl-5-methyl-2-hexene-1-al	10% pet.	1			
2-isopropyl-5-methyl-2-hexene-1-ol	10% pet.	5			
2-isopropyl-5-methyl-2-hexene-1-yl acetate	10% pet.	20			
4-isopropyl-1-methyl-2-propenylbenzene	6% pet.				
isopropyl myristate (IPM)	20% pet.	100	10% alc. 2% pet.	+	*See* § 5.20
6-isopropyl-2-(1H)-octahy-dronaphthalenone	10% pet.				
isopropyl palmitate	8% pet.	120	2% pet.	+	*See* § 5.20
p-isopropyl phenylacetalde-hyde	4% pet.	1			
isopropyl quinoline	2% pet.	1	pure		
isopropyl tiglate	10% pet.	1			
isopulegol	8% pet.	3			
isopulegol acetate	8% pet.	2			
isosafrole	8% pet.	1			Carcinogenic (?)
isovaleric acid	1% pet.	1			

(continued)

§ 30.7 *(continuation)*

Name	Non-irritating patch test conc. (RIFM) (§ 30.6)	Quant. use (§ 30.6)	Patch test conc. & veh. (§ 30.1)	Cont. all. (§ 30.3)	Comment (N: § 30.6)
jasmine absolute	3% pet.	1	jasmin oil 2% pet.	+	N. *See* § 5.14
juniper berry oil	8% pet.	2	2% pet.	+	N. *See* § 30.2, [23]
juniperus phoenicea oil	1% pet.		1% alc./2% pet. [7], 1% pet. [17]		N. Not to be confused with the oil of *Juniperus sabina* L
karo karounde absolute	1% pet.				N
labdanum oil	8% pet.	5	1% alc./2% pet. [7] 1% pet. [17]		
lactoscatone	4% pet.				Test concentration weakly irritating
laevulinic acid	4% pet.	1			
laurel leaf oil	10% pet.		laurel oil 2% pet.	+	*See* § 5.14
lavandin oil	5% pet.	500	2% pet.	+	N. *See* § 30.2, [23]. Derived from *Lavendula angustifolia* (Labiatae)
lavandulyl acetate	10% pet.	1			
lavender absolute	10% pet.	5			N
lavender oil	16% pet.	100	2% pet.	+	N. *See* § 5.14. *See also* § 30.2, [23]. Derived from *Lavendula officinalis* (Labiatae)
lavender (spike lavender) oil	8% pet.	100	2% pet.		N
lemon grass oil East Indian	4% pet.	50	lemon grass oil 2% pet.	+	N. *See* § 5.14. Derived from *Cymbopogon citratus* (Gramineae)
lemon grass oil West Indian	4% pet.	250	lemon grass oil 2% pet.	+	N. *See* § 5.14
lemon oil distilled	10% pet.		2% pet.	+	N. *See* § 5.14 *under* lemon oil. Derived from *Citrus limon* (Rutaceae)
lemon oil expressed	10% pet.	150	1-2% pet.	+	N. *See* § 5.14 *under* lemon oil. Phototoxic; (IFRA, October 1975, June 1992). Derived from *Citrus limon* (Rutaceae)

(continued)

§ **30.7** *(continuation)*

Name	Non-irritating patch test conc. (RIFM) (§ 30.6)	Quant. use (§ 30.6)	Patch test conc. & veh. (§ 30.1)	Cont. all. (§ 30.3)	Comment (N: § 30.6)
lemon petitgrain oil	10% pet.	1			N
lilial	1% pet.		1% pet.	+	*See* § 5.14
lilial-methylanthranilate (Schiff base)	12% pet.				
lime oil distilled	15% pet.	50	1% alc./2% pet. [7], 1% pet. [17]		N
lime oil expressed	no test concentration	50	1% alc./2% pet. [7], 1% pet. [17]		N. Contains bergapten; (IFRA, October 1975, June 1992)
D-limonene	8% pet.	150	2% pet.	+	*See* § 5.38 *under* thyme oil and § 13.14
L-limonene	4% pet.	1	2% pet.	+	*See* § 5.38 *under* thyme oil and § 13.14
linaloe wood oil	8% pet.	1	1% alc./2% pet. [7], 1% pet. [17]		N
linalool	20% pet.	200	30% pet.	+	*See* § 5.14
linalyl anthranilate	8% pet.	1			
linalyl benzoate	8% pet.	3			
linalyl butyrate	8% pet.	1			
linalyl cinnamate	8% pet.	3			
linalyl formate	10% pet.	1			
linalyl isobutyrate	8% pet.	1			
linalyl isovalerate	20% pet.	1			
linalyl methyl ether	5% pet.	1			
linalyl phenylacetate	4% pet.	1			
linalyl propionate	8% pet.	10			
litsea cubeba oil	8% pet.	<1	2% pet.	+	N. *See* § 30.2 [23]
longifolene	10% pet.				
lovage oil	2% pet.	1			N. Derived from *Levisticum officinale* (Umbelliferae)
mace oil	8% pet.	2	1% alc./2% pet. [7], 1% pet. [17]		N

(continued)

§ **30.7** *(continuation)*

Name	Non-irritating patch test conc. (RIFM) (§ 30.6)	Quant. use (§ 30.6)	Patch test conc. & veh. (§ 30.1)	Cont. all. (§ 30.3)	Comment (N: § 30.6)
mandarin oil, expressed	8% pet.		1% alc./2% pet. [7], 1% pet. [17]		N
maltol	10% pet.				
marjoram oil, Spanish	6% pet.	2	1% alc./2% pet. [7] 1% pet. [17] 1% alc./2% pet. [7]		N. Derived from *Origanum majorana* (Labiatae)
marjoram oil sweet	6% pet.	1	1% pet. [17]		N. Derived from *Origanum majorana* (Labiatae)
mastic absolute	8% pet.				N. Weak sensitizer in HMT
matricaria oil					*See* chamomile oil
mentha citrata oil	8% pet.		1% alc./2% pet. [7], 1% pet. [17]		N
menthadiene-7-methylformate	10% pet.				Sensitizer in HMT (IFRA, February 1986)
L-(*p*-menthen-6-yl)-1-propanone	4% pet.	50			
L-menthol	8% pet.	50	menthol 2% pet.		*See* § 5.37
menthol racemic	8% pet.	5	menthol 2% pet.		*See* § 5.37
menthone racemic	8% pet.	1			
L-menthyl acetate	8% pet.	3			
menthyl acetate racemic	8% pet.	3			
menthyl acetoacetate	8% pet.	<1			
menthyl isovalerate	1% pet.	<1			
2-menthyl phenylacetate	6% pet.				
p-methoxyacetophenone	6% pet.	2			
o-methoxybenzaldehyde	4% pet.	1			
o-methoxycinnamic aldehyde	4% pet.	1	4% pet.	+	*See* § 5.14
methoxycitronellal	10% pet.		1% pet.	+	*See* § 5.14

(continued)

§ **30.7** *(continuation)*

Name	Non-irritating patch test conc. (RIFM) (§ 30.6)	Quant. use (§ 30.6)	Patch test conc. & veh. (§ 30.1)	Cont. all. (§ 30.3)	Comment (N: § 30.6)
7-methoxycoumarin	8% pet.				Sensitizer and photosensitizer; should not be used in fragrances (IFRA recommendation, June 1979, April 1989). *See also* § 6.5
methoxydicyclopentadiene carboxaldehyde	25% alc.				
p-methoxyhydratropaldehyde	2% pet.				
p-methoxyphenylacetone	4% pet.	1			
4-(*p*-methoxyphenyl) butan-2-one	5% pet.	1			
methyl abietate	2% pet.	25			
methyl acetate	10% pet.				
methyl acetoacetate	8% pet.	1			
p-methylacetophenone	6% pet.	30			
methyl *n*-amyl ketone	4% pet.	1			
α-methylanisalacetone	8% pet.	1			Sensitizer in HMT. Test conc. may be irritating; should not be used in fragrances (IFRA recommendation, November 1977, May 1980)
methyl anisate	4% pet.	1	4% pet.	+	*See* § 5.14
methyl anthranilate	10% pet.	50			
methyl benzoate	4% pet.	15	1% pet.		
4-methylbenzylacetate	5% pet.				
methylbenzylcarbinyl acetate	6% pet.	<1			
5-methyl-3-butyltetrahydropyran-4-yl acetate	8% pet.	1			
2-methyl butyraldehyde	1% pet.	<1			
3-methyl butyraldehyde	1% pet.				
methyl butyrate	8% pet.	<1			

(continued)

§ **30.7** *(continuation)*

Name	Non-irritating patch test conc. (RIFM) (§ 30.6)	Quant. use (§ 30.6)	Patch test conc. & veh. (§ 30.1)	Cont. all. (§ 30.3)	Comment (N: § 30.6)
methyl caproate	4% pet.	<1			
methyl chavicol	3% pet.	4			
methyl cinnamate	10% pet.	25			
methylcinnamic alcohol	2% pet.	5			
α-methylcinnamic aldehyde	8% pet.	5			
6-methylcoumarin	4% pet.	1	1% pet.	+	*See* § 30.2 [4] and § 5.14; should not be used in fragrances (IFRA recommendation, October 1978, February 1980)
7-methylcoumarin	8% pet.				Should not be used in fragrances (IFRA recommendation, February 1979, May 1983)
methyl crotonate	6% pet.	1			Sensitizer in HMT; should not be used in fragrances (IFRA recommendation, March 1978, May 1980)
1-methylcylododecyl-methylether (madrox)	20% pet.				
methylcyclooctyl carbonate (jasmacyclat)	10% pet.				
3-methylcyclopentade-canone	30% pet.	1			
methyl cyclopentenolone	3% pet.	1			
γ-methyl decalactone	2% pet.				
methyl diphenyl ether	2% pet.	2			
methyl dihydrojasmonate (hedione)	20% pet.				
methyl ester of rosin (partially hydrogenated)	10% pet.	200			
4-methyl-7-ethoxycoumarin					Photosensitizer; should not be used in fragrances (IFRA recommendation, June 1979)

(continued)

§ **30.7** *(continuation)*

Name	Non-irritating patch test conc. (RIFM) (§ 30.6)	Quant. use (§ 30.6)	Patch test conc. & veh. (§ 30.1)	Cont. all. (§ 30.3)	Comment (N: § 30.6)
methyl ethyl ketone	20% pet.	50	pure		
methyl eugenol	8% pet.	50			
5-methylfurfural	2% pet.	<1			
methyl furoate	10% pet.	1			
5-methyl-3-heptanone oxime (stemone)	6% pet.				
methyl heptenol	2% pet.	1			
methyl heptanoate	6% pet.				
methyl heptenone	3% pet.	2			
methyl heptine carbonate	2% pet.	3	0.5% pet.	+	*See* § 5.14. Sensitizer in HMT; (IFRA, October 1976, June 1992)
methylhexylacetaldehyde	10% pet.	<1			
methyl hexyl ketone	4% pet.	6			
p-methyl hydratropaldehyde	4% pet.	7			
α-methylionol	8% pet.				
methylionone	10% pet.	250	10% pet.	+	*See* § 5.14
methyl isoeugenol	8% pet.	3			
methyl isopropyl ketone	10% pet.				
methyl-*o*-methoxybenzoate	10% pet.				
α-methyl naphthyl ketone	2% pet.	5			
β-methyl naphthyl ketone	2% pet.	50			
3-methyl-2(3)-nonenenitrile	10% pet.				Sensitizer in HMT. (IFRA, February 1980, May 1983)
methyl nonylenate	20% pet.	1			
methyl nonyl ketone	5% pet.				
3-methyloctan-3-ol	10% pet.				
3-methyl-1-octen-3-ol	10% pet.				Weak sensitizer in HMT

(continued)

§ **30.7** *(continuation)*

Name	Non-irritating patch test conc. (RIFM) (§ 30.6)	Quant. use (§ 30.6)	Patch test conc. & veh. (§ 30.1)	Cont. all. (§ 30.3)	Comment (N: § 30.6)
methyl octine carbonate	2% pet.	1	1% MEK	+	Sensitizer (IFRA, March 1988, June 1992). *See* § 5.14
methyl octyl acetaldehyde	10% pet.				
2-methylpentanoic acid	2% pet.				
methyl phenylacetate	8% pet.	5			
methylphenylcarbinyl acetate	4% pet.	10			
methyl propionate	2% pet.	<1			
p-methylquinoline	2% pet.	1			
methyl salicylate	8% pet.	90	1-2% pet.	+	*See* § 5.41
methyl tiglate	5% pet.				
methyl *p*-toluate	8% pet.	1			
2-methylundecanal dimethylacetal	8% pet.				
methyl undecylenate	12% pet.	<1			
mimosa absolute	1% pet.	1			N
musk ambrette	20% pet.	100	5% pet.	+	*See* § 5.14. Photosensitizer (IFRA, June 1981, October 1985)
musk ketone	5% pet.	50	5% pet.		
musk tibetene	2% pet.	1			
musk xylol	5% pet.	150			
β-myrcene	4% pet.	2	1% pet.		
myrcenol	4% pet.				
myrcenyl acetate	4% pet.	10			
myrrh oil	8% pet.	5	myrrh 10% alc.		N
myrrh absolute	8% pet.				N
myrtenol	8% pet.				
myrtenyl acetate	10% pet.				
β-naphthyl ethyl ether	2% pet.	10			

(continued)

§ **30.7** *(continuation)*

Name	Non-irritating patch test conc. (RIFM) (§ 30.6)	Quant. use (§ 30.6)	Patch test conc. & veh. (§ 30.1)	Cont. all. (§ 30.3)	Comment (N: § 30.6)
β-naphthyl methyl ether	4% pet.	5			
β-naphthyl isobutyl ether	4% pet.				
narcissus absolute	2% pet.	1			N
neral	1% pet.		1% pet.	+	Sensitizer in HMT. *See* § 5.14
nerol	4% pet.	20			
neroli oil Tunesian	4% pet.	1	neroli oil 2% pet.		N. *See also* § 5.14
nerolidol	4% pet.	1			
nerolidyl acetate	12% pet.	1			
nerol oxide	10% pet.				20% pet. produced 1 sensitization reaction in HMT (n=25) and 1 irritation reaction
neryl acetate	10% pet.	2			
neryl formate	6% pet.	1			
neryl isobutyrate	5% pet.				
neryl isovalerate	6% pet.	1			
neryl propionate	6% pet.	1			
nitrobenzene (mirbane oil)	–		10% pet.		Dermatotoxic, should not be used in fragrances (IFRA recommendation, June 1974)
2,6-nonadienal	2% pet.	1			
2,6-nonadienol	1% pet.				
γ-nonalactone	10% pet.	7			
δ-nonalactone	10% pet.	1			
1,3-nonanediol acetate (mixed esters)	8% pet.	50			
2-nonanone	5% pet.				
3,5,7-nonatrien-2-one	2% pet.				
2-nonenal	4% pet.	1			
cis-6-nonenal	1% pet.	<0.1			

(continued)

§ **30.7** *(continuation)*

Name	Non-irritating patch test conc. (RIFM) (§ 30.6)	Quant. use (§ 30.6)	Patch test conc. & veh. (§ 30.1)	Cont. all. (§ 30.3)	Comment (N: § 30.6)
2-nonyn-1-al dimethylacetal	4% pet.				
nootkatone	–				Sensitizer (IFRA, October 1980, June 1981) (not if highly purified)
nopol	8% pet.	10			
nopyl acetate	10% pet.	200			
nutmeg oil East Indian	2% pet.	10	1% alc./2% pet. [7], 1% pet. [17]		N. Derived from *Myristica fragrans* (Myristicaceae)
oakmoss concrete	10% pet.	75	2% pet.	+	N. *See* § 5.14; (IFRA, September 1988, June 1992)
ocimene	5% pet.	3			
ocimenol	4% pet.				
ocimenyl acetate	4% pet.	1			
ocotea cymbarum oil	20% pet.		1% alc./2% pet. [7], 1% pet. [17]		N. Derived from *Sassafras Brazilian* (Lauraceae)
octahydrocoumarin	8% pet.	<1			
γ-octalactone	12% pet.				
δ-octalactone	12% pet.	<1			
octanol-3	12% pet.	5			
octyl isobutyrate	2% pet.	1			
octyl formate	2% pet.	1			
octyl salicylate	5% pet.		2% pet.		
oil lavandin acetylated	10% pet.	20	1% alc./2% pet. [7], 1% pet. [17]		N
olibanum absolute	8% pet.				N
olibanum gum	8% pet.	10	olibanum 2% pet.		N
opoponax	–				N. Sensitizer (not the alcoholic extract) (IFRA, March 1978, December 1981)

(continued)

§ **30.7** *(continuation)*

Name	Non-irritating patch test conc. (RIFM) (§ 30.6)	Quant. use (§ 30.6)	Patch test conc. & veh. (§ 30.1)	Cont. all. (§ 30.3)	Comment (N: § 30.6)
orange flower absolute	20% pet.	4			N
orange (bitter orange) oil	10% pet.	20	2% pet.	+	N. *See* § 5.14. Phototoxic. For Sweet orange oil *see* § 30.2, [23]
orange oil expressed	8% pet.	200	2% pet.	+	N. *See* § 5.14. Derived from *Citrus cinensis* (Rutaceae)
origanum oil	2% pet.	6	origanum 2% pet.		N
orris absolute	3% pet.	1			N
10-oxahexadecanolide	10% pet.				
11-oxahexadecanolide	10% pet.	<3			
12-oxahexadecanolide	10% pet.	3			
palmarosa oil	8% pet.	30	1% alc./2% pet. [7], 1% pet. [17]		N
parsley seed oil	2% pet.	1	1% alc./2% pet. [7], 1% pet. [17]		N. Derived from *Petroselinum sativum* (Umbelliferae)
patchouly oil	10% pet.	300	2% pet.		N. *See* § 5.14
pelargonic acid	12% pet.				
pennyroyal oil Eurafrican	6% pet.	11	1% alc./2% pet. [7], 1% pet. [17]		N
1,1,3,3,5-pentamethyl-4,6-dinitroindane	10% pet.	50			
pentylcyclopen-tanonepropanone	20% pet.				
pentylidene cyclohexanone	10% pet.	1			Strong sensitizer in HMT; should not be used in fragrances (IFRA recommendation, February 1979, May 1983)
perilla aldehyde	4% pet.				Sensitizer in HMT (IFRA, October 1979, May 1989)
perilla oil	4% pet.		1% alc./2% pet.[7], 1% pet. [17]		N. Weak sensitizer ?

(continued)

§ **30.7** *(continuation)*

Name	Non-irritating patch test conc. (RIFM) (§ 30.6)	Quant. use (§ 30.6)	Patch test conc. & veh. (§ 30.1)	Cont. all. (§ 30.3)	Comment (N: § 30.6)
Peru balsam oil	8% pet.	14	1% alc./2% pet. [7], 1% pet. [17]		N. (IFRA, October 1974, December 1991)
petitgrain bigarade oil	8% pet.		1% alc./2% pet. [7], 1% pet. [17]	+	Cross reactions to some balsams, *See* § 5.14
petitgrain Paraguay oil	7% pet.	300	5% pet.		N. Sensitizer in HMT *See* § 5.14
α-phellandrene	4% pet.	12			
phenoxyacetaldehyde	4% pet.	1			
phenoxyacetic acid	2% pet.				
phenoxyethyl isobutyrate	4% pet.	4			
phenoxyethyl propionate	10% pet.	4			
phenylacetaldehyde	2% pet.	18	0.5% pet.	+	*See* § 5.14. Sensitizer in HMT; (IFRA, October 1975, February 1980)
phenylacetaldehyde 2,4-dihydroxy-2-methylpentane acetal (reseda body)	1% pet.				
phenylacetaldehyde dimethyl acetal	2% pet.	6			
phenylacetaldehyde ethyleneglycol acetal	6% pet.				
phenylacetaldehyde glyceryl acetal	3% pet.	6			
phenylacetic acid	2% pet.	7			
phenyl acetyl nitrile	2% pet.	1			
phenylethyl acetate	10% pet.	50	1% pet. [7]		
phenylethyl alcohol	8% pet.	1000	5% pet.	+	*See* § 5.14
phenylethyl anthranilate	10% pet.	1			
phenylethyl benzoate	8% pet.	1			
phenylethyl butyrate	8% pet.	2			
phenylethyl cinnamate	2% pet.	3			
phenylethyl formate	6% pet.	1			
phenylethyl isobutyrate	2% pet.	20			

(continued)

§ **30.7** *(continuation)*

Name	Non-irritating patch test conc. (RIFM) (§ 30.6)	Quant. use (§ 30.6)	Patch test conc. & veh. (§ 30.1)	Cont. all. (§ 30.3)	Comment (N: § 30.6)
phenylethyl isovalerate	2% pet.	1			
phenylethyl methacrylate	6% pet.				
phenylethyl-2-methyl-butyrate	4% pet.				
phenylethyl methyl ether	8% pet.	<1			
phenylethyl methyl ethyl carbinol	10% pet.	1			
phenylethyl methylethyl-carbinyl acetate	10% pet.				
phenylethyl phenylacetate	2% pet.	10			
phenylethyl propionate	8% pet.	5			
phenylethyl salicylate	8% pet.	10			
phenylethyl tiglate	6% pet.	1			
phenylpropyl acetate	8% pet.	10			
phenylpropyl alcohol	8% pet.	5			
phenylpropyl aldehyde	8% pet.	10			
phenylpropyl cinnamate	4% pet.	3			
phenylpropyl formate	8% pet.	1			
3-phenylpropyl isobutyrate	8% pet.	1			
phenylpropyl propionate	8% pet.	<1			Weak sensitizer in HMT
phenyl salicylate	6% pet.	1	1% pet.	+	*See* § 27.16
phytol	10% pet.	1			Weak sensitizer in HMT
pimenta berry oil	8% pet.	1	1% alc./2% pet. [7], 1% pet. [17]		N
pimenta leaf oil	12% pet.	5	1% alc./2% pet. [7], 1% pet. [17]		N
pinacol	8% pet.	1			
cis-2-pinanol	20% pet.				
α-pinene	10% pet.	6	15% pet.	+	*See* § 5.38 *under* turpentine *and* § 5.39
β-pinene	12% pet.	15	1% pet.	+	Toxic. *See* § 5.14

(continued)

§ **30.7** *(continuation)*

Name	Non-irritating patch test conc. (RIFM) (§ 30.6)	Quant. use (§ 30.6)	Patch test conc. & veh. (§ 30.1)	Cont. all. (§ 30.3)	Comment (N: § 30.6)
pinus pumilio oil	12% pet.	1	pine oil 5% pet.		N. For contact allergy to pine needle oil, *see* § 30.2, [23]. Derived from *Pinus* sp. (Pinaceae)
pinus sylvestris oil	12% pet.	1	pine oil 5% pet.		
piperitone	10% pet.	1			
piperonal					*See under* heliotropine
piperonyl acetate	8% pet.	1			
piperonyl acetone	4% pet.	1			
prenol	10% pet.				
prenyl acetate	20% pet.	<1			
prenyl benzoate	20% pet.	<1			
prenyl salicylate	20% pet.	<10			
n-propyl acetal	10% pet.	1			
3-propylbicyclo [2.2.1] hept-5-ene-2-carboxalde-hyde	6% pet.				Test concentration slightly irritant
propyloctanoate	2% pet.				
propylidene phthalide	4% pet.	1	20% pet.	+	Sensitization at 4%; (IFRA, May 1977, May 1978, February 1979) *See* § 5.14
propyl phenylethyl acetal	5% pet.				Test concentration weakly irritating
propyl propionate	20% pet.	1			
pseudo linalyl acetate	12.5% m.o., 5% DMP				
d-pulegone	10% pet.	1			
rhodinol	5% pet.				
rhodinyl acetate	12% pet.	2			
rhodinyl butyrate	12% pet.	1			
rhodinyl formate	4% pet.	2			
rhodinyl isobutyrate	4% pet.	1			

(continued)

§ **30.7** *(continuation)*

Name	Non-irritating patch test conc. (RIFM) (§ 30.6)	Quant. usc (§ 30.6)	Patch test conc. & veh. (§ 30.1)	Cont. all. (§ 30.3)	Comment (N: § 30.6)
rhodinyl phenylacetate	4% pet.				
rhodinyl propionate	4% pet.	1			
rose absolute French	2% pet.	4			N
rosemary oil	10% pet.	50	1% alc./2% pet. [7], 1% pet. [17]		N. Derived from *Rosmarinus officinalis* (Labiatae)
rose oil Bulgarian	2% pet.	2	rose oil 2% pet.	+	N. *See* § 5.14. Derived from *Rosa* sp. (Rosaceae)
rose oil Moroccan	2% pet.	2	rose oil 2% pet.	+	N. *See* § 5.14. Derived from *Rosa* sp. (Rosaceae)
rose (oil rose) Turkish	2% pet.	2	rose oil 2% pet.	+	N. *See* § 5.14. Derived from *Rosa* sp. (Rosaceae)
rose oxide levo	2% pet.	5			
rue oil	1% pet.	1	1% alc./2% pet. [7], 1% pet. [17]		N. Phototoxic (IFRA, November 1974, October 1978). Derived from *Ruta graveolens* (Rutaceae)
safrole	8% pet.	50			Carcinogenic (?); should not be used in fragrances (IFRA recommendation, October 1976, July 1987, September 1987)
sage clary oil, Russian	8% pet.	<3	1% alc./2% pet. [7], 1% pet. [17]		N. Derived from *Salvia sclareae* (Labiatae)
sage oil, Dalmatian	8% pet.	20	1% alc./2% pet. [7], 1% pet. [17]		N. Derived from *Salvia officinalis* (Labiatae)
sage oil, Spanish	8% pet.	4	1% alc./2% pet. [7], 1% pet. [17]		N. Derived from *Salvia officinalis* (Labiatae)
salicylaldehyde	2% pet.	1			
sandalwood oil, East Indian	10% pet.	48	2% pet.	+	N. *See* § 5.14 *See also* § 30.2, [23] Derived from *Santalum album* (Santalaceae)
α-santalol	20% pet.	4			
santalyl acetate	20% pet.	1			

(continued)

§ **30.7** *(continuation)*

Name	Non-irritating patch test conc. (RIFM) (§ 30.6)	Quant. use (§ 30.6)	Patch test conc. & veh. (§ 30.1)	Cont. all. (§ 30.3)	Comment (N: § 30.6)
sassafras oil	4% pet.		1% pet.		N. *See* § 5.14. Derived from *Sassafras albidum* (Lauraceae)
savin oil	–		1% alc./2% pet. [7], 1% pet. [17]		N. Plant origin determines sensitizing capacity (IFRA, May 1980, June 1982)
savory oil (summer variety)	6% pet.	1	1% alc./2% pet. [7], 1% pet. [17]		N
sclareol	10% pet.				Weak sensitizer depending on purity (IFRA, 1986)
schinus molle oil	4% pet.	1	1% alc./2% pet. [7], 1% pet. [17]		N
skatole	2% pet.	1			
snakeroot oil Canadian	4% pet.	1	1% alc./2% pet. [7], 1% pet. [17]		N
spearmint oil	4% pet.	25	2% pet.	+	N. *See* § 13.3. Derived from *Mentha spicata* (Labiatae)
spruce oil (hemlock oil, picea oil, tsuga oil)	1% pet.		1% alc./2% pet. [7], 1% pet. [17]	+	N. *See* § 5.14
stearic acid	7% pet.		5% pet.	+	*See also* § 30.2 [19]
styrallyl alcohol	8% pet.	10			
styrax (= storax)	–		2% pet.	+	N. *See* § 5.38. Sensitizer (not if purified with alkali) (IFRA, May 1980, June 1982)
sucrose octaacetate	4% pet.				
sweet birch oil	4% pet.	1	1% alc./2% pet. [7], 1% pet. [17]		N
tagetes oil	2% pet.		1% alc./2% pet. [7], 1% pet. [17]	+	N. Derived from *Tagetes patula* (§ 30.2 [16])
tangelo oil	8% pet.		1% alc./2% pet. [7], 1% pet. [17]		N
tangerine oil	5% pet.	16	1% alc./2% pet. [7], 1% pet. [17]		N

(continued)

§ **30.7** *(continuation)*

Name	Non-irritating patch test conc. (RIFM) (§ 30.6)	Quant. use (§ 30.6)	Patch test conc. & veh. (§ 30.1)	Cont. all. (§ 30.3)	Comment (N: § 30.6)
tansy oil	4% pet.	1	1% alc./2% pet. [7], 1% pet. [17]		N
tea tree oil	1% pet.		pure	+	N. Derived from *Melaleuca alternifolia* (Myrtaceae)
α-terpinene	5% pet.	1			
γ-terpinene	5% pet.	1			
terpineol	5% pet.	10			
terpineol	12% pet.	1000	α-terpineol 5% pet.	+	*See* § 5.14 *and* § 5.38
terpinolene	20% pet.	50	1% pet.		
terpinyl acetate	5% pet.	1000			
terpinyl formate	2% pet.	1			
terpinyl isobutyrate	10% pet.				
terpinyl propionate	4% pet.	10			
tetrahydrogeranial (dihydrocitronellal)	4% pet.				
tetrahydrolinalool	4% pet.	1			
tetrahydro-4-methyl-2-(2-methylpropen-1-yl) pyran (rose oxide, rosoxide)	2% pet. 1.25% alc.				5% DMP produced 5 reactions (n=51)
tetrahydromuguol	4% pet.	35			
tetrahydromugyl acetate	4% pet.	1			
tetrahydro-pseudo-ionone	8% pet.				Irritating when tested 8% in alc./DMP (3/1); sensitizer in HMT
3,3,5,5-tetramethyl-4-ethoxyvinyl-cyclohexanone	10% pet.	1			
thyme oil red	8% pet.	7	1–5% alc.	+	N. *See* § 5.38. *See also* § 30.2, [23]
tiglic acid	1% pet.	<1			
tobacco leaf absolute	1% pet.				N

(continued)

§ 30.7 *(continuation)*

Name	Non-irritating patch test conc. (RIFM) (§ 30.6)	Quant. use (§ 30.6)	Patch test conc. & veh. (§ 30.1)	Cont. all. (§ 30.3)	Comment (N: § 30.6)
tolualdehyde	4% pet.	3			
tolualdehyde glyceryl acetal	10% pet.				
p-tolyl acetaldehyde	2% pet.	1			
p-tolyl alcohol	4% pet.	<1			
tonka absolute	8% pet.	1			N
tree moss concrete	10% pet.	35			N. Sensitization (IFRA, April 1991, June 1992)
triacetin	20% pet.	20			
trichlormethylphenylcarbinyl acetate	1% pet.	40			
tricyclodecen-4-yl 8-acetate	8% pet.	50			
tricyclodecenyl propionate	20% pet.				
4-tricyclodecylidene butanal (dupical)	6% pet.				
2-tridecanal	4% pet.				
triethyl citrate	20% pet.				
triethylene glycol	20% pet.	10			
triethyl orthoformate	4% pet.				
3,5,5-trimethylcyclohexanol	4% pet.	2			
(mixture of:) 1,2,4 and 1,3,5-trimethyl-3-cyclohexene-1-methanol	10% pet.				
3,6,10-trimethyl-3,5,9-undecatrien-2-one (methylisopseudoionone)	8% pet.				Sensitizer in HMT
4-(2,6,6-trimethyl-2(and/or 3)-cyclohexen)-2-methylbutanal (cetonal)	10% pet.				
4-(2,4,6-trimethyl-3-cyclohexen-1-yl)-3-buten-2-one (iritone)	2% pet.				
2,6,10-trimethyl-9-undecenal (farenal)	12% pet.				

(continued)

§ **30.7** *(continuation)*

Name	Non-irritating patch test conc. (RIFM) (§ 30.6)	Quant. use (§ 30.6)	Patch test conc. & veh. (§ 30.1)	Cont. all. (§ 30.3)	Comment (N: § 30.6)
3,5,5-trimethylhexanal	4% pet.	1			
3,5,5-trimethylhexyl acetate	4% pet.	15			
γ-undecalactone	2% pet.	15			
δ-undecalactone	2% pet.				
1,3,5-undecatriene	1% pet.				
undecylenic acid	4% pet.	1	2-5% pet.	+	*See* § 5.30
undecylenic aldehyde digeranyl acetal	10% pet.	<1			
undecylenic aldehyde (mixed isomers)	5% pet.	<10			
n-valeraldehyde	2% pet.	1			
γ-valerolactone	10% pet.	<1			
vanilla tincture	10% pet.	160			N
vanillin	2% pet.	250	10% pet.		
veratraldehyde	15% pet.				
verbena absolute	2% pet.				N. Weak sensitization when tested 12% pet. (IFRA, 1987)
verbena oil	12% pet.		1% alc./2% pet. [7], 1% pet. [17]		N. Sensitizer in HMT; should not be used in fragrances (IFRA, 1981)
vetiver acetate	20% pet.	75			Sensitizer in HMT to impurities of technical product
vetiver oil	8% pet.	75	2% pet.	+	N. *See* § 30.2 [23]
vetiverol	8% pet.	3			
violet leaf absolute	2% pet.	1			N
ylang-ylang oil	10% pet.	76	2% pet.	+	N. *See* § 5.14
zingerone	8% pet.				

COLOURS

30.8 This section contains the following information on colours:
- Conversion of CTFA/FDA names to Color Index numbers (§ 30.9)
- Tabulation of colours (§ 30.10)
- Tabulation of colour ingredients of hair dye preparations (§ 30.11)

Color Index numbers refer to the *Color Index, 3rd Edition,* 1971.

Colours permitted in the EEC: Colours marked * in the 'Comment' column of § 30.10 are permitted colours for cosmetics in the EEC, as defined in the *EEC Cosmetic Directive* of 27 July 1976 (76/768/EEC) and subsequent amendments up until the 15th Commission Directive 92/86/EC (21/10/1992)

30.9 Conversion of CTFA/FDA names to Color Index numbers (CI)

CTFA/FDA name	CI	CTFA/FDA name	CI
Acid black 1	CI 20470	Acid Red 33	CI 17200
Acid Blue 1	CI 42045	Acid Red 51	CI 45430
Acid Blue 3	CI 42051	Acid Red 52	CI 45100
Acid Blue 9	CI 42090	Acid Red 73	CI 27290
Acid Blue 9 Aluminum lake	CI 42090:2	Acid Red 87	CI 45380 (Sodium salt)
		Acid Red 92	CI 45410 (Sodium salt)
Acid Blue 9 Amonium salt	CI 42090 (ammonium salt)	Acid Red 95	CI 45425
Acid Blue 74	CI 73015	Acid Violet 43	CI 60730
Acid Blue 74 Aluminum lake	CI 73015:Al lake	Acid Yellow 1	CI 10316
		Acid Yellow 3	CI 47005
Acid Green 1	CI 10020	Acid Yellow 3 Aluminum lake	CI 47005:1
Acid Green 25	CI 61570		
Acid Green 50	CI 44090	Acid Yellow 23	CI 19140
Acid Orange 3	CI 10385	Acid Yellow 23 Aluminum lake	CI 19140:1
Acid Orange 6	CI 14270	Acid Yellow 73	CI 45350
Acid Orange 7	CI 15510	Acid Yellow 73 Sodium salt	CI 45350 Sodium salt
Acid Orange 24	CI 20170		
Acid Red 14	CI 14720	Acid Yellow 104 Aluminum lake	CI 15985:1
Acid Red 18	CI 16255		
Acid Red 27	CI 16185	Alumina	CI 77002
		Aluminum Powder	CI 77000
Acid Red 27 Aluminum lake	CI 16185:1	Annatto	CI 75120

(continued

§ **30.9** *(continuation)*

CTFA/FDA name	CI	CTFA/FDA name	CI
Barium Sulfate	CI 77120	DC Orange 5	CI 45370:1
Basic Blue 26	CI 44045	DC Orange 10	CI 45425:1
Basic Blue 99	CI 56059	DC Orange 11	CI 45425 (Sodium salt)
Basic Red 76	CI 12245	DC Red 6	CI 15850
Basic Violet 1	CI 42535	DC Red 7	CI 15850:1 (Ca salt)
Basic Violet 3	CI 42555	DC Red 17	CI 26100
Basic Violet 10	CI 45170	DC Red 21	CI 45380:2
Basic Violet 14	CI 42510	DC Red 22	CI 45380 (Sodium salt)
Bismuth Oxychloride	CI 77163	DC Red 27	CI 45410:1
Bronze Powder	CI 77400	DC Red 28	CI 45410 (Disodium salt)
		DC Red 30	CI 73360
Calcium Carbonate	CI 77220	DC Red 31	CI 15800:1 (Ca salt)
Calcium Sulfate	CI 77231	DC Red 33	CI 17200
Carbon Black	CI 77266	DC Red 34	CI 15880:1 (Ca salt)
Carmine	CI 75470	DC Red 36	CI 12085
Chlorophyllin–Copper complex	CI 75810	DC Violet 2	CI 60725
		DC Yellow 7	CI 45350:1
Chromium Hydroxide Green	CI 77289	DC Yellow 8	CI 45350 (Sodium salt)
Chromium Oxide Greens	CI 77288	DC Yellow 10	CI 47005
Copper Powder	CI 77400	DC Yellow 11	CI 47000
		Direct Black 51	CI 27720
DC Blue 1 Aluminum lake	CI 42090 Aluminum lake	Direct Blue 86	CI 74180
DC Blue 4	CI 42090 (Ammonium salt)		
DC Brown 1	CI 20170	Ext. DC Violet 2	CI 60730
DC Green 3 Aluminum lake	CI 42053	Ext. DC Yellow 7	CI 10316
DC Green 5	CI 61570	Fast Green FCF	CI 42053
DC Green 6	CI 61565	FDC Blue 1	CI 42090
DC Green 8	CI 59040	FDC Blue 1 Aluminum lake	CI 42090:2
DC Orange 4	CI 15510	FDC Green 3	CI 42053
DC Orange 4 Aluminum lake	CI 15510	FDC Red 4	CI 14700

(continued

§ 30.9 *(continuation)*

CTFA/FDA name	CI	CTFA/FDA name	CI
FDC Red 40	CI 16035	Pigment Red 63:1	CI 15880:1 (Ca salt)
FDC Yellow 5	CI 19140	Pigment Red 64:1	CI 15800:1 (Ca salt)
FDC Yellow 5 Aluminum lake	CI 19140:1	Pigment Red 68	CI 15525
		Pigment Red 83	CI 58000:1
FDC Yellow 6	CI 15985	Pigment Red 112	CI 12370
Ferric Ferrocyanide	CI 77510/CI 77520	Pigment Red 172 Aluminum lake	CI 45430:1
Iron Oxides	CI 77489	Pigment Yellow 1	CI 11680
	CI 77491	Pigment Yellow 3	CI 11710
	CI 77492	Pigment Yellow 13	CI 21100
	CI 77499		
		Silver	CI 77820
Kaolin	CI 77004	Solvent Blue 35	CI 61554
		Solvent Green 3	CI 61565
Magnesium Carbonate	CI 77713	Solvent Green 7	CI 59040
Magnesium Oxide	CI 77711	Solvent Orange 1	CI 11920
Manganese Violet	CI 77742	Solvent Red 1	CI 12150
Mica	CI 77019	Solvent Red 3	CI 12010
		Solvent Red 23	CI 26100
Pigment Blue 15	CI 74160	Solvent Red 24	CI 26105
Pigment Blue 15:2	CI 74160:2	Solvent Red 49:1	CI 45170:1 (Stearate)
Pigment Green 7	CI 74260	Solvent Red 73	CI 45425:1
Pigment Orange 5	CI 12075	Solvent Violet 13	CI 60725
Pigment Red 4	CI 12085	Solvent Yellow 29	CI 21230
Pigment Red 5	CI 12490	Solvent Yellow 33	CI 47000
Pigment Red 48:4	CI 15865:4		
Pigment Red 53	CI 15585	Talc	CI 77718
Pigment Red 53:1	CI 15585:1 (Ba salt)	Titanium Dioxide	CI 77891
Pigment Red 57	CI 15850		
Pigment Red 57:1	CI 15850:1 (Ca salt)	Ultramarines	CI 77007
Pigment Red 57:2 Barium lake	CI 15850:2		
		Zinc Oxide	CI 77947

30.10 Colours

Color Index no. (§ 30.8)	Common name/Color Index name	Lakes or salts	USA-FDA name for certified batches	EEC colour no.	Freq. use (§ 30.3)	Patch test conc. & vch. (§ 30.1)	Cont. all. (§ 30.3)	Comment (* § 30.8)
Nitroso and nitro dyes								
10006	Pigment Green 8							*
10020	Acid Green 1		Ext. DC-green 1		17	1% aqua†		*
10316	Acid Yellow 1		Ext. DC-yellow 7		22			*
		aluminum lake						*
10385	Acid Orange 3				45			
Azo-dyes								
11390	Yellow OB®		Solvent Yellow 6			1% pet. [9]	+	*See* § 4.3
11680	Pigment Yellow 1		Pigment Yellow 1			1% pet.	+	**See* § 30.2 [26]
11710	Pigment Yellow 3		Pigment Yellow 3					*
11720	Pigment Yellow 9					2% pet.†		
11725	Pigment Orange 1							*
11920	Solvent Orange 1		Solvent Orange 1			2% pet.†		*
12010	Solvent Red 3		Solvent Red 3			1% pet.	+	**See* § 30.2 [26]
12055	Solvent Yellow 14, Sudan I					0.1% pet. [9]	+	*See* § 4.3
12075	Pigment Orange 5		DC Orange 17			1% pet.	+	*See* § 27.16; EC Annex II; no. 397 (prohibited)
		lake						
12085	Pigment Red 4, Flaming Red		DC Red 36		83	1% pet.	+	**See* § 27.6 *and* § 27.16
		lake			18	20% aqua [8]		*
		barium lake			13			*
12100	Solvent Orange 2		Ext. DC Orange 4			1% pet. [9]	+	See § 4.3
12120	Pigment Red 3, Toluidine Red					1% pet. [9]	+	**See* § 30.2 [26]

(continued)

§ 30.10 *(continuation)*

Color Index no. (§ 30.8)	Common name/Color Index name	Lakes or salts	USA-FDA name for certified batches	EEC colour no.	Freq. use (§ 30.3)	Patch test conc. & veh. (§ 30.1)	Cont. all. (§ 30.3)	Comment (* § 30.8)
12140	Solvent Orange 7, Sudan II					1% pet. [9]	+	*See* § 4.3
12150	Solvent Red 1		Solvent Red 1			0.5% pet.†	+	**See* 30.2 [15]
12175	Solvent Orange 8, Vacanceine Red					1% pet. [9]	+	*See* § 4.3
12245	Basic Red 76				6			
12250	Basic Brown 16				28	0.5% pet.†		
12251	Basic Brown 17				5	0.5% pet.†		
12370	Pigment Red 112							*
12420	Pigment Red 7					1% pet.	+	**See* § 30.2 [26]
12480	Pigment Brown 1					2% pet.†		*
12490	Pigment Red 5		Pigment Red 5			2% pet.†		*
12700	Disperse Yellow 16							*
12719	Basic Yellow 57				17			
13015	Acid Yellow 9					1% aq.†		*
14270	Acid Orange 6							*
14700	Food Red 1, Ponceau SX		FDC Red 4		1006	2% pet.†		*
14720	Acid Red 14, Azorubin			E-122		5% aqua;2% pet.†		*
14815	Scarlet GN			E-125		1% pet.†		*
15510	Acid Orange 7		DC Orange 4		382	1% pet.†		*
		aluminum lake	DC Orange 4		16			*
15525	Pigment Red 68		Pigment Red 68			2% pet.†		*
15575	Acid Orange 8							*
15580	Pigment Red 51							*
15585	Pigment Red 53		DC Red 8			1% pet.	+	EC Annex II; no. 401 (prohibited) *See* § 30.2 [26]

(continued)

§ **30.10** *(continuation)*

Color Index no. (§ 30.8)	Common name/Color Index name	Lakes or salts	USA-FDA name for certified batches	EEC colour no.	Freq. use (§ 30.3)	Patch test conc. & veh. (§ 30.1)	Cont. all. (§ 30.3)	Comment (* § 30.8)
		sodium salt	DC Red 8			20% aqua [8]		
		barium salt (15585:1)	DC Red 9					
		barium lake	DC Red 9			2% pet.		
		barium/ strontium lake	DC Red 9					
		zirconium lake	DC Red 9					
15620	Acid Red 88							*
15630	Pigment Red 49, Lithol red		DC Red 10			1% pet. [9]	+	* § 30.2 [26]
		aluminum lake	DC Red 10			20% aqua [8]		*
		sodium salt	DC Red 10					*
		calcium salt (15630:2)	DC Red 11					*
		calcium lake	DC Red 11			20% aqua [8]		*
		barium salt (15630:1)	DC Red 12					*
		barium lake	DC Red 12			20% aqua [8]		*
		strontium salt (15630:3)	DC Red 13					*
		strontium lake	DC Red 13			20% aqua [8]		*
15685	Acid Red 184							*

(continued)

§ 30.10 *(continuation)*

Color Index no. (§ 30.8)	Common name/Color Index name	Lakes or salts	USA-FDA name for certified batches	EEC colour no.	Freq. use (§ 30.3)	Patch test conc. & veh. (§ 30.1)	Cont. all. (§ 30.3)	Comment (* § 30.8)
15800	Pigment Red 64, Brilliant Lake Red R		DC Red 31			1% pet.	+	*See § 27.6 and § 27.16
		calcium salt (15800:1)	DC Red 31					*
15850	Pigment Red 57, Lithol Rubin B		DC Red 6		54	20% aqua [8]		*
		aluminum lake	DC Red 6					*
		barium lake	DC Red 6		644	10% pet.†		*
		barium/ strontium lake	DC Red 6		45			*
		calcium/ strontium lake	DC Red 6		9			*
		zirconium lake	DC Red 6					*
		calcium salt (15850:1)	DC Red 7		68			*
		aluminum lake	DC Red 7		4			*
		barium lake (15850:2)	DC Red 7		12			*
		calcium lake	DC Red 7		974	5% pet.†		*
		zirconium lake	DC Red 7					*
15865	Pigment Red 48:4		Pigment Red 48:4			1% pet.	+	*See § 30.2 [26]
15880:1	Pigment Red 63, calcium salt		DC Red 34		13	2% pet.†		*
15980	Food Orange 2			E-111				*

(continued)

§ **30.10** *(continuation)*

Color Index no. (§ 30.8)	Common name/Color Index name	Lakes or salts	USA-FDA name for certified batches	EEC colour no.	Freq. use (§ 30.3)	Patch test conc. & veh. (§ 30.1)	Cont. all. (§ 30.3)	Comment (* § 30.8)
15985	Food Yellow 3, Sunset Yellow		FDC Yellow 6	E-110	719	2% pet.	+	*See § 30.2 [26]
		aluminum lake	FDC Yellow 6		164			*
		aluminum lake	DC Yellow 6		54			*
16035	Allura Red		FDC Red 40		249			*
16185	Acid Red 27, Food Red 9, Amaranth		FDC Red 2	E-123		1% pet.	+	*See § 30.2 [26]
		aluminum lake (16185:1)	FDC Red 2					*
		aluminum lake	DC Red 2					*
16230	Food Orange 4					1% pet.	+	*See § 30.2 [26]
16255	Food Red 7, Acid Red 18, Cochenille Red A			E-124		1% pet.	+	*See § 30.2 [26]
16290	Food Red 8			E-126				*
17200	Food Red 12, Acid Red 33		DC Red 33		767	1% pet.†		*
18050	Food Red 10							*
18130	Acid Red 155							*
18690	Acid Yellow 121							*
18736	Acid Red 180							*
18820	Acid Yellow 11							*
18965	Acid Yellow 17							*
19140	Food Yellow 4, Tartrazine, Acid Yellow 23		FDC Yellow 5	E-102	2025	2% pet.	+	*See § 30.2 [26]
		aluminum lake	FDC Yellow 5		408	20% aqua [8]		*
		aluminum lake	DC Yellow 5		188			*

(continued)

§ 30.10 *(continuation)*

Color Index no. (§ 30.8)	Common name/Color Index name	Lakes or salts	USA-FDA name for certified batches	EEC colour no.	Freq. use (§ 30.3)	Patch test conc. & veh. (§ 30.1)	Cont. all. (§ 30.3)	Comment (* § 30.8)
		zirconium lake	DC Yellow 5		83			*
20170	Acid Orange 24		DC Brown 1		31	1% pet.†		*
20470	Acid Black 1					2% aqua†		*
21100	Pigment Yellow 13		Pigment Yellow 13					*
21108								*
21230	Solvent Yellow 29		Solvent Yellow 29			1% pet.†		*
24790	Acid Red 163							*
26100	Solvent Red 23, Sudan III, Toney Red		DC Red 17		181	1% pet. [9]	+	*See* § 27.6, § 27.11 and § 27.16
26105	Solvent Red 24		Solvent Red 24			1% pet.	+	EC Annex II, no. 379 (prohibited) *See* § 30.2 [26]
27290	Acid Red 73							*
27720	Direct Black 51		Direct Black 51		25			
27755	Food Black 2			E-152				*
28440	Food Black 1, Brilliant Black BN			E-151				*
Stilbene Dyes								
40215	Direct Orange 34							*
Carotenoid dyes								
40800	β-Carotene				69			*
40820	Apocarotenal (red)			E-160e				*
40825	Ethyl ester of apocarotenal			E-160f				*
40850	Canthaxanthin (red)			E-160g				*

(continued)

§ **30.10** *(continuation)*

Color Index no. (§ 30.8)	Common name/Color Index name	Lakes or salts	USA-FDA name for certified batches	EEC colour no.	Freq. use (§ 30.3)	Patch test conc. & veh. (§ 30.1)	Cont. all. (§ 30.3)	Comment (* § 30.8)
Triarylmethane dyes								
42045	Acid Blue 1					2% pet.†		*
42051	Acid Blue 3, Food Blue 5, Patent Blue V			E-131		2% pet.†		*
42053	Food Green 3		FDC Green 3, Fast Green FCF		158	2% pet.†		*
42080	Acid Blue 7							*
42090	Acid Blue 9, Brilliant Blue FCF		FDC Blue 1		1706	2% pet.†		*
		aluminum lake	FDC Blue 1		403			*
		aluminum lake	DC Blue 1		10			*
		ammon-ium salt	DC Blue 4		28			*
42100	Acid Green 9							*
42170	Acid Green 22							*
42510	Basic Violet 14							*
42520	Basic Violet 2							*
42535	Basic Violet 1, Gentian Violet		Basic Violet 1			1-2% aqua	+	*See* § 5.7; EC Annex II, no. 388 (prohibited)
42555	Basic Violet 3, Crystal Violet		Basic Violet 3		6	1-2% aqua	+	*See* § 5.7; EC Annex II, no. 380 (prohibited)
42640	Acid Violet 49		(formerly) FDC-Violet 1					EC Annex II, no. 386 (prohibited)
42735	Acid Blue 104							*
44045	Basic Blue 26							*
44090	Food Green 4, Wool Green BS			E-142				*

(continued)

§ 30.10 *(continuation)*

Color Index no. (§ 30.8)	Common name/Color Index name	Lakes or salts	USA-FDA name for certified batches	EEC colour no.	Freq. use (§ 30.3)	Patch test conc. & veh. (§ 30.1)	Cont. all. (§ 30.3)	Comment (* § 30.8)
Xanthene dyes								
45100	Acid Red 52							*
45160	Basic Red 1							*
45170	Basic Violet 10, Rhodamine B		DC Red 19			1% pet.	+	*See* § 27.16; to be discontinued in the USA; EC Annex II; no. 398 (prohibited)
		aluminum lake	DC Red 19					
		barium lake	DC Red 19					
		zirconium lake	DC Red 19					
		stearate (CI 45170:1)	DC Red 37, Solvent Red 49:1					
45220	Acid Red 50							*
45350	Acid Yellow 73, Uranin (acid)		DC Yellow 7		12	2% pet.[†]		*
		sodium salt	DC Yellow 8		22	1% alcohol[†]		*
45370	Acid Orange 11 (acid)		DC Orange 5		125	5% pet.[†]		*
		aluminum lake	DC Orange 5		18			*
		zirconium lake	DC Orange 5		107			*
45376	Acid dye							*
45380	Acid Red 87, Eosin yellowish (acid)		DC Red 21		161	50% aqua; 2% pet.	+	**See* § 27.16
		aluminum lake	DC Red 21		115			*

(continued)

§ **30.10** *(continuation)*

Color Index no. (§ 30.8)	Common name/Color Index name	Lakes or salts	USA-FDA name for certified batches	EEC colour no.	Freq. use (§ 30.3)	Patch test conc. & veh. (§ 30.1)	Cont. all. (§ 30.3)	Comment (* § 30.8)
		aluminum benzoate lake	DC Red 21		3			*
		zirconium lake	DC Red 21		66			*
		aluminum lake	DC Red 22		9			*
		sodium salt	DC Red 22		10	50% aqua		*
45405	Acid Red 98, Phloxine							*
45410	Acid Red 92, Phloxine B (acid)		DC Red 27		97			*
		aluminum lake	DC Red 27		304	20% aqua [8]		*
		zirconium lake	DC Red 27		126	20% aqua [8]		*
		sodium salt	DC Red 28		35			*
		aluminum lake	DC Red 28		9			*
45425	Acid Red 95 (acid)		DC Orange 10					*
45430	Acid Red 51, Food Red 14, Erythrosine		DC Red 3			2% pet.†		*
		aluminum lake	DC Red 3		84			*
		erythro-sine	FDC Red 3	E-127		2% pet.		*
		aluminum lake	FDC Red 3					*
Quinoline dyes								
47000	Solvent Yellow 33		DC Yellow 11		193	0.1% pet.	+	**See* § 27.6, § 27.11 and § 27.16

(continued)

§ 30.10 *(continuation)*

Color Index no. (§ 30.8)	Common name/Color Index name	Lakes or salts	USA-FDA name for certified batches	EEC colour no.	Freq. use (§ 30.3)	Patch test conc. & veh. (§ 30.1)	Cont. all. (§ 30.3)	Comment (* § 30.8)
47005	Acid Yellow 3, Quinoline Yellow		DC Yellow 10	E-104	544	0.1% pet.	+	*See § 27.11 *under* D&C Yellow no. 11
		aluminum lake	DC Yellow 10		41			*
Azine dyes								
50325	Acid Violet 50							*
50420	Acid Black 2		Acid Black 2					
Oxazine dyes								
51319	Pigment Violet 23					1% aqua[†]		*
Aminoketone and hydroxyketone dyes								
56059	Basic Blue 99				26	0.5% pet.[†]	+	*See* § 26.6
Anthraquinone dyes								
58000	Mordant Red 11		Pigment Red 83 (CI 58000:1)					*
59040	Solvent Green 7, Pyranine		DC Green 8		40			*
60724	Disperse Violet 27							*
60725	Solvent Violet 13		DC Violet 2		177	2% pet.[†]		*
60730	Acid Violet 43		Acid Violet 43					*
			Ext. DC Violet 2		226			*
61554	Solvent Blue 35		Solvent Blue 35					EC Annex II; no. 389 (prohibited)
61565	Solvent Green 3		DC Green 6		151	2% pet.[†]		*
61570	Acid Green 25		DC Green 5		349	2% pet.[†]		*
61585	Acid Blue 80							*
69800	Vat Blue 4, Indanthrone			E-130				*

(continued)

§ **30.10** *(continuation)*

Color Index no. (§ 30.8)	Common name/Color Index name	Lakes or salts	USA-FDA name for certified batches	EEC colour no.	Freq. use (§ 30.3)	Patch test conc. & veh. (§ 30.1)	Cont. all. (§ 30.3)	Comment (* § 30.8)
69825	Vat Blue 6		DC Blue 9			1% pet.	+	**See* § 30.2 [26]
71105	Pigment Orange 43					1% pet.†		*
Indigoid dyes								
73000	Vat Blue 1		DC Blue 6			1% pet.	+	**See* § 30.2 [26]
73015	Food Blue 1, Indigotine		FDC Blue 2	E-132	4	2% pet.†		*
73360	Vat Red 1, Helindone Pink		DC Red 30		66	2% pet.†	+	**See* § 30.2 [26]
		lake	DC Red 30		237			
73385	Vat Violet 2							*
73900	Pigment Violet 19							*
73915	Pigment Red 122							*
Phthalocyanine dyes								
74100	Pigment Blue 16							*
74160	Pigment Blue 15		Pigment Blue 15		15	1% pet.	+	**See* § 30.2 [26]
74180	Direct Blue 86		Direct Blue 86					*
74260	Pigment Green 7		Pigment Green 7			2% pet.†		*
Natural Dyes								
75100	Natural Yellow 6, Crocetin							*
75120	Natural Orange 4, Bixine, Norbixine, Anatto		Anatto	E-160b	4	5% pet.		*
75125	Natural Yellow 27, Lycopene			E-160d				*
75130	Natural Yellow 26, β-Carotene, Carotene			E-160a	69	50% pet.		*

(continued)

§ 30.10 *(continuation)*

Color Index no. (§ 30.8)	Common name/Color Index name	Lakes or salts	USA-FDA name for certified batches	EEC colour no.	Freq. use (§ 30.3)	Patch test conc. & veh. (§ 30.1)	Cont. all. (§ 30.3)	Comment (* § 30.8)
75135	Natural Yellow 27, Rubixanthin			E-160d				*
75170	Natural White 1, Guanine				55	pure	+	*See § 28.2
75300	Natural Yellow 3, Curcumine			E-100				
75470	Natural Red 4, Carminic acid			E-120				*
		aluminum lake	Carmine		569	pure; 5% pet.†		*
75480	Natural Orange 6, Lawsone (from Henna leaves)					1% aqua, prick test	+	*
75810	Natural Green 3		Chlorophyl		6	2% pet.†		*
			Chlorophyllin	E-140	12			*
			Chlorophyllin copper complex	E-141	14			*
Inorganic pigments								
77000	Aluminum powder		Aluminum powder	E-173	168	50% pet.†	+	*See* § 29.13
77002	Alumina (aluminum oxide)		Alumina		5	2% pet.†		*
77004	Kaolin, China clay		Kaolin		796	5% pet.†		*
77007	Ultramarine		Ultramarine blue		1246	2% pet.†		*
			Ultramarine red		12	2% pet.†		
			Ultramarine violet		292			
			Ultramarine pink		255			
77015	CI Pigment Red 101 & 102 (Aluminum silicate + ferric oxide)					50% pet.†		*

(continued)

§ **30.10** *(continuation)*

Color Index no. (§ 30.8)	Common name/Color Index name	Lakes or salts	USA-FDA name for certified batches	EEC colour no.	Freq. use (§ 30.3)	Patch test conc. & veh. (§ 30.1)	Cont. all. (§ 30.3)	Comment (* § 30.8)
77019	Mica		Mica		1469	5% pet.†		*
77120	Barium sulfate, blanc fixe		Barium sulfate		9			*
77163	Bismuth oxychloride		Bismuth oxychloride		689	pure†	+	**See* § 30.2, [19]
77220	Calcium carbonate		Calcium carbonate	E-170	121	2% pet.†		*
77231	Calcium sulfate				19			*
77266	Graphite (Carb-on black)		Graphite (carbon black)			50% pet.†		*
77268:1	CI Pigment Black 8 (carbon)			E-153				*
77288	Chrome oxide green		Chromium oxide greens		354	0.5% pet.†		*
77289	Chrome hydroxide		Chromium hydroxide		407	Bichromate 0.5% pet.	+	*See* § 4.4
77343	Chrome-cobalt-aluminum oxide (bluish green)							
77346	Cobalt aluminate (blue)							*
77400	Bronze powder		Bronze powder		23			*
77400	Copper powder		Copper powder		30			
77480	Gold powder			E-175				*
77489	Iron (II) oxide (black)		Iron oxide	E-172		50% pet.†		*
77491	Iron (III) oxide (red-brown)		Iron oxide	E-172		20% aqua [8]		*
77492	Hydrated iron (III) oxide, (yellow)		Iron oxide	E-172				*
77499	Iron (II-III) oxide (black)		Iron oxide	E-172		2% pet.†		*
	All iron oxides				2489			

(continued)

§ 30.10 *(continuation)*

Color Index no. (§ 30.8)	Common name/Color Index name	Lakes or salts	USA-FDA name for certified batches	EEC colour no.	Freq. use (§ 30.3)	Patch test conc. & veh. (§ 30.1)	Cont. all. (§ 30.3)	Comment (* § 30.8)
77510	Ferric ferrocyanide, Prussian blue		Ferric ferrocyanide		305	2% aqua†		*
77520	Ammonium ferric ferrocyanide							*
77713	Magnesium carbonate		Magnesium carbonate		413	pure†		*
77718	Talc		Talc		2195	pure†		*
77742	Manganese ammonium pyrophosphate		Manganese Violet		505	2% pet.†		*
77745	Manganese phosphate (pink)							*
77820	Silver		Silver	E-174	82			*
77891	Titanium dioxide		Titanium dioxide	E-171	3446	pure†		*
77947	Zinc oxide		Zinc oxide		283	pure	+	*See § 5.20
Colours without Color Index numbers								
	Acid Black 107				61			Syn: Irgalan Black BGL®
	Acid Black 131					1% pet.†		Syn: Irgalan Black BGL®
	Acid Blue 168				19			Syn: Irgalan Blue BL®
	Acid Blue 170				16			Syn: Irgalan Blue BRL®
	Acid Brown 45				37			Syn: Irgalan Brown 3BL®
	Acid Orange 87				17			Syn: Irgalan Orange RL®
	Acid Red 195							*
	Acid Red 211				16			Syn: Irgalan Red 2GL®

(continued)

§ 30.10 *(continuation)*

Color Index no. (§ 30.8)	Common name/Color Index name	Lakes or salts	USA-FDA name for certified batches	EEC colour no.	Freq. use (§ 30.3)	Patch test conc. & veh. (§ 30.1)	Cont. all. (§ 30.3)	Comment (* § 30.8)
	Acid Red 252				17			Syn: Irgalan Brilliant Red BL®
	Acid Red 259				46			Syn: Irgalan Red 4GL®
	Acid Yellow 127				12			Syn: Irgalan Brilliant Yellow 3GLS®
	Aluminum, zinc, magnesium and calcium stearates							*
	Anthocyanes			E-163				*
	Azulene (blue)				45	1% pet.	+	*See* § 27.16
	Bromocresol green							*
	Bromothymol blue							*
	Calamine							
	Capsanthine (orange-red)			E-160c				*
	Caramel (brown)			E-150	88	2% aqua†		*
	Disodium EDTA-copper (green)				25			
	Disperse Black 9				84			Syn: Amacel Black 3G®
	Lactoflavin (yellow), Vitamin B2			E-101				*
	Vegetable black			E-153				*

30.11 Colour ingredients of hair dye preparations

Ingredient	Synonym; CI number	Patch test conc. & veh. (§ 30.1)	Freq. use (§ 30.3)	Cont. all. (§ 30.3)	Comment (§ 30.3)
Acid Blue 62	CI 62045				
Acid Orange 3	CI 10385		45		*See* § 30.10
Acid Red 35	CI 18065				
2-amino-6-chloro-4-nitrophenol			3		
2-amino-6-chloro-4-nitrophenol hydrochloride			104		‡
2-amino-2-hydroxytoluene	4-amino-*o*-cresol	1% pet.†	257		
p-aminodiphenylamine					See *N*-phenyl-*p*-phenylenediamine
2-amino-4-nitrophenol		2% pet.	19		‡EC Annex II, 383 (prohibited)
2-amino-5-nitrophenol	CI 76535	2% pet.			EC Annex II, 384 (prohibited)
4-amino-2-nitrophenol	*o*-nitro-*p*-aminophenol; CI 76555	2% pet.			
m-aminophenol	MAP; CI 76545; 3-aminophenol	2% pet.	551	+	*See* § 26.6
m-aminophenol HCL	3-aminophenol hydrochloride		17		
o-aminophenol	OAP; CI 76520; 2-aminophenol	2% pet.	86		
p-aminophenol	PAP; CI 76550; 4-aminophenol	2% pet.	672	+	*See* § 26.6
Basic Blue 9	CI 52015; Methylene Blue	2% pet.			
Basic Blue 99	CI 65059; Arianor Steel Vlue 306004®	0.5% pet.†	26	+	*See* § 26.6
Basic Brown 16	CI 12250; Arianor Mahogany 306002®	0.5% pet.†	28		
Basic Brown 17	CI 12251; Arianor Sierra Brown 306001®	0.5% pet.†	5		
Basic Violet 1	CI 42535; Gentian Violet				*See* § 30.10 *and* § 5.7 EC Annex II, 388 (prohibited)

(continued)

§ **30.11** *(continuation)*

Ingredient	Synonym; CI number	Patch test conc. & veh. (§ 30.1)	Freq. use (§ 30.3)	Cont. all. (§ 30.3)	Comment (§ 30.3)
Basic Violet 3	CI 42555; Crystal Violet		6		*See* § 30.10 *and* § 5.7; EC Annex II, 380 (prohibited)
N,N-bis-(2-hydroxyethyl)-*p*-phenylenediamine sulfate			257		
bismuth citrate					
2-chloro-*p*-phenylenediamine	CI 76065; 2-chloro-1,4-benzenediamine	2% pet			
2-chloro-*p*-phenylenediamine sulfate	2-chloro-1,4-benzenediamine sulfate		33		
4-chlororesorcinol	CI 76510; 4-chloro-1,3-benzene diol	2% aqua†	33		
2,4-diaminoanisole					‡*See* methoxy-phenylenediamine
2,4-diaminodiphenylamine					
4,4′-diaminodiphenylamine					
2,4-diaminophenol		2% pet.	9		
2,4-diaminophenol HCl					
2,4-diamino-phenylethanol					‡EC Annex II, no. 407 (prohibited)
2,4-diamino-phenoxyethanol HCl			108		
2,6-diaminopyridine	2,6-pyridinediamine				
Disperse Black 9	Amacel Black 3G®		84		*See* § 30.10
DC Green 5	CI 61570		349		
DC Orange 4	CI 15510		382		
DC Red 19	CI 45170			+	‡to be discontinued in the USA; *See* § 30.10 *and* § 27.16
DC Red 33	CI 17200		767		*See* § 30.10
DC Yellow 10	CI 47005		544		
Disperse Black 9			84		

(continued)

§ **30.11** *(continuation)*

Ingredient	Synonym; CI number	Patch test conc. & veh. (§ 30.1)	Freq. use (§ 30.3)	Cont. all. (§ 30.3)	Comment (§ 30.3)
Disperse Blue 1	CI 64500	1% pet.	112	+	*See* § 30.2 [26]
Disperse Blue 3	CI 61505	1% pet.	12	+	*See* § 30.2 [26]
Disperse Violet 1	1,4-diamino-9,10-anthracenedione		115		
Disperse Violet 4	CI 61105				
4-ethoxy-*m*-phenylenediamine					EC Annex II, no. 406 (prohibited)
Ext. DC Violet 2	CI 60730		226		
Ext. DC Yellow 7	CI 10316		22		*See also* § 30.10
FDC Blue 1	CI 42090	2% pet.	1706		*See also* § 30.10
FDC Red 4	CI 14700	2% pet.	1006		*See also* § 30.10
FDC Yellow 5	CI 19140	2% pet.	2025	+	*See also* § 30.10
FDC Yellow 6	CI 15985; Sunset Yellow	1% pet and 2% pet.	719		*See* § 30.2 [26]
HC Blue 1	N′,N′-bis(2-hydroxyethyl)-N′- methyl-2-nitro-*p*-phenylenediamine				For percutaneous penetration under usage conditions. *See* § 26.7
HC Blue 2	*N,N,N*-tris(2-hydroxyethyl)-2-nitro-*p*-phenylene-diamine		118		
HC Blue 4					
HC Blue 5					
HC Orange 1	2-nitro-4′-hydroxy-diphenylamine		43		
HC Red 1	4-amino-2-nitrodiphenylamine		28		
HC Red 3	N′-(2-hydroxyethyl)-2-nitro-*p*-phenylenediamine		105		
HC Yellow 2	*N*-(2-hydroxyethyl)-2-nitroaniline		91		
HC Yellow 4	*N,N*-bis(2-hydroxyethyl)-2-amino-5-nitrophenol		87		
HC Yellow 5	*N*1-(2-hydroxyethyl)-4-nitro-*o*-phenylenediamine		24		

(continued)

§ **30.11** *(continuation)*

Ingredient	Synonym; CI number	Patch test conc. & veh. (§ 30.1)	Freq. use (§ 30.3)	Cont. all. (§ 30.3)	Comment (§ 30.3)
henna (dried leaves of *Lawsonia alba*)		10 mg in 100 ml aqua-ether-ethanol		+	*See* § 26.6
hydroquinone	1,4-benzenediol-*p*-hydroxyphenol	1% pet.	208	+	*See* § 29.11
2-hydroxy-1,4-benzo-morpholine	3,4-dihydro-2H-1,4-benzoxazin-6-ol		46		
hydroxynapthoquinone					*See* lawsone
lawsone	2-hydroxy-1,4-naphthoquinone				
lead acetate		1% aqua	9	+	*See* § 26.6
4-methoxy-*m*-phenyle-nediamine	4-MMPD; 2,4-diaminoanisole; 24-DAA	2% pet.			*See* § 26.7. EC Annex II, 376 (prohibited)
4-methoxy-*m*-phenyle-nediamine sulfate	4-MMPD-sulfate	2% pet.			EC Annex II, 376 (prohibited)
5-methoxy-*p*-phenyle-nediamine	5-MPPD; 2,5-diaminoanisole: 25-DAA				‡EC Annex II, 377 (prohibited)
4-methoxytoluene-2,5-diamine					
p-methylaminophenol sulfate	metol	1% pet.	52		
1,5-naphthalenediol			26		‡
2,3-naphthalenediol			40		
2,7-naphthalenediol			3		
1-naphthol	α-naphthol	5% o.o.; 0.1% pet.; 1% alc.	372		
2-nitro-*p*-phenyle-nediamine	2-NPPD; CI 76070	1% pet.	27	+	*See* § 26.6
4-nitro-*m*-phenyle-nediamine	CI 76030	2% pet.			
4-nitro-*o*-phenyle-nediamine	4-NOPD; CI 76020	2% pet.	62		*See* § 26.7
m-phenylenediamine	MPD; CI 76125	2 % pet.	133		*See* § 26.7
– sulfate			63		

(continued)

§ **30.11** *(continuation)*

Ingredient	Synonym; CI number	Patch test conc. & veh. (§ 30.1)	Freq. use (§ 30.3)	Cont. all. (§ 30.3)	Comment (§ 30.3)
o-phenylenediamine	OPD	1% pet.			*See* § 30.2 [26]
p-phenylenediamine	PPD; CI 76060	1% pet.	761	+	*See* § 26.6 *and* § 26.7
– HCl	CI 76061				
– sulfate					
phenylmethylpyrazolone			158		
N-phenyl-*p*-phenylenediamine	CI 76085; *p*-aminodiphenylamine	0.25% pet.	7	+	*See* § 26.6
– HCl			12		
– sulfate					
phloroglucinol	1,3,5-trihydroxybenzene		6		
picramic acid (sodium salt)	2-amino-4,6-dinitrophenol; CI 76540		111		
pyrocatechol	catechol; pyrocatechin; CI 76500	2% pet.	38	+	EC Annex II, no. 408 (prohibited). *See* § 22.28
pyrogallol	1,2,3-trihydroxybenzene; CI 76515	1% pet.	29	+	EC Annex II, no. 409 (prohibited)
resorcinol		2% pet.	799	+	*See* § 26.6, § 5.37 *and* § 26.14
sodium picramate					*See* picramic acid
toluene-2,4-diamine	*m*-toluenediamine; 24TDA	1% pet.		+	*See* § 26.6
toluene-2,5-diamine and sulfate	*p*-toluenediamine; 25TDA; CI 76042	2% pet.	131	+	*See* § 26.6

SUNSCREENS

30.12 Sunscreens (UV-absorbers) are tabulated in § 30.13.
Sunscreens permitted in the USA and the EEC are indicated in the 'Comment' column:

a = permitted in the USA (*Cat. 1, OTC Sunscreen Drugs, Federal Register, 25* August 1978)

b = permitted in the EC (Council Directive 76/768/EC and subsequent amendments up until the 15th Commission Directive (92/86/EC) of 21.11.1992)

30.13 Sunscreens (UV-absorbers)

Sunscreen	Synonym®	Patch test con. & veh. (§ 30.1)	Freq. use (§ 30.3)	Cont. all. (§ 30.3)	Comment (a b: § 30.12 and § 30.3)
PABA series					
(*p*-aminobenzoic acid)					
allantoin-PABA	Alpaba	5% pet.			
ethyl dihydroxypropyl PABA	Amerscreen P, *N*-propoxylated ethyl PABA	5% pet.	46		a
ethyl *N*-dimethyl PABA		5% pet.			‡
ethyl-*N*-ethoxylated PABA	Lusanthan 25	5% pet.			‡b
glyceryl PABA	Escalol 106	5% pet.	23	+	a. *See* § 29.15
octyl dimethyl PABA	Escalol 507, Padimate 0	5% pet.	520	+	a,b. *See* § 29.15
PABA	*p*-aminobenzoic acid	2% pet.	46	+	a,b. *See* § 29.19
PEG-25 PABA	Polyoxyethylene PABA				
pentyl dimethyl PABA	Escalol 506, Padimate A	5% pet.	10	+	a. *See* § 29.19 EC Annex II, no. 381 (prohibited)
Anthranilates series					
(*o*-aminobenzoic acid)					
glyceryl-3-(glyceroxy)anthranilate (= α-glycerol ester of orthoamino-meta (2,3-dihydroxypropoxy) benzoic acid	UV-A filter in Contralum cream	5% pet.		+	‡*See* § 29.19
homomenthyl *N*-acetyl anthranilate	in Parsol Ultra	2% pet.			‡
menthyl anthranilate			9		a
Salicylates series					
isopropylbenzylsalicylate					b
benzyl salicylate		2% pet.		+	*See* § 29.19
homosalate (= homomenthyl salicylate)	Filtrosol A	2% pet.	95	+	a,b. *See* § 29.19

(continued)

§ 30.13 *(continuation)*

Sunscreen	Synonym®	Patch test con. & veh. (§ 30.1)	Freq. use (§ 30.3)	Cont. all. (§ 30.3)	Comment (a b: § 30.12 and § 30.3)
menthyl salicylate	Filtrol				
octyl salicylate	Sunarome WMO	2% pet.	73		a,b
phenyl salicylate		2% pet.		+	*See* § 29.19, § 27.16 *and* § 13.3
PPG-2 salicylate			5		
TEA salicylate	Sunarome		16		a
Cinnamates series					
cyclohexyl-*p*-methoxycinnamate	in Parsol Ultra				‡
DEA methoxycinnamte			30		a
cinoxate	GivTan F; 2-ethoxyethyl-*p*-methoxycinnamate	1% pet.		+	*See* § 29.19
ethyldiisopropyl cinnamate	in Neo Heliopan	1% pet.†			
isopropyl methoxycinnamate	in Neo Heliopan	2% pet.†			
octocrylene	Uvinul N-539, 2-octyl-a-cyano-b-phenyl-cinnamate (= 2-ethylhexyl-2-cyano-3,3-diphenylacrylate)	1% pet.†	5		a
octyl methoxycinnamate	Neo Heliopan AV, Parsol MCX	2% pet.†	451		a,b
potassium cinnamate					‡
potassium *p*-methoxycinnamate	Solprotex II				‡
n-propyl *p*-methoxycinnamate	Solprotex I, II, III				‡
Benzophenone series					
benzophenone 1 (= 2,4-dihydroxy-)	Uvinul 400	1% pet.†	161		
benzophenone 2 (= 2,2′,4,4′-tetrahydroxy-)	Uvinul D-50	1% pet.†	460		

(continued)

§ **30.13** *(continuation)*

Sunscreen	Synonym®	Patch test con. & veh. (§ 30.1)	Freq. use (§ 30.3)	Cont. all. (§ 30.3)	Comment (a b: § 30.12 and § 30.3)
benzophenone 3 (= 2-hydroxy-4-methoxy-)	Uvinul M-40, Eusolex 4360, oxybenzone	2% pet.	308	+	a,b. *See* § 29.19
benzophenone 4 (= 2-hydroxy-4-methoxy-5-sulfonic acid)	sulisobenzone, Uvinul MS-40, Uvistat 1121	2% pet.	384	+	a,b. *See* § 29.19
benzophenone 5 (= sodium salt of benzophenone 4)			8		b
benzophenone 6 (= 2,2′-dihydroxy-4,4′-dimethoxy-)	Uvinul D-49	2% pet.†	24		
benzophenone 7 (= 5-chloro-2-hydroxy-)	Dow HCB				
benzophenone 8 (= 2,2′-dihydroxy-4-methoxy-)	Dioxybenzone, Uvistat 24	2% pet.	9	+	a. *See* § 29.19 *under* dioxybenzone
benzophenone 9 (= 2,2′-dihydroxy-4,4′-dimethoxy-5-sulfonate soldium)	Uvinul DS-49		29		
benzophenone 10 (= 2-hydroxy-4-methoxy-4′-methyl-)	Mexenone, Uvistat 2211	2% pet.		+	*See* § 29.19
benzophenone 11 (= mixture of benzophenone 6 and 2)	Uvinul 490	2% pet.†	18		
benzophenone 12 (= 2-hydroxy-4-*n*-octoxy-)	Cyasorb UV 531				
benzophenone, 4-phenyl-	Eusolex 3490				‡
benzophenone, 4′-phenyl-2-octyl-carboxylate	Eusolex 3573				‡
Camphor series					
3-benzylidene camphor	Ultracyd, Ultren BK				b
4-methylbenzylidene camphor	Eusolex 6300	2% pet.	8	+	b. *See* § 29.19
3-(4′-sulfobenzylidene) camphor					‡b
3-(3′-sulfo-4′-methylbenzylidene) camphor					‡

(continued)

§ 30.13 *(continuation)*

Sunscreen	Synonym®	Patch test con. & veh. (§ 30.1)	Freq. use (§ 30.3)	Cont. all. (§ 30.3)	Comment (a b: § 30.12 and § 30.3)
3-(4-trimethylammoniumbenzyl-idene) camphor methosulfate					‡b
Other UV-absorbers					
bornelone	Prosolol S9, 5-(3,3-dimethyl-2-norbornylidene)-3-pentene-2-on	5% pet.		+	*See* § 27.3
butylmethoxydibenzoyl methane	Parsol 1789	2%pet.	25	+	b. *See* § 27.16 *and* § 29.19
dianisoyl methane	Parsol DAM	10% pet.			‡
dibenzalazine	Eusolex 6653				‡
digalloyl trioleate	in Solprotex 1	3.5% pet.	4	+	a,b. *See* § 29.19
drometrizole	Tinuvin P	5% pet.	44	+	*See* § 27.3 *and* § 29.19
guanine		pure	55	+	*See* § 28.2
isopropyl dibenzoylmethane	Eusolex 8020	2% pet.		+	b. *See* § 27.16
methoxy benzylidene cyanic acid *n*-hexyl ester					‡
octyltriazone	Uvinul T-150				b
phenyl-benzimidazole sulfonic acid	Eusolex 232, Novantisol	1% aqua	18	+	a,b. *See* § 29.19
3,3′-(1,4-phenylene-di-methylidyne)bis-(7,7-dimethyl-2-oxo-bicyclo-(2,2,1) heptane-1-methane sulfonic acid	Mexoryl SX				‡b
2-phenyl-5-methyl benzoxazole	Witisol	1% pet.		+	‡ *See* § 29.19
1-phenyl-3-(3-pyridyl)-1,3-propanedione					‡
red petrolatum		pure			a
sodium 3,4-dimethoxyphenyl glyoxilate	Eusolex 161				‡
p-tolyl benzoxazole					‡
urocanic acid ethyl ester					b

LIPIDS AND SURFACTANTS

30.14 In the following paragraphs, tabulations are given of:
- Lipids (§ 30.15.1)
- Anionic surfactants (§ 30.15.2)
- Cationic surfactants (§ 30.15.3)
- Non-ionic surfactants (§ 30.15.4)
- Amphoteric surfactants (§ 30.15.5)
- Amines — aminoalkanols (§ 30.15.6)
- Diols and polyols (§ 30.15.7)

30.15.1 Lipids (hydrocarbons, fatty acids, fatty alcohols, esters and silicones)

Name	Synonym®	Patch test conc. & veh. (§ 30.1)	Freq. use (§ 30.3)	Cont. all. (§ 30.3)	Comment (§ 30.3)
acetylated lanolin		30% pet.	215	+	*See* § 27.16
acetylated lanolin alcohol		30% pet.	522		
almond oil, sweet		pure			‡
apricot kernel oil			65		
arachidonic acid		5% aq.† after neutralisation	31		
arachidyl alcohol			5		‡
arachidyl propionate			33		
avocado oil		pure	284	+	*See* § 29.19
beeswax, white		30% pet.	1428	+	*See* § 5.38 *and* § 27.3
beeswax, yellow		30% pet	181		
behenic acid		5% pet.†	8		
behenyl alcohol		30% pet.†	66		
butyl myristate			5		
butyl stearate		5% pet.†	76		
C 12-16 alcohols			12		
C 12-15 alcohols lactate			22		
C 10-11 isoparaffin			8		
C 10-13 isoparaffin			14		
C 11-12 isoparaffin		30% pet.†	13		
C 11-13 isoparaffin			11		

(continued)

§ **30.15.1** *(continuation)*

Name	Synonym®	Patch test conc. & veh. (§ 30.1)	Freq. use (§ 30.3)	Cont. all. (§ 30.3)	Comment (§ 30.3)
C 12-14 isoparaffin			3		
C 13-14 isoparaffin			3		
C 30-46 piscine oil			3		
candelilla wax		41% m.o.	866		
caprylic/capric triglyceride			522		
carnauba		50% m.o.	452		
castor oil		pure	1029	+	*See* § 5.20
ceresin		30% pet.-pure	389		
cetearyl alcohol		20% pet.†	27		
cetearyl alcohol + sodium cetearyl sulfate (90 + 10)	Lanette N	20% pet.		+	‡*See* § 5.20
cetearyl octanoate		30% pet.†	273		
cetyl alcohol		20% pet.	2882	+	*See* § 5.20
cetyl lactate		5% aqua	107		
cetyl octanoate			19		
cetyl palmitate		20% pet.†	273		
cetyl ricinoleate			53		
cetyl stearate		20% pet.†	3		
cholesterol		10% pet.†	215		
cocoa butter			178		
coconut acid			72		
coconut oil		pure	200		
cod liver oil			8		
corn oil		30% pet.†	214		
cottonseed oil		pure	5		
cyclomethicone		pure†	718	+	*See* § 27.3
decyl oleate		1% pet.	176	+	*See* § 5.20
dibutyl phthalate		5% pet.	262	+	*See* § 5.20
diethyl phthalate		5% pet.	64		

(continued)

§ **30.15.1** *(continuation)*

Name	Synonym®	Patch test conc. & veh. (§ 30.1)	Freq. use (§ 30.3)	Cont. all. (§ 30.3)	Comment (§ 30.3)
dihydroabietyl alcohol	Abitol	10% pet.	13	+	*See* § 5.14
diisobutyl adipate			8		
diisopropyl adipate			61		
diisopropyl dilinoleate			8		
diisostearyl dilinoleate			16		
dimethicone		10% pet.†	1568		
dimethicone copolyol		5% pet.†	460		
dimethyl phthalate		5% pet.	27		
emulsifying wax		30% pet.	97		‡Contact allergy to ingredients has been reported (*See* § 5.20)
ethyl linoleate		10% pet.†	33		
glyceryl erucate					
glyceryl isostearate		30% pet.†	36	+	*See* § 27.16
glyceryl linoleate		30% pet.†	19		
glyceryl myristate			16		
glyceryl oleate		30% pet.	10	+	*See* § 5.20
glyceryl palmitate			6		‡
glyceryl ricinoleate			30	+	*See* § 29.13
glyceryl stearate		30% pet.	1894	+	*See* § 5.20
glyceryl stearate SE		30% pet.†	269		
glyceryl triacetyl ricinoleate			39		
glycol distearate		50% m.o.			
glycol stearate		30% pet.†	407		
glycol stearate SE			22		
grape seed oil			59		
hexamethyldisiloxane			5		
hexyl laurate			6		
hybrid safflower oil		30% pet.†	47		

(continued)

§ 30.15.1 *(continuation)*

Name	Synonym®	Patch test conc. & veh. (§ 30.1)	Freq. use (§ 30.3)	Cont. all. (§ 30.3)	Comment (§ 30.3)
hydroabietyl alcohol	Abitol	10% pet.		+	‡ *See* § 5.14 *under* dihydroabietyl alcohol
hydrogenated castor oil		30% pet.†	181	+	*See* § 27.16
hydrogenated coconut oil		30% pet.†	72		
hydrogenated cottonseed oil			98		
hydrogenated jojoba wax			4		
hydrogenated lanolin		30% pet.	221		
hydrogenated lard glyceride			11		
hydrogenated menhaden acid			4		
hydrogenated palm glyceride			13		‡
hydrogenated palm kernel glyceride		30% pet.†	14		‡
hydrogenated palm kernel oil			24		
hydrogenated palm oil		30% pet.†	15		
hydrogenated peanut oil		30% pet.†	15		
hydrogenated rice bran wax			13		
hydrogenated soy glyceride			92		
hydrogenated soybean oil			11		
hydrogenated tallow			36		
hydrogenated tallow glyceride			23		
hydrogenated tallow glycerides		30% pet.†	17		
hydrogenated vegetable glycerides			40		
hydrogenated vegetable oil		30% pet.	355		
hydroxylated lanolin		30% pet.	136		
isocetyl alcohol		20% pet.†	35		
isocetyl linoleyl stearate			8		‡
isocetyl myristate			5		
isocetyl stearate			81		
isocetyl stearoyl stearate			23		

(continued)

§ **30.15.1** *(continuation)*

Name	Synonym®	Patch test conc. & vch. (§ 30.1)	Freq. use (§ 30.3)	Cont. all. (§ 30.3)	Comment (§ 30.3)
isodecyl isononanoate			3		
isodecyl laurate			3		
isodecyl neopentanoate			30		
isodecyl oleate		pure	66		
iso-octyl hydroxystearate			107		
iso-octyl palmitate			72		‡
iso-octyl stearate			18		‡
isopropyl isostearate		5% pet.†	120		
isopropyl lanolate		20% pet.	598		
isopropyl linoleate			15		
isopropyl myristate		5-10% pet.	1368	+	*See* § 5.20
isopropyl palmitate		2% pet.	618	+	*See* § 5.20
isopropyl stearate			29		
isostearic acid			161		
isostearyl alcohol		5% alc., pure	34	+	*See* § 29.13
isostearyl behenate			3		‡
isostearyl erucate			6		
isostearyl isostearate			21		
isostearyl neopentanoate		5% pet.†	104		
Japan wax		25% m.o.†	190		
jojoba oil		20% pet.†	19	+	*See* index
jojoba wax					
lanolin		pure	1021	+	*See* § 5.20
lanolin acid		5% pet.†	112		
lanolin alcohol (wool alcohols)		30% pet.	519	+	*See* § 5.20
lanolin oil		30% pet.	756	+	*See* § 27.8
lanolin wax		30% m.o.†	148		
lard glyceride			10		
lauric acid		5% pet.†	51		

(continued)

§ 30.15.1 *(continuation)*

Name	Synonym®	Patch test conc. & veh. (§ 30.1)	Freq. use (§ 30.3)	Cont. all. (§ 30.3)	Comment (§ 30.3)
lauryl alcohol		5% pet.	12		
lauryl lactate			14		
lauryl palmitate			3		
linoleic acid		2.5% aqua†	55		
linolenic acid			43		
linseed oil		pure	11		
methyl oleate					
microcrystalline wax		pure†	468	+	*See* § 30.2 [19] *and* § 27.16
mineral oil, heavy		pure	1431	+	‡*See* § 27.16
mineral oil, light		pure	2532	+	‡*See* § 27.16
mink oil		30% pet.†	160		
montan wax		5% pet.†	26		
myristic acid			48		
myristyl alcohol		20% pet.	28	+	*See* § 5.20
myristyl lactate		13.8% pet.	158		
myristyl myristate		30% pet.†	225		
octyldodecanol	Eutanol G®	30% pet.	606	+	*See* § 5.20
octyl isononanoate			6		
octyl octanoate			9		‡
octyl palmitate		20% pet.†	513		
octyl stearate		20% pet.†	90		
oleic acid		5% pet.†	864		
oleyl alcohol		30% pet.	437	+	*See* § 5.20
oleyl oleate			30		
olive oil		pure	150	+	*See* § 5.20
ozokerite		pure	766		
palm kernel oil			23		
palm oil			49		

(continued)

§ **30.15.1** *(continuation)*

Name	Synonym®	Patch test conc. & veh. (§ 30.1)	Freq. use (§ 30.3)	Cont. all. (§ 30.3)	Comment (§ 30.3)
palm oil glycerides			4		
palmitic acid		5% pet.†	67		
paraffin		pure	676	+	*See* § 5.20
peach kernel oil			14		
peanut oil		30% pet.†	52		
penta-erythrityl rosinate			6		
penta-erythrityl tetraabietate			12		
penta-erythrityl tetrabehenate			6		
penta-erythrityl tetracaprylate/caprate			9		‡
penta-erythrityl tetraoctanoate			9		
penta-erythrityl tetrapelargonate			3		‡
penta-erythrityl tetrastearate			54		
petrolatum, white		pure	698	+	‡*See* § 5.20
petrolatum, yellow		pure	689	+	‡ *See* § 5.20
petrolatum wax			23		‡ *See under* paraffin *or* microcrystalline wax
petroleum destillate			76		
phenyl dimethicone			111		‡
phenyl trimethicone			52		
polybutene		30% pet.	245		
propylene glycol		2-20% aqua	4896	+	*See* § 5.20
propylene glycol dicaprylate/dicaprate			250		
propylene glycol dioctanoate			13		
propylene glycol diperlargonate			44		
propylene glycol hydroxystearate			4		
propylene glycol isostearate			15		‡
propylene glycol laurate		10% pet.†	159		
propylene glycol myristate		20% pet.†	7		

(continued)

§ **30.15.1** *(continuation)*

Name	Synonym®	Patch test conc. & veh. (§ 30.1)	Freq. use (§ 30.3)	Cont. all. (§ 30.3)	Comment (§ 30.3)
propylene glycol oleate			7		
propylene glycol ricinoleate		10% pet.†	42		
propylene glycol stearate		10% pet.†	214		
propylene glycol stearate SE		5% pet.†	73		
ricinoleic acid		30% pet. and pure	9	+	*See* § 5.20
safflower oil			132		
sesame oil		pure	287	+	*See* § 5.20
shea butter			171		
simethicone		5% pet.†	241		
soybean oil		pure†	111		
spermaceti		pure	36		‡
squalane		20% pet.	551		
squalene		pure	23		
stearic acid		5% pet.	2579	+	*See* § 27.3
stearoxy dimethicone			79		
stearoxy trimethylsilane			9		
stearyl alcohol		30% pet.	811	+	*See* § 5.20
stearyl dimethicone			9		‡
stearyl heptanoate		20% pet.†	137		
stearyl stearate			13		
stearylstearoyl stearate			5		
stearyl urecate			3		‡
sunflower seed oil			80		
sunflower seed oil glyceride			6		
synthetic beeswax		30% pet.†	99		
synthetic wax		pure†	142		
tall oil acid			3		
tall oil glycerides			11		

(continued)

§ **30.15.1** *(continuation)*

Name	Synonym®	Patch test conc. & veh. (§ 30.1)	Freq. use (§ 30.3)	Cont. all. (§ 30.3)	Comment (§ 30.3)
tallow			3		
tallow acid			4		
tallow glyceride			24		
tallow glycerides			10		
trihydroxystearin		20% pet.†	65		
triisostearyl trilinoleate			7		
trilaurin		30% pet.†	129		
trilinolein			4		
tristearin			52		
turtle oil			18		‡
undecylenic acid		2-5% pet.	8	+	*See* § 5.30
vegetable oil		pure†	40		
wheat germ glycerides		2% pet.	224		
wheat germ oil		20% pet.†	325		

30.15.2 Anionic surfactants

Anionic surfactants are salts that dissociate in solution to form an anion with a negatively charged hydrophilic end and a lipophilic tail. They lower the surface tension between two immiscible substances. This property makes them suitable as cleansing agents and they are widely used in shampoos and bath foams. They are also used as (auxiliary) emulsifier and solubilizer. The best known example is sodium lauryl sulfate.

Name	Synonym®	Patch test conc. & veh. (§ 30.1)	Freq. use (§ 30.3)	Cont. all (§ 30.3)	Comment (§ 30.3)
ammonium laureth sulfate			100		
ammonium laureth-12 sulfate			15		
ammonium lauryl sulfate		0.1% aqua†	285		

(continued)

§ 30.15.2 *(continuation)*

Name	Synonym®	Patch test conc. & veh. (§ 30.1)	Freq. use (§ 30.3)	Cont. all (§ 30.3)	Comment (§ 30.3)
ammonium lauryl sulfosuccinate			3		
ammonium nonoxynol-4 sulfate			20		
ammonium xylene sulfonate			50		
DEA-cetyl phosphate			110		
DEA-lauryl sulfate			17		
DEA-oleth-3 phosphate			15		
DEA-oleth-10 phosphate			10		
DEA-tallowate			4		
dioctyl sodium sulfosuccinate	Aerosol OT	5% aqua	45		test concentration irritant
disodium cocamido MIPA-sulfosuccinate			18		
disodium laureth sulfosuccinate		2% aqua†	62		
disodium lauryl sulfosuccinate			9		
disodium monooleamido sulfosuccinate			11		‡
disodium oleamido MEA-sulfosuccinate			6		
disodium oleamido MIPA-sulfosuccinate			11		
disodium oleamido PEG-2 sulfosuccinate			24		
disodium ricinoleamido MEA-sulfosuccinate		0.1% aq.†	11		
disodium undecylenamido MEA-sulfosuccinate		5% aq.†	4		
dodecylbenzene sulfonic acid			4		
magnesium laureth sulfate			17		
magnesium lauryl sulfate			3		
MIPA-laureth sulfate			4		
potassium cocoate			14		
potassium laurate			6		
potassium lauryl sulfate			11		
potassium myristate			12		
potassium octoxynol-12 phosphate		0.1% aq.†	17		

(continued)

§ **30.15.2** *(continuation)*

Name	Synonym®	Patch test conc. & vch. (§ 30.1)	Freq. use (§ 30.3)	Cont. all (§ 30.3)	Comment (§ 30.3)
potassium oleate			13		
potassium palmitate			10		
sodium C12-15 alkyl sulfate			12		
sodium C14-16 olefin sulfonate		0.1% aq.†	92		
sodium C14-17 alkyl SEC sulfonate			3		
sodium cetearyl sulfate		0.2% aqua†	40		
sodium cetyl sulfate		0.1% aqua†	6		
sodium cocoate		1% aqua†	99		
sodium cocoyl isethionate			70		
sodium dodecylbenzenesulfonate		0.1% aq.†	13		
sodium lauramino dipropionate			25		
sodium laureth sulfate		1-2% aqua	550	+	*See* § 26.2
sodium laureth sulfosuccinate		0.5% aq.†	4		‡
sodium lauroyl sarcosinate		2% aqua	82		Test concentration irritant
sodium lauryl sulfate		0.1% aqua	863	+	*See* § 5.20
sodium lauryl sulfoacetate			33		
sodium methyl cocoyl taurate			50		
sodium methyl oleyl taurate			7		
sodium myreth sulfate		0.1%-1% aqua†	41		
sodium myristate			9		
sodium myristal sulfate			3		
sodium nonoxynol-9 phosphate					
sodium octoxynol-3 sulfonate			5		‡
sodium oleate			11		
sodium palmitate			11		
sodium polynaphthalene sulfonate			59		
sodium soap			6		‡
sodium stearate		1% aq.†	210		

(continued)

§ **30.15.2** *(continuation)*

Name	Synonym®	Patch test conc. & veh. (§ 30.1)	Freq. use (§ 30.3)	Cont. all (§ 30.3)	Comment (§ 30.3)
sodium tallowate		1% aq.†	85		
sodium trideceth sulfate			19		
sodium xylenesulfonate			16		
sulfated castor oil		1% o.o/2% aqua	91	+	2% aqua is irritant. *See* index
TEA-dodecylbenzenesulfonate			58		
TEA-laureth sulfate			14		
TEA-lauryl sulfate		0.1% aqua†	371		
TEA-stearate		5% pet.	50	+	*See* § 5.20
trideceth-7 carboxylic acid			37		

30.15.3 Cationic surfactants

Cationic surfactants are quaternary ammonium compounds. Their structure is essentially a positively charged tetra substituted nitrogen, the substituents often being aliphatic, but also carrying additional substituents. Because the substituents are generally lipophilic, cationics act as surfactants. They are not used for cleansing, however. Their main application is hair conditioning, because the positive charge makes them substantive to the negatively charged proteins of the hair. Polymeric quats also find application in hair setting and styling products, while several quats are useful as antimicrobial agents (see § 30.5).

Quaternary ammonium compounds are generally irritant. They may usually be tested 0.1% and 0.01% aqua.

Name	Synonym®	Patch test conc. & veh. (§ 30.1)	Freq. use (§ 30.3)	Cont. all. (§ 30.3)	Comment (§ 30.3)
behentrimonium chloride (behenyl-trimethylammoniumchloride)		0.1% aq.†	10		
benzalkonium chloride (alkyl dimethyl benzyl ammonium chloride)		0.01% and 0.1% aqua	100	+	See § 5.7 under quaternary ammonium compounds

(continued)

§ **30.15.3** *(continuation)*

Name	Synonym®	Patch test conc. & veh. (§ 30.1)	Freq. use (§ 30.3)	Cont. all. (§ 30.3)	Comment (§ 30.3)
benzethonium chloride	Hyamine 1622	0.01% and 0.1% aqua	77	+	*See* § 5.7 under quaternary ammonium compounds
cetrimonium bromide (cetyl trimethyl ammonium bromide; cetrimide)		0.01% and 0.1% aqua	37	+	*See* § 5.7 under quaternary ammonium compounds
cetrimonium chloride (cetyl trimethyl ammonium chloride)		0.05% aq.†	138		
cetylpyridinium chloride		0.01% and 0.1% aqua	18	+	*See* § 5.7 under quaternary ammonium compounds
denatonium benzoate	Bitrex	2% pet.†	14		
dicetyldimonium chloride (quaternium-31)			124		
distearyldimonium chloride (quaternium-5)	Dehyquart DAM		58		
domiphen bromide (dodecyldimethyl-2-phenoxyethylammonium bromide)		0.01% and 0.1% aqua	8	+	*See* § 5.7 *under* quaternary ammonium compounds
guar hydroxypropyltrimonium chloride			75		
hexadimethrine chloride	Mexamere PO		97		
hydroxyethyl cetyldimonium chloride (quaternium-44)			36		
isostearamidopropyl ethyldimonium ethosulfate	Schercoquat IAS		17		
isostearyl ethylimidonium ethosulfate (quaternium-32)			20		
lapyrium chloride	Emcol E 6071		21		
laurtrimonium chloride (lauryl trimethyl ammonium chloride)			4		
lauryl isoquinolinium bromide	Dodecin		3		
methyl benzethonium chloride	Hyamine 10X		6		

(continued)

§ 30.15.3 *(continuation)*

Name	Synonym®	Patch test conc. & veh. (§ 30.1)	Freq. use (§ 30.3)	Cont. all. (§ 30.3)	Comment (§ 30.3)
myristalkonium chloride (myristyl dimethyl benzyl ammonium chloride)		0.05% aq.†	5		
myristalkonium saccharinate (quaternium-3)			3		
myrtrimonium bromide (myristyl trimethyl ammonium bromide)		0.05% aq.†	3		
olealkonium chloride (oleyl dimethyl benzyl ammonium chloride)		0.1% aq.†	35		
PEG-15 cocomonium chloride	Ethoquad C/25		5		
PEG-15 stearmonium chloride			38		
polyquaternium-2	Mirapol A-15	0.1% aq.†	56		
polyquaternium-4 (diallyldimonium chloride/hydroxyethylcellulose copolymer)	Celquat H-100	0.05% pet.†	100		
polyquaternium-6 (poly(dimethyl diallyl ammonium chloride))	quaternium-40;Merquat 100	0.1% aq.†	52		
polyquaternium-7 (quaternium-41)	Merquat s	0.1% aq.†	109		
polyquaternium-10 (quaternium-19)		0.05% aq.†	388		
polyquaternium-11 (quaternium-23)	Gafquat 734	0.05% aq.†	276		
polyquaternium-12 (quaternium-37)			3		
PPG-9 diethylmoniumchloride (quaternium-6; polyoxypropylene (9) methyl diethyl ammonium chloride)			22		
quaternium-3	Onyxide 3300		3		‡*See* myristalkonium saccharinate
quaternium-11			14		‡
quaternium-15 (chloroallyhexaminium chloride)	Dowicil 200	1% pet.	885	+	*See* § 5.7 and § 27.3
quaternium-18 (dimethyl dihydrogenated tallow ammonium chloride)	Varisoft DHT		80		
quaternium-18 bentonite	Bentone 34	0.5% pet.†	76		
quaternium-18 hectorite	Bentone 38	pure	213		
quaternium-22 (gluconamidopropyldimethyl-2-hydroxyl ammonium chloride)			86		

(continued)

§ **30.15.3** *(continuation*

Name	Synonym®	Patch test conc. & veh. (§ 30.1)	Freq. use (§ 30.3)	Cont. all. (§ 30.3)	Comment (§ 30.3)
quaternium-26 (minkamidopropyl dimethyl-2-hydroxyethyl ammonium chloride)		0.1% aq.†	61		
quaternium-27	Varisoft 475; Rewoquat W 90		6		
quaternium-31 (dicetyl dimethyl ammonium chloride)			15		‡ *See*: dicetyl-dimonium chloride
quaternium-47			30		‡*See* dilauryl-dimonium chloride
quaternium-51	Takanal		5		
quaternium-52	Dehyquart SP		13		
quaternium-61	Schercoquat DAS		9		
quaternium-70 (stearamidopropyl dimethyl-(myristyl acetate) ammonium chloride)			5		
steapyrium chloride (quaternium-7)			46		
stearalkonium chloride		0.01% and 0.1% aqua	387		
stearalkonium hectorite	Bentone 27	1% pet.†	258		
steartrimonium hydrolyzed collagen		0.05% aq.†	61		‡
tallowdimonium propyltrimonium dichloride	Duoquat T-50		4		

30.15.4 Non-ionic surfactants

Non-ionic surfactants do not dissociate in solution. They carry both hydrophilic and lipophilic groups that give an uneven charge distribution on the molecule, which accounts for their surfactant properties. They are used as cleansing agents, foam boosters, emulsifiers and in a number of other applications.

Non-ionic surfactants can be classified into chemical subgroups, which roughly correspond to their uses. The various categories are listed in the following tables (§ 30.15.4–30.15.4.6).

30.15.4.1 Alkanolamides

Alkanolamides are condensation products of fatty acids with primary or secondary alkanolamines (mono- and diethanolamine; MEA, DEA). Their main application is as foam boosters in shampoos and bath foams.

Name	Synonym®	Patch test conc. & veh. (§ 30.1)	Freq. use (§ 30.3)	Cont. all. (§ 30.3)	Comment (§ 30.3)
capramide DEA	Alrosol C	1% aqua			Test concentration may be irritant
cocamide DEA		0.5% pet. or aqua†	711	+	*See* § 29.3 and § 26.2
cocamide MEA		0.5% aqua	193		
isostearamide DEA			15		
lauramide DEA		1% aqua	748	+	*See* § 26.2
lauramide MEA		1% aqua†			
lauramide MIPA			22		
linoleamide DEA			120		
myristamide DEA			16		
oleamide DEA			120		
oleamide MIPA			6		
ricinoleamide DEA		0.5% aqua†	3		
stearamide DEA			26		
stearamide MEA			19		
undecylenamide MEA			4		

30.15.4.2 Alkoxylated alcohols

Alkoxylated alcohols are formed from the reaction of alcohols with alkylene oxides, generally ethylene oxide or propylene oxide. The number of alkylene oxide molecules used in the reaction varies, resulting in molecules of widely different length and character.

Alkoxylated alcohol used in cosmetics may function as surfactants, emulsifiers and solubilizers. The table summarizes those alkoxylated alcohols that are primarily used for these purposes. Some compounds of this category are also employed as skin and hair conditioners; these are listed in § 30.17.

Name	Synonym®	Patch test conc. & veh. (§ 30.1)	Freq. use (§ 30.3)	Cont. all. (§ 30.3)	Comment (§ 30.3)
ceteareth-3	Procol CS-3		3		
ceteareth-5	Unicol CSA 5		30		
ceteareth-6	Marlowet TA 6	5% pet.†	9		
ceteareth-10		5% pet.†			
ceteareth-12	Eumulgin B1: Procol CS-12	20% pet.†	69		
ceteareth-15	Hetoxol nonionic CS15		3		
ceteareth-17	Atlas G-70147		3		
ceteareth-20	Brij 68; Emulgin B-2	20% pet.†	260		
ceteareth-25	Cremophor A 25		31		
ceteareth-30	Lipocol CS-30; Unimul B3	20% pet.†	18		
ceteth-1			3		
ceteth-2	Brij 52	10% pet.†	38		
ceteth-10	Brij 56		11		
ceteth-12			3		
ceteth-16		10% pet.†			
ceteth-20	Brij 58		200		
ceteth-24			20		
ceteth-30	Lipocol C 30		16		
ceteth-60		10% aqua†			‡
choleth-24	Fancol CH-24	5% pet.	97		
C-12-15 pareth-12	Alkasurf LA-12		17		
dodoxynol-9		5% aqua†			
isoceteth-20	Arlasolve 200	20% pet.†	13		
isolaureth-6	Tergotol TMN-6		9		
isosteareth-2			3		
isosteareth-10	Arosurf 66E10; Hexetol IS-10		17		
isosteareth-20			14		
laneth-5	Aqualose W5		46		
laneth-15	Polychol 15	30% pet.†	15		
laneth-16	Ethoxyol 1690	10% pet.†	60		
laneth-25			4		
laneth-40	Polychol 40		3		
laureth-3		10% aqua†			
laureth-4	Dehydol LS4	5% aqua†	141		
laureth-7	Akypo MB 1169		17		
laureth-9	Atlas G-4829		5		

(continued)

§ 30.15.4.2 *(continuation)*

Name	Synonym®	Patch test conc. & veh. (§ 30.1)	Freq. use (§ 30.3)	Cont. all. (§ 30.3)	Comment (§ 30.3)
laureth-10	Dehydo 100	5% aqua†	5		
laureth-11	Marlipal 24/110		6		
laureth-12	Alkasurf LAN-12		10		
laureth-20		10% pet.†			
laureth-23	Brij 35	20% pet.†	417		
nonoxynol-1	Alkasurf NP-1		55		
nonoxynol-4	Alkasurf NP-4	5% aqua	428		
nonoxynol-6	Triton N-60	0.5% aqua	12		
nonoxynol-7	Elfapur N-70	5% aqua	3		
nonoxynol-9	Elfapur N-90	1% aqua	94		irritant reactions at 1% aqua
nonoxynol-10	Eumilgin 286	5% aqua	165		
nonoxynol-12	Alkasurf NP-12	5% aqua	22		
nonoxynol-14	Makon-14	5% aqua	37		
nonoxynol-15	Triton N-150		119		
nonoxynol-30	Witconol NP 300		4		
nonoxynol-40	Hodag Nonionic E-40		14		
nonyl nonoxynol-10	Hetoxide DNP-10		4		
nonyl nonoxynol-49			4		
octoxynol-1	Triton X-15		217		
octoxynol-5	Alkasurf OP-5; Triton X-45	0.1% aqua	3		
octoxynol-9	Triton X-100	1% aqua	234		Test concentration may be irritant
octoxynol-11	Oxypol-11		19		
octoxynol-13	Triton X102		71		
oleth-2	Brij-92		29		
oleth-3	Brox Ol-3	20% pet.†	16		
oleth-5	Eumulgin 05	20% pet.†	19		
oleth-8	Atlas G-3908S		8		
oleth-10	Brij 96	25% pet.†	79		
oleth-16	Solulan 16	10% pet.†			
oleth-20	Brij 98	20% pet.†	192		
oleth-25	Lipocol O-25		3		
oleth-30	Marlowet OA 30		86		
PEG-6 caprylic/capric glycerides	Softigen 767		27		

(continued)

§ **30.15.4.2** *(continuation)*

Name	Synonym®	Patch test conc. & veh. (§ 30.1)	Freq. use (§ 30.3)	Cont. all. (§ 30.3)	Comment (§ 30.3)
PEG-9 castor oil	Etocas 9		3		
PEG-30 castor oil	Emulphor CO 30		13		
PEG-36 castor oil	Arlaton 650		4		
PEG-40 castor oil	Eumulgin RO 40	30% pet.†	81		
PEG-50 castor oil		20% pet.†			
PEG-7 glyceryl cocoate	Cetiol HE	20% pet.†	147		
PEG-30 glyceryl cocoate	Rewoderm LI 63		3		
PEG-20 glyceryl oleate		20% pet.†			
PEG-20 glyceryl ricinoleate		30% pet.†	5		
PEG-5 glyceryl stearate	Arlatone 983S	20% pet.†	11		
PEG-20 glyceryl stearate		20% pet.†			
PEG-30 glyceryl stearate	Tagat S		10		
PEG-200 glyceryl tallowate		10% aqua†			
PEG-7 hydrogenated castor oil	Arlacel 989	30% pet.†	24		
PEG-25 hydrogenated castor oil	Arlatone G	30% pet.†			
PEG-30 hydrogenated castor oil	Crodaret 30		5		
PEG-40 hydrogenated castor oil	Cremophor RH40	30% pet.†	201		
PEG-45 hydrogenated castor oil	Arlatone 975	30% pet.†			
PEG-60 hydrogenated castor oil	Eumulgin HRE60	30% pet.†	65		
PEG-20 hydrogenated lanolin			6		
PEG-24 hydrogenated lanolin	Lipolan 31		9		
PEG-5 lanolin			7		
PEG-20 lanolin	Laneto 20		5		
PEG-24 lanolin			3		
PEG-25 lanolin		20% pet.†			‡

(continued)

§ **30.15.4.2** *(continuation)*

Name	Synonym®	Patch test conc. & veh. (§ 30.1)	Freq. use (§ 30.3)	Cont. all. (§ 30.3)	Comment (§ 30.3)
PEG-27 lanolin	Laneto 27		14		
PEG-40 lanolin	Ethoxygel 1683		9		
PEG-50 lanolin	Laneto 49	30% pet.†	6		
PEG-60 lanolin	Solan		14		
PEG-75 lanolin	Solulan 75	30% pet.†	144		
PEG-85 lanolin	Lanogel 61		9		
PEG-75 lanolin oil	Rewolan AWS		42		
PEG-120 methyl glucose dioleate	Glucamate DOE 120	20% pet.†	63		
PEG-55 propylene-glycol oleate		10% aqua†	3		
PEG-25 propylene-glycol stearate	Atlas G 2162	10% aqua†	18		
PEG-5 soya sterol	Generol 122 E 5	20% pet.†	65		
PEG-10 soya sterol	Generol 122 E 10		51		
PEG-16 soya sterol	Generol 122 E 16		9		
PEG-25 soya sterol	Generol 122 E 25		11		
PPG-12-buteth-16			51		
PPG-26-buteth-26	Witconol APEB		4		
PPG-24 glycereth-24	Polyglycol 15-200		10		
PPG-27 glycerylether	Witconol CD-18		4		
PPG-2-isodeceth-12	Sandoxylate SX-424		5		
ricinoleth-40	Polyglicoleum		11		
steareth-2	Brij 72	20% pet.†	136		
steareth-4	Procol SA-4; Nikkol BS-4		3		
steareth-6		20% pet.†	5,		
steareth-7	Emulgator E 2149	20% pet.†			
steareth-10	Brij 76	5% aqua†	21		
steareth-16		10% pet.†			
steareth-20	Brij 78	5% aqua†	195		
steareth-21	Brij 721	5% aqua†	59		
steareth-100	Brij 700		11		
trideceth-6	Hexetol TD-6		8		
trideceth-9		20% pet.†			

30.15.4.3 Alkoxylated carboxylic acids

Alkoxylated carboxylic acids result from the reaction between a carboxylic acid and an alkylene oxide (often ethylene oxide). The resulting non ionic surfactants are either monoesters or diesters, depending on the reaction conditions. At the same time they are ethers. Alkoxylated carboxylic acids function as emulsifier, solubilizer and suspending agent. They are also used as emollients.

Name	Synonym®	Patch test conc. & veh. (§ 30.1)	Freq. use (§ 30.3)	Cont. all. (§ 30.3)	Comment (§ 30.3)
PEG-4 dilaurate	Cithrol 2DL		11		
PEG-8 dilaurate	Alkamuls 400DL		22		
PEG-8 dioleate	Alkamuls 400DO		6		
PEG-2 distearate			5		
PEG-3 distearate	Cutina TS	20% pet.†	12		
PEG-4 distearate	Hodag 22S		10		
PEG-8 distearate		20% pet.†	62		
PEG-12 distearate	Elfacos PEG 6000		9		
PEG-100 distearate		20% pet.†			‡
PEG-150 distearate	Atlas G1821		133		
PEG-2 laurate		20% pet.†			
PEG-4 laurate	Hodag 20L		14		
PEG-8 laurate	Hodag 42S		8		
PEG-3 oleate			6		
PEG-5 oleate	Ethofat 015	5% pet.†			
PEG-6 oleate	Olepal 1		9		
PEG-8 oleate	Elfacos PEG 400 MD		5		
PEG-12 oleate	Alkamuls 600 MO		5		
PEG-6 palmitate			3		
PEG-2 stearate	Tegin D6100	20% pet.†	106		
PEG-2 stearate SE			25		Self emulsifying: contains some sodium/potassium stearate
PEG-4 stearate	Crodet Sa		18		
PEG-5 stearate	Ethofat 60/15		9		

(continued)

§ **30.15.4.3** *(continuation)*

Name	Synonym®	Patch test conc. & veh. (§ 30.1)	Freq. use (§ 30.3)	Cont. all. (§ 30.3)	Comment (§ 30.3)
PEG-9 stearate		20% pet.†			
PEG-10 stearate	Ethofat 60/20		256		
PEG-12 stearate	Crodet S12		18		
PEG-20 stearate	Myrj 51	30% pet.†	49		
PEG-23 stearate		20% pet.†			‡
PEG-30 stearate	Myrj 51		3		
PEG-32 stearate	Hodag 154-S	20% pet.†	12	+	*See* § 27.3
PEG-40 stearate	Myrj 52	20% aqua†	159		
PEG-50 stearate	Myrj 53	20% pet.†	29		
PEG-75 stearate			3		
PEG-100 stearate		10% aqua†			
PEG-150 stearate	Hodag CSA 102		22		
PEG-6-32 stearate	Hodag 150-S	20% pet.†	62		‡

30.15.4.4 Sorbitan derivatives

Esters and ethers of sorbitan, a heterocyclic ether and polyalcohol derived from sorbitol by dehydration. Spans and Tweens are members of this group of surfactants. Sorbitan derivatives are widely used as emulsifiers, stabilizers and suspending agents in foods, drugs and cosmetics.

Name	Synonym®	Patch test conc. & veh. (§ 30.1)	Freq. use (§ 30.3)	Cont. all. (§ 30.3)	Comment (§ 30.3)
PEG-6 sorbitan beeswax	Atlas G 1702		6		
PEG-20 sorbitan beeswax	Atlas G-1726	10% pet.†	46		
PEG-20 sorbitan isostearate	Isoixol	5% pet.†			
PEG-40 sorbitan lanolate	Atlas G-1441		3		

(continued)

§ **30.15.4.4** *(continuation)*

Name	Synonym®	Patch test conc. & veh. (§ 30.1)	Freq. use (§ 30.3)	Cont. all. (§ 30.3)	Comment (§ 30.3)
PEG-10 sorbitan laurate	Atlas G-7606J		15		
PEG-44 sorbitan laurate	Hetsorb L-44		8		
PEG-80 sorbitan laurate	Emsorb 2721		11		
PEG-40 sorbitan peroleate	Arlatone T	10% pet.†	12		
PEG-20 sorbitan stearate		5% pet.†			‡
polysorbate 20	Tween 20	5% aqua	843		irritant reactions at 5% aqua [2]
polysorbate 21	Tween 21		4		
polysorbate 40	Tween 40	10% pet.	65	+	*See* § 5.20
polysorbate 60	Tween 60	5% aqua†	474	+	*See* § 5.20
polysorbate 61	Tween 61		14		
polysorbate 65	Tween 65		4		
polysorbate 80	Tween 80	10% pet.	246	+	*See* § 5.20
polysorbate 81	Tween 81		7		
polysorbate 85	Tween 85		39		
polysorbate 80 acetate	Solulan 97		3		
sorbitan isostearate	Arlacel 987	5% pet.†	41		
sorbitan laurate	Arlacel 20; Span 20	5% aqua or o.o.	101		*See* § 5.20; 5% o.o. may be irritant
sorbitan oleate	Span 80	5% aqua or o.o.	108	+	*See* § 5.20; 5% o.o. may be irritant
sorbitan palmitate		5% aqua†			
sorbitan sesquiisostearate			13		
sorbitan sesquioleate	Dehymuls SSO Arlacel 83	20% pet.	272	+	*See* § 5.20
sorbitan stearate	Span 60	5% aqua or pet.†	388	+	*See* § 5.20; 5% pet. may be irritant
sorbitan trioleate	Span 85		18		
sorbitan tristearate	Span 65	5% m.o.†	23		

30.15.4.5 Amine oxides

Amine oxides are derived from tertiary amines by oxidation. They are nonionic surfactants with mildly cationic properties at acid pH, which are used as detergents and emulsifiers.

Name	Synonym®	Patch test conc. & veh. (§ 30.1)	Freq. use (§ 30.3)	Cont. all. (§ 30.3)	Comment (§ 30.3)
cocamidopropylamine oxide		1% aqua†			
cocamine oxide			4		
lauramine oxide	Ammonyx L O	3.7% aqua		+	*See* § 29.3
myristamine oxide			17		
oleamine oxide			7		
palmitamine oxide			3		
stearamine oxide			41		

30.15.4.6 Miscellaneous nonionic surfactants

This table lists nonionic surfactants not belonging to one of the chemical categories described in the previous tables. Included are amines, amides, ethers, esters and sucrose derivatives used as surfactants in cosmetic products.

Name	Synonym®	Patch test conc. & veh. (§ 30.1)	Freq. use (§ 30.3)	Cont. all. (§ 30.3)	Comment
cocamide	Fancol CH-24	0.5% aqua†	5		
cocamidopropyl dimethylamine propionate			15		
laneth-10 acetate	Lipolan 98	10% pet.†	109		
methyl glucose dioleate	Glucolate DO	5% aqua†; 5% pet.			
methyl glucose sesquioleate	Glucate SS		3		
methyl glucose sesquistearate		5% pet.	115	+	*See* index
oleth-3 phosphate			8		

(continued)

§ **30.15.4.6** *(continuation)*

Name	Synonym®	Patch test conc. & veh. (§ 30.1)	Freq. usc (§ 30.3)	Cont. all. (§ 30.3)	Comment
PEG-2 cocamide			3		
PEG-5 cocamide	Eumulgin C4	1% aqua†			
PEG-2 cocamine		5% aqua†	3		
PEG-3 cocamine			11		
PEG-15 cocamine		1% aqua†	28		
PEG-20 cocamine			43		
PEG-8 hydrogenated tallow-amine			68		
PEG-5 soyamine			10		
PEG-5 tallow amide			29		
PEG-50 tallow amide	Ethomid HT/60		93		
PEG-5 tallow amine			29		
PEG-8 tallow amine			68		
PEG-15 tallow polyamine		1% aqua†	51		
Poloxamer 105			3		
Poloxamer 182			4		
Poloxamer 184		pure†	22		
Poloxamer 188			14		
Poloxamer 237			3		
Poloxamer 238			5		
Poloxamer 282			63		
Poloxamer 333			8		
Poloxamer 407		pure†	18		
polyglyceryl-10 decaoleate			12		
polyglyceryl-3 diisostearate		5% pet.†	46		
polyglyceryl-3 hydroxy-laurylether			6		
polyglyceryl-4 oleate			3		
polyglyceryl-2 oleyether		5% aqua†	64		

(continued)

§ **30.15.4.6** *(continuation*

Name	Synonym®	Patch test conc. & veh. (§ 30.1)	Freq. use (§ 30.3)	Cont. all. (§ 30.3)	Comment
polyglyceryl-4 oleyether		5% aqua†	61		
polyglyceryl-2 sesquiisostearate		5% pet.†	4		
polyglyceryl-3 stearate		20% pet.†			
PPG-2 myristyl ether propionate			25		
stearamide DIBA-stearate			21		
stearamide MEA-stearate			30		
sucrose cocoate			8		
sucrose distearate			8		
sucrose laurate			3		
trilaureth-4 phosphate		0.5%-1% pet.	8	+	*See* § 29.3

30.15.5 Amphoteric surfactants

Amphoteric surfactants dissociate in solution, but are special in that they can be both anionic and cationic. At extreme pH they can behave like anionic or cationic surfactants, but at normal pH they may be present as zwitterion. They are mainly used as detergents and foam boosters in shampoos and bath foams. Examples are betaines and cocoamphodiacetates and -dipropionates.

Name	Synonym®	Patch test conc. & veh. (§ 30.1)	Freq. use (§ 30.3)	Cont. all. (§ 30.3)	Comment (§ 30.3)
amphoteric-2					‡ *See* cocoamphodipropionic acid
amphoteric-6	Miranol 2 MCA mod.	1% aqua	4		‡*See* disodium cocoamphodiacetate and sodium laurylsulfate and hexylene glycol

(continued)

§ **30.15.5** *(continuation)*

Name	Synonym®	Patch test conc. & veh. (§ 30.1)	Freq. usc (§ 30.3)	Cont. all. (§ 30.3)	Comment (§ 30.3)
amphoteric-14	Miranol 2 MHT mod.	1% aqua	6		‡*See* disodium lauramphodiacetate and sodium trideceth sulfate and hexylene glycol
cocamidopropyl betaine		1% aqua	521	+	*See* § 26.2
cocamidopropyl hydroxysul-taine	Rewoteric AM CAS	2% aqua	62		
cocoamphocarboxyglycinate					‡ *See* disodium cocoamphodiacetate
cocoamphodipropionic acid	Miranol C2M	1% aqua	39		
cocoamphoglycinate					‡*See* sodium cocoamphoacetate
coco-betaine	Tegobetaine	1-2% aqua	93	+	*See* § 26.2
disodium cocoamphodiacetate		1% aqua	65		
disodium cocoamphodipropion-ate		1% aqua	34		
disodium isostearoam-phodipropionate			12		
disodium lauroamphodiacetate		1-2% aqua	15		2% may be irritant; patch test sensitization at 3% (§ 30.7)
disodium lauroam-phodipropionate			51		
hydrogenated tallow betaine			7		
lauramidopropyl betaine			16		
lauroamphocarboxyglycinate					‡*See* disodium lauroamphodiacetate
lauroamphoglycinate					‡*See* sodium lauroamphoacetate
lauryl betaine		1% aqua†	11		
oleyl betaine		1% aqua†	14		
sodium cocoamphoacetate		1% aqua†	7		
sodium lauroamphoacetate		1% aqua†	3		

30.15.6 Amines — aminoalkanols

Name	Synonym®	Patch test conc. & veh. (§ 30.1)	Freq. use (§ 30.3)	Cont. all. (§ 30.3)	Comment (§ 30.3)
aminoethyl propanediol					
aminomethyl propanediol			14		
aminomethyl propanol		2% aqua†	421		
behenamidopropyl dimethylamine	Schercodine B	0.5% aqua†	14	+	antistatic agent; *See* § 29.3
cocamidopropyl dimethylamine	Lexamine C13	0.1% aqua†		+	antistatic agent; *See* § 29.3
diethanolamine	DEA	0.1% aqua	131		
diisopropanolamine	DIPA	1% aqua	36	+	*See* § 27.6
3-dimethylaminopropylamine		1% pet.			‡
dimethyl stearamine			67		antistatic agent
ethanolamine	MEA (monoethanolamine)	2% aqua†	294		
ethanolamine HCl			3		*See also* ethanolamine
ethylenediamine		1% pet.		+	‡*See* § 5.20. Hardly, if at all, used in cosmetics
ethylenediamine HCl		1% pet.		+	‡*See* § 5.20
isopropanolamine	monoisopropanolamine	1% aqua†	40	+	*See* index
isostearamidopropyl dimethylamine	Schercodine I	0.3% aqua†	4	+	antistatic agent; *See* § 29.3
lauramidopropyl dimethylamine	Lexamine L13	0.2% aqua†		+	antistatic agent; *See* § 29.3
minkamidopropyl dimethylamine	Foamole B	0.1% aqua†	5		antistatic agent
mixed isopropanolamines					*See* isopropanolamine: mixture of isopropanolamines
monoethanolamine	MEA		294		‡*See* ethanolamine
morpholine		1% pet.	16		

(continued)

§ **30.15.6** *(continuation)*

Name	Synonym®	Patch test conc. & veh. (§ 30.1)	Freq. use (§ 30.3)	Cont. all. (§ 30.3)	Comment (§ 30.3)
oleamidopropyl dimethylamine	Lexamine 013	0.1%-0.3% aqua (phosphate)	44	+	test dilution of 0.3% aq. slightly irritating [18]: antistatic agent; *See* § 29.3
palmitamidopropyl dimethylamine		0.025% aqua†		+	antistatic agent: *see* § 29.3
stearamidoethyl diethylamine		0.4% aqua	10	+	antistatic agent; *See* § 29.3
stearamidopropyl dimethylamine	Lexamine S13	0.3% aqua	98	+	antistatic agent; *See* § 29.3
tallowamidopropyl dimethylamine	Schercodine T	0.3% aqua†		+	antistatic agent; *See* § 29.3
triethanolamine	TEA	2.5% pet.	3377	+	*See* § 5.20
triisopropanolamine	TIPA		40		
tromethamine	Tris (hydroxymethyl) aminomethane	0.5% aqua†	23		

30.15.7 Diols and polyols, including polyethyleneglycols (PEGs) and polypropyleneglycols (PPGs)

Name	Synonym®	Patch test conc. & veh. (§ 30.1)	Freq. use (§ 30.3)	Cont. all. (§ 30.3)	Comment (§ 30.3)
butylene glycol	1,3-butanediol	10% aqua†	402	+	*See* § 5.20
diethylene glycol	diglycol	2.5–10% aqua	14		
dipropylene glycol		20% pet.	180		
ethyl hexanediol	ethohexadiol	5% o.o.			
glucose		10% aqua†	26		
glycerin	glycerol	1–10% aqua	2603	+	*See* § 5.20
glycol	1,2-ethanediol	1–5% aqua or alc.			

(continued)

§ 30.15.7 *(continuation)*

Name	Synonym®	Patch test conc. & veh. (§ 30.1)	Freq. use (§ 30.3)	Cont. all. (§ 30.3)	Comment (§ 30.3)
1,2,6-hexanetriol		5% aqua†			
hexylene glycol		5% aqua†	193	+	*See* § 5.20
inositol		10% aqua†	9		
lactose	milk sugar		9		
maltitol			26		
mannitol			4		
PEG	polyethyleneglycol (carbowax)	pure			‡ degree of ethoxy-lation not specified
PEG-4	polyethyleneglycol 200	pure	20		
PEG-5 M	PEG 5000	pure	13		
PEG-6	polyethyleneglycol 300	pure	28		
PEG-6-32		pure	46		‡
PEG-7 M	PEG 7000	pure	8		
PEG-8	polyethyleneglycol 400	pure	177		
PEG-12	polyethyleneglycol 600	pure	7		
PEG-14	polyethyleneglycol (14)	pure	4		
PEG-14 M	PEG 14000	pure	58		
PEG-16	polyethyleneglycol (16)	pure	3		
PEG-18	polyethyleneglycol (18)	pure			
PEG-20	polyethyleneglycol (20)	pure	32		
PEG-20 M		pure			‡
PEG-30		pure			‡
PEG-32	polyethyleneglycol (32)	pure	24		
PEG-40	polyethyleneglycol 2000	pure			
PEG-45 M	PEG 45000	pure	13		
PEG-75	polyethyleneglycol 4000	pure	34		
PEG-100	polyethyleneglycol (100)	pure			
PEG-150	polyethyleneglycol 6000	pure	12		
PEG/PPG-17/6 copolymer			3		

(continued)

§ **30.15.7** *(continuation)*

Name	Synonym®	Patch test conc. & veh. (§ 30.1)	Freq. use (§ 30.3)	Cont. all. (§ 30.3)	Comment (§ 30.3)
polypropylene glycol					‡ degree of propoxylation not specified
PPG-9	polypropyleneglycol (9)		8		
PPG-26	polypropyleneglycol (26)	30% pet.†	8		
propylene glycol		2% aqua	4896	+	*See* § 5.20
sorbitol		10% aqua†	524		
sucrose		10% aqua†	43		
triethylene glycol		20% pet.	6		
tris(hydroxymethyl)nitromethane		1% pet.			

BOTANICAL INGREDIENTS

Botanical ingredients in cosmetics are tabulated in § 30.16. Contact allergy refers to the ingredients as such. No reference is made to reactions from their botanical sources.

30.16 Botanical ingredients

Name	Source	Patch test conc. & veh. (§ 30.1)	Freq. use (§ 30.3)	Cont. all. (§ 30.3)	Comment (§ 30.3)
acacia (gum arabic, gum acacia)	exudation of the stems and branches of *Acacia species*, Leguminosae	50% aqua; pure	34		viscosity increasing agent
agrimony extract	*Agrimonia eupatoria*, Rosaceae		3		
alfalfa extract	*Medicago sativa, Papilionaceae*		14		use as colourant prohibited in USA
algae extract	Algae		98		
aloe	*Aloe species*, Liliaceae				
aloe extract	*Aloe species*, Liliaceae	10% alc.†	283		

(continued)

§ 30.16 *(continuation)*

Name	Source	Patch test conc. & veh. (§ 30.1)	Freq. use (§ 30.3)	Cont. all. (§ 30.3)	Comment (§ 30.3)
aloe, powdered	leaves of *Aloe species*, Liliaceae	10% pet.			‡
aloe vera gel	mucilago obtained from *Aloe barbadensis* Miller, Liliaceae				
althea extract	roots of *Althea officinalis*, Malvaceae		13		
annatto	seeds of *Bixa orellana*, Bixaceae				*See* § 30.10 (colours)
apple extract	fruits from *Pyrus malus*, Rosaceae		4		
apricot extract	fruits from *Prunus armeniaca*, Rosaceae	10% aqua†	7		‡
apricot kernel	*Prunus armeniaca*, Rosaceae		4		‡ Skin abrasive
arnica extract	dried flower heads of *Arnica montana*, Compositae	20% pet.		+	*See* § 5.38 (*Arnica montana*)
arnica oil	*Arnica montana*, Compositae		4		‡
asafoetida extract	*Ferula asafoetida*, Umbelliferae		3		
avocado extract	fruits from *Persea americana*, Lauraceae		9		
balm mint extract	leaves and flower tops of *Melissa officinalis*, Labiatae	5-10% aqua†	21		
balm mint oil	leaves and flower tops of *Melissa officinalis*, Labiatae	1% pet.	6		
balm oil, lemon	*Melissa officinalis, Labiatae*		6		‡ *See* Balm Mint Oil
barley flour	ground seed of *Hordeum species*, Gramineae		5		
basil extract	leaves and flowers of *Ocimum basilicum*, Labiatae	4% pet.	4		
bay oil	volatile oil from leaves of *Pimenta acris*, Myrtaceae				*See* § 30.7 *under* bay oil
bayberry wax	berries of *Myrica cerifera*, Myricaceae		3		
benzoin extract	extract of resin obtained from *Styrax benzoin*, Hamamelidaceae	benzoin gum: 2-10% pet. or alc.	4	+	*See* § 5.38

(continued)

§ **30.16** *(continuation)*

Name	Source	Patch test conc. & veh. (§ 30.1)	Freq. use (§ 30.3)	Cont. all. (§ 30.3)	Comment (§ 30.3)
bergamot oil	volatile oil obtained from *Citrus bergamia,* Rutaceae		10		CTFA listed oil is psoralen free; *See also* § 30.7 *under* Bergamot oil
bilberry extract	fruits and leaves of *Vaccinium myrtillus,* Ericaceae		9		
bioflavonoids	flavonoids obtained from *Citrus species,* Rutaceae		4		
birch bark extract	bark of *Betula alba,* Cupuliferae		5		
birch extract	leaves and bark of *Betula alba,* Cupuliferae		5		
birch leaf extract	leaves of *Betula verrucosa,* Cupuliferae	10% alc.†	23		*See also under* birch extract
birch sap	liquid obtained by tapping *Betula verrucosa,* Cupuliferae		6		*See also under* birch extract
bitter almond oil	volatile oil obtained from kernels of *Prunus amygdalus amara,* Rosaceae		13		*See* § 30.7 *under* Almond oil, bitter
black current extract	fruits from *Ribes nigrum,* Ribesiaceae		3		
bladderwrack extract	dried thallus of *Fucus vesiculosus,* Algae	5% aqua†			
borage extract	herb of *Borago officinalis,* Boraginaceae		6		
buckthorn extract	dried bark of *Rhamnus frangula,* Rhamnaceae	10% aqua†			
burdock root extract	roots of *Arctium minus,* Compositae		4		
butcherbroom extract	rhizome of *Ruscus aculeatus,* Liliaceae	10% aqua†			
calendula	flowers of *Calendula officinalis,* Compositae			+	
calendula extract	flowers of *Calendula officinalis,* Compositae	10% alc.†	123	+	
calendula oil	flowers of *Calendula officinalis,* Compositae	10% pet.†	35		
camellia oil	leaves of *Thea sinensis,* Ternstroemiaceae		3		

(continued)

§ **30.16** *(continuation)*

Name	Source	Patch test conc. & veh. (§ 30.1)	Freq. use (§ 30.3)	Cont. all. (§ 30.3)	Comment (§ 30.3)
cananga oil	*Cananga odorata,* Anonaceae		5		‡
capsicum	fruits of *Capsicum frutescens,* Solanaceae	0.5% pet.	3		Cayenne pepper
capsicum extract	fruits of *Capsicum frutescens,* Solanaceae	1% alc.: 0.5% pet.†	18		
capsicum oleoresin	resinous extract from the fruits of *Capsicum frutescens,* Solanaceae	1% alc.			
cardamon oil	volatile oil obtained from the seeds of *Elettaria cardamomum,* Zingiberaceae		14		*See* § 30.7 *under* cardamon oil
carline thistle extract	*Carlina species,* Compositae		3		‡
carob oil	*Ceratonia siliqua,* Leguminosae	20% pet.†			‡
carrot oil	seeds of *Daucus carota,* Umbelliferae	4% pet.†		+	‡ phototoxicty from carrot seed oil [2]
carrot seed extract	seeds of *Daucus carota,* var. sativa, Umbelliferae				
cassia oil	volatile oil obtained from leaves and twigs of *Cinnamomum cassia,* Lauraceae				‡ *See* § 30.7 *under* cinnamon oil and § 5.14
celandine extract	*Chelidonium majus*		14		
chamomile extract	flowers of *Anthemis nobilis,* Compositae	5% aqua†	150		
chamomile oil	volatile oil obtained from the dried flowerheads of *Anthemis nobilis* (or *Matricaria chamomilla*), Compositae		39		*See* § 30.7 *under* Chamomile oil (German, Roman)
chinese tea extract	*Thea sinensis,* Ternstroemiaceae		12		
cinchona extract	bark of *Cinchona species,* Rubiaceae	5% aqua†	16		
cinnamon	*Cinnamomum zeylanicum / loureirii,* Lauraceae				cinnamon bark oil is a sensitizer due to cinnamic aldehyde [2]
clove oil	volatile oil obtained by steam distillation of the flower buds of *Eugenia caryophyllus,* Myrtaceae		49	+	*See* § 30.7 *under* clove bud oil

(continued)

§ **30.16** *(continuation)*

Name	Source	Patch test conc. & veh. (§ 30.1)	Freq. usc (§ 30.3)	Cont. all. (§ 30.3)	Comment (§ 30.3)
clover blossom extract	flowers of *Trifolium pratense*, Papilionaceae		7		*See also* Trifolium extract
coconut water	*Cocos nucifera*, Palmae		4		‡
colocynth	fruits of *Citrullus colocynthis*, Cucurbitaceae		6	+	Colocynth in alcoholic hair tonics and brillantines has caused eczema [2]
colocynth extract	fruits of *Citrullus colocynthis*, Cucurbitaceae		3		
coltsfoot leaf extract	leaves of *Tussilago farfara*, Compositae	1% alc.	12		
comfrey	*Symphytum officinale*, Boraginaceae		6		‡
comfrey extract	roots and rhizomes of *Symphytum officinale*, Boraginaceae		63		
coneflower extract	*Echinacea pallida*, Compositae	10% alc.†	7		
coriander extract	leaves and fruits of *Coriandrum sativum*, Umbelliferae		5		
corn cob meal	milled cobs of *Zea mays*, Graminae		4		
corn flour	seed of *Zea mays*, Graminae		8		
corn poppy extract	petals of *Papaver rhoeas*, Papaveraceae		8		
corn starch	*Zea mays*, Graminae	pure†			
cornflower	dried flowers of *Centaurea cyanus*, Compositae				
cornflower extract	flowers of *Centaurea cyanus*, Compositae	10% alc.†	47		
crataegus extract	berries of *Crataegus oxyacantha*, Pomaceae		23		
cucumber extract	*Cucumus sativus*, Cucurbitaceae	10% aqua†	62		
cucumber juice	*Cucumus sativus*, Cucurbitaceae		7		
cypress extract	leaves and twigs of *Cupressus sempervirens*, Coniferae	Cypress oil: 5% pet.	21		

(continued)

§ 30.16 *(continuation)*

Name	Source	Patch test conc. & veh. (§ 30.1)	Freq. use (§ 30.3)	Cont. all. (§ 30.3)	Comment (§ 30.3)
dandelion extract	rhizome and roots of *Taraxatum officinale,* Compositae		6		
dandelion root	dried rhizoma and roots of *Taraxatum officinale,* Compositae			+	
elder water	*Sambucus nigra,* Caprifoliaceae	10% aqua†			‡
ephedra extract	herb of *Ephedra vulgaris/sinica,* Ephedraceae		3		
escin	*Aesculus hippocastanum,* Hippocastanaceae	1% pet.†	32		
eucalyptus extract	fresh leaves of *Eucalyptus globulus* and other species, Myrtaceae	2% pet.	7		
eucalyptus oil	volatile oil obtained from fresh leaves of *Eucalyptus species,* Myrtaceae		58	+	*See* § 30.7 *under* eucalyptus oil
euphrasia extract	*Euphrasia officinalis,* Scrophulariaceae		7		eyebright extract
fennel extract	fruits of *Foeniculum vulgare,* Umbelliferae		17		
fenugreek extract	*Trigonella foenumgraceum,* Papilionaceae		4		
garlic	*Allium sativum,* Liliaceae			+	‡
garlic extract	bulb of *Allium sativum,* Liliaceae		5		*See also*: garlic
gentian extract	rhizome and roots of *Gentiana species,* Gentianaceae		4		
geranium extract	*Geranium species,* Geraniaceae		12		
geranium oil	volatile oil obtained from *Geranium species,* Geraniaceae		89		*See* § 30.7 *under* Geranium oil (Algerian, Bourbon, Moroccan)
ginger extract	*Zingiber officinale,* Zingiberaceae	Ginger oil 4% pet.	9		‡ *Ginger oil* is irritant and allergenic; weakly phototoxic [2]
gingko extract	*Gingko biloba,* Ginkoaceae	10% aqua†	14		

(continued)

§ **30.16** *(continuation)*

Name	Source	Patch test conc. & veh. (§ 30.1)	Freq. use (§ 30.3)	Cont. all. (§ 30.3)	Comment (§ 30.3)
ginseng	dried roots of *Panax ginseng,* Araliaceae		10		
ginseng extract	dried roots of *Panax ginseng,* Araliaceae		106		
grape extract	fruits of *Vitis vinifera,* Vitaceae		6		
grapefruit extract	fruits of *Citrus decumana, Citrus paradisi,* Rutaceae	10% alc.†			
grapefruit oil	volatile oil obtained from the peels of the fruits of *Citrus paradisi,* Rutaceae		7		*See* § 30.7 *under* grapefruit oil, expressed
grapefruit pulp extract	*Citrus paradisi,* Rutaceae		6		‡
grapefruit seed extract	seeds of the fruits of *Citrus paradisi,* Rutaceae		5		
hayflower extract	extract of hay flowers		6		
hazelnut oil	nuts of *Corylus species,* Cupiliferae	30% pet.†	94		
henna extract	dried leaves, flowers and fruits of *Lawsonia inermis,* Lythraceae	10% aqua†, 10mg powder in 100ml water, ether and alcohol	19		Extract of *Lawsonia inermis,* prepared to remove most colouring matter
honeysuckle oil	*Lonicera* species, Caprifoliaceae	2% pet.†	4		‡
hops extract	dried strobiles of *Humulus lupulus,* Cannabaceae	10% alc.†	59		
horse chestnut extract	*Aesculum hippocastanum,* Hippocastanaceae	20% aqua†	82	+	Dermatitis from ointment and pills containing horse chestnut extract [2]; *See also* § 5.38 *under*: esculin
horsetail extract	sterile caules of *Equisetum arvense,* Equisetaceae	10% alc.†	128		
hydrocotyl extract	leaves or roots of *Hydrocotyle asiatica,* Umbelliferae		25		
hypericum extract (St. John's wort extract)	flowers, leaves and stem heads of *Hypericum perforatum,* Hypericaceae	10% m.o.†			

(continued)

§ **30.16** *(continuation)*

Name	Source	Patch test conc. & veh. (§ 30.1)	Freq. use (§ 30.3)	Cont. all. (§ 30.3)	Comment (§ 30.3)
hypericum oil	*Hypericum perforatum,* Hypericaceae	10% pet.†	22		‡
ivy	powdered dry leaves and stems of *Hedera helix,* Araliaceae				
ivy extract	leaves and branches of *Hedera helix,* Araliaceae	10% alc.†	76		
jasmine extract	leaves and flowers of *Jasminum officinale/grandiflorum,* Oleaceae		7		
jasmine oil	volatile oil obtained from *Jasminum officinale,* Oleaceae	2% pet. 10% pet.	19		
juniper extract	ripe fruits of *Juniperus communis,* Cupressaceae		22		
juniper oil	berries of *Juniperus communis,* Cupressaceae	2% pet.			Irritant to the skin and respiratory tract [2]; *See also* § 30.7 *under* juniper berry oil
juniper tar (cade oil)	volatile oil obtained from the wood of *Juniperus oxycedrus,* Cupressaceae	3% pet.†	10		*See* § 30.7 under cade oil rectified
karaya gum	dried exudate of the tree of *Sterculia urens,* Sterculiaceae	pure	8	+	*See* § 5.38
kelp	*Macrocystis pyriferae*		19		
krameria extract	*Krameria triandra,* Krameriaceae	5% alc. (tincture)	6	+	Allergic dermatitis, also from topical preparations containing *krameria* [2]
lady's mantle extract	*Alchemilla vulgaris,* Rosaceae	5% aqua†			
lappa extract	roots of *Arctium lappa,* Compositae				Giant burdock
laurel extract	leaves of *Laurus nobilis,* Lauraceae				Laurel oil is a sensitizer (§ 5.14)
lavandin oil	*Lavandula angustifolia,* Labiatae		3	+	‡*See* § 30.7 under lavandin oil
lavender	*Lavandula officinale,* Labiatae		9		‡
lavender extract	*Lavandula officinalis,* Labiatae	10% pet.†			

(continued)

§ **30.16** *(continuation)*

Name	Source	Patch test conc. & veh. (§ 30.1)	Freq. use (§ 30.3)	Cont. all. (§ 30.3)	Comment (§ 30.3)
lavender oil	volatile oil obtained from *Lavandula officinalis,* Labiatae		164	+	*See* § 30.7 under lavender oil
lemon extract	fruits of *Citrus limon,* Rutaceae	5% alc.†	48		
lemon juice	fruits of *Citrus limon,* Rutaceae		12		has caused dermatitis [2]
lemon oil	*Citrus limon,* Rutaceae		91	+	*See* § 30.7 under lemon oil, distilled/ expressed and § 5.14 under lemon oil
lemongrass oil	oil obtained by steam distillation of the fresh grass of *Cymbopogon citratus,* Gramineae		16	+	*See* § 30.7 under lemongrass oil, East Indian and West Indian and § 5.14
lettuce extract	*Lactuca species,* Compositae		5		
licorice extract	*Glycyrrhiza glabra,* Papilionaceae		10		
lime juice	*Citrus aurantifolia,* Rutaceae		9		‡
lime oil	*Citrus aurantifolia,* Rutaceae		9		‡ *See* § 30.7 under lime oil expressed/ distilled
linden distillate	*Tilia cordate,* Tilaceae	20% aqua†			‡
linden extract	flowers of *Tilia cordata,* Tiliaceae	20% aqua†	70		
lotus extract	*Lotus species,* Papilionaceae	10% m.o.†	6		‡
macadamia nut oil	*Macadamia ternifolia*	5% pet.†	48		
mallow extract	leaves and flowers of *Malva silvestris,* Malvaceae	10% alc.†	85		
marjoram oil, sweet	*Origanum majorana,* Labiatae				‡ *See* § 30.7 under marjoram oil sweet
matricaria	*Matricaria chamomilla,* Compositae		11	+	‡ *See also* § 5.38 under chamomile oil
matricaria extract	flower heads of *Matricaria chamomilla,* Compositae	10% aqua †	88	+	*See matricaria*

(continued)

§ **30.16** *(continuation)*

Name	Source	Patch test conc. & veh. (§ 30.1)	Freq. use (§ 30.3)	Cont. all. (§ 30.3)	Comment (§ 30.3)
matricaria oil	volatile oil distilled from the flower heads of *Matricaria chamomilla*, Compositae	25% o.o.	13		
meadowsweet extract	*Filipendula ulmaria,* Rosaceae		14		
melissa extract	*Melissa officinalis,* Labiatae				‡*See* balm mint extract
mistletoe	*Viscum alba,* Loranthaceae				
mugwort extract	flowering herb of *Artemisia absinthium,* Compositae				
mulberry extract	dried leaves of *Morus species,* Urticaceae	10% aqua†			
mullein leaf	*Verbascum thapsis,* Scrophulariaceae		3		‡
myrrh	*Commiphora species,* Burseraceae	myrrh oil: 8% pet.	5		‡
myrrh extract	*Commiphora species,* Burseraceae	10% alc.	18		
myrtle oil	*Myrtus communis,* Myrtaceae		8		‡
nettle extract	*Urtica dioica,* Urticaceae	5% aqua†	33		
nutmeg oil	oil extracted from the kernel of *Myristica fragrans,* Myristicaceae				*See* § 30.7 under nutmeg oil, East Indian
oak bark extract	bark of *Quercus,* Fagaceae	5% aqua†	3		*Bark*: allergic contact dermatitis; irritant dermatitis [2]
oak root extract	roots of *Quercus*, Fagaceae		29		
oat extract	seeds of *Avena sativa,* Graminae		6		
oat flour	*Avena sativa,* Graminae	pure†	84		
oatmeal	coarsely milled kernels of *Avena sativa,* Graminae		8		
olive extract	leaves or fruits of *Olea europaea,* Oleaceae		11		
orange extract	fruits of *Citrus sinensis,* Rutaceae	10% alc.†	8		

(continued)

§ **30.16** *(continuation)*

Name	Source	Patch test conc. & veh. (§ 30.1)	Freq. use (§ 30.3)	Cont. all. (§ 30.3)	Comment (§ 30.3)
orange flower extract	flowers of *Citrus sinensis,* Rutaceae		4		
orange flower oil	flowers of *Citrus sinensis,* Rutaceae		17		*See* § 30.7 under neroli oil
orange flower water	aqueous solution of the odoriferous principles of the flower of *Citrus sinensis,* Rutaceae		9		
orange oil	fresh peel of *Citrus sinensis,* Rutaceae		39		*See* § 30.7 under orange oil, expressed
orange peel extract	peels of the fruits of *Citrus sinensis,* Rutaceae		3		
orris root extract	*Iris florentina,* Iridaceae		7		
orris root oil	*Iris florentina,* Iridaceae		4		‡
orris root, powder	*Iris florentina,* Iridaceae	pure			‡
palmarosa oil	*Andropogon schoenanthus,* Gramineae		16		‡ *See* § 30.7 under palmarosa oil
pansy extract	*Viola tricolor,* Violaceae		17		
papaya extract	fruits of *Carica papaya,* Caricaceae		10		
parsley extract	*Petroselinum sativum,* Umbelliferae		4		
passionflower extract	*Passiflora carnata,* Passifloraceae		8		
peach extract	*Prunus persica,* Amygdalaceae		10		
pellitory extract	leaves and stem of *Parietaria officinalis,* Urticaceae				
peppermint	*Mentha piperita,* Labiatae		3		‡ Contact allergy to oil of peppermint in perfumes and toothpastes (§ 13.3)
peppermint extract	leaves of *Mentha piperita,* Labiatae		7		*See also* peppermint
peppermint oil	volatile oil obtained from leaves of *Mentha piperita,* Labiatae	1% pet.†	99	+	Contact allergy to oil of peppermint in perfumes and toothpastes (§ 13.3)

(continued)

§ 30.16 *(continuation)*

Name	Source	Patch test conc. & veh. (§ 30.1)	Freq. use (§ 30.3)	Cont. all. (§ 30.3)	Comment (§ 30.3)
pine needle extract	needles of *Pinus species*, Pinaceae		5		
pine oil	volatile oil obtained by distillation of *Pinus species*, Pinaceae	5% pet.†	30		See § 30.7 under pinus pumilio oil and pinus sylvestris oil and § 30.2 [23]
pine tar (pix liquida)	obtained by destructive distillation of the wood of Pinaceae species	3% pet.	5		*See* § 5.37
pine tar oil	volatile oil obtained by steam distillation of pine tar		5		
pineapple extract	fruits of *Ananas comosus*, Bromeliaceae		15		
plantain extract	*Plantago* sp., Plantaginaceae		12		
pollen extract	extract of flower pollen		4		
pumpkin seed oil	*Cucurbita pepo*, Cucurbitaceae		3		‡
quince seed	seeds of *Cydonia oblonga*, Pomaceae	pure	3		
ratanhia tincture	*Krameria triandra*, Krameriaceae	5% alc.			‡ *See* Krameria extract
red raspberry extract	fruits of *Rubus ideaus*, Rosaceae		7		
rice bran wax	wax obtained from *Oryza sativa*, Graminae		5		
rice hulls	*Oryza sativa*, Graminae		3		
rice starch	*Oryza sativa*, Graminae	pure†	33		
rose extract	*Rosa species*, Rosaceae		16		
rose hips extract	fruits of *Rosa canina*, Rosaceae		3		
rosemary	*Rosmarinus officinalis*, Labiatae		8		‡ Irritancy and allergic dermatitis from rosemary oil; photosensitivity from the oil [2]
rosemary extract	leaves of *Rosmarinus officinalis*, Labiatae	10% aqua†	101		

(continued)

§ **30.16** *(continuation)*

Name	Source	Patch test conc. & veh. (§ 30.1)	Freq. usc (§ 30.3)	Cont. all. (§ 30.3)	Comment (§ 30.3)
rosemary oil	volatile oil obtained from the flowers of *Rosmarinus officinalis,* Labiatae		132		*See* § 30.7 under rosemary oil, and rosemary
rose oil	volatile oil obtained from the flowers of *Rosa species,* Rosaceae		15	+	*See* § 30.7 under Rose oil (Bulgarian, Moroccan, Turkish) and § 5.14
rose petal	*Rosa species,* Rosaceae		8		‡
rose water	aqueous solution of the odoriferous principles of the flowers of *Rosa centifolia,* Rosaceae	10% aqua†	67		
rosin (colophony)	*Pinus palustrus,* Pinaceae	20% pet.	22	+	*See* § 5.38 under colophony, and index
rye flour	*Secale cereale,* Graminae		4		
sage	*Salvia officinalis,* Labiatae		6	+	‡ Allergic dermatitis due to alantolactone [10]
sage extract	herb of *Salvia officinalis,* Labiatae	10% alc.†	105		
sage leaf extract	leaves of *Salvia officinalis,* Labiatae		11		‡
sage oil	volatile oil obtained from *Salvia officinalis,* Labiatae		67		*See* § 30.7 under sage oil (Dalmation, Spanish)
sambucus (elder)	*Sambucus species,* Caprifoliaceae		3		‡
sambucus extract	*Sambucus species,* Caprifoliaceae	10% alc.†			
sandalwood oil	volatile oil obtained from the heartwood of *Santalum album,* Santalaceae		27	+	*See* § 30.7 under Sandalwood oil, East Indian
sanguinaria extract	rhizomes and roots of *Sanguinaria canadensis,* Papaveraceae		3		
sassafras oil	roots of *Sassafras albidum,* Lauraceae		5		*See* § 30.7 under sassafras oil and § 5.14

(continued)

§ 30.16 *(continuation)*

Name	Source	Patch test conc. & veh. (§ 30.1)	Freq. use (§ 30.3)	Cont. all. (§ 30.3)	Comment (§ 30.3)
soybean extract	*Glycine max.*, Papillionaceae		8		
spearmint extract	*Mentha spicata,* Labiatae		3		
spearmint oil	volatile oil obtained from the dried tops and leaves of *Mentha spicata,* Labiatae; mainly carvone		26	+	*See* § 30.7 under spearmint oil and § 13.3
St. John's wort oil	*Hypericum perforatum,* Hypericaceae		22		‡ *See* hypericum oil
strawberry extract	*Fragaria chiloensis,* Rosaceae		3		
sunflower seed extract	*Helianthus annuus,* Compositae				*Seed*: allergic contact dermatitis [2]
sweet clover extract	*Melilotus species,* Papilionaceae				
sweet marjoram extract	*Origanum majorana,* Labiatae		3		
tea tree oil	volatile oil obtained from the leaves of *Melaleuca alternifolia,* Myrtaceae	pure	7	+	*See* § 5.38
thyme	*Thymus vulgaris,* Labiatae		4	+	‡ Cheilitis and glossitis from toothpaste containing thymol (§ 13.3)
thyme extract	leaves and flowers of *Thymus vulgaris,* Labiatae	10% aqua†	12		
thyme oil	volatile oil obtained from the leaves and flowers of *Thymus vulgaris,* Labiatae		75	+	*See* § 30.7 under thyme oil red
tormentil extract	roots of *Potentilla erecta,* Rosaceae		9		
trifolium (clover blossom)	*Trifolium pratense,* Papilionaceae				‡
turmeric extract	rhizomes of *Curcuma longa*, Zingiberaceae		3		
turpentine	terpene hydrocarbons obtained from *Pinus species,*, Coniferae		4		
vanilla	unripe fruits of *Vanilla planifolia, Vanilla tahitensis*	pure†			

(continued)

§ **30.16** *(continuation)*

Name	Source	Patch test conc. & veh. (§ 30.1)	Freq. use (§ 30.3)	Cont. all. (§ 30.3)	Comment (§ 30.3)
veronica extract (speedwell extract)	leaves, flowers and stems of *Veronica officinalis*, Scrophulariaceae		4		
walnut extract	husks and shells of *Juglans* species, Juglandaceae	20% aqua†			
walnut oil	oil from the nutmeat of *Juglans* species, Juglandaceae	30% pet.†	5		
walnut shell powder	ground shells of *Juglans regia*, Juglandaceae	50% pet.†	12	+	
watercress extract	leaves and flowers of *Nasturtium officinale*, Cruciferae		11		
wheat bran	*Triticum aestivum*, Graminae		6		
wheat flour	*Triticum aestivum*, Graminae		3		
wheat germ	*Triticum aestivum*, Graminae		11		
wheat germ extract	*Triticum aestivum*, Graminae	10% aqua†	46		
wheat gluten	*Triticum aestivum*, Graminae		4		
wheat starch	*Triticum aestivum*, Graminae		17		
white lily extract	*Lilium candidum*, Liliaceae		24		
wild thyme extract	*Thymus serpyllum*, Labiatae		8		
wild thyme oil	*Thymus serpyllum*, Labiatae			+	Thyme oil has caused contact allergy in biogaze (§ 5.38)
witch hazel	*Hamamelis virginiana*, Hamamelidaceae	pure; 10% alc.†	67		
witch hazel distillate	aqueous solution of tannins and volatile oils of twigs of *Hamamelis virginiana*, Hamamelidaceae	10% aqua†	116		Contains hamamelitannin
witch hazel extract	twigs, barks and leaves of *Hamamelis virginiana*, Hamamelidaceae	20% aqua†	47		Contains hamamelitannin
witch hazel leaf extract	*Hamamelis virginiana*, Hamamelidaceae		38		‡ *See also* § 5.17 under Hamamelis
yarrow extract	*Achillea millefolium*, Compositae		42		

30.17 Miscellaneous cosmetic ingredients

Name	Class	Patch test conc. & veh. (§ 30.1)	Freq. use (§ 30.3)	Cont. all. (§ 30.3)	Comment (§ 30.3)
acetamide MEA	humectant; antistat		117		
acetanilid	chemical additive; peroxide stabilizer	5% pet.; 2% pet.†	10		
acetic acid	pH adjuster, acidic; solvent	3% aqua	12		
acetone	solvent	10% o.o.	53		
acrylamides copolymer	film former; hair fixative	1% pet.			
acrylamide/sodium acrylate copolymer	hair fixative	1% pet.†	7		
acrylates/acrylamide copolymer	film former		13		
acrylates/C10-30 alkyl acrylate crosspolymer (Carbopol 1342®)	viscosity increasing agent		22		
acrylates copolymer	binder	1% pet.†	215		
acrylates/steareth-20 methacrylate copolymer	viscosity increasing agent		19		
adenosine triphosphate	skin conditioning agent		37		
adipic acid/dimethyl-aminohydroxypropyl diethylenetriamine copolymer	filmer former; hair fixative		19		
alanine	amino acid; skin conditioning agent	2% pet.; 2% aqua†	40		
albumen	skin conditioning agent		5		
alcloxa (aluminum chlorohydroxy allantoinate)	skin conditioning agent	1% aqua†	44		
alcohol (ethanol, ethyl-alcohol)	solvent; adstringent	10% aqua; pure	2605	+	*See* § 5.7
aldioxa (aluminum dihy-droxy allantoinate)	antiperspirant; pH adjuster	1% pet.†	53		
algin (sodium alginate)	viscosity increasing agent; binder	pure	35		
allantoin	skin conditioning agent	0.5% aqua; 5% pet.†	1069	+	*See* § 30.2 [19]
allantoin acetyl methionine	skin conditioning agent		13		

(continued)

§ **30.17** *(continuation)*

Name	Class	Patch test conc. & veh. (§ 30.1)	Freq. use (§ 30.3)	Cont. all. (§ 30.3)	Comment (§ 30.3)
allantoin ascorbate	skin conditioning agent		3		
allantoin galacturonic acid	skin conditioning agent		4		
allantoin glycine	skin conditioning agent		6		‡
allantoin glycyrrhetinic acid	skin conditioning agent		6		
allantoin polygalacturonic acid	skin conditioning agent		36		
almond meal	abrasive		19		
aluminum chloride	antiperspirant	2% aqua	10	+	*See* § 29.13
aluminum chlorohydrate	antiperspirant	10% aqua	140		
aluminum chlorohydrex	antiperspirant		3		
aluminum dichlorohydrate	adstringent; antiperspirant		3		
aluminum distearate	vicosity increasing agent; anticaking agent		18		
aluminum hydroxide	opacifying agent		69		
aluminum sesquichlorohydrate	antiperspirant		5		
aluminum silicate	abrasive ; absorbent; anticaking; bulking agent	5% pet.†	10		
aluminum starch octenylsuccinate	anticaking agent; absorbent	1% m.o.†	66		
aluminum stearate	anticaking; viscosity increasing agent (for hydrocarbons)	5% pet.†	69		
aluminum sulfate	antiperspirant	2% aqua			
aluminum tristearate	anticaking; viscosity increasing agent (for hydrocarbons)	5% pet.†	17		
aluminum zirconium tetrachlorohydrex GLY	antiperspirant		111		
ammoniated mercury	skin lightening agent	1% pet.		+	*See* § 29.11; EC Annex II, no. 221 (prohibited)
ammonium acetate	pH adjuster; buffering agent	2% aqua†	61		

(continued)

§ 30.17 *(continuation)*

Name	Class	Patch test conc. & veh. (§ 30.1)	Freq. use (§ 30.3)	Cont. all. (§ 30.3)	Comment (§ 30.3)
ammonium acrylates copolymer	film former; hair fixative		23		
ammonium alum	adstringent		11		
ammonium bicarbonate	pH adjuster; buffering agent		53		
ammonium carbonate	pH adjuster; buffering agent	5% aqua	9		
ammonium chloride	pH adjuster; buffering agent		104		
ammonium hydroxide	pH adjuster; alkaline		948		
ammonium persulfate	oxidizing agent	2.5% pet.	25	+	*See* § 26.14
ammonium sulfate	reducing agent		16		
ammonium sulfite	hair waving/depilating agent; reducing agent		3		
ammonium thioglycolate	hair waving/depilating agent	2.5% pet.	232	+	*See* § 26.14
amniotic fluid	biological additive		26		
amyl acetate	solvent	5% pet.†	21		
arginine	amino acid; skin conditioning agent	2% pet.†	43		
ascorbic acid	vitamin C; antioxidant	pure	267	+	*See* § 30.2 [25]
aspartic acid	amino acid; skin conditioning agent	5% pet.†	38		
attapulgite	bulking agent, viscosity increasing agent; sorbent		3		
azulene	antiinflammatory agent	1% pet.	45	+	*See* § 27.16
barium sulfide	depilating agent	2% aqua, freshly prepared	5		
beer	hair/skin conditioning agent		3		*See* § 26.3 under alcohol
bentonite	viscosity increasing agent; absorbent	5% aqua†	141		
benzocaine	local anaesthetic; counterirritant	5% pet.	12	+	‡*See* § 5.18; EC Annex II, no. 167 (prohibited)

(continued)

§ **30.17** *(continuation)*

Name	Class	Patch test conc. & veh. (§ 30.1)	Freq. use (§ 30.3)	Cont. all. (§ 30.3)	Comment (§ 30.3)
benzoyl peroxide	antiacne agent	1% pet.			test substance not stable [17]; EC Annex II, no. 380 (prohibited)
biotin	vitamin H	1% aqua†	53		
bisabolol	skin conditioning agent	5% pet.†	165		
boric acid	preservative; buffering agent	3% aqua; 5% glyc.	128		
boron nitride	abrasive		3		
brucine sulfate	alcohol denaturant	1% pet. (brucine)			EC Annex II, no. 62 (prohibited)
butane	aerosol propellant		319		
butoxyethanol (Butyl cellosolve®)	solvent	2% aqua†	114		
butyl acetate	solvent	25% o.o; 5% pet.†	286	+	*See* § 30.2 [21]
n-butyl alcohol	solvent	70% aqua	67		
t-butyl alcohol	solvent	70% aqua	11		
butyl benzoic acid/phthalic anhydride/trimethylolethane copolymer	film former		7		
butyl ester of PVM/MA copolymer (Gantrez ES 425®)	film former; hair fixative	10% alc.†	57		
calcium chloride	viscosity increasing agent		24		
calcium hydroxide	pH adjuster, alkaline	pure, 10% pet.†	36		Irritant reactons when tested pure
calcium oxide	pH adjuster, alkaline	do not test	3		
calcium pantothenate	vitamin B5, calcium salt; hair conditioning agent	5% aqua†	30		
calcium silicate	absorbent; buling agent	5% pet.†	188		
calcium stearate	anticaking agent	pure	44		
calcium thioglycolate	depilating agent	5% aqua	123		
calfskin extract	biological additive		4		

(continued)

§ **30.17** *(continuation)*

Name	Class	Patch test conc. & veh. (§ 30.1)	Freq. use (§ 30.3)	Cont. all. (§ 30.3)	Comment (§ 30.3)
carbomer	viscosity increasing agent				
carbomer 934	viscosity increasing agent	10% aqua†, pure† [CIR] [6]	728		‡
carbomer 940	viscosity increasing agent	10% aqua†, pure† [CIR] [6]	894		‡
carbomer 941	viscosity increasing agent	10% aqua†, pure† [CIR] [6]	464		‡
carbomer 980	viscosity increasing agent	10% aqua, pure [CIR] [6]	3		‡
carboxymethyl hydroxyethylcellulose	viscosity increasing agent		3		
carboxyvinyl polymer	viscosity increasing agent	pure†	32		‡
carrageenan	viscosity increasing agent	pure; 25% aqua†	64		
caviar extract	biological additive	10% aqua†			‡
cellulose	absorbent; bulking agent	pure	22		
cellulose acetate butyrate	film former		4		
cellulose gum	film former; binder	10% aqua†	393		
chamazulene	antiinflammatory agent		6		‡
chick embryo extract	biological additive		6		‡
chitin	viscosity increasing agent		8		
chitin extract	viscosity increasing agent		6		‡
chitosan	deacylated chitin; film former	pure†	3		
chlorofluorocarbon 11	aerosol propellant	pure		+	‡ *See* § 5.20
chlorofluorocarbon 12	aerosol propellant	pure		+	‡ *See* § 5.20
chlorofluorocarbon 113	aerosol propellant	pure		+	‡ *See* § 5.20
chloroform	flavour (toothpaste)	40% o.o.			‡ EC Annex II, no. 335 (prohibited)
p-chlorotoluene	solvent	2% pet.†			‡
cholecalciferol	vitamin D3; hair conditioning agent		46		EC Annex II, no. 335 (prohibited)
C8-9 isoparaffin	solvent	pure†	6		

(continued)

§ **30.17** *(continuation)*

Name	Class	Patch test conc. & veh. (§ 30.1)	Freq. use (§ 30.3)	Cont. all. (§ 30.3)	Comment (§ 30.3)
citric acid	pH adjuster; acidic	1% aqua	2073		
clay	absorbent (masks)		13		‡
collagen	skin conditioning agent	10% aqua†	178		
collagen amino acids	skin conditioning agent		47		
collagen amino acids, animal	skin conditioning agent		26		‡
colloidal sulfur	skin conditioning agent	1–5% pet.	6		
copper gluconate			11		
cupric sulfate	inorganic salt	1% aqua			
cyanoacrylate monomer	adhesive	pure, allow to dry before testing; 1–5–10% pet. [27]		+	‡*See* § 28.2
cysteine	amino acid; antioxidant; skin conditioning agent		16		*See* § 30.5.1
cysteine HCl	amino acid; antioxidant; skin conditioning agent		11		*See* § 30.5.1
cystine	amino acid; skin conditioning agent		22		
deodorized kerosene (Deobase®)	solvent	12% pet.	3		
desamido collagen	skin conditioning agent	10% aqua†			
dextrin	viscosity increasing agent; bulking agent	10% aqua†	27		
diacetone alcohol	solvent in nail polish removers		6		
diammonium dithio-diglycolate	chemical additive in hair conditioner and perm waves	1% aqua†	94		
diatomaceous earth	adsorbent; abrasive		18		
dicalcium phosphate	abrasive (dentrifices)		23		
dicalcium phosphate dihydrate	abrasive (dentrifices)		11		
diethylene glycolamine/ epichlorhydrine/ piperazine copolymer	film former; hair fixative	0.5% pet.†			

(continued)

§ **30.17** *(continuation)*

Name	Class	Patch test conc. & veh. (§ 30.1)	Freq. use (§ 30.3)	Cont. all. (§ 30.3)	Comment (§ 30.3)
diethyl toluamide (DEET)	insect repellant	5% alc.			
dihydroxyacetone	skin tanning agent	10% aqua or alc.	62		
dimethyl ether	solvent		36		
dimethylol ethylene thiourea (Ineral®)	biocide	10% aqua; 10% pet.		+	*See* index
dimethyl phthalate	plasticizer	5% pet.	27		
diphenhydramine HCl	antihistaminic agent	1% pet.	4	+	‡ *See* § 5.30; EC Annex II, no. 339 (prohibited)
dipotassium EDTA	chelating agent	1% pet.†	18		
dipotassium phosphate	pH adjuster; corrosion inhibitor	2% aqua†			
disodium adenosine triphosphate	skin conditioning agent		5		
disodium phosphate	pH adjuster; buffering agent; corrosion inhibitor	1% aqua†	85		
disodium pyrophosphate	buffering agent; corrosion inhibitor		3		
DMHF (dimethylhydantoin formaldehyde resin)	film former	1% alc. 95% or pet.	18		
DM hydantoin	chemical additive	1% aqua†	13		
egg	natural ingredient; skin conditioning agent		14		Contact urticaria (*See* § 30.2 [14])
egg oil	natural ingredient; skin conditioning agent		14		
egg yolk	natural ingredient; skin conditioning agent	pure			‡
egg yolk extract	biological additive; skin conditioning agent		3		
ergocalciferol	vitamin D2; hair conditioning agent		56		EC Annex II, no. 335 (prohibited)
estrone	hormone		4		‡ EC Annex II, no. 260 (prohibited)

(continued)

§ **30.17** *(continuation)*

Name	Class	Patch test conc. & veh. (§ 30.1)	Freq. use (§ 30.3)	Cont. all. (§ 30.3)	Comment (§ 30.3)
ethanolamine thioglycolate	hair waving/depilating agent		13		
ethoxydiglycol (Carbitol®)	solvent	20% pet; 10% pet.†	302		
ethoxyethanol (Cellosolve®)	solvent	2% pet.†			
ethyl acetate	solvent	10% pet; 5% MEK	307		
ethyl carbonate	solvent	2% aqua†			‡
ethylcellulose (Ethocel®)	film former; viscosity increasing agent; binder		13		
ethylene dichloride	solvent	50% o.o.			
ethylene/MA copolymer	film former; hair fixative		4		
ethylene/VA copolymer	film former; hair fixative		13		
ethyl ester of PVM/MA copolymer	film former; hair fixative		152		
ethyl hydroxymethyl oleyl oxazoline	solvent		10		
ethyl nicotinate	rubefacient		3		‡
etidronic acid	chelating agent		5		
fructose	humectant; flavour	10% aqua†	18		
fullers earth	abrasive		4		
gelatin	viscosity increasing agent	pure†	57	+	*See* § 5.41
glucose	humectant; flavour	10% aqua†	26		
glucose glutamate	amino acid; humectant	5% aqua†	29		
glutamic acid	amino acid; humectant	5% pet.†			
glutathione	biological additive		4		‡
glycereth-7	humectant		3		
glycereth-26	humectant		75		
glyceryl phthalate resin	resin	10% pet.		+	‡ *See* § 28.2
glyceryl rosinate	film former	10% alc.†			
glyceryl thioglycolate	hair waving agent (in acid perms)	2.5% pet.	29	+	*See* § 26.14

(continued)

§ 30.17 *(continuation)*

Name	Class	Patch test conc. & veh. (§ 30.1)	Freq. use (§ 30.3)	Cont. all. (§ 30.3)	Comment (§ 30.3)
glycine	amino acid; skin conditioning agent	2% aqua†	60		
glycolic acid	pH adjuster, acidic		25		
glycyrrhetinic acid	biological additive		69		
glyoxylic acid	pH adjuster, acidic	0.05% aqua†			
guaiazulene	skin conditioning agent	1% pet.	33		
guanidine carbonate	pH adjuster		17		
guanosine	skin conditioning agent	5% aqua†	4		
guar gum	viscosity increasing agent		38		
hectorite	viscosity increasing agent		9		
heptane	solvent		5		
hexyl nicotinate	skin conditioning agent	1% aqua†	8		
hinokitiol (= β-thujaplicin)	antiseborrheic agent	0.1% alc.	6	+	*See* § 26.14
histidine	amino acid; humectant		39		
honey	secration of *apis mellifera*; humectant	pure†	187		
human placental protein	skin conditioning agent	30% aqua†	6		
hyaluronic acid	viscosity increasing agent; skin conditioning agent	2% aqua†	138		
hyaluronidase	enzym		4		‡
hydrated silica	viscosity increasing agent; abrasive	pure†	100		
hydrochloric acid	pH adjuster, acidic	1% aqua	57		Do not test
hydrochlorofluorocarbon 22	aerosol propellant		35		
hydrochlorofluorocarbon 142b	aerosol propellant		16		
hydrocortisone	hormone	2.5% alc.	3	+	‡*See* § 5.36; EC Annex II, no. 300 (prohibited)
hydrofluorocarbon 152a	aerosol propellant		50		
hydrogenated honey	humectant		4		
hydrogenated lecithin	skin conditioning agent	2% pet.†	8		

(continued)

§ **30.17** *(continuation)*

Name	Class	Patch test conc. & veh. (§ 30.1)	Freq. use (§ 30.3)	Cont. all. (§ 30.3)	Comment (§ 30.3)
hydrogenated menhaden oil	solvent		4		
hydrogenated polyisobutene	emollent	5% pet.†	90		
hydrogenated starch hydrolysate	humectant		8		
hydrogen peroxide	oxidizing agent	3% aqua	227		
hydrolyzed animal collagen	skin conditioning agent		13		‡
hydrolyzed animal protein	skin conditioning agent		1316		
hydrolyzed collagen	skin conditioning agent	5%/50% aqua†	1316		
hydrolyzed elastin	skin conditioning agent	10% aqua†	187		
hydrolyzed keratin	skin conditioning agent		193		
hydrolyzed milk protein	skin conditioning agent		20		
hydrolyzed reticulin	skin conditioning agent		19		
hydrolyzed silk protein	skin conditioning agent		39		‡
hydrolyzed vegatable protein	skin conditioning agent	5–50% aqua†	15		
hydrolyzed yeast	skin conditioning agent		9		
hydrolyzed yeast protein	skin conditioning agent		27		
hydroquinone (= 1,4-benzenediol; *p*-hydroxyphenol)	skin bleaching agent/hair dye	1% pet.	208	+	*See* § 29.11
hydroquinone monoethylether	skin bleaching agent				‡ EC Annex II, no. 178 (prohibited)
hydroquinone monomethylether	skin bleaching agent				‡ EC Annex II, no. 178 (prohibited)
Hydroviton® (mixture of amino acids and other ingredients)	skin conditioning agent	10% aqua†			‡
hydroxyethylcellulose	viscosity increasing agent; film former	10% aqua†			
hydroxyethyl ethylcellulose	viscosity increasing agent; film former	10% aqua†	740		

(continued)

§ 30.17 *(continuation)*

Name	Class	Patch test conc. & veh. (§ 30.1)	Freq. use (§ 30.3)	Cont. all. (§ 30.3)	Comment (§ 30.3)
hydroxylated lecithin	suspending agent; surfactant		28		
hydroxylysine	amino acid; skin/hair conditioning agent		3		‡
hydroxymethylcellulose	viscosity increasing agent	10% aqua†			‡
hydroxyproline	amino acid; skin/hair conditioning agent		15		
hydroxypropylcellulose	viscosity increasing agent; film former		67		
hydroxypropyl guar	film former	20% pet.†	8		
hydroxypropyl methyl-cellulose	viscosity increasing agent; film former	5% aqua†	291		
ichthammol	antidandruff agent	5% aqua	3	+	*See* index
iron gluconate	chemical additive		3		‡
isobutane	aerosol propellant		487		
isoleucine	amino acid; skin conditioning agent		16		
isopropyl acetate	solvent		3		
isopropyl alcohol	solvent	10% aqua;pure	1105	+	*See* § 5.20
isopropyl ester of PVM/MA copolymer	film former; binder; hair fixative	10% alc.†			
keratin	skin conditioning agent	pure†	21		
keratin amino acids	skin conditioning agent	10% aqua†	43		
lactic acid	pH adjuster, acidic; humectant	3% aqua	325		
lactose	humectant		9		
lauryl aminopropylglycine	skin conditioning agent		5		
lauryl diethylenediamino-glycine	skin conditioning agent		3		
lecithin	skin conditioning agent; emulsifier	5% pet.†	627		
lecithinamide DEA	viscosity increasing agent; hair conditioning agent		5		
lecithin, soybean	skin conditioning agent	5% pet.†	3		‡

(continued)

§ **30.17** *(continuation)*

Name	Class	Patch test conc. & veh. (§ 30.1)	Freq. use (§ 30.3)	Cont. all. (§ 30.3)	Comment (§ 30.3)
leucine	amino acid; skin conditioning agent	2% aqua†			
lidocaine (= xylocaine; lignocaine)	local anaesthetic	2% pet.	5	+	‡*See* § 5.18; EC Annex II, no. 399 (prohibited)
linoleamide DEA	viscosity increasing agent; hair conditioning agent		120		
Lipacide-cas®	skin conditioning agent	10% pet.†		+	‡*See* § 30.2
lithium hydroxide	pH adjuster, alkaline		7		
lithium stearate	anticaking agent		51		
lysine	amino acid; skin conditioning agent	2% aqua†	21		
lysine carboxymethyl cysteinate			5		‡
lysine hydrochloride	amino acid; skin conditioning agent		19		‡
magnesium aluminum silicate (Veegum)	suspending agent; viscosity increasing agent	5% aqua†	788		
magnesium aspartate	skin conditioning agent		10		
magnesium carbonate (CI 77713)	absorbent; bulking agent; colour	pure	413		
magnesium chloride	inorganic salt	0.6% aqua†	64		
magnesium hydroxide	pH adjuster, alkaline; absorbent		3		
magnesium myristate	anticaking agent	10% pet.†	69		
magnesium oxide	pH adjuster, alkaline; absorbent	pure	10		
magnesium silicate	adsorbent; anticaking agent		17		
magnesium stearate	anticaking agent	pure†	148		
magnesium sulfate	skin conditioning agent	1% aqua†	139		
magnesium trisilicate	adsorbent; abrasive		8		
maleic acid	pH adjuster, acidic				
malic acid	pH adjuster, acidic	1% aqua†	51		

(continued)

§ 30.17 *(continuation)*

Name	Class	Patch test conc. & veh. (§ 30.1)	Freq. use (§ 30.3)	Cont. all. (§ 30.3)	Comment (§ 30.3)
maltodextrin	film former; absorbent		7		
MEK (methyl ethyl ketone)	solvent	pure (open test)	4		
methionine	amino acid; skin conditioning agent	2% pet.†	23		
methoxycypropanol	solvent		8		‡
methyl alcohol (methanol)	solvent	pure	3		
methyl cellulose (Methocel A®)	viscosity increasing agent	pure; 2% aqua†	53		
methylene chloride (dichloromethane)	solvent		4		‡
methyl gluceth-10	skin conditioning agent; humectant		40		
methyl gluceth-20	skin conditioning agent; humectant		77		
methyl gluceth-20 sesquistearate	emollient; emulsifier	5% aqua†	110		‡
methylstyrene/vinyl-toluene copolymer	viscosity increasing agent (non aqueous)		18		
methyl nicotinate	rubefacient	0.1% pet.†			‡
milk powder	skin conditioning agent		6		‡
milk protein	skin conditioning agent	1% aqua†	22		
mineral spirits	solvent	3% pet.†	8		
mineral waters	natural ingredient; solvent		8		‡
minoxidil	hairgrowth stimulant	2% alc. (70%) with 10% propylene glycol		+	‡*See* § 5.41; EC Annex II, no. 372 (prohibited)
monobenzone (hydroquinone monobenzylether)	skin lightening agent	1% pet.		+	‡*See* § 5.41 and § 29.11; EC Annex II, no. 178 (prohibited)
monoethanolamine (MEA)	pH adjuster, alkaline		294		‡*See* ethanolamine § 30.15.6
montmorrilonite	absorbent; bulking agent		23		

(continued)

§ **30.17** *(continuation)*

Name	Class	Patch test conc. & veh. (§ 30.1)	Freq. use (§ 30.3)	Cont. all. (§ 30.3)	Comment (§ 30.3)
myreth-3-myristate	emollient	5% pet.†	46		
niacin (nicotinic acid)	hair conditioning agent	1% aqua	4		
niacinamide	vitamin PP; skin conditioning agent		13		
nitrocellulose	film former (nail polishes and enamels)	10% aqua; 10% aceton, cave irrit. vehic.	226	+	*See* § 30.2 [19] and § 28.2
nitrogen	aerosol propellant		3		
non-fat dry milk	skin conditioning agent		76		
nylon	bulking agent	pure†	154		‡
nylon-12	opacifying agent; bulking agent		38		
octylacrylamide/acrylates/butylaminoethyl methacrylate copolymer (Amphomer®)	film former; hair fixative		92		
octylacrylamide/acrylates copolymer	film former; hair fixative		9		
octyldodeceth-20	hair conditioning agent		6		
oleamide DEA	hair conditioning agent	0.5% aqua†	120		
oleamide MIPA	hair conditioning agent		6		
oleamidopropyl dimethylamine hydrolyzed collagen	hair conditioning agent		7		
oleostearine	skin conditioning agent		5		
oryzanol	biological additive		28		
oxyquinoline sulfate	biocide		13		*See* § 30.5.7
palmitoyl animal collagen amino acids	hair/skin conditioning agent	10% pet.		+	*See* index
palmitoyl hydrolyzed animal protein	hair/skin conditioning agent; surfactant	10% pet.†			
palmitoyl hydrolyzed collagen	hair/skin conditioning agent		11		
palmitoyl hydrolyzed milk protein	surfactant; hair conditioning agent	10% pet.		+	*See* index
pantetheine	biological additive		14		‡

(continued)

§ **30.17** *(continuation)*

Name	Class	Patch test conc. & veh. (§ 30.1)	Freq. use (§ 30.3)	Cont. all. (§ 30.3)	Comment (§ 30.3)
pantethine	antihyperlipoproteinemic agent		66		
panthenol	hair conditioning agent	30% pet.	1025		
panthenyl ethyl ether	hair conditioning agent	30% pet.	120		*See* § 26.14
pantothenic acid	Vitamin B5; hair conditioning agent		14		
PCA	humectant		26		
pectin	viscosity increasing agent		56		
PEG-16 hydrogenated castor oil	emollient		5		
pentasodium aminotrimethylene phosphate	chelating agent		8		
pentasodium triphosphate	chelating agent		30		
pentetic acid	chelating agent	1% aqua†	51		*See also* §30.5.1
petroleum destillate	solvent	pure; 25% o.o.;3% pet.†			Irritant when tested undiluted†
phenacetin	hydrogen peroxide stabilizer	1% pet.	35		
phenyl methyl pyrazolone (2,4-dihydro-5-methyl-2-phenyl-3h-pyrazol-3-one)	hydrogen peroxide stabilizer; hair colour	1% pet.†	158		
phosphoric acid	pH adjuster, acidic	0.5% aqua†	386		
phthalic anhydride/ glycerin/glycidyl decanoate copolymer	film former; hair fixative		7		
phytol	biological additive	10% pet.		‡	
pigskin extract	biological additive		17		
placental enzymes	biological additive		8		
placental extract, animal	biological additive	20% aqua†	29	‡	
placental extract, human, lyophilized	biological additive		33		
placental lipids	biological additive	10% pet.†			

(continued)

§ **30.17** *(continuation)*

Name	Class	Patch test conc. & veh. (§ 30.1)	Freq. use (§ 30.3)	Cont. all. (§ 30.3)	Comment (§ 30.3)
plankton extract	biological additive	10% aqua†	49		
polyacrylamide	film former; hair fixative		57		
polyacrylamidomethyl-propane sulfonic acid	film former; hair fixative		10		
polyacrylic acid	film former; binder	0.1% aqua†	20		
polyamino sugar condensate	humectant		25		
polybeta-analine	skin conditioning agent	10% aqua†			
polybutene	binder; viscosity increasing agent	30% pet.†	245		
polyester resin	film former	10% pet.†			‡
polyethylacrylate	film former; hair fixative	5% pet.†			
polyethylene	film former; hair fixative	pure†	354		
polyglycerylmethyl-acrylate	chemical additive	1% pet.†	41		
polyisoprene	viscosity increasing agent, non aqueous		7		
polymethylmeth-acrylate	synthetic polymer	pure	44		
polyoxymethylene urea (urea/formaldehyde resin)	bulking agent	10% pet.	40	+	Allergen in textile finishes
polypentene	synthetic polymer	5% pet.†			
polypropylene	synthetic polymer		16		
polystyrene	film former		10		
polyvinyl acetate	film former; hair fixative	10% pet.†	4		
polyvinyl alcohol	film former		42		
polyvinyl butyral	film former; hair fixative		14		
polyvinyl laurate	film former	5% pet.†			
potassium alum	adstringent	10% aqua	6		
potassium aspartate	amino acid; skin conditioning agent		6		
potassium bicarbonate	pH adjuster; buffering agent		3		

(continued)

§ 30.17 *(continuation)*

Name	Class	Patch test conc. & veh. (§ 30.1)	Freq. use (§ 30.3)	Cont. all. (§ 30.3)	Comment (§ 30.3)
potassium carbomer-934	viscosity increasing agent		4		‡
potassium carbomer-941	viscosity increasing agent		16		‡
potassium carbonate	pH adjuster, alkaline	1% aqua	12		
potassium chloride	inorganic salt; viscosity increasing agent		74		
potassium cocoyl hydrolyzed animal protein	surfactant; hair conditioning agent	5% pet.†	155		
potassium hydroxide	pH adjuster, alkaline	do not test	160		
potassium persulfate	oxidizing agent	0.5–5% aqua	32		
potassium phosphate	buffering agent	2% aqua†	21		
potassium sulfate	viscosity increasing agent		4		
potassium undecylenoyl hydrolyzed collagen	hair conditioning agent; surfactant		13		
potato starch	binder; absorbent; viscosity increasing agent	pure†			
PPG-2 methyl ether	solvent		9		
procaine hydrochloride	local anaesthetic	1% pet.		+	‡*See* § 5.18. EC Annex II, no. 167 (prohibited)
procollagen	skin conditioning agent		20		
proline	amino acid; skin conditioning agent		42		
propane	aerosol propellant		458		
propanol					‡ *See* propyl alcohol
propantheline bromide	anticholinergic agent; antiperspirant	5% pet.		+	‡ *See* § 29.13
propolis	natural ingredient	10% pet.	14	+	‡ *See* § 5.41
propolis extract	biological additive	5% aqua†	30		‡
propyl acetate	solvent		3		‡
propyl alcohol	solvent	10% aqua; pure	6		
propylene carbonate	solvent	2% aqua†	126		
pumice	abrasive (skin)		15		

(continued)

§ **30.17** *(continuation)*

Name	Class	Patch test conc. & veh. (§ 30.1)	Freq. use (§ 30.3)	Cont. all. (§ 30.3)	Comment (§ 30.3)
PVM/MA copolymer	film former; hair fixative	pure†	5		
PVP	film former; hair fixative	pure	454		
PVP/dimethylamino-ethylmethacrylate copolymer	film former; hair fixative		51		
PVP/eicosene copolymer	film former; hair fixative	10% pet.†	38		
PVP/hexadecene copolymer	film former; hair fixative	pure†; 5% pet.	49	+	*See* § 27.3
PVP/VA copolymer	binder; film former	pure†	191		
pyridoxine	vitamin B6; skin conditioning agent	10% pet.	3		
pyridoxine dioctenoate	skin conditioning agent; antiseborrhoeic agent	1% pet.		+	*See* § 26.14
pyridoxine dipalmitate	vitamin B6 derivate; skin conditioning agent		5		
pyridoxine HCl	vitamin B6 hydrochloride; skin conditioning agent	10% pet.		+	*See* § 26.14
pyrocton olamine	antidandruff agent	1% pet.†			‡
quartz particles	abrasives		3		‡
rayon	bulking agent	pure†	5		
resorcinol acetate	keratolytic agent	5% aqua		+	*See* § 5.37
retinol	vitamin A; skin conditioning agent	0.1% pet.	81	+	*See* index
retinyl acetate	vitamin A derivative; skin conditioning agent		5		
retinyl palmitate	vitamin A derivative; skin conditioning agent	pure	355	+	*See* index
riboflavin	vitamin B2		6		
RNA (ribonucleic acid)	skin conditioning agent		30		
royal jelly	skin conditioning agent		42		
royal jelly extract	skin conditioning agent		3		
rutin	capillary protectant		6		‡
saccharide isomerate	skin conditioning agent		22		
saccharin	sweetener	pure	212		‡

(continued)

§ **30.17** *(continuation)*

Name	Class	Patch test conc. & veh. (§ 30.1)	Freq. use (§ 30.3)	Cont. all. (§ 30.3)	Comment (§ 30.3)
saponins	biological additive	1% aqua†			
SD alcohol 40	solvent	10% aqua†			Denatured with brucine (sulfate) or quassin and *t*-butyl alcohol, or with denatonium benzoate and *t*-butyl alcohol
SD alcohol 39-C	solvent	10% aqua†			denatured with diethyl phthalate
sea salt	natural ingredient	0.9% aqua†	4		‡
sea urchin extract	biological additive		3		‡
sea water	natural ingredient	pure†	17		‡
selenium sulfide	antidandruff agent	2% pet.		+	‡ *See* § 26.2
serine	amino acid; skin conditioning agent	1% aqua†			
serum albumin	skin conditioning agent		29		
serum protein	skin conditioning agent		42		
shellac	natural ingredient; secration of *Laccifer (tachardia) lacca*	20% alc; pure	47		Irritant when tested pure
silica	abrasive; anticaking agent	pure†	539		
silica aerogel			3		‡
silica silylate	bulking agent; emollient		29		
silk amino acids	amino acids; skin conditioning agent		134		
silk powder	skin conditioning agent		82		Silk has caused contact urticaria (§ 30.2 [13])
sodium acetate	pH adjuster; buffering agent		4		
sodium aluminum chlorohydroxy lactate	antiperspirant		3		

(continued)

§ **30.17** *(continuation)*

Name	Class	Patch test conc. & veh. (§ 30.1)	Freq. use (§ 30.3)	Cont. all. (§ 30.3)	Comment (§ 30.3)
sodium bicarbonate	pH adjuster; buffering agent	10% aqua†	49		
sodium bisulfate	pH adjuster		3		
sodium bisulfite	hair waving agent; reducing agent	2% pet.	160	+	*See* § 26.14
sodium borate	pH adjuster, alkaline	sat. aqua. sol.	525		
sodium bromate	oxidizing agent	1–5% aqua	61		
sodium carbomer-934	viscosity increasing agent		4		‡
sodium carbonate	pH adjuster, alkaline	10% aqua	34		
sodium carrageenan	viscosity increasing agent; film former; hair fixative		18		
sodium caseinate	skin conditioning agent	5% aqua	5		
sodium chloride	viscosity increasing agent; salt	0.9% aqua†	871		
sodium chondroitin sulfate	skin conditioning agent		15		
sodium citrate	pH adjuster; buffering agent	1% aqua†	163		
sodium C4-12 olefin/ maleic acid copolymer	binder; suspending agent	10% aqua†	7		
sodium DNA	skin conditioning agent		11		
sodium fluoride	anticaries agent	0.5% aqua	9		
sodium gluconate	skin conditioning agent		3		
sodium glutamate	amino acid; skin conditioning agent		10		
sodium hexametaphos-phate	chelating agent; corrosion inhibitor	1% aqua†	42		
sodium hyaluronate	skin conditioning agent	2% aqua†	154		
sodium hydrosulfite	reducing agent		7		
sodium hydroxide	pH adjuster, alkaline	do not test	406		
sodium hypochlorite		0.5% aqua			‡
sodium isethionate	pH adjuster; hair conditioning agent		8		
sodium lactate	humectant	3% aqua†	82		

(continued)

§ **30.17** *(continuation)*

Name	Class	Patch test conc. & veh. (§ 30.1)	Freq. use (§ 30.3)	Cont. all. (§ 30.3)	Comment (§ 30.3)
sodium metabisulfite	antioxidant; reducing agent	1–5% pet.	77		*See also* § 30.5.1
sodium metasilicate	chelating agent; corrosion inhibitor		80		
sodium monofluorophosphate	anticaries agent	0.5% aqua	8		
sodium PCA	humectant	2% aqua†	371		*See* § 27.3
sodium perborate	oxidizing agent	10% pet.	11		
sodium persulfate	oxidizing agent		13		
sodium phosphate	pH adjuster; buffering agent	2% aqua†	52		
sodium polymethacrylate	film former; binder		12		
sodium pyrithione (Sodium omadine®)	antidandruff agent	0.1% pet.	3		EC Annex II, no. 369 (prohibited)
sodium ribonucleic acid	skin conditioning agent		7		‡
sodium saccharin	sweetener	10% aqua†	98		
sodium sesquicarbonate	CO_2-releasing agent; pH adjuster		62		
sodium silicate	viscosity increasing agent		42		
sodium sulfate	viscosity increasing agent		56		
sodium sulfite	antioxidant; depilating agent	2% aqua†	624		
sodium thiosulfate	reducing agent	1% aqua	12		‡
sodium zinc citrate			3		‡
soluble animal collagen (soluble collagen)	skin conditioning agent		99		‡
soluble animal keratin	skin conditioning agent		24		‡
soluble collagen	skin conditioning agent	10% aqua†	169		
solutio carbonis detergens (coal tar solution)	antidandruff agent			+	‡*See* § 5.37 *under* tar, coal
sorbitol solution	humectant	10% sorbitol aqua	122		‡
spent grain wax	natural ingredient	30% pet.†			

(continued)

§ **30.17** *(continuation)*

Name	Class	Patch test conc. & veh. (§ 30.1)	Freq. use (§ 30.3)	Cont. all. (§ 30.3)	Comment (§ 30.3)
spleen extract	biological additive	10% aqua†			
stannic chloride		10% aqua	9		
stannous chloride			3		
starch diethylaminoethyl ether	film former; hair fixative		3		
stearamide MEA	hair conditioning agent		19		
strontium hydroxide	pH adjuster, alkaline	do not test	3		
styrene/acrylamide copolymer	opacifying agent		11		
styrene/acrylates copolymer	opacifying agent		138		
styrene/PVP copolymer	film former; opacifying agent	10% aqua†	62		
succinic acid	pH adjuster, acidic		4		
sucrose	humectant; sweetener	10% aqua†	43		
sucrose acetate isobutyrate	plasticizer; denaturant	5% alc/aqua†	36		
sucrose benzoate	plasticizer	5% aqua†	18		
sucrose octaacetate	denaturant	4% pet.	3		
sulfur	antiacne agent; antidandruff agent	1–5% pet.	46	+	*See* § 5.37
sulfur precipitated	antiacne agent; antidandruff agent		7		‡
sulfuric acid	pH adjuster, acidic	do not test	22		
tartaric acid	pH adjuster, acidic	1% aqua†	58		
TEA-lactate	humectant		7		
p-tert-butylphenolresin	resin	1% pet.		+	Sensitizer in glues
tetrahydroxypropyl ethylenediamine	chelating agent		17		
tetrapotassium pyrophosphate	pH adjuster; buffering agent; corrosion inhibitor		4		
tetrasodium pyrophosphate	chelating agent		17		

(continued)

§ 30.17 *(continuation)*

Name	Class	Patch test conc. & veh. (§ 30.1)	Freq. use (§ 30.3)	Cont. all. (§ 30.3)	Comment (§ 30.3)
theophylline	bronchodilator	5% pet.	3		
thiamine HCl	vitamin B1; skin conditioning agent	10% pet.		+	*See* § 5.43
thioglycerin	hair waving/depilating agent	10% aqua		+	*See* § 26.14
thioglycolic acid	antioxidant; hair waving agent	1% aqua†	59		
thiolactic acid	antioxidant; hair waving agent	1% pet; 1% aqua†	38		
threonine	amino acid; skin conditioning agent		17		
thymus extract	biological additive	10% aqua†	6		
tin oxide	bulking agent	2% pet.†	44		
tioxolone	antiseborrheic agent	0.5% alc.		+	*See* § 26.14
toluene	solvent	50% pet.	262		
toluenesulfonamide/ formaldehyde resin (Santolite®)	film former (nail polishes and enamels)	10% pet.	219	+	*See* § 28.2
tragacanth gum	viscosity increasing agent; film former	1% aqua	22		
tretinoin (retinoic acid; vitamin A acid)	vitamin A; antiacne agent	0.005% alc.		+	‡ *See* § 5.37; EC Annex II no. 375 (prohibited)
triacetin (glyceryl triacetate)	solvent; plasticizer	pure; 1–10% alc; 20% pet; 5% alc†	14		
tricalcium phosphate	abrasive (dentrifices)		12		
tricresyl ethyl phtalate	plasticizer	5% pet.		+	‡ *See* § 28.2
triisononanoin	solvent	10% alc†	6		
trioctyl citrate	skin conditioning agent		8		
tris(hydroxymethyl) nitromethane	antimicrobial	1% pet.			
tromethamine	pH adjuster		23		
tromethamine magnesium aluminum silicate	viscosity increasing agent	1% aqua†			

(continued)

§ **30.17** *(continuation)*

Name	Class	Patch test conc. & veh. (§ 30.1)	Freq. use (§ 30.3)	Cont. all. (§ 30.3)	Comment (§ 30.3)
tryptophan	amino acid; skin conditioning agent		15		
tyrosine	amino acid; believed to promote tanning	2% pet.†	60		
urea	humectant	10% aqua	214		
urea/formaldehyde resin					‡ *See* polyoxymethylene urea
uric acid	pH adjuster, acidic; skin conditioning agent	1% aqua	4		
VA/crotonates copolymer	binder; filmer former; hair fixative	10% pet.†	30		
VA/crotonates/vinyl neodecanoate copolymer	film former; hair fixative		95		
valine	amino acid; skin conditioning agent		20		
vinegar	natural ingredient		9		*See also* acetic acid
vinyl acetate	monomer	2% pet.†			
vinyl acetate/allylstearate copolymer	synthetic polymer	pure†			‡
vinylpyrrolidone/styrene copolymer	synthetic polymer		59		‡
vinyl pyrrolidone/vinyl-acetate copolymer	synthetic polymer	10% pet.†			‡
water	solvent	pure	13014		
whey	skin conditioning agent		4		‡
xanthan gum	viscosity increasing agent	10% aqua†	522		
xylene	solvent	30–50% o.o.			
yeast	natural ingredient		4		
yeast extract	biological additive	10% aqua†	36		
zinc chloride	adstringent; oral care	2% aqua	6		
zinc gluconate			6		
zinc laurate	anticaking agent		4		

(continued)

§ 30.17 *(continuation)*

Name	Class	Patch test conc. & veh. (§ 30.1)	Freq. use (§ 30.3)	Cont. all. (§ 30.3)	Comment (§ 30.3)
zinc myristate	anticaking agent		21		
zinc phenolsulfonate	adstringent	1% alc; 5% aqua	33		
zinc stearate	anticaking agent	10% pet.	819		
zinc sulfate	adstringent; oral care	5% aqua	16		

Index

Index